Campylobacter jejuni

Current Status and Future Trends

Campylobacter jejuni
Current Status and Future Trends

Editors

Irving Nachamkin
University of Pennsylvania School of Medicine
Philadelphia, Pennsylvania 19104

Martin J. Blaser
Vanderbilt University School of Medicine
and Department of Veterans Affairs Medical Center
Nashville, Tennessee 37232

Lucy S. Tompkins
Stanford University School of Medicine
Stanford, California 94305

American Society for Microbiology
Washington, D.C.

1325 Massachusetts Ave., N.W.
Washington, DC 20005

Library of Congress Cataloging-in-Publication Data

Campylobacter jejuni: current status and future trends / co editors,
Irving Nachamkin, Martin J. Blaser, Lucy S. Tompkins.
p. cm.
Includes bibliographical references and index.
ISBN 1-55581-042-X
1. Campylobacter infections. 2. Campylobacter jejuni.
I. Nachamkin, Irving. II. Blaser, Martin J. III. Tompkins, Lucy S.
[DNLM: 1. Campylobacter Infections. 2. Campylobacter jejuni. QW
154 C1991]
QR201.C25C36 1992
616'.0145–dc20

Printed in the United States of America

CONTENTS

IV. PATHOGENESIS OF CAMPYLOBACTER INFECTIONS

In Vivo Models

In Vitro Models

V. IMMUNE RESPONSES AND ANTIGENIC ANALYSIS

VI. MOLECULAR PATHOGENESIS

CONTRIBUTORS

RICHARD A. ALM, Department of Biochemistry and Microbiology, University of Victoria, Victoria, British Columbia, Canada V8W 3P6

G. O. ASPINALL, Department of Chemistry, York University, North York, Toronto, Ontario, Canada M3J 1P3

CAROLYN N. BAKER, Nosocomial Pathogens Laboratory Branch, Hospital Infections Program, National Center for Infectious Diseases, Centers for Disease Control, Atlanta, Georgia 30333

ROBERT E. BLACK, Department of International Health, Johns Hopkins School of Hygiene and Public Health, Baltimore, Maryland 21205

MARTIN J. BLASER, Division of Infectious Diseases, Department of Medicine, Vanderbilt University School of Medicine, Nashville, Tennessee 37232-2605, and Infectious Disease Section, Department of Veterans Affairs Medical Center, Nashville, Tennessee 37203

JEFFREY L. BROWN, Science and Technology, Food Safety and Inspection Service, U.S. Department of Agriculture, Washington, D.C. 20250

DONALD H. BURR, Enteric Diseases Program, Naval Medical Research Institute, Bethesda, Maryland 20889-5055

JEAN-PAUL BUTZLER, WHO Collaborating Center for Enteric Campylobacter, St. Pieters University Hospital, 1000 Brussels, Belgium

JUAN J. CALVA, Department of Infectious Diseases, National Institute of Nutrition, Mexico City 14000 D.F., Mexico

LUZ ELENA CERVANTES, Department of Infectious Diseases, National Institute of Nutrition, Mexico City 14000 D.F., Mexico

WITOLD CIEPLAK, JR., Laboratory of Vectors and Pathogens, National Institute of Allergy and Infectious Diseases, Rocky Mountain Laboratories, Hamilton, Montana 59840

MARY LOU CLEMENTS, Department of International Health, Johns Hopkins School of Hygiene and Public Health, Baltimore, Maryland 21205

MICHAEL P. DOYLE, Department of Food Science and Technology, Georgia Experiment Station, University of Georgia, Griffin, Georgia 30223

PETER D. ECHEVERRIA, U.S. Medical Component, Armed Forces Research Institute of Medical Sciences, Bangkok, Thailand

RICHARD T. ELLISON III, Medical and Research Services, Department of Veterans Affairs Medical Center, and Division of Infectious Diseases, Department of Medicine, University of Colorado School of Medicine, Denver, Colorado 80220

GUODONG FANG, Division of Geographic Medicine, University of Virginia School of Medicine, Charlottesville, Virginia 22908

J.-L. FAUCHÈRE, Microbiologie A, CHRU, 86021 Poitiers, France

C. FENDRI, Hôpital Charles Nicolle, Tunis, Tunisia

CYNTHIA L. FENNELL, Department of Medicine, Harborview Medical Center, Seattle, Washington 98104

JAMES G. FOX, Division of Comparative Medicine, Massachusetts Institute of Technology, Cambridge, Massachusetts 02139

HERMAN GOOSSENS, WHO Collaborating Center for Enteric Campylobacter, St. Pieters University Hospital, 1000 Brussels, Belgium

RICHARD L. GUERRANT, Division of Geographic Medicine, University of Virginia School of Medicine, Charlottesville, Virginia 22908

PATRICIA GUERRY, Enteric Diseases Program, Naval Medical Research Institute, Bethesda, Maryland 20814

RALPH W. JOHNSTON, Science and Technology, Food Safety and Inspection Service, U.S. Department of Agriculture, Washington, D.C. 20250

DENNIS M. JONES, Department of Clinical Bacteriology, Public Health Laboratory Service, Withington Hospital, Manchester M20 8LR, United Kingdom

BERTIL KAIJSER, Department of Clinical Bacteriology, University of Göteborg, Göteborg, Sweden

M. Kervella, Laboratoire de Bacteriologie, CHU Necker-Enfants Malades, 75730 Paris Cédex, France

Michael E. Konkel, Laboratory of Vectors and Pathogens, National Institute of Allergy and Infectious Diseases, Rocky Mountain Laboratories, Hamilton, Montana 59840

L. A. Kurjanczyk, Department of Microbiology, University of Toronto, Toronto, Ontario, Canada M5G 1L5

Myron M. Levine, Center for Vaccine Development, Division of Geographic Medicine, Department of Medicine, University of Maryland School of Medicine, Baltimore, Maryland 21201

Yves Lobet, Laboratory of Vectors and Pathogens, National Institute of Allergy and Infectious Diseases, Rocky Mountain Laboratories, Hamilton, Montana 59840

Yolanda Lopez-Vidal, Department of Infectious Diseases, National Institute of Nutrition, Mexico City 14000 D.F., Mexico

A. G. McDonald, Department of Chemistry, York University, North York, Toronto, Ontario, Canada M3J 1P3

Francis Mégraud, Laboratoire de Bactériologie, Hôpital des Enfants, University of Bordeaux II, Bordeaux, France

S. D. Mills, Department of Microbiology, University of Toronto, Toronto, Ontario, Canada M5G 1L5

Ban Mishu, Division of Infectious Diseases, Department of Medicine, Vanderbilt University School of Medicine, Nashville, Tennessee 37232-2605

Irving Nachamkin, Department of Pathology and Laboratory Medicine, University of Pennsylvania School of Medicine, Philadelphia, Pennsylvania 19104-4283

David S. Newburg, Department of Biochemistry, E. K. Shriver Center for Mental Retardation, Waltham, Massachusetts 02154

Diane G. Newell, Central Veterinary Laboratory, Ministry of Agriculture, Fisheries and Food, New Haw, Weybridge, Surrey KT15 3NB, United Kingdom

Marvin A. Norcross, Science and Technology, Food Safety and Inspection Service, U.S. Department of Agriculture, Washington, D.C. 20250

Piet J. M. Nuijten, Department of Bacteriology, Institute of Infectious Diseases and Immunology, University of Utrecht, 3508 TD Utrecht, The Netherlands

J. M. Pagès, Centre National de la Recherche Scientifique, Marseilles, France

Charlotte M. Patton, Enteric Diseases Branch, Division of Bacterial and Mycotic Diseases, National Center for Infectious Diseases, Centers for Disease Control, Atlanta, Georgia 30333

Zhiheng Pei, Division of Infectious Diseases, Department of Medicine, and Department of Microbiology and Immunology, Vanderbilt University School of Medicine, Nashville, Tennessee 37232-2605

Richard D. Pearson, Division of Geographic Medicine, University of Virginia School of Medicine, Charlottesville, Virginia 22908

J. L. Penner, Department of Microbiology, University of Toronto, Toronto, Ontario, Canada M5G 1L5

Ross A. Pennie, Division of Geographic Medicine, University of Virginia School of Medicine, Charlottesville, Virginia 22908

Guillermo I. Perez-Perez, Division of Infectious Diseases, Department of Medicine, Vanderbilt University School of Medicine, Nashville, Tennessee 37232-2605

Daniel Perlman, University Park Medical Clinic, Denver, Colorado

Mary E. Power, Department of Biochemistry and Microbiology, University of Victoria, Victoria, British Columbia, Canada V8W 3P6

T. S. Raju, Department of Chemistry, York University, North York, Toronto, Ontario, Canada M3J 1P3

David M. Rollins, Enteric Diseases Program, Naval Medical Research Institute, Bethesda, Maryland 20889-5055

A. Rosenau, Faculté des Sciences, Université de Tours, 37200 Tours, France

Guillermo M. Ruiz-Palacios, Department of Infectious Diseases, National Institute of Nutrition, Mexico City 14000 D.F., Mexico

Robert G. Russell, Department of Pathology and Program of Comparative Medicine, School of Medicine, University of Maryland, Baltimore, Maryland 21201

CAROLINE A. RYAN, Children's Hospital and Medical Center, Seattle, Washington 98105
MARTIN B. SKIRROW, Public Health Laboratory, Gloucestershire Royal Hospital, Gloucestershire GL1 3NN, United Kingdom
NORMAN J. STERN, U.S. Department of Agriculture–Agricultural Research Service, Richard Russell Research Center, Athens, Georgia 30613
ROBERT V. TAUXE, Enteric Diseases Branch, Division of Bacterial and Mycotic Diseases, National Center for Infectious Diseases, Centers for Disease Control, Atlanta, Georgia 30333
DIANE E. TAYLOR, Department of Medical Microbiology and Infectious Diseases and Canadian Bacterial Diseases Network, University of Alberta, Edmonton, Alberta, Canada T6G 2H7
DAVID N. TAYLOR, Enteric Infections Branch, Walter Reed Army Institute of Research, Washington, D.C. 20307-5100
FRED C. TENOVER, Nosocomial Pathogens Laboratory Branch, Hospital Infections Program, National Center for Infectious Diseases, Centers for Disease Control, Atlanta, Georgia 30333
LUCY S. TOMPKINS, Department of Medicine (Infectious Diseases) and Department of Microbiology and Immunology, Stanford University Medical Center, Stanford, California 94305
TREVOR J. TRUST, Department of Biochemistry and Microbiology, University of Victoria, Victoria, British Columbia, Canada V8W 3P6
BERNARD A. M. VAN DER ZEIJST, Department of Bacteriology, Institute of Infectious Diseases and Immunology, University of Utrecht, 3508 TD Utrecht, The Netherlands
I. KAYE WACHSMUTH, Enteric Diseases Branch, Division of Bacterial and Mycotic Diseases, National Center for Infectious Diseases, Centers for Disease Control, Atlanta, Georgia 30333
RICHARD I. WALKER, Enteric Diseases Program, Naval Medical Research Institute, Bethesda, Maryland 20889-5055
TRUDY M. WASSENAAR, Department of Bacteriology, Institute of Infectious Diseases and Immunology, University of Utrecht, 3508 TD Utrecht, The Netherlands
XIAO-HE YANG, Department of Pathology and Laboratory Medicine, University of Pennsylvania School of Medicine, Philadelphia, Pennsylvania 19104-4283

Preface

During the past decade, *Campylobacter jejuni* has become recognized as probably the most common cause of sporadic bacterial diarrheal illness in the United States and as being of considerable importance worldwide. Several hundred investigators have studied various aspects of *Campylobacter* infections during this time, and major advances in understanding the clinical disease and epidemiology of infections have occurred. In more recent years, scientists have begun to examine the biology and pathogenesis of *C. jejuni* infection, and with the development of newer genetic approaches, significant progress should follow in the years to come.

Although *Campylobacter* is well known to many clinicians and scientists, it has remained obscure to the lay public. With a more health-conscious population, however, there has been much written about *Campylobacter* in the lay press during 1991. In addition to articles in food magazines and newspapers, television news in at least one major metropolitan area (Washington, D.C.) has had a significant impact in educating the consumer about *Campylobacter* infections. Our congressional representatives have also conducted hearings related to the safety of poultry products produced for human consumption, a major vehicle for dissemination of *Campylobacter* infections to the general population. Thus, *Campylobacter* may be coming from obscurity into the limelight during the 1990s.

Workers in the field of *Campylobacter* research have been meeting regularly over the past 10 years at biannual international workshops to present new findings and discuss recent progress. The present text arises from a recent symposium sponsored by the National Institute of Allergy and Infectious Diseases, organized to bring together the clinicians and scientists most deeply involved in the field to summarize the current understanding of various topics and to discuss future needs.

The topics discussed here include a review of the clinical and epidemiologic characteristics of *Campylobacter* infections in the United States and worldwide, animal reservoirs of infection and the importance of campylobacters to the food industry, clinical microbiology and antimicrobial resistance mechanisms, pathogenesis of infection, host immune responses, and molecular pathogenesis. Each of the sections in this volume begins with an editorial summary of the particular field to provide perspective to the topic.

We hope that this text will serve as a source of information for persons already working in the field of *Campylobacter* research and will help to stimulate those outside the field to help solve the important issues in the prevention and treatment of *Campylobacter* disease.

Irving Nachamkin
Martin J. Blaser
Lucy S. Tompkins

Acknowledgments

We would like to express our great appreciation to Dale Spriggs, Enteric Diseases Branch, National Institute of Allergy and Infectious Diseases, for providing major support for the conference. We also extend our thanks to the Proctor and Gamble Company, and in particular Bruce McCarty, for their support for the conference. The assistance of Loretta Borko at the University of Pennsylvania in helping to organize the conference is also gratefully acknowledged.

I. CLINICAL AND EPIDEMIOLOGIC ASPECTS

CHAPTER 1

Clinical and Epidemiologic Considerations

MARTIN B. SKIRROW AND MARTIN J. BLASER

CAMPYLOBACTER JEJUNI INFECTIONS IN THE UNITED STATES AND OTHER DEVELOPED COUNTRIES

Campylobacter enteritis is caused by the two closely related species, *Campylobacter jejuni* and *Campylobacter coli,* but *C. jejuni* is predominant and the name is commonly used to include both species, as in the title to this volume. In this account, the anglicized term "campylobacters" refers to the two species unless otherwise specified.

Incidence

Precise measurement of the incidence of *Campylobacter* enteritis is probably not possible, any more than it is for salmonellosis or other acute bacterial infections of the gut that can be diagnosed only by identification of the causative organism in the laboratory. Laboratory reports represent only a small proportion of all infections and are dependent on the availability of medical and laboratory services and on the scope and reporting policies of the testing laboratories.

In the United States, voluntary laboratory reporting to the Centers for Disease Control has yielded fairly constant *Campylobacter* incidences of 6 to 7/100,000 over several years (18), but active local surveillance has given much higher incidences, in the range of 30 to 60/100,000 (8, 9). In the United Kingdom, where most clinical laboratories regularly report to the Public Health Laboratory Service Communicable Disease Surveillance Centre, the incidence in 1990 was 87/100,000. This represents a fourfold rise since 1980, which is thought to be due mainly to increased ascertainment. There are two especially valuable sources of incidence data. The first is a survey in a single general practice in England which permitted a calculated incidence of 11/1,000 (1.1% per year) (10). The second is a waterborne outbreak of *Campylobacter* enteritis in the United States in which it was found that 1 in 18 of victims consulted their doctors and that stool cultures were performed for 1 in 80 (14). Applying these ratios to laboratory isolation rates gives an incidence of 10/1,000 (1% per year), a figure very similar to the British one. If this estimation is correct, the total number of cases of *Campylobacter* enteritis in the United States would be in the neighborhood of 2.4 million per year, which is similar to that calculated for *Salmonella* enteritis (4).

Morbidity and Cost

The usual manifestation of *Campylobacter* enteritis is a very unpleasant attack of acute diarrhea lasting about 5 days. The pathology is that of an acute inflammatory enterocolitis; stool microscopy almost invariably shows the presence of cellular exudate, and frank blood is visible in the stools of about one-quarter of patients. Fever and other signs of acute infection are common in the early stages of the disease.

Complications are uncommon. Abdominal pain can be sufficiently severe for patients to be hospitalized with suspected appendicitis, and some undergo unnecessary appendectomy. About 1% of patients suffer from reactive (aseptic) arthritis arising 7 to 10 days after onset of illness; although benign, it may cause pain and incapacity for several weeks or even months. More serious, but uncommon, is Guillain-Barré

Martin B. Skirrow, Public Health Laboratory, Gloucestershire Royal Hospital, Gloucestershire GL1 3NN, United Kingdom. **Martin J. Blaser,** Division of Infectious Diseases, Department of Medicine, Vanderbilt University School of Medicine, Nashville, Tennessee 37232–2605, and Infectious Disease Section, Department of Veterans Affairs Medical Center, Nashville, Tennessee 37203.

syndrome (postinfective polyneuropathy), which can cause severe and sometimes fatal paralysis (11). In general, the infection is not as dangerous to infants and old people as is salmonellosis. Although serious complications are rare, even a tiny percentage of 2.4 million cases is a substantial number. Deaths attributable to *Campylobacter* infection in the United States are estimated to be 120 to 360 per year.

Perhaps a more telling statistic is the cost of the disease. A detailed study of 53 routinely diagnosed sporadic cases in the United Kingdom gave a figure of £273 (ca. $480) per case for health care and lost productivity and more than twice this sum if allowance was made for "pain and suffering" (16). Costs in the United States are likely to be at least as high, so *Campylobacter* enteritis is clearly a multimillion-dollar disease.

Age and Sex

In developed countries, persons of all ages are affected, but the age distribution differs from that of other bacterial infections of the gut in that incidence peaks in young adults as well as in young children (8, 9, 15, 18). Moreover, a slight male predominance is accentuated in this age group, e.g., 1.7:1 in a British survey (15). The reasons for this phenomenon are unknown, but the consumption of poorly prepared and undercooked chicken was found to be a major factor among male students preparing food while residing in university housing in the United States (5).

Pattern of Infection and Seasonal Variation

Most *Campylobacter* infections occur as sporadic single cases or as part of small family outbreaks. Community outbreaks are exceptional, but when they do occur they can be devastating. Outbreaks affecting several thousand people have arisen from the consumption of polluted water and raw milk in the United States, Scandinavia, and the United Kingdom (2).

In temperate regions, the incidence of *Campylobacter* enteritis is more than twice as high in summer than in winter. In the United Kingdom the rise occurs with remarkable precision each May (15), and recent evidence indicates that a small part of this rise is due to the seasonal pecking of doorstep-delivered bottles of fresh milk by birds of the crow family (17). However, this cannot be the reason for the summer rise in most other countries, because milk is not usually delivered in this way. In the United States there is a difference between the annual distribution of sporadic cases and those associated with outbreaks: sporadic cases peak in summer, whereas outbreak cases peak in the spring and fall (18). The reasons for these seasonal patterns are unknown, but studies in Sweden and the United States showed that *Campylobacter* carriage rates in chickens, a major source of sporadic cases, were much higher in summer than in winter. Other likely reasons are the summer activities of eating barbecue-prepared meals and drinking untreated water from streams and other natural sources when hiking and camping, both of which are known to be high-risk activities.

Sources of Infection

The fact that campylobacters live as commensals in the intestinal tracts of a wide range of birds and mammals, including the domestic animals most widely used for food production and as pets, means that there are many potential pathways of infection. Campylobacters can survive in the environment for several weeks at temperatures around 4°C and cause infection when consumed in untreated water and milk. Infection can also be acquired by direct contact with infected animals, mainly in specialized occupations, but pet dogs and cats can also be sources. A survey in Seattle showed that about 6% of sporadic infections were attributable to pets. Case-control studies in the United States have associated contact with cats with a substantially increased risk of infection, a finding that requires confirmation and explanation. Patients with *Campylobacter* enteritis are seldom a source of infection, except young children, who sometimes infect those in close contact with them.

Yet all of these sources are minor compared with food. *Campylobacter* enteritis is essentially a food-borne disease, and the principal vehicle of infection is raw or undercooked meat. Any raw meat is likely to be contaminated with campylobacters, and poultry is by far the most important source, especially broiler chickens, as they are consumed in such prodigious quantities. Retailed chickens have contamination rates of 60 to 80%, with *Campylobacter* counts in the region of 10^6 per fresh chicken carcass (about 2 $\log_{10}$ lower in frozen birds). Eating chicken carries a risk of infection only if it is undercooked, as campylobacters are killed by modest heat. Another problem is that of cross-contamination from raw chickens (and, to a lesser extent, other raw meats) to other foods during storage and preparation. Case-control studies in the United States attributed 48 to 70% of sporadic infections to consumption of chicken (5, 7). The figure of 48% was obtained in a major community survey in King County, Wash., and is probably representative of many developed countries. The higher figure of 70% was in a university campus and may be less applicable. Results of a major case-control study in the United Kingdom are currently being analyzed.

Campylobacter enteritis is also a cause of traveler's diarrhea. About 5 to 10% of infections in the United States are acquired abroad. The proportion is similar in the United Kingdom, but is about 50% in Scandinavia.

CAMPYLOBACTER JEJUNI INFECTIONS IN DEVELOPING COUNTRIES

In developing countries, *Campylobacter* enteritis is virtually limited to young children. Asymptomatic and multiple infections are common, so much so that it was once suspected that some of the *Campylobacter* strains were nonpathogenic; but it is now thought likely that any strain is capable of causing disease in nonimmune subjects. In general, watery diarrhea is a more common manifestation of the infection in children in these areas, but the strains typically isolated from such children, whether symptomatic or not, produce acute inflammatory disease in nonimmune visitors from developed countries; the manifestations of infection in United States servicemen were observed to be the same whether they acquired the infection in Thailand or Kentucky.

The explanation for the different age distribution and disease expression in developing and developed countries is the early acquisition of immunity by children exposed to hyperendemic infection. This is clearly shown by the decreasing ratio of symptomatic to asymptomatic infection consistently observed during the first 2 years of life and the rising concentrations of specific antibody, especially immunoglobulin A, that parallels this trend (1, 3). Under these conditions it is probable that congenital immunity from immune mothers mitigates the effects of disease in children under 6 months old. Studies in Algeria showed that breast-fed infants were less likely to suffer *Campylobacter* diarrhea than were formula-fed infants, although there was no great difference in infection rates (12).

These hyperendemic conditions characterized by a predominance of asymptomatic infections are stable and might appear to have some advantages. Unfortunately, prevalence is so high that even the small proportion of symptomatic infections constitute major infant morbidity, even though the *Campylobacter* enteritis is possibly less severe than are rotavirus and some other infectious diarrheas. However, it is important to realize that measures taken to reduce transmission could result in increased morbidity, at least until there is substantial control. As exposure decreased, maternal and infant immunity would fall and symptomatic infection would begin to affect older children and adults. Therefore, in any diarrheal disease control program it is imperative that long-term surveillance be established to detect such trends. Ironically, mesoendemic conditions are probably the worst. For example, in rural Yugoslavia the annual incidence of *Campylobacter* enteritis in children under the age of 1 year is 25/1,000, yet the disease is at least as common in adults as in the United Kingdom and the United States (13). Even that high childhood rate, albeit well below the rates in developing countries, was insufficient to produce immunity in the general population.

Seasonal trends are much less evident in tropical and subtropical countries. In general, higher incidences have been observed during rainy seasons. One reason for this lack of seasonality relative to *Shigella* and rotavirus infections is that campylobacters, like salmonellas, are transmitted largely in food and water rather than through personal contact. Known risk factors for infection are a lack of pipe-borne water and the presence of chickens in the household. However, much work must be done to define more precisely the pathways of infection and hence suitable preventive interventions. There is a great need for the development and wider use of molecular methods for the investigation of sources and modes of transmission in developing countries.

In many developing countries, such as the Central African Republic, Chile, and Hong Kong, *C. coli* accounts for a higher proportion of infections than elsewhere. Although *C. coli* is particularly associated with pigs, this association is not exclusive, and in some areas *C. coli* is commonly found in chickens.

IMPORTANCE OF OTHER CAMPYLOBACTERS IN HUMAN DISEASE

The genus *Campylobacter* contains 11 species, most of which have been found in humans at some time. Other species are of much less importance than *C. jejuni* or *C. coli,* although the status of several has yet to be properly ascertained. The type species, *C. fetus,* is an important cause of abortion in sheep and cattle, but it is infrequently recognized to cause disease in humans, and when it does, the persons are usually immunodeficient. The typical manifestation is that of a low-grade septicemic disease, sometimes with focal infection such as meningitis or peritonitis or infection at an endovascular site. In the United States *Campylobacter* bacteremia reported to the Centers for Disease Control is almost as often due to *C. fetus* as to *C. jejuni,* but in the United Kingdom *C. jejuni* and *C. coli* bacteremias, mostly associated with acute diarrhea, outnumber those due to *C. fetus* by 10:1. These differences are almost certainly due to differences in sampling and reporting; the U.S. numbers show that *C. fetus* bacteremias occur three times more often in men than women. AIDS is now recognized as a risk factor for *C. fetus* as well as other extraintestinal *Campylobacter* infections.

Among the other *Campylobacter* species that have been isolated from the feces of patients with diarrhea, *C. upsaliensis* stands out as the most important; however, even for this organism evidence of pathogenicity, although strong, is incomplete (6).

With the exception of *C. lari,* which accounts for only about 0.1% of infections, all of these other campylobacters require special filtration methods for their isolation from feces, as they do not grow reliably, or at all, on the conventional antibiotic-containing media used for the isolation of *C. jejuni* and *C. coli.* Their relative infrequency and unknown pathogenicity may not justify the cost of routine culture; it is more important that laboratories include culture for conventional campylobacters in their routine protocols than that they look for other campylobacters. However, the fact that the other species have been found more frequently in children in developing countries, notably Thailand, indicates geographic variation, and it is suggested that laboratories with a special interest in campylobacters might survey for these organisms to determine their regional prevalence.

CONTROL MEASURES AND RESEARCH NEEDS

General Measures

The basic measures for the control of any intestinal infection are applicable to *Campylobacter* enteritis. These are the provision of purified water supplies, the hygienic disposal of sewage, and the heat treatment of all milk sold to the public. To this may be added the hygienic handling of animals, especially hand washing after animal contact and before eating.

Food

More specifically, there is the problem of campylobacters contaminating foods originating from food-producing animals. The occurrence of campylobacters as commensals of a wide range of warm-blooded animals makes control of the reservoir of the organisms impractical. Red meat carcasses become heavily contaminated from intestinal contents at slaughter, but because many campylobacters are destroyed by the drying effect of conventional forced-air chilling, few remain on the product sold at retail markets. Offal, such as liver and kidneys, are likely to be more heavily contaminated.

Colonization of Poultry

The main problem is with poultry, which not only harbors many campylobacters in the cecum, but also becomes heavily cross-contaminated during mass-mechanized processing. Although improvements can be achieved at the processing stage, the consensus is that the best way to obtain *Campylobacter*-free poultry is to prevent or reduce infection while the birds are growing. It is our strong view that more resources and effort should be put into researching the epizootiology of *Campylobacter* colonization of broiler chickens and finding interventions that reduce or eliminate contamination. This will have to be a long-term undertaking requiring close cooperation between microbiologists, veterinarians, private industry, and government.

Public Education

Education of the public about the correct handling of poultry and other raw meats in the kitchen should be promulgated more energetically through television and other mass media. There is no reason why such education should be detrimental to what is a sensitive and highly competitive industry if it is done sensibly and as a cooperative venture. This cannot be the complete solution, so the main thrust should still be to control colonization in poultry.

Assessment of Sources and Risk

Although there is no doubt that chickens are a major source of food-borne *Campylobacter* enteritis, we need to measure more accurately the proportion of infections attributable to them and to assess the risk factors in their preparation and handling. In addition, the importance of other potential food sources, such as offal and seafood, must be properly assessed, and the apparent risk of cat ownership must be resolved. Case-control studies are probably the best means of obtaining such data.

Surveillance of Human Infection

One of the more surprising facts to emerge recently was that many clinical microbiology laboratories looked for campylobacters in diarrheal stools only when specifically asked to do so, for reasons of cost. This suggests a general lack of awareness by general physicians and microbiologists of the frequency and importance of *Campylobacter* enteritis. This deficiency highlighted the need for more accurate assessments of incidence, morbidity, and mortality, particularly in the United States, but also in other developed and developing countries. Prospective surveillance should be established to achieve this. Analysis of the economic costs to society of *Campylobacter* infection is also valuable in that it brings a salutary economic perspective to the disease and thus encourages political awareness and resource allocation.

SUMMARY OF PRINCIPAL RESEARCH NEEDS

The principal research needs may be summarized as follows. They include (i) prospective surveillance of incidence, morbidity, mortality, and cost of infection in both developed and developing countries; (ii) surveillance of targeted complications, such as Guillain-Barré syndrome, to more completely assess the impact of this infection; (iii) case-control and other studies to define more precisely the risk factors for the acquisition of sporadic infection and to measure the proportion of infections attributable to each; and (iv) studies to determine how chicken flocks become colonized and how this can be prevented or reduced.

REFERENCES

1. **Blaser, M. J., D. N. Taylor, and P. Echeverria.** 1986. Immune response to *Campylobacter jejuni* in a rural community in Thailand. *J. Infect. Dis.* **153:**249–254.
2. **Blaser, M. J., D. N. Taylor, and R. A. Feldman.** 1983. Epidemiology of *Campylobacter jejuni* infections. *Epidemiol. Rev.* **5:**157–176.
3. **Calva, J. J., G. M. Ruiz-Palacios, A. B. Lopez-Vidal, A. Ramos, and R. Bojalil.** 1988. Cohort study of intestinal infection with *Campylobacter* in Mexican children. *Lancet* **i:**503–506.
4. **Chalker, R., and M. J. Blaser.** 1988. A review of human salmonellosis. III. Magnitude of salmonellosis in the United States. *Rev. Infect. Dis.* **110:**111–124.
5. **Deming, M. S., R. V. Tauxe, P. A. Blake, S. E. Dixon, B. S. Fowler, T. S. Jones, E. A. Lockamy, C. M. Patton, and R. O. Sikes.** 1987. *Campylobacter* enteritis at a university: transmission from eating chicken and from cats. *Am. J. Epidemiol.* **126:**526–534.
6. **Goossens, H., L. Vlaes, M. De Boeck, B. Pot, K. Kersters, J. Levy, P. De Mol, J.-P. Butzler, and P. Vandamme.** 1990. Is *Campylobacter upsaliensis* an unrecognised cause of human diarrhoea? *Lancet* **335:**584–586.
7. **Harris, N. V., N. S. Weiss, and C. M. Nolan.** 1986. The role of poultry and meats in the etiology of *Campylobacter jejuni/coli* enteritis. *Am. J. Public Health* **76:**407–411.
8. **Hopkins, R. S., and R. N. Olmsted.** 1985. *Campylobacter jejuni* infection in Colorado: unexplained excess of cases in males. *Public Health Rep. Wash.* **100:**333–336.
9. **Johnson, K. E., and C. M. Nolan.** 1985. Community-wide surveillance of *Campylobacter jejuni* infection. *Diagn. Microbiol. Infect. Dis.* **3:**389–396.
10. **Kendall, E. J. C., and E. I. Tanner.** 1982. *Campylobacter* enteritis in general practice. *J. Hyg.* (Cambridge) **88:**155–163.
11. **Kuroki, S., T. Haruta, M. Yoshioka, Y. Kobayashi, M. Nukina, and H. Nakanishi.** 1991. Guillain-Barre syndrome associated with *Campylobacter* infection. *Pediatr. Infect. Dis.* **10:**149–151.
12. **Megraud, F., G. Boudraa, K. Bessaoud, S. Bensid, F. Dabis, R. Soltana, and M. Touhami.** 1990. Incidence of *Campylobacter* infection in infants in western Algeria and the possible protective role of breast feeding. *Epidemiol. Infect.* **105:**73–78.
13. **Popovic-Uroic, T.** 1989. *Campylobacter jejuni* and *Campylobacter coli* diarrhoea in rural and urban populations in Yugoslavia. *Epidemiol. Infect.* **102:**59–67.
14. **Sacks, J. J., S. Lieb, L. M. Baldy, S. Berta, C. M. Patton, M. C. White, W. J. Bigler, and J. J. Witte.** 1986. Epidemic campylobacteriosis associated with a community water supply. *Am. J. Public Health* **76:**424–429.
15. **Skirrow, M. B.** 1987. A demographic survey of *Campylobacter, Salmonella* and *Shigella* infections in England. *Epidemiol. Infect.* **99:**647–657.
16. **Sockett, P. N., and A. D. Pearson.** 1988. Cost implications of human *Campylobacter* infections, p. 261–264. *In* B. Kaijser and E. Falsen (ed.), *Campylobacter IV.* University of Göteborg, Göteborg, Sweden.

17. **Southern, J. P., R. M. M. Smith, and S. R. Palmer.** 1990. Bird attack on milk bottles: possible mode of transmission of *Campylobacter jejuni* to man. *Lancet* **336:**1425–1427.

18. **Tauxe, R. V., N. Hargrett-Bean, C. M. Patton, and I. Wachsmuth.** 1988. *Campylobacter* isolates in the United States, 1982–1986. *Morbid. Mortal. Weekly Rep.* **37:**1–13.

CHAPTER 2

Epidemiology of *Campylobacter jejuni* Infections in the United States and Other Industrialized Nations

ROBERT V. TAUXE

Campylobacter organisms have long been recognized as a cause of diarrhea in cattle and of septic abortion in both cattle and sheep, but they have been recognized as an important cause of human illness for only the last 20 years. *Campylobacter* organisms may have been what Escherich observed in the stools of infants with diarrhea in Germany in 1880 (13). However, *Campylobacter* was thought to be a rare and perhaps opportunistic human pathogen when it was isolated from blood cultures of humans in the 1950s (29). The most commonly identified species, *Campylobacter jejuni,* was first isolated from human diarrheal stools in 1972 by a filtration technique developed for veterinary diagnosis (9). The subsequent development of selective *Campylobacter* stool culture media led to the recognition that *C. jejuni* was a common cause of human diarrheal illness in many countries.

NATIONAL *CAMPYLOBACTER* SURVEILLANCE IN THE UNITED STATES

To learn more about the epidemiology of *Campylobacter* infections, the Centers for Disease Control (CDC) began national *Campylobacter* surveillance in 1982 (14, 43, 58, 59). Reports of isolates are mailed to the CDC by state health departments, using the same format used for *Salmonella* and *Shigella* surveillance in the United States. The reported data include the *Campylobacter* species isolated, the date of reporting to CDC, the age and sex of the person from whom the isolate came, the person's county of residence, and the clinical source of the culture. No other clinical information is included, and deaths are not reported. Unlike for *Salmonella* species, *Campylobacter* isolates are not routinely referred for serotyping or confirmation except in the outbreak setting or for an unusual isolate. We are dependent largely on species identification by the local laboratory. Many clinical laboratories may not routinely culture for *Campylobacter* species, and others may not use optimal culture methods. Participating states vary widely in their internal reporting requirements for *Campylobacter* species, which is reflected in the number of *Campylobacter* isolations reported.

Since 1982 the total number of reported isolates has increased, but the isolation rate has not changed markedly (Table 1). The increase from 1982 to 1983 is related to an increase in the number of reporting states. In 1989 isolates were reported from 45 states; 15 states accounted for 79% of isolates. These reported annual isolation rates of 5 to 6/100,000 are close to that of *Shigella* species (7 to 8/100,000) and considerably lower than that of *Salmonella* species (18 to 20/100,000). As discussed below, *Campylobacter* infections are actually likely to be more common than *Salmonella* infections. The lower reported isolation rates for *Campylobacter* species than *Salmonella* species reflect the limitations of surveillance.

The species was reported for 91% of isolates, and *C. jejuni* represented 99% of the reported species. Reported isolations of *Campylobacter* organisms in general and of *C. jejuni* specifically have shown a consistent seasonal distribution (Fig. 1). The number of *C. jejuni* isolates is low in the first 4 months of the year, and then there is a marked surge beginning in May and June,

Robert V. Tauxe, Enteric Diseases Branch, Division of Bacterial and Mycotic Diseases, National Center for Infectious Diseases, Centers for Disease Control, Atlanta, Georgia 30333.

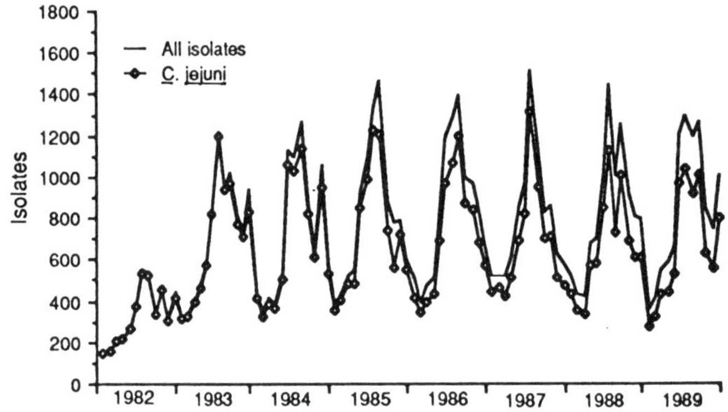

FIGURE 1. Reported *Campylobacter* isolates by month, United States, 1982 to 1989.

a peak in July and August, and a sustained plateau or second peak in the rest of the year.

The age- and sex-specific incidence of total reported *Campylobacter* isolates shows a pattern unique among bacterial infections (Fig. 2). The relatively high isolation rates in young adults may reflect specific exposures in that age group. The isolation rates were higher for males than for females. The male predominance extended from infancy to age 45, above which the infection rates were equal for both sexes. It is difficult to explain this difference entirely by a sex-specific behavior difference, such as a greater willingness on the part of males to eat undercooked chicken. The highest isolation rate was in infancy, approximately 14/100,000.

The vast majority of *Campylobacter* isolates came from stool specimens. During 1982 to 1989, only 0.3% overall of reported *C. jejuni* isolates came from blood, in contrast to *Salmonella* isolates, 3% of which came from blood.

Host factors play a major role in the risk of *C. jejuni* bacteremia. The proportion of isolates from blood did not vary by sex, but did vary by age, increasing with increasing age (Fig. 3). The proportion of bacteremias rose abruptly above age 70, to 1.2%. As of 1989, there is no increase in bacteremia in men aged 25 to 49, the group most affected by AIDS, suggesting that AIDS does not predispose patients with *Campylobacter* gastroenteritis to bacteremia.

TABLE 1. Reported isolates and isolation rate, national *Campylobacter* surveillance system, United States, by year

Year	No. of isolates	Isolation rate per 100,000
1982	4,027	7.2
1983	8,630	4.9
1984	8,770	5.0
1985	9,753	5.7
1986	10,063	5.9
1987	9,552	5.5
1988	10,024	5.8
1989	10,179	5.9

COMMON-SOURCE OUTBREAKS

CDC receives reports of food-borne and waterborne disease outbreaks, including those caused by *Campylobacter* species, as part of the national food-borne and waterborne disease surveillance systems. The first reported *Campylobacter* outbreak, in 1978, was also the largest. A contaminated community water supply affected an estimated 3,000 persons (64). Between 1978 and 1986, 57 outbreaks of *Campylobacter* infections were reported, including 11 waterborne outbreaks, 45 food-borne outbreaks, and 1 outbreak in a tourist group for which the source was unclear (Table 2). A species was reported for 43 outbreaks; 42 outbreaks were due to *C. jejuni,* including one raw-milk-associated outbreak due to both *C. jejuni* and a thermotolerant strain of *C. fetus* subsp. *fetus* (31); and 1 outbreak was due to a cluster of *C. fetus* subsp. *fetus* infections in cancer patients (6). The median number of cases was 22 in waterborne outbreaks and 14 in food-borne outbreaks. Two outbreak-associated fatalities were reported, one occurring during a food-borne outbreak of *C. jejuni* infections at a nursing home and one occurring in a patient with metastatic melanoma as part of the cluster

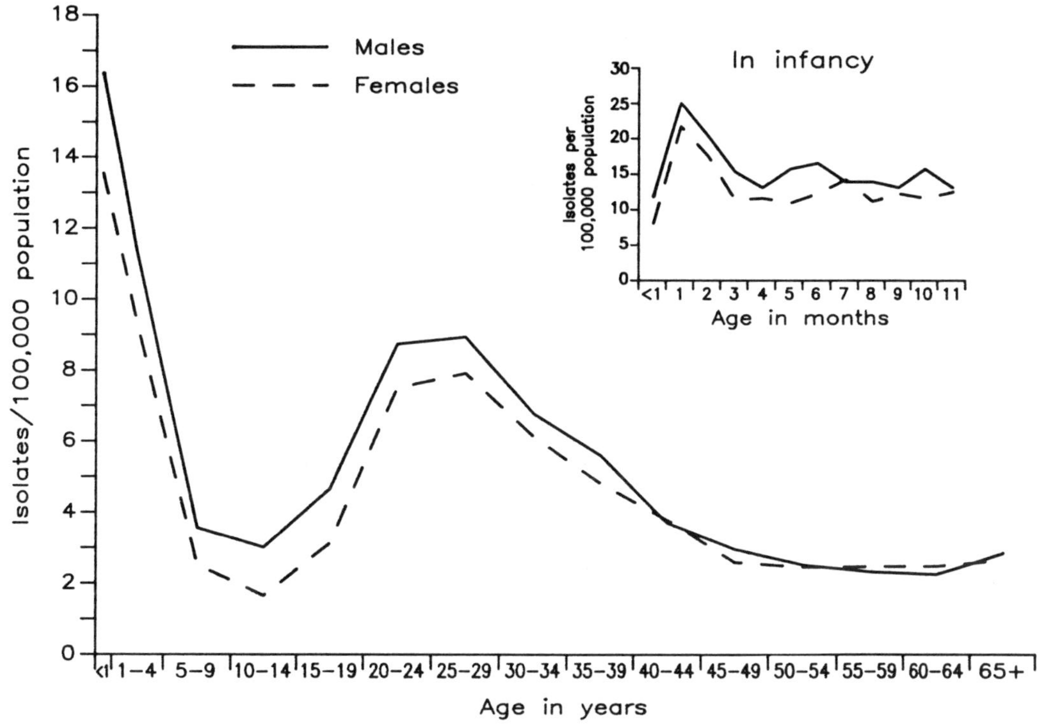

FIGURE 2. Reported *Campylobacter* isolates by age and sex, United States, 1982 to 1986.

of *C. fetus* subsp. *fetus* infections (6). The case-fatality ratio for outbreak-associated *Campylobacter* infections was 2/6,441 or 3/10,000. A vehicle was determined for 80% of the food-borne outbreaks; of these, 70% were caused by raw milk and 8% were associated with poultry. The waterborne outbreaks were all related to drinking untreated surface water or water supplies with inadequate chlorination, which may have been contaminated by bird droppings.

There is little evidence for sustained person-to-person transmission. Occasional secondary cases in contacts have been documented, and nosocomial transmission has been reported (27). However, no outbreaks have been reported in the United States in day-care centers or institutions for the mentally retarded, settings where person-to-person transmission has been common for other enteric pathogens such as *Giardia* and *Shigella* species.

It is important to recognize that the vast majority of *Campylobacter* infections are sporadic cases that are not associated with recognized outbreaks. Major differences exist between the epidemiology of outbreaks and that of the sporadic cases. The seasonality of common-source outbreaks of *Campylobacter* infection differs markedly from that of *Campylobacter* isolates reported through the national *Campylobacter* surveillance system (Fig. 4). The seasonal distribution of outbreaks is bimodal,

TABLE 2. Reported common-source outbreaks of *Campylobacter* infections by vehicle of transmission, United States, 1978 to 1986

Vehicle	No. of outbreaks	No. of ill persons
Food	45	1,308
Raw milk	26	829
Poultry	3	27
Egg	1	26
Other	6	87
≥Unknown	9	339
Water	11	4,983
Community water supply	7	4,930
Other	4	53
Travel associated	1	150
Total	57	6,441

with peaks in May and October and a low point in summer. In marked contrast, reported isolates, which are largely sporadic cases, peak in the summer months. This suggests that the vehicles and circumstances of outbreaks are quite different from those of sporadic cases. As discussed below, most sporadic cases are associated with poultry. Most outbreaks are due to contaminated raw milk or water, so there may be a bimodal seasonality to surface water contamination and to infection in dairy herds. This seasonality difference suggests that there are important differences in the ecology of the poultry reservoir and that of the bovine reservoir for *Campylobacter* species. It also means that universal pasteurization of milk and proper treatment of all drinking water could prevent 90% of the outbreak-associated cases in the United States, but would have only a limited effect on the much more frequent sporadic cases.

ESTIMATES OF INCIDENCE

The annual incidence of infection with *C. jejuni* in the United States is much greater than the reported isolation rate of 5/100,000. Surveillance data are incomplete for all infections; for example, it has been estimated that *Salmonella* infections are underreported by at least a factor of 20 (8). One important reason is that many laboratories do not routinely culture specifically for *Campylobacter* species in diarrheal stool specimens and many states do not require of isolates. To determine the relative frequency of diagnosed infection with *C. jejuni* compared with other enteric pathogens, CDC conducted a study in 1980 at eight hospitals whose microbiology laboratories cultured *Campylobacter* species routinely from diarrheal stool specimens along with *Salmonella* and *Shigella* species (3). The percentage of stool cultures that yielded *Campylobacter, Salmonella,* and *Shigella* species varied with the ages of the patients (Table 3). In children less than 1 year old, *Salmonella* species were isolated more than four times as frequently as *Campylobacter* species. For all age groups combined, *Campylobacter* species were isolated twice as frequently as *Salmonella* species and 4.5 times more frequently than *Shigella* species. This was good evidence that *Campylobacter* infections are more common than *Salmonella* infections if they are sought with equal frequency. Since the reported isolation rate of *Salmonella* species is 20/100,000 and that of *Shigella* species is 8/100,000, the reported incidence of *Campylobacter* infections would be 36 to 40/100,000 if they were diagnosed and reported in parallel with *Salmonella* and *Shigella* infections.

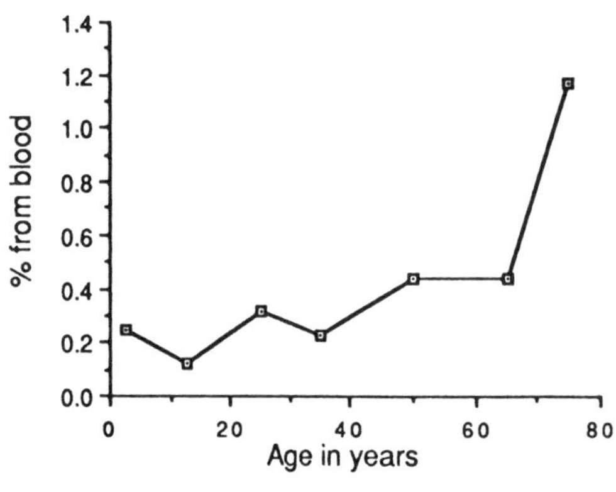

FIGURE 3. Proportion of reported *C. jejuni* isolates which were isolated from blood, by age, United States, 1982 to 1989.

Data from a Seattle health maintenance organization (HMO) provide a second estimate of the actual *Campylobacter* isolation rate when it is looked for routinely in all diarrheal stools. At this HMO the isolation rate was 71/100,000 in 1981 to 1982 (52). In a more recent survey in 1985 at the same HMO, it was 50/100,000 (32). This rate was much higher than the contemporaneous rates for *Salmonella* (21/100,000) and *Shigella* (7/100,000) isolation (32). These data suggest that when laboratories routinely look for *Campylobacter* organisms along with other enteric pathogens in diarrheal stools, the isolation rate is an order of magnitude greater than the reported isolation rate obtained through the national surveillance system.

Underreporting also occurs because physicians do not order diagnostic laboratory studies for all patients who consult them for a diarrheal illness. In 1975, the proportion of such visits that resulted in a stool culture was estimated to be as low as 33% (48). This indicates that the number of persons ill with campylobacteriosis who consult physicians is greater than the number whose infections are diagnosed, even when *Campylobacter* cultures are ordered routinely along with *Salmonella* and *Shigella* cultures. If we conservatively assume that cultures are done for 67% of patients presenting with gastroenteritis, the actual incidence of illness bringing patients to physicians can be estimated to be 54 to 60/100,000.

In addition, many *Campylobacter* infections are likely to go undiagnosed because a person may not consult a physician for the illness.

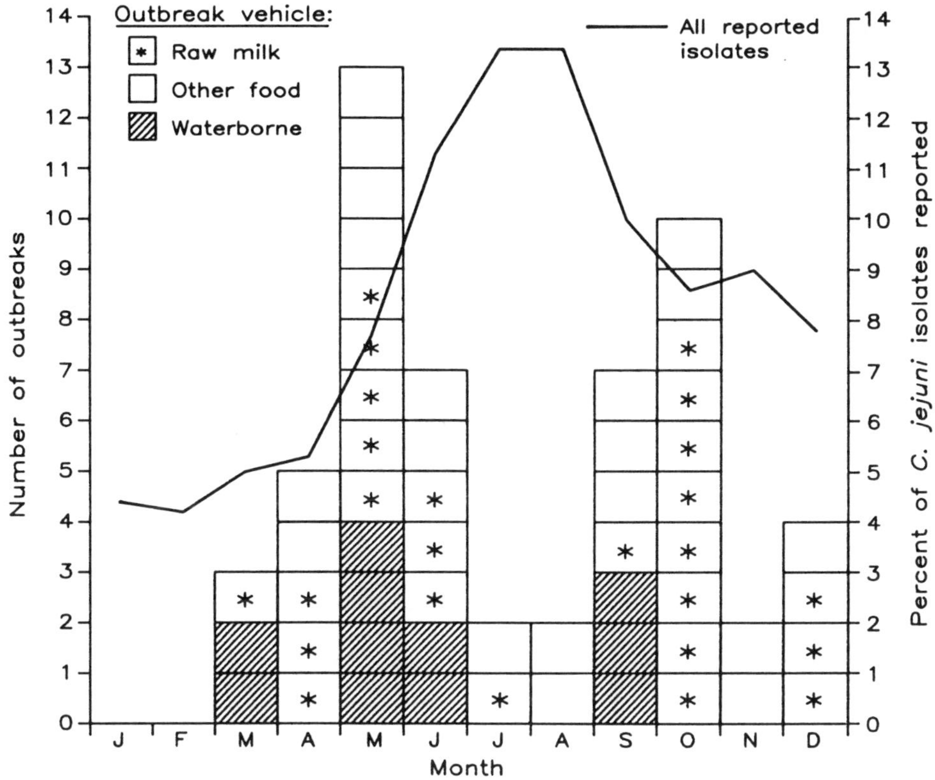

FIGURE 4. Distribution by month of reported outbreaks of *Campylobacter* infection and of *Campylobacter* isolates, United States, 1978 to 1986.

son may not consult a physician for the illness. No cultures would be obtained from these persons, and they could not be reported even to the best surveillance system. The number of milder infections is likely very large, both for sporadic cases and in the outbreak setting. A community-wide outbreak of *Campylobacter* infections related to a contaminated public water supply provided an opportunity to measure the number of illnesses that occur in addition to those that bring someone to see a physician (49). The investigation included a door-to-door search for cases, which identified a total of 865 persons with a compatible illness defined as diarrhea lasting for at least a day. Of all the ill patients, 4 (0.5%) were hospitalized, or 1 of every 200 ill. Of these 865 patients, only 47 (ca. 5.4%) had consulted the physician in town (1 of every 18 ill). This ratio of 18:1 is an estimate of the number of milder infections caused by *Campylobacter* species that may be present in a community compared with those that led to consultation with a physician.

These figures can be used to directly estimate an infection rate of *C. jejuni* for the United States. The estimated isolation rate, if all laboratories tested for *Campylobacter* species whenever they tested for *Salmonella* and *Shigella* species, is approximately 36 to 40/100,000; the actual incidence of illness bringing patients to a physician's office is 54 to 60/100,000; and the estimated proportion of milder infections for every patient that visits a physician is 18:1. The estimated infection rate for the United States for *C. jejuni* infections is thus approximately 960 to 1,080/100,000, some 2,160,000 to 2,430,000 infections per year, or 1% of the U.S. population per year. This estimate, which does not include asymptomatic infections, is close to an estimate of 1.1% for the annual incidence of *Campylobacter* infections in a general practice population in Great Britain (28).

The mortality associated with *Campylobacter* infections in the United States can be roughly estimated as well. *Campylobacter* deaths are not reported to the CDC. Because the current *International Classification of Disease (ICD-9) Ninth*

TABLE 3. Frequency of enteric bacterial pathogens in stool cultures of diarrheal patients, by age group, at eight hospitals in the United States, 1980 to 1981[a]

Age (yr)	% of cultures with: *Campylobacter* spp.	*Salmonella* spp.	*Shigella* spp.	Ratio of *Campylobacter* spp. to: *Salmonella* spp.	*Shigella* spp.
<1	1.1	4.6	0	0.2	
1–4	4.8	3.0	2.4	1.6	2.0
5–9	2.0	5.9	5.9	0.3	0.3
10–19	8.3	2.3	3.0	3.6	2.8
20–29	10.5	2.6	1.1	4.0	9.5
30–39	4.4	1.7	0	2.6	
40–49	4.6	0	0		
50–59	3.0	0	0		
≥60	2.3	0.9	0	2.5	
Total	4.6	2.3	1.0	2.0	4.6

[a] From reference 3.

Revision code (8a) does not specify *Campylobacter* infections, *Campylobacter* is not reported as a cause of death on death certificates either. However, deaths are reported in the common-source outbreak surveillance systems. In the series of common-source *Campylobacter* outbreaks reported to the CDC described above, two deaths were reported among 6,000 cases, giving a case-fatality rate of 3/10,000 outbreak-associated illnesses, which includes many milder illnesses. Applying this rate to the above estimates of all illness yields an estimate of between 680 and 730 *Campylobacter* deaths per year in the United States. Smith and Blaser have reported two *Campylobacter* deaths among 600 culture-confirmed cases in Colorado, giving a case-fatality rate of 24/10,000 culture-confirmed cases (56). Applying this rate to the estimated number of infections that are culture confirmed yields an estimate of approximately 200 deaths a year as a result of *Campylobacter* infection.

Campylobacter infections are also common in other developed countries. Typically, between 4 and 15% of diarrheal stool cultures yield *Campylobacter* organisms (60). The age range of affected individuals is similarly broad, and males usually predominate, although the prominent young-adult peak is sometimes absent, as, for example, in France (33). In 21 studies from developed countries comparing the yield of cultures from diarrheal stools for *Campylobacter* and for *Salmonella* species, 12 found *Campylobacter* infection to be more frequent than *Salmonella* infection, including studies conducted in the United Kingdom, the Netherlands, France, Italy, Sweden, the United States, and Australia (60). A smaller number of studies have reported isolations among definable population denominators, yielding annual isolation rates. In the United Kingdom, *Campylobacter* organisms were reported to be isolated at a rate of 58/100,000 (54). In a region around Freiburg, Federal Republic of Germany, largely served by a single laboratory, the isolation rate was reported to be 20/100,000 (30). Substantially higher rates have been reported from some areas. A national isolation rate of 86/100,000 has been reported from New Zealand, and a rate of 179/100,000 for Christchurch itself (5). In two districts of Ontario, an annual isolation rate of 290/100,000 was reported, ranging from 240/100,000 in urban areas to 1,092/100,000 in rural farm areas, where raw milk is often consumed (63). Among urban dwellers of Haifa, Israel, the isolation rate was 170/100,000, higher among Jews than non-Jews and higher in households with more education; exposure to raw milk was uncommon (44).

Outbreaks of *Campylobacter* infections have been reported in other industrialized nations. For example, recent waterborne outbreaks have been reported in Finland, Norway, and New Zealand (7, 34, 42). Raw-milk-associated outbreaks of campylobacteriosis have been relatively common in the United Kingdom (55).

The infectious dose of *C. jejuni* for humans appears to be low. Robinson reported his own experience following ingestion of 500 organisms (45). He developed an acute febrile diarrheal illness that lasted for 3 days. Human volunteer studies at the University of Maryland have shown that *Campylobacter* organisms can produce infection at a variety of doses ranging from 800 organisms, the lowest dose tested, to 10^6 organisms (2). The attack rates did not vary importantly with the dose, being generally in the neighborhood of 10%. Therefore, it is difficult to determine the lowest dose capable of causing disease or what dose is required to make 50% of the exposed persons ill. However, these data clearly show that relatively low doses, on the order of 500 to 800 organisms, are sufficient to cause illness.

SOURCES OF INFECTION

The sources of *Campylobacter* infection have been studied extensively in the United States. Four sources appear to account for nearly all cases: poultry, raw milk, untreated surface water, and pets. A small percentage of cases are associated with foreign travel; although no data are available concerning the specific sources of these infections, they are likely to include these same four. As noted above, most common-source outbreaks of *C. jejuni* infection are related to consumption of raw milk or untreated surface water. A typical outbreak occurs after a school class visit to a dairy farm, when children are given raw milk to drink. This practice is hazardous and should be discouraged. The mechanisms by which raw milk becomes contaminated are likely to include fecal contamination of the milk, perhaps related to long-term biliary carriage in the bovine (65). It can also be the result of asymptomatic bovine mastitis caused by *C. jejuni;* this has been documented to be the source of human infection on two occasions (21, 22). Neither mechanism is totally avoidable, even with exemplary dairy technique, and illness has been associated with "certified" raw milk produced under particularly hygienic conditions (40). Only pasteurization will reliably prevent such outbreaks. The means by which dairy animals become infected is unclear, although the similarity in seasonality of these outbreaks and waterborne outbreaks suggests that the two types may be related.

Waterborne transmission of *Campylobacter* organisms has occurred because of drinking unboiled surface water, contamination of groundwater with surface water, faulty disinfection, and contamination by wild-bird feces. In remote mountain wilderness areas, the infection is associated with drinking surface water from cold mountain streams; it can be more common than giardiasis in this setting (61). The presence of *Campylobacter* organisms in surface water appears to be seasonally dependent, affected by both temperature and sunlight, and is lowest in the summer, which could explain the paucity of waterborne outbreaks in the summer (4).

Sporadic cases of *Campylobacter* infection are far more common than outbreak-associated cases, have a different seasonal distribution, and appear to be associated largely with eating or handling poultry meat. Calculating the etiologic fraction with data from case-control studies provides an estimate of the proportion of cases attributable to various exposures (50). A large case-control study conducted at a Seattle HMO showed that eating poultry, including chicken, turkey, and Cornish game hens, accounted for over 50% of all of the cases (17, 52). Five percent of the cases were attributed to raw milk, including both cow and goat milk; 6% of the cases could be attributed to contact with pets; 9% were related to exposure during overseas travel; and 8% could be attributed to drinking contaminated surface water.

In a second study, conducted among students at a Georgia university, 70% of cases were attributed to eating chicken and the other 30% were related to contact with cats (10). No cases were related to drinking raw milk, traveling overseas, or drinking untreated surface water. In a case-control study of sporadic cases in Colorado, the identified risk factors were drinking untreated water or raw milk, contact with cats, and eating undercooked chicken, although their independence was not assessed (19). In a second study conducted in Colorado, handling raw chicken, as opposed to eating it, emerged as a risk factor (20). In some rural parts of the country where drinking raw milk remains popular, raw milk can be an important source of sporadic cases as well as of outbreaks. In a study of sporadic cases in Dubuque, Iowa, an etiologic fraction of 47% can be calculated for raw-milk exposure, and this was the only risk factor identified (51).

Case-control studies of sporadic campylobacteriosis in the Netherlands showed a marked association with eating chicken prepared in the home (37). A similar investigation in Sweden showed that most cases were associated with holiday travel to other countries without further clarifying the type of exposure; however, domestically acquired cases were significantly associated with preparing and eating chicken in the home (35).

These studies also provide information on how home-prepared poultry causes these infections. The case-control study in Seattle also identified an association between infection and not washing down the kitchen cutting board with soap, an indicator of potential cross-contamination. In the Swedish investigation, seven of nine infected persons who ate the chicken also prepared it and thus presumably had contact with raw poultry. In the second case-control study in Colorado, infection was specifically associated with handling the raw chicken meat; illness occurred in the preparers, rather than the eaters, of chicken. The person who prepared the chicken in the kitchen was the one most likely to become infected. In studies at the University in Georgia, we noted three ways in which poultry can easily cause *C. jejuni* infections. The first was eating chicken raw. The second was eating chicken undercooked, defined operationally as still bloody and pink near the bone. This is a relatively common exposure, particularly among male college students. The third was using a knife or cutting board for cutting up a raw chicken and then, without washing the utensil, using it to prepare other food. This mode of transmission also appeared to be common.

These relatively simple errors in food handling are consistent with the low infectious dose. The quantity of *Campylobacter* organisms in raw chicken juice has been estimated to be 10^6 per chicken in one study in the United Kingdom (18). Ingestion of a small drop of raw chicken juice could easily provide the infectious dose. The low infectious dose means that reducing the proportion of carcasses that are contaminated could have a greater impact on public health than reducing the number of *Campylobacter* organisms on each carcass. Unlike for *Salmonella* infection, eating food which has been left out for many hours and not reheated has not emerged as a common food-handling error leading to campylobacteriosis. Campylobacters are sensitive to drying and ambient atmosphere and may not grow rapidly on poultry at ambient temperatures; this may explain the rarity of large outbreaks related to solid foods (15).

Ample laboratory evidence supports a dominant role for poultry as a source of *C. jejuni* infections. Many studies have shown high levels of contamination of poultry with *C. jejuni* at the point of sale; typically more than 50% of carcasses have such contamination (15, 16, 38, 47, 53). In Seattle, the seasonality of contamination of poultry carcasses with *C. jejuni* also shows a summer peak, consistent with the summer peak in sporadic human cases (16). Jones et al. conducted an exhaustive survey of environmental isolates for 1 year in Lancaster, United Kingdom, collecting specimens from surface waters, sewage sludge, and fresh liquid sewage (23–25). *Campylobacter* organisms were rarely isolated in surface water in late spring and summer, when human illness was at its peak, making that an unlikely source. Sampling of various points in the sewage system identified the highest counts in the effluent from abattoirs and a poultry-processing plant, with a seasonal distribution that matched human illness rates, suggesting that slaughter animals and poultry were the primary sources of infection.

The isolates from sporadic human cases and those from retail poultry have been compared in several laboratory studies. In Belgium, comparison of serotypes showed that those isolated from humans strongly resembled those isolated from poultry, rather than those isolated from other animals (36). In Israel, the most common serogroup of *C. jejuni* isolated from humans was also the most common serogroup isolated from chicken meat (46). In the Netherlands, comparison of biotypes and serotypes of human and animal isolates of *C. jejuni* showed that five of the six most common types present in human isolates were also common in chicken isolates, whereas there was little overlap in types isolated from humans compared with those from swine (1), even though the Dutch population consumes more than four times as much pork as poultry. In Ontario, the serotypes of *C. jejuni* found in chickens were those commonly found in humans (41). In the United States, comparison of serotypes, plasmid profiles, and antibiotic resistance patterns showed substantial similarity between human and poultry isolates (39). The tetracycline resistance plasmid was strikingly similar in the two groups (62). More recently, the appearance of fluoroquinolone resistance in poultry and human isolates indicates that the two groups are connected (12). Whole-cell DNA restriction digest patterns were used in New Zealand to characterize thermophilic *Campylobacter* strains from a variety of sources; 50% of human isolates had patterns that were indistinguishable from those isolated from poultry (26).

Although many chicken flocks do not have *Campylobacter* infections, the organism can rapidly spread horizontally in chickens, presumably through a common water source or fecal contact (53). Uncontaminated birds easily become contaminated at slaughter. Important points of contamination are likely to be water used in the defeathering process and in the final chill tank (53). Cleaning practices at the plant may influence the contamination rate: a progressive increase in contamination in poultry carcasses slaughtered from Monday through Wednesday after a weekend cleanup has been reported (52). Other meats, and nonmeat foods such as mushrooms, have been shown to yield *Campylobacter* organisms on culture (11). Their role in producing human illness remains to be epidemiologically clarified.

A smaller proportion of human cases have been associated with pet animal contact. The Seattle study documented an association with diarrheic kittens (52). Deming et al. found that 30% of the cases in university students were associated with healthy cats (10). Brieseman suggested that the *Campylobacter* infections in Christchurch, New Zealand, may be associated with dog ownership (5). The nature of the contact with an infected dog or cat that transmits the illness remains to be defined, as do the means by which the pets become infected in the first place.

An unusual combination of exposures has recently been reported from the United Kingdom. A study of sporadic cases showed an association with drinking pasteurized milk from bottles attacked by birds (57). A remarkable 80% of infected persons reported drinking milk from bottles whose lids had been visibly pecked through by birds, usually jackdaws and magpies.

SUMMARY

C. jejuni is the most common bacterial enteric pathogen in the United States. Although usually not invasive, infection is occasionally fatal. Diagnostic laboratories should routinely screen diarrheal stools for *Campylobacter* species. The vast bulk of infections are sporadic, and most are poultry associated. Raw milk, untreated surface water, and pet animals are also important sources of the infection. The infectious dose is as low as several hundred organisms, making exposure through simple contact with raw and undercooked chicken an easy route of infection. In addition to pasteurizing milk and disinfecting drinking water, further control of this infection will depend on understanding the ecology of the organism in flocks and slaughter plants and on reducing the level of contamination in retail raw chicken.

REFERENCES

1. **Banferr, J. R. J.** 1985. Biotypes and serotypes of *Campylobacter jejuni* and *Campylobacter coli* strains isolated from patients, pigs and chicken in the region of Rotterdam. *J. Infect.* **10:**277–281.
2. **Black, R. E., M. D. Levine, M. L. Clements, T. P. Hughes, and M. J. Blaser.** 1988. Experimental *Campylobacter jejuni* infection in humans. *J. Infect. Dis.* **157:**472–479.
3. **Blaser, M. J., J. G. Wells, R. A. Feldman, R. A. Pollard, J. R. Allen, and the Collaborative Diarrheal Disease Study Group.** 1983. *Campylobacter* enteritis in the United States: a multicenter study. *Ann. Intern. Med.* **98:**360–365.
4. **Bolton, F. J., D. Coates, D. N. Hutchinson, and A. F. Godfree.** 1987. A study of thermophilic campylobacters in a river system. *J. Appl. Bacteriol.* **62:**167–176.
5. **Brieseman, M. A.** 1990. A further study of the epidemiology of *Campylobacter jejuni* infections. *N.Z. Med. J.* **103:**207–209.
6. **Centers for Disease Control.** 1981. *Campylobacter* sepsis associated with "nutritional therapy"—California. *Morbid. Mortal. Weekly Rep.* **30:**294–295.
7. **Centers for Disease Control.** 1991. *Campylobacter* enteritis—New Zealand, 1990. *Morbid. Mortal. Weekly Rep.* **40:**116–123.
8. **Chalker, R. B., and M. J. Blaser.** 1988. A review of human salmonellosis. III. Magnitude of *Salmonella* infection in the United States. *Rev. Infect. Dis.* **10:**111–124.

8a. **Commission on Professional and Hospital Activities.** 1978. *International Classification of Diseases, 9th Revision, Clinical Modification.* Commission on Professional and Hospital Activities, Ann Arbor, Mich.

9. **Dekeyser, P. J., M. Gossuin-Detrain, J. P. Butzler, and J. Sternon.** 1972. Acute enteritis due to related *Vibrio:* first positive stool cultures. *J. Infect. Dis.* **125:**390–392.
10. **Deming, M. S., R. V. Tauxe, P. A. Blake, S. E. Dixon, B. S. Fowler, T. S. Jones, E. A. Lockamy, C. M. Patton, and R. O. Sikes.** 1987. *Campylobacter* enteritis at a university: transmission from eating chicken and from cats. *Am. J. Epidemiol.* **126:**526–534.
11. **Doyle, M. P., and J. L. Schoeni.** 1986. Isolation of *Campylobacter jejuni* from retail mushrooms. *Appl. Environ. Microbiol.* **51:**449–450.
12. **Endtz, H., R. P. Mouton, T. vander Ryden, G. J. Ruijs, M. Biever, and B. van Klingeren.** 1989. Fluoroquinolone resistance in *Campylobacter* spp. isolated from human stools and poultry products. *Lancet* **335:**787.
13. **Escherich, T.** 1881. Beitrage zur Kenntniss der Darmbacterien. III. Ueber das vorkommen von Vibrionen in Darmcanal und den Stuhlgaengen der Saeuglinge. *Muench. Med. Wochenschr.* **33:**815–817.
14. **Finch, M. J., and L. W. Riley.** 1984. *Campylobacter* infections in the United States. Results of an 11-state surveillance. *Arch. Intern. Med.* **144:**1610–1612.
15. **Franco, D. A.** 1988. *Campylobacter* species: considerations for controlling a food-borne pathogen. *Food Prot.* **51:**145–153.
16. **Harris, N. V., D. Thompson, D. C. Martin, and C. M. Nolan.** 1986. A survey of *Campylobacter* and other bacterial contaminants of pre-market chicken and retail poultry and meats, King County Washington. *Am. J. Public Health* **76:**401–406.
17. **Harris, N. V., N. S. Weiss, and C. M. Nolan.** 1986. The role of poultry and meats in the etiology of

Campylobacter jejuni/coli enteritis. *Am. J. Public Health* **76**:407–411.
18. **Hood, A. M., A. D. Pearson, and M. Shahamat.** 1988. The extent of surface contamination of retailed chickens with *Campylobacter jejuni* serogroups. *Epidemiol. Infect.* **100**:17–25.
19. **Hopkins, R. S., R. Olmsted, and G. R. Istre.** 1984. *Campylobacter jejuni* infection in Colorado: identified risk factors. *Am. J. Public Health* **74**:249–250.
20. **Hopkins, R. S., and A. B. Scott.** 1983. Handling raw chicken as a source for sporadic *Campylobacter jejuni* infections. *J. Infect. Dis.* **148**:770. (Letter.)
21. **Hudson, P. J., R. L. Vogt, J. Brondum, and C. M. Patton.** 1984. Isolation of *Campylobacter jejuni* from milk during an outbreak of campylobacteriosis. *J. Infect. Dis.* **150**:789.
22. **Hutchinson, D. N., F. J. Bolton, P. M. Hinchliffe, et al.** 1985. Evidence of udder excretion of *Campylobacter jejuni* as the cause of milk-borne *Campylobacter* outbreak. *J. Hyg.* (Cambridge) **94**:205–215.
23. **Jones, K., M. Betaieb, and D. R. Telford.** 1990. Thermophilic campylobacters in surface waters around Lancaster, UK: negative correlation with *Campylobacter* infections in the community. *J. Appl. Bacteriol.* **69**:758–764.
24. **Jones, K., M. Betaieb, and D. R. Telford.** 1990. Seasonal variation of thermophilic campylobacters in sewage sludge. *J. Appl. Bacteriol.* **69**:185–189.
25. **Jones, K., M. Betaieb, and D. R. Telford.** 1990. Correlation between environmental monitoring of thermophilic campylobacters in sewage effluent and the incidence of *Campylobacter* infection in the community. *J. Appl. Bacteriol.* **69**:235–240.
26. **Kakoyiannis, C. K., P. J. Winter, and R. B. Marshall.** 1988. The relationship between intestinal *Campylobacter* species isolated from animals and humans as determined by Brenda. *Epidemiol. Infect.* **100**:379–387.
27. **Karmali, M. A., B. Norrish, H. Lior, B. Heyes, A. Monthealth, and H. Montgomery.** 1984. *Campylobacter* enterocolitis in a neonatal nursery. *J. Infect. Dis.* **149**:874–877.
28. **Kendall, E. J., and E. I. Tanner.** 1982. *Campylobacter* enteritis in general practice. *J. Hyg.* (Cambridge) **88**:155–163.
29. **King, E. O.** 1962. The laboratory recognition of *Vibrio fetus* and closely related *Vibrio* species isolated from cases of human vibriosis. *Ann. N.Y. Acad. Sci.* **98**:700–711.
30. **Kist, M., and D. G. Newell.** 1982. *Campylobacter enteritidis:* epidemiological and clinical data from recent isolations in the region of Freiburg West Germany, p. 138–143. *In* D. G. Newell (ed.), *Epidemiology, Pathogenesis, and Biochemistry.* MTP Press, Lancaster, U.K.
31. **Klein, B. S., J. M. Vergeront, M. J. Blaser, et al.** 1986. *Campylobacter* infection associated with raw milk: an outbreak of gastroenteritis due to *Campylobacter jejuni* and thermotolerant *Campylobacter fetus* subsp *fetus*. *JAMA* **255**:361–364.
32. **MacDonald, K. L., M. J. O'Leary, M. L. Cohen, P. Edmonds, D. J. Brenner, D. Janssen, and J. P. Davis.** 1988. *Escherichia coli* O157:H7, an emerging gastrointestinal pathogen. *JAMA* **259**:3567–3570.
33. **Megraud, F.** 1989. Reseau de surveillance national des infections a *Campylobacter.* Bilan de l'annee 1988. *Bull. Epidemiol. Hebd.* **51**:215–216.
34. **Melby, K., O. P. Dahl, L. Crisp, and J. L. Penner.** 1990. Epidemiology. Clinical and serological manifestations in patients during a waterborne epidemic due to *Campylobacter jejuni. J. Infect.* **21**:309–316.
35. **Norkrans, G., and A. Svedhem.** 1982. Epidemiological aspects of *Campylobacter jejuni* enteritis. *J. Hyg.* (Cambridge) **89**:163–170.
36. **Oosterom, J., J. R. J. Banffer, S. Lauwers, and A. E. Busschbach.** 1985. Serotyping of and hippurate hydrolysis by *Campylobacter jejuni* isolates from human patients, poultry and pigs in the Netherlands. *Antonie van Leeuwenhoek* **51**:65–70.
37. **Oosterom, J., C. H. Den Uyl, J. R. J. Banffer, and J. Huisman.** 1984. Epidemiological investigations on *Campylobacter jejuni* in households with a primary infection. *J. Hyg.* (Cambridge) **92**:325–332.
38. **Park, C. E., Z. K. Stankiewicz, J. Lovett, J. Hunt, and D. W. Francis.** 1983. Effect of temperature, duration of incubation, and pH of enrichment culture on the recovery of *Campylobacter jejuni* from eviscerated market chickens. *Can. J. Microbiol.* **29**:803–806.
39. **Patton, C. M., T. J. Barrett, and G. K. Morris.** 1985. Comparison of the Penner and Lior methods for serotyping *Campylobacter* spp. *J. Clin. Microbiol.* **22**:558–565.
40. **Potter, M. E., M. J. Blaser, R. K. Sikes, A. F. Kaufman, and J. G. Wells.** 1983. Human *Campylobacter* infection associated with certified raw milk. *Am. J. Epidemiol.* **117**:475–483.
41. **Prescott, J. F., and O. S. Gellner.** 1984. Intestinal carriage of *Campylobacter jejuni* and *Salmonella* by chicken flocks at slaughter. *Can. J. Comp. Med.* **48**:329–331.
42. **Rautelin, H., K. Koota, R. vonEssen, M. Jahkola, A. Siitonen, and T. U. Kosunen.** 1990. Waterborne *Campylobacter jejuni* epidemic in a Finnish hospital for rheumatic diseases. *Scand. J. Infect. Dis.* **22**:321–326.
43. **Riley, L. W., and M. J. Finch.** 1985. Results of the first year of national surveillance of *Campylobacter* infections in the United States. *J. Infect. Dis.* **151**:956–959.
44. **Rishpon, S., L. M. Epstein, M. Shmilovitz, B. Kretzer, A. Tamir, and N. Egoz.** 1984. *Campylobacter jejuni* infections in Haifa Subdistrict, Israel, summer 1981. *Int. J. Epidemiol.* **13**:216–220.
45. **Robinson, D. A.** 1981. Infective dose of *Campylobacter jejuni* in milk. *Br. Med. J.* **282**:1584.
46. **Rogol, M., and I. Sechter.** 1987. Serogroups of thermophilic campylobacters from humans and from non-human sources, Israel 1982–1985. *Epidemiol. Infect.* **99**:175–182.
47. **Rogol, M., I. Sechter, Z. Greenberg, R. Mizrachi, Y. Shtark, and S. Alfi.** 1985. Contamination of

chicken meat and environment with various serogroups of *Campylobacter jejuni/coli*. *Int. Food Microbiol.* **1**:271–276.

48. **Rosenberg, M. L., J. S. Marr, E. J. Gangarosa, R. A. Pollard, M. Wallace, and O. Brolnitsky.** 1977. CDC news: *Shigella* surveillance in the United States, 1975. *J. Infect. Dis.* **136**:458–460.
49. **Sacks, J. J., S. Lieb, L. M. Baldy, et al.** 1986. Epidemic campylobacteriosis associated with a community water supply. *Am. J. Public Health* **76**:424–428.
50. **Schlesselman, J. J.** 1982. *Case-Control Studies: Design, Conduct, Analysis.* Oxford University Press, New York.
51. **Schmid, G. P., R. E. Schaefer, and B. D. Plikaytis.** 1987. A one-year study of endemic campylobacteriosis in a midwestern city: association with consumption of raw milk. *J. Infect. Dis.* **156**:218–222.
52. **Seattle – King County Department of Public Health.** 1984. *Surveillance of the Flow of Salmonella and Campylobacter in a Community.* Communicable Disease Control Section, Seattle-King County Department of Public Health, Seattle.
53. **Shane, S. M.** 1991. Environmental factors associated with *Campylobacter jejuni* colonization of poultry, p. 29–46. *In* L. C. Blankenship and S. M. Shane (ed.), *Colonization Control of Human Bacterial Enteropathogens in Poultry.* Academic Press, Inc., San Diego, Calif.
54. **Skirrow, M. B.** 1987. A demographic survey of *Campylobacter, Salmonella* and *Shigella* infections in England. A public health laboratory service survey. *Epidemiol. Infect.* **99**:647–657.
55. **Skirrow, M. B.** 1990. Food-borne illness. *Campylobacter. Lancet* **336**:921–923.
56. **Smith, G. S., and M. J. Blaser.** 1985. Fatalities associated with *Campylobacter jejuni* infections. *JAMA* **253**:2873–2875.
57. **Southern, J. P., R. M. M. Smith, and S. R. Palmer.** 1990. Bird attack on milk bottles: possible mode of transmission of *Campylobacter jejuni* to man. *Lancet* **336**:1425–1427.
58. **Tauxe, R. V., N. Hargrett-Bean, C. M. Patton, and I. K. Wachsmuth.** 1988. *Campylobacter* isolates in the United States, 1982–1986. CDC Surveillance Summaries, June 1988. *Morbid. Mortal. Weekly Rep.* **37**(SS-2):1–14.
59. **Tauxe, R. V., D. A. Pegues, and N. H. Bean.** 1987. *Campylobacter* infections: the emerging national pattern. *Am. J. Public Health* **77**:1219–1221.
60. **Taylor, D. N., and M. J. Blaser.** 1991. *Campylobacter* infections, p. 151–172. *In* A. S. Evans and P. S. Brachman (ed.), *Bacterial Infections in Humans,* 2nd ed. Plenum Publishing Corp., New York.
61. **Taylor, D. N., K. T. McDermott, J. R. Little, J. G. Wells, and M. J. Blaser.** 1983. *Campylobacter* enteritis from untreated water in the Rocky Mountains. *Ann. Intern. Med.* **99**:38–40.
62. **Tenover, F. C., S. Williams, K. P. Gordon, C. Nolan, and J. J. Plorde.** 1985. Survey of plasmids and resistance factors in *Campylobacter jejuni* and *Campylobacter coli*. *Antimicrob. Agents Chemother.* **27**:37–41.
63. **Thompson, J. S., F. E. Cahoon, and D. S. Hodge.** 1986. Rate of *Campylobacter* spp. isolation in three regions of Ontario, Canada, from 1978 to 1985. *J. Clin. Microbiol.* **24**:876–878.
64. **Vogt, R. L., H. E. Sours, T. Barrett, et al.** 1982. *Campylobacter* enteritis associated with contaminated water. *Ann. Intern. Med.* **96**:292–296.
65. **Warner, D. P., J. H. Bryner, and G. W. Beran.** 1986. Epidemiologic study of campylobacteriosis in Iowa cattle and the possible role of unpasteurized milk as a vehicle of infection. *Am. J. Vet. Res.* **47**:254–258.

CHAPTER 3

Campylobacter Infections in Developing Countries

DAVID N. TAYLOR

INTRODUCTION

Campylobacter species occur in the animal food chain of humans from the most to the least economically developed cultures. Although *Campylobacter* species are recognized as among the most common causes of diarrhea worldwide, the epidemiology of *Campylobacter* infections in the developing world differs markedly from that in the developed world. Given the differences in climate, population density, and ethnic background of the inhabitants of the developing world from those in the developed world, it is not surprising that there are geographic differences in the disease patterns. However, there are also great geographic and cultural diversities among the developing countries of Asia, Africa, and Latin America, yet a definite developing world pattern of disease has emerged. The explanation for the pattern in the developing world is not immediately obvious and has been the subject of investigation for the past decade. The epidemiologic differences in developed and developing countries described in this paper are best explained by increased exposure and high infection rates early in life in developing world populations, which in turn induce high levels of immunity early in life.

At the outset, it is important to acknowledge the contributions of a number of international agencies that have been instrumental in allowing investigators to go beyond the initial descriptive phase to more comprehensive studies of *Campylobacter* infections in the developing world. The World Health Organization supported many laboratories in the developing world with Lior serotyping antisera provided by the Public Health Service of Canada and also provided grants for epidemiologic studies. The Rockefeller Masters in Epidemiology program at McMaster University and the Centers for Disease Control Field Epidemiology Training Program brought better-trained epidemiologists to the developing world. The Applied Diarrheal Disease Research program funded by U.S. Aid for International Development and World Health Organization provides grants for use in the developing world to study diarrheal disease. These agencies supplied the tools, the funds, and the educational resources that allowed a second wave of research in the field in the form of well-designed, prospective studies, which also contributed much to our general understanding of diarrheal disease.

MAGNITUDE OF INFECTION

Most, if not all, of the many differences in the epidemiology of *Campylobacter* infection can be traced to the concept that the incidence of disease in developing countries is higher by several orders of magnitude than in developed countries. In England and the United States, the annual incidence of *Campylobacter* enteritis is approximately 50/100,000 population and about 300/100,000 for children 1 to 4 years old (28, 38) (Table 1). In Yugoslavia, a country intermediate in its economic development, the incidence of disease is about 90/100,000 per year and increases to 2,500/100,000 in children 1 to 4 years old (31).

The incidence of *Campylobacter* enteritis in Mexico and Thailand is much higher: 0.4 episode per child per year, or 40,000/100,000 for children younger than 5 years old (9, 47) (Table 2). Although these rates seem extraordinarily high, they are substantiated by *Campylobacter* diarrhea rates in travelers to these countries of 2–3% per month (or 27,000 to 38,000/100,000

David N. Taylor, Enteric Infections Branch, Walter Reed Army Institute of Research, Washington, D.C. 20307–5100.

TABLE 1. Incidence of *Campylobacter* enteritis by country[a]

Location	Age group (yr)	Incidence/100,000
United States	All ages	50
England	All ages	60
	1–4	300
Yugoslavia	All ages	90
	1–4	2,500
Mexico	0–4	40,000
Thailand	0–4	40,000

[a] Data from references 9, 28, 31, 38, and 47.

per year) (14, 46, 51). For children in Mexico and Thailand the rate of asymptomatic infection is three to four times the rate of symptomatic infections. Although the diarrhea rates in young children of the developing world are over 100 times greater than those seen in England, the rates of symptomatic illness in school-age children and adults in developing countries are lower than in England. Thus, the incidence of *Campylobacter* enteritis for all age groups in the developing world may not be much higher than for Yugoslavia.

ASYMPTOMATIC INFECTIONS

In surveys of diarrheal disease in England and the United States *Campylobacter* species are isolated from about 5% of patients with diarrhea. The isolation rates are considerably higher than for *Salmonella* species, isolated from 2 to 3% of patients, and *Shigella* species, isolated from 1% of patients (7, 38). *Campylobacter* species are rarely isolated from healthy persons in developed countries (5, 43).

In developing parts of Asia, Africa, and Latin America *Campylobacter* isolation rates have ranged from 10 to 20% in surveys performed in children with diarrhea (43). *Campylobacter* species are commonly isolated as often as rotavirus and enterotoxigenic *Escherichia coli* and are frequently more common than nontyphoidal *Salmonella* and *Shigella* species (12, 47, 48).

From the first studies in the developing world, it was recognized that *Campylobacter* species could be isolated from children who were well as often as from children who had diarrhea. In 1979 Bokkenheuser et al. (8) found that after the age of 9 months, there was no difference in the isolation rate of *Campylobacter* species in South African children. When cultures were made from samples isolated from schoolchildren over a 16-month period, 6 of 73 children apparently excreted the organism for over 9 months without signs of illness (33). A high rate of asymptomatic carriage was also found in Bangladesh (20). Not all enteropathogens were isolated so frequently from healthy children in the developing world. In surveys in Thailand rotavirus and *Shigella* species were infrequently found in asymptomatic controls, whereas *Campylobacter* and *Salmonella* species were isolated nearly as often in children without diarrhea as in those with diarrhea (12, 48). Although frequent isolation from asymptomatic persons is a typical feature of *Campylobacter* infection throughout the developing world, some studies did find a difference in isolation rates of *Campylobacter* species in children with and without diarrhea who were less than 6 months old (8, 11, 12). However, a number of studies have found no difference in rates in any age group (17, 19, 20, 54).

The dynamics of *Campylobacter* infection were studied by Calva et al. (9) in 1985 to 1986 in a cohort of 179 children under 5 years old in San Pedro Martir, a low-income area on the outskirts of Mexico City. For 1 year these children were visited twice a week and cultured for *Campylobacter* species. Typical of many developing countries, there were 2.7 episodes of diarrhea per child-year, but only 0.4 of these episodes was associated with *Campylobacter* species. Over the year 66% of the cohort had a *Campylobacter* infection and 30% had an illness associated with *Campylobacter* infection. *Campylobacter* infections occurred at an early age; they peaked at 18 months of age and declined steadily thereafter. The illness-to-infection ratio was highest in the first 6 months of age, with half of the infections being symptomatic.

Another cohort study was performed in Bangui, Central African Republic, among 127 infants monitored from birth to 6 months of age (19). There were 82 *Campylobacter* infections observed in 42% of the children, but there was no difference in isolation rates between children with and without diarrhea.

TABLE 2. Episodes of *Campylobacter* infection and disease in Mexican and Thai children[a]

	No. of episodes/child-year		
Country	Total	Symptomatic	Asymptomatic
Mexico	2.1	0.4	1.7
Thailand	1.5	0.4	1.1

[a] Data from references 9 and 47.

POLYMICROBIAL INFECTIONS AND DURATION OF EXCRETION

In the developed world, infections with multiple enteric pathogens are infrequent and the mean duration of convalescent-phase excretion of *Campylobacter* organisms after an acute infection is 2 to 3 weeks (24, 42). In Thailand the average duration of convalescent-phase excretion of *Campylobacter* organisms was 14 days for children under 1 year old and 8 days for children 1 to 5 years old, a significant difference ($P < 0.02$) (47). In Mexico the median duration of excretion in cases of *Campylobacter* diarrhea was 3 days (range, 1 to 29 days) (9). When infections were asymptomatic the duration of excretion was 7 days.

Campylobacter species were isolated from 18% of Thai children with diarrhea, with a peak isolation rate in children 8 months of age (47). Another enteric pathogen was isolated from half of the cases in which *Campylobacter* was isolated. This is typical of studies throughout the developing world, and the proportion of mixed infections may be more dependent on the number of pathogens looked for than on any true differences in proportion. In Thailand children were repeatedly infected with new *Campylobacter* serotypes during a 12-week convalescent-phase surveillance period. About 10% of a cohort of Thai children under 5 years old acquired a new *Campylobacter* infection each week, and over 1.5 infections per child could be estimated in a year.

In Mexico, children were repeatedly infected with new serotypes when follow-up cultures were taken, and multiple *Campylobacter* serotypes were isolated from 42% of 62 patients (37). There was no difference between the serotypes isolated from symptomatic and asymptomatic infections (37). These studies in Thailand and Mexico, which have examined serotype-specific excretion rates, have demonstrated that frequent isolation of *Campylobacter* species from healthy persons in the developing world is not a function of prolonged carriage, as was postulated previously (33), but of constant reinfection. The average length of excretion for Thai and Mexican children is actually shorter than children in developed countries, probably because the children in developing countries are partially immune.

CLINICAL ILLNESS

In the developed world, *Campylobacter* enteritis can be quite severe. The most prominent features among patients presenting to medical attention are diarrhea, abdominal pain, and fever (3, 7, 24, 42). Grossly bloody stools are common and are often the reason for seeking medical attention. Abdominal pain is the most characteristic manifestation of illness. In hospital surveys bloody diarrhea occurs in about half of the patients.

In developing countries, *Campylobacter jejuni* infection is milder than in patients in developed countries (17, 20, 47). In Thailand, about one-third of symptomatic infections were bloody, one-third were watery, and one-third were mucoid (Table 3). In the developing world, bloody diarrhea is most often seen with *Shigella* infections. In Thailand, *Shigella* organisms were

TABLE 3. Clinical features of diarrheal disease in Thai children infected with a single enteric pathogen, Bangkok, Thailand[a]

	No. of patients with disease						
Organism	Total no. (%)	No. with single pathogen	No. with fever >38°C	No. with bloody stool	No. with >10 leukocytes	No. given i.v. fluid[b]	No. hospitalized
Shigella spp.	155 (13)	94	42[c]	37	67	3	2
EIEC[d]	19 (2)	11	45	18	36	9	0
Salmonella spp.	151 (12)	81	27	26	27	3	4
Campylobacter spp.	163 (13)	80	28	14	24	4	0
Rotavirus	220 (20)	141	28	5	6	19	4
ETEC[d]	112 (9)	48	17	4	6	6	2

[a] Adapted from reference 12.
[b] i.v., intravenous.
[c] Expressed as percentage of single-pathogen infection.
[d] EIEC, enteroinvasive *E. coli*; ETEC, enterotoxigenic *E. coli*.

associated with grossly bloody diarrhea in 37% of cases in which only one pathogen was detected, whereas *Campylobacter* and *Salmonella* organisms were associated with bloody stools in 14 and 26%, respectively (Table 4). More than 10 fecal leukocytes per high-power microscopic field, an indicator of invasive diarrheal disease, were present in 67% of patients infected with *Shigella* species and in 24 to 36% of patients infected with enteroinvasive *E. coli*, *Salmonella* species, or *Campylobacter* species. Similar to rates in Thailand, *Campylobacter* organisms were isolated from 14 and 12% of children with diarrhea in Bangladesh and the Central African Republic, respectively (17, 20).

OTHER EPIDEMIOLOGIC TRENDS

In the developed world, *Campylobacter* isolations typically increase during the summer and fall months (15, 38) and, although most cases appear to be sporadic, epidemics do occur (5). In the developing world, there is less seasonal variation and epidemics are not reported. The lack of seasonality might be explained by the lack of seasons in tropical climates, and the apparent lack of epidemics might be explained by poor surveillance. However, the combination of the milder illness, the high rates of asymptomatic illness, and the high rates of infections with multiple pathogens suggests a different epidemiologic process. These epidemiologic differences suggest that *Campylobacter* species may not be pathogens in the developing world at all.

TABLE 4. Clinical symptoms of patients with diarrhea associated with *C. jejuni*, *Shigella* spp., and enterotoxigenic *E. coli*, Bangladesh, 1980[a]

	No. of patients with symptom due to:		
Symptom	*C. jejuni* (n = 164)	*Shigella* spp. (n = 413)	ETEC[b] (n = 624)
Watery diarrhea	66	30	78
Abdominal pain	45	69	54
Bloody stool	17	55	10
Mucoid stool	61	86	46
Vomiting	66	37	67
Fever	50	52	42
Dehydration	20	13	26

[a] Adapted from reference 20.
[b] ETEC, enterotoxigenic *E. coli*.

CAMPYLOBACTER INFECTION AS A CAUSE OF TRAVELER'S DIARRHEA

Studies on diarrhea in travelers to the developing world have shown that *Campylobacter* species can be an important cause of traveler's diarrhea (Tables 5 and 6). The severity of illness in travelers is similar to the illness encountered in their native developed country.

In Sweden over 70% of cases of *Campylobacter* enteritis were acquired outside the country (42). Thus, some studies from developed countries may reflect the symptoms associated with *C. jejuni* strains acquired in the developing world. When a group of 380 Finnish tourists went to Morocco in January and February 1989, *C. jejuni* was isolated from 29% of 80 persons with diarrhea (35). Studies done by the same group of investigators at different times of the year have yielded much lower rates, suggesting seasonal variation in Morocco (30a). Similarly, rates of *C. jejuni* isolation have been high (39%) in U.S. military personnel on maneuvers in Thailand (51). The rates in Thailand may have been increased because the soldiers received doxycycline (tetracycline) daily for malaria prophylaxis. However, doxycycline was shown to have decreased the number of cases of diarrhea due to enterotoxigenic *E. coli*, rather than to have increased the number of cases due to *C. jejuni*.

Among Japanese travelers, *C. jejuni* enteritis was more common in travelers to the Indian subcontinent than in travelers to other countries in the Far East (45). The Japanese studies, as well as studies of travelers to Bangladesh and Nepal, have consistently indicated that over 10% of diarrhea in travelers to South Asia is caused by *C. jejuni* (39, 45, 49).

Most *Campylobacter* infections in travelers cause symptoms. Asymptomatic infections were found in only 2% of 313 Finnish tourists who went to Morocco (35). The symptoms associated with *C. jejuni* infections acquired by travelers in the developing world were similar to the symptoms associated with domestically acquired infections (Table 7). The symptoms of *Campylobacter* infections in travelers were generally more severe than the symptoms associated with *Campylobacter* infections in children from the developing world.

STRAIN DIFFERENCES

Strain differences have been cited as one possible explanation for the epidemiologic dif-

TABLE 5. Isolation rates of *Campylobacter* spp. and other enteric pathogens from travelers in the developing world[a]

Origin	Travel location	% Isolation of: *Campylobacter* spp.	ETEC[b]	*Salmonella* spp.
Finland	Morocco	29	5	10
United States	Egypt	0	57	2
Switzerland	The Gambia	1	42	4
United States	Thailand	39	6	18
Japan	Asia	5	34	11
Japan	Far East	5	33	15
Japan	India	11	39	6
Western	Bangladesh	15	ND[c]	0
Western	Nepal	14	27	3
United States	Mexico	3	20	1
United States	Mexico	1	24	1

[a] Data from references 35, 39, 45, 46, 49, and 52.
[b] ETEC, enterotoxigenic *E. coli*.
[c] ND, not determined.

ferences in developed and developing countries. These differences could include differences in serotype, in virulence factors, or in *Campylobacter* species. *Campylobacter* strains isolated in developing countries are biochemically and serotypically similar to strains isolated in developed countries (27, 47). Most *Campylobacter* strains isolated in the developing world can be typed by using typing antisera from the developed world (Table 8). There is little evidence that serotype differences can account for these markedly different clinical and epidemiologic patterns (37). There may be differences in other virulence factors such as enterotoxicity, but for *E. coli* there is a good correlation between serotype and virulence features. Furthermore, as described above, the spectrum of illness in travelers is similar to the illness observed in the developed world.

Although *C. jejuni* is the species most commonly associated with diarrhea, other species associated with diarrhea include *C. coli, C. lari, C. hyointestinalis, C. fetus* subsp. *fetus, C. cinaedi, C. fennelliae,* and *C. upsaliensis* (13, 26, 36). These species can be distinguished from *C. jejuni* by their inability to hydrolyze hippurate.

Many of the hippurate-negative species are not isolated by using standard methods for *C. jejuni* isolation. An alternative isolation method uses a cellulose acetate filter (pore size, 0.45 or 0.65 μm) placed directly on a non-antibiotic-containing agar medium (16, 21, 40, 41, 44, 53). The isolation rates of *C. jejuni* by this method appear comparable to those obtained with antibiotic-containing media, but the number of hippurate-negative *Campylobacter* species is greatly increased.

The proportion of infections due to *C. coli* or other hippurate-negative strains can be much higher in developing than developed countries (Table 9). In Europe and the United States *C. coli* infections account for less than 5% of all *Campylobacter* infections. *C. coli* was as often isolated from cases as from controls and was not associated with bloody diarrhea in Thailand, whereas *C. jejuni* was associated with bloody diarrhea in about one-third of cases. Thus, the spectrum of *Campylobacter* infections appears to be milder in areas where *C. coli* is frequently isolated. *C. coli* was isolated from 12% of children with *Campylobacter* infections in Thailand, but accounted for 41 and 39% of isolates in Hong Kong and the Central African Republic, respectively (18, 23).

TABLE 6. Incidence of *Campylobacter* enteritis in travelers to Mexico and Thailand[a]

Destination	No. of travelers	Survey time (wk)	No. of cases	Rate/100	Rate 10^5/yr
Mexico	227	6	7	3.1	27,000
Thailand	2,500	3	56	2.2	38,000

[a] Data from reference 14 and unpublished results.

TABLE 7. Symptoms associated with *Campylobacter* infections among U.S. military personnel during an outbreak in Fort Knox, Kentucky, and a field maneuver in Thailand

Symptom	% of individuals with symptoms in: Kentucky (*n* = 34)	Thailand (*n* = 43)
Diarrhea	88	100
Cramps	76	75
Fever	68	–[a]
Headache	65	70
Vomiting	59	51
Bloody diarrhea	26	30

[a]–, data not collected.

By using the membrane filter technique, *C. jejuni* was isolated from 10%, *C. coli* from 2%, and atypical campylobacters from 3% of 631 Thai children with diarrhea (50) (Table 10). In this study 15 of 17 atypical strains were aerotolerant strains, designated group 2 aerotolerant *Campylobacter* species or "*Campylobacter butzleri*" (25). Atypical campylobacters were also isolated in Australia from persons returning from India or Indonesia, suggesting that atypical strains may be more common in developing countries in general, and possibly also more common in Asian countries (53). However, they have also been isolated in European studies (21). Determination of the importance of these organisms in developed countries awaits large-scale studies involving nonselective isolation methods.

The clinical illness associated with hippurate-negative *Campylobacter* infections was milder than that associated with *C. jejuni* infections in children of the same age (50). This supports our conclusions, and those of others who found that *C. coli* infections tended to be milder than *C. jejuni* infections (47).

IMMUNE RESPONSE

The hyperendemicity of *Campylobacter* species appears to be the most important factor in defining the epidemiologic pattern of infection in the developing world. Healthy children in Bangladesh, Thailand, and the Central African Republic develop serum antibodies to *Campylobacter* species very early in life and have much higher level of *Campylobacter*-specific antibodies than do children in the United States (4, 6, 29). In Thai children there is an early rise in the level of antibodies to *Campylobacter* species that parallels the peak in isolation rate (47). In the Central African Republic the rise in the level of antiflagellar antibody inversely correlated with rates of *Campylobacter* enteritis (29).

The development of immunity to these or other antigens appears to play an important role in the age-related decreases in the case-to-infection ratio and the duration of convalescent-phase excretion (47). Further exposure to *Campylobacter* species probably continues to stimulate gut immunity and prevent tissue involvement and subsequent symptomatic infection, but has less effect on asymptomatic infections. In Thailand, *Campylobacter* infection was most often associated with bloody diarrhea in the first year of life, most probably as a result of a primary infection (47). These observations suggest that immunity may prevent bloody diarrhea from developing and eventually prevents any disease from occurring. This is supported by volunteer studies which have found that rechallenge with the same organism led to infection but not to disease (1).

These studies clearly demonstrate that the expression of the illness is influenced by preexisting immunity. The role of *Campylobacter* species in polymicrobial infections is unclear, and the presence of asymptomatic *Campylobacter* infections suggested that in an immune host *Campylobacter* species were nonpathogenic. In a second study, we examined the effect of age, symptoms, excretion pattern, and coinfection

TABLE 8. Isolation of Lior serotypes from children in Mexico, Thailand, and Nigeria[a]

Lior type	% isolated in: Mexico (*n* = 31)	Thailand (*n* = 104)	Nigeria (*n* = 79)
21	32	0	0
2	26	1	4
36	16	43	20
4	7	12	15
11	7	4	3
13	3	0	0
1	3	3	4
20	3	2	3
12	3	0	0
28	0	13	1
53	0	0	13
Untypable	0	3	–[b]

[a]Data from references 37 and 47.
[b]–, not reported.

TABLE 9. Relative isolation rates of *C. jejuni* by geographic location[a]

Location (yr)	Proportion of infection due to: *C. jejuni*	*C. coli*
Mexico (1985)	90	10
Thailand (1985)	87	13
Thailand (1988)	87	7
Algeria	85	15
France	83	17
Nigeria	81	19
Thailand (1987)	67	15
Yugoslavia	64	35
Hong Kong (1982)	59	41
Chile (1990)	56	44
Central African Republic	56	44

[a]Adapted from references 9, 18, 23, 30, 31, 41, 47, and 48.

with other enteric pathogens on the immune response to *Campylobacter* infection and on the quantitative excretion of the organism in Thai children (30b). In theory, nonpathogenic organisms might not cause a serum immune response and might be excreted for shorter periods or in smaller numbers.

For 6 months, children under 5 years of age who came to the Bangkok Childrens Hospital with diarrhea were cultured. Any patient whose stool culture was positive for *Campylobacter* species or *Shigella* species was seen at 2 and 4 weeks after the initial visit. Serum samples were collected at the initial presentation and at the time of the two home visits. *Campylobacter* species were isolated by using the membrane filter method. *Campylobacter* organisms were isolated from 19% of children under 1 year old, 12% of children from 1 to 2 years old, and 10% of children from 3 to 5 years old. In 35 cases *Campylobacter* species were the only pathogens found, and in 26 cases there was a mixed infection. Compared with the United States, where bloody diarrhea was seen in 50% of patients with *Campylobacter* infection, in Thailand only 25% of patients had bloody diarrhea, and most of these children were less than 2 years old. There were no differences between the illnesses in children with *Campylobacter* species as the sole pathogens and those due to mixed infection. Children shed from 1 to 8 logs of campylobacters. Quantitative fecal shedding was inversely related to age.

Campylobacter antibody production is age dependent. As the age increases, baseline levels of antibody also increase. During the first 6 months of life, immunoglobulin A (IgA) and IgM, and to a lesser extent IgG, levels in serum did not appear to rise in response to infection. After that, rises were seen in all Ig subclasses. Antibody response was not dependent on symptoms or the presence of coinfections. A poor seroresponse in the first 6 months of life may occur because it is a primary response to *Campylobacter* species and/or because maternal antibodies are present from placental transfer or breast feeding. Previous studies in the same population have shown that 38% of children under 1 year old receive breast milk.

PROTECTIVE EFFECT OF MATERNAL ANTIBODY AND BREAST-FEEDING

In Mexico, where 98 infants were monitored from birth to 2 years of age, breast-feeding was shown to decrease the number of episodes and the duration of diarrhea (34). The diarrhea rate caused by *C. jejuni* was significantly greater for non-breast-fed infants than for breast-fed infants. Secretory IgA antibody titers to *Campylobacter* surface antigens were highest in colostrum but persisted throughout lactation. Human milk consumed by children with *Campylobacter* diarrhea did not contain secretory *Campylobacter* antibodies. This study provided the first direct association of *Campylobacter* antibodies in human milk and prevention of *Campylobacter* diarrhea.

In Algeria, *Campylobacter* species were isolated from 58 infants less than 6 months old (30); 35 had diarrhea, and 23 did not. The difference in isolation rate was not significant. Only 4 (15%) children with diarrhea were exclusively breast-fed, whereas 10 (40%) children without diarrhea were exclusively breast-fed. This study suggested that exclusively breast-fed infants had fewer

TABLE 10. Isolation rates of *Campylobacter* species in Thailand[a]

Location and yr	Proportion of infections due to: *C. jejuni*	*C. coli*	Other hippurate-negative spp.
Thailand (1985)	87	13	0
Thailand (1987)	67	15	18
Thailand (1988)	87	7	7

[a]Data from references 46, 47, and 50.

symptomatic *Campylobacter* infections than did infants who were both breast- and bottle-fed.

A cohort of 127 African infants were monitored from birth until 6 months of age (19). None of 11 *Campylobacter* infections in the first month of life was associated with symptoms, compared with 13 (20%) of 71 infections in children 2 to 6 months old. The presence of maternal antibody was suggested as one reason for the lack of symptoms in children less than 1 month old. In this study, infants who were exclusively breast-fed were actually more likely to have a symptomatic *Campylobacter* infection than were infants who were both breast- and bottle-fed.

SOURCES AND MODES OF TRANSMISSION

In developed countries, outbreaks of *Campylobacter* enteritis are most frequently traced to contaminated milk and water (5). Eating undercooked chicken appears to be the most common cause of sporadic cases of *Campylobacter* enteritis (10). In general, the transmission is similar to that of *Salmonella* infection.

In the developing world, *Campylobacter* species are frequently isolated in populations at every stage of economic development. *Campylobacter* species appear to be part of the fecal flora of domestic animals, particularly poultry, regardless of how the animals are reared. Close direct contact with animals was reported to be an important risk factor in rural areas (2, 11, 22). In Lima, Peru, exposure to living chickens in the household was a significant risk factor for *Campylobacter* infection (2, 22). This is in contrast to *Salmonella* infections, which are very rare in less developed countries such as India and Africa, except in institutional settings such as orphanages. *Salmonella* species are not common in the least developed areas of the world, where livestock are not mass produced.

In more developed countries, *Campylobacter* infection is much more likely to be food borne. In Bangkok, Thailand, *Campylobacter* and *Salmonella* species are now well established in the food chain (32). In a recent study of foods in Bangkok open-air markets, *Salmonella* species were isolated from 30% of beef and pork samples and *Campylobacter* species were isolated from 40% of chicken samples (32). The serotypes of these organisms were similar to the ones isolated from humans. It appears that food-associated pathogens can be acquired very early in life from the foods themselves, from other humans who are excreting the organisms, or from environmental contamination. This may explain why there is no seasonality associated with infections due to these organisms. In contrast, *Shigella* species and rotavirus were not detected in foods, were not associated with a high rate of asymptomatic infections, and showed seasonality. Since *Campylobacter* organisms do not multiply at ambient temperatures and oxygen concentrations, recontamination of cooked foods, theoretically, should not occur.

ANTIBIOTIC RESISTANCE

In Thailand, *Campylobacter* strains are frequently resistant to tetracycline and erythromycin (44). For example, 11% of 114 community-acquired *C. jejuni* strains and 46% of *C. coli* strains were resistant to erythromycin in a 1987 survey. In an orphanage where *Campylobacter* infections were hyperendemic, over 50% of *C. jejuni* strains were resistant to erythromycin. Only 5% of *C. jejuni* strains isolated from rural Thailand were resistant to erythromycin, whereas all strains were resistant to tetracycline. Resistance to ciprofloxacin has not been observed in strains isolated prior to treatment, but has occurred as a result of ciprofloxacin treatment in 2 of 59 cases of *Campylobacter* enteritis in travelers (42a).

CONCLUSIONS

Both strain and host factors play important roles in the divergent clinical and epidemiologic features of *Campylobacter* infections in the developed and developing world. In the developing world, where *Campylobacter* infections are endemic, the peak isolation rate occurs in children less than 2 years old and is associated with a humoral response to *C. jejuni* antigens. The development of immunity to these antigens plays an important role in decreasing the case-to-infection ratio and the duration of convalescent-stage excretion. Further *Campylobacter* exposure continues to stimulate gut immunity and prevent tissue involvement and subsequent symptomatic infection, but does not prevent asymptomatic infection. The most well-defined strain difference is the increase in the proportion of hippurate-negative strains in some parts of the developing world. These strains appear to be less pathogenic than *C. jejuni*. The role of other virulence factors in the clinical illness is as yet unclear.

REFERENCES

1. **Black, R. E., M. M. Levine, M. L. Clements, T. P. Hughes, and M. J. Blaser.** 1988. Experimental *Campylobacter jejuni* infection in humans. *J. Infect. Dis.* **157:**472–479.
2. **Black, R. E., G. Lopez de Romana, K. H. Brown, N. Bravo, O. G. Bazalar, and H. C. Kanashiro.** 1989. Incidence and etiology of infantile diarrhea and major routes of transmission in Huascar, Peru. *Am. J. Epidemiol.* **129:**785–799.
3. **Blaser, M. J., I. D. Berkowitz, F. M. LaForce, F. M. Cravens, L. B. Reller, and W. L. L. Wang.** 1979. *Campylobacter* enteritis: clinical and epidemiologic features. *Ann. Intern. Med.* **91:**179–185.
4. **Blaser, M. J., R. E. Black, D. J. Duncan, and J. Amer.** 1985. *Campylobacter jejuni*-specific serum antibodies are elevated in healthy Bangladeshi children. *J. Clin. Microbiol.* **21:**164–167.
5. **Blaser, M. J., and L. B. Reller.** 1981. *Campylobacter* enteritis. *N. Engl. J. Med.* **305:**1444–1452.
6. **Blaser, M. J., D. N. Taylor, and P. Echeverria.** 1986. Immune response to *Campylobacter jejuni* in a rural community in Thailand. *J. Infect. Dis.* **153:**249–254.
7. **Blaser, M. J., J. G. Wells, R. A. Feldman, R. A. Pollard, J. R. Allen, and the Collaborative Diarrheal Disease Study Group.** 1983. *Campylobacter* enteritis in the United States: a multicenter study. *Ann. Intern. Med.* **98:**360–365.
8. **Bokkenheuser, V. D., N. J. Richardson, J. H. Bryner, D. J. Roux, A. B. Schutte, H. J. Koornhof, I. Freiman, and E. Hartman.** 1979. Detection of enteric campylobacteriosis in children. *J. Clin. Microbiol.* **9:**227–232.
9. **Calva, J. J., G. M. Ruiz-Palacios, A. B. Lopez-Vidal, A. Ramos, and R. Bojalil.** 1988. Cohort study of intestinal infection with *Campylobacter* in Mexican children. *Lancet* **i:**503–506.
10. **Deming, M. S., R. V. Tauxe, P. A. Blake, S. E. Dixon, B. S. Fowler, T. S. Jones, E. A. Lockamy, C. M. Patton, and R. O. Sikes.** 1987. *Campylobacter* enteritis at a university: transmission from eating chicken and from cats. *Am. J. Epidemiol.* **126:**526–534.
11. **De Mol, P., D. Brasseur, W. Hemelhof, T. Kalala, J. P. Butzler, and H. L. Vis.** 1983. Enteropathogenic agents in children with diarrhoea in rural Zaire. *Lancet* **i:**516–518.
12. **Echeverria, P., D. N. Taylor, U. Lexsomboon, M. Bhaibulaya, N. R. Blacklow, and R. Sakazaki.** 1989. Case-control study of endemic diarrheal disease in Thai children under 5 years old. *J. Infect. Dis.* **159:**543–548.
13. **Edmonds, P., C. M. Patton, P. M. Griffin, T. J. Barrett, G. P. Schmid, C. N. Baker, M. A. Lambert, and D. J. Brenner.** 1987. *Campylobacter hyointestinalis* associated with human gastrointestinal disease in the United States. *J. Clin. Microbiol.* **25:**685–691.
14. **Ericsson, C. D., H. L. DuPont, J. J. Mathewson, M. S. West, P. C. Johnson, and J. M. Bitsura.** 1990. Treatment of traveler's diarrhea with sulfamethoxazole and trimethoprim and loperamide. *JAMA* **263:**257–261.
15. **Finch, M. J., and L. W. Riley.** 1984. *Campylobacter* infections in the United States: results of an 11-state surveillance. *Arch. Intern. Med.* **144:**1610–1612.
16. **Fongsiri, K., O. Suthienkul, D. N. Taylor, S. Saiborisuth, S. Sricharmorn, S. Kongvisaisook, and P. Echeverria.** 1989. A comparison of methods for the isolation of *Campylobacter* species from stool specimens. *Southeast Asian J. Trop. Med. Public Health* **20:**139–146.
17. **Georges, M. C., I. K. Wachsmuth, D. M. V. Meunier, N. Nebout, F. Didier, M. R. Siopathis, and A. J. Georges.** 1984. Parasitic, bacterial, and viral enteric pathogens associated with diarrhea in the Central African Republic. *J. Clin. Microbiol.* **19:**571–575.
18. **Georges-Courbot, M. C., C. Baya, A. M. Beraud, D. M. Y. Meunier, and A. J. Georges.** 1986. Distribution and serotypes of *Campylobacter jejuni* and *Campylobacter coli* in enteric *Campylobacter* strains isolated from children in the Central African Republic. *J. Clin. Microbiol.* **23:**592–594.
19. **Georges-Courbot, M. C., A. M. Beraud-Cassel, I. Gouandjika, and A. J. Georges.** 1987. Prospective study of enteric *Campylobacter* infections in children from birth to 6 months in the Central African Republic. *J. Clin. Microbiol.* **25:**836–839.
20. **Glass, R. I., B. J. Stoll, M. I. Huq, M. J. Struelens, M. J. Blaser, and A. K. G. Kibriya.** 1983. Epidemiology and clinical features of endemic *Campylobacter jejuni* infection in Bangladesh. *J. Infect. Dis.* **148:**292–296.
21. **Goossens, H., M. De Boeck, H. Coignau, L. Vlaes, C. van den Borre, and J.-P. Butzler.** 1986. Modified selective medium for isolation of *Campylobacter* spp. from feces: comparison with Preston medium, a blood-free medium, and a filtration system. *J. Clin. Microbiol.* **24:**840–843.
22. **Grados, O., N. Bravo, R. E. Black, and J. P. Butzler.** 1988. Paediatric *Campylobacter* diarrhoea from household exposure to live chickens in Lima, Peru. *Bull. W.H.O.* **66:**369–374.
23. **Ho, D. D., and W. T. Wong.** 1985. A one-year survey of *Campylobacter* enteritis and other forms of bacterial diarrhoea in Hong Kong. *J. Hyg.* (Cambridge) **94:**55–60.
24. **Karmali, M. A., and P. C. Fleming.** 1979. *Campylobacter* enteritis in children. *J. Pediatr.* **94:**527–533.
25. **Kiehlbauch, J. A., D. J. Brenner, M. A. Nicholson, C. N. Baker, C. M. Patton, A. G. Steigerwalt, and I. K. Wachsmuth.** 1991. *Campylobacter butzleri* sp. nov. isolated from humans and animals with diarrheal illness. *J. Clin. Microbiol.* **29:**376–385.
26. **Klein, B. S., J. M. Vergeront, M. J. Blaser, P. Edmonds, D. J. Brenner, D. Janssen, and J. P. Davis.** 1986. *Campylobacter* infection associated with raw milk: an outbreak of gastroenteritis due to *Campylobacter jejuni* and thermotolerant *Campylobacter fetus* subsp. *fetus*. *JAMA* **255:**361–364.

27. **Lior, H., D. L. Woodward, J. A. Edgar, L. J. Laroche, and P. Gill.** 1982. Serotyping of *Campylobacter jejuni* by slide agglutination based on heat-labile antigenic factors. *J. Clin. Microbiol.* **15:**761–768.
28. **MacDonald, K. L., M. J. O'Leary, M. L. Cohen, P. Norris, J. G. Wells, E. Noll, J. M. Kobayashi, and P. A. Blake.** 1988. *Escherichia coli* O157:H7: an emerging gastrointestinal pathogen: results of a one-year, prospective, population-based study. *JAMA* **259:**3567–3570.
29. **Martin, P. M. V., J. Mathiot, J. Ipero, M. Kirimat, A. J. Georges, and M. C. Georges-Courbot.** 1989. Immune response to *Campylobacter jejuni* and *Campylobacter coli* in a cohort of children from birth to 2 years of age. *J. Clin. Microbiol.* **57:**2542–2546.
30. **Megraud, F., G. Boudraa, K. Bessaoud, S. Bensid, F. Dabis, R. Soltana, and M. Touhami.** 1990. Incidence of campylobacter infection in infants in western Algeria and the possible protective role of breast feeding. *Epidemiol. Infect.* **106:**73–78.
30a. **Peltola, H.** Personal communication.
30b. **Perlman, D., University of Colorado Medical Center, Denver.** Unpublished data.
31. **Popovic-Uroic, T.** 1989. *Campylobacter jejuni* and *Campylobacter coli* diarrhoea in rural and urban populations in Yugoslavia. *Epidemiol. Infect.* **102:**59–67.
32. **Rasrinaul, L., O. Suthienkul, P. D. Echeverria, D. N. Taylor, J. Seriwatana, and A. Bangtrakulnonth.** 1988. Foods as a source of antibiotic resistant enteropathogens causing childhood diarrhea in Thailand. *Am. J. Trop. Med. Hyg.* **39:**97–102.
33. **Richardson, N. J., H. J. Koornhoff, and V. D. Bokkenheuser.** 1981. Long-term infections with *Campylobacter fetus* subsp. *jejuni*. *J. Clin. Microbiol.* **13:**846–849.
34. **Ruiz-Palacios, G. M., J. J. Calva, L. K. Pickering, Y. Lopez-Vidal, P. Volkow, H. Pezzarossi, and M. S. West.** 1990. Protection of breast-fed infants against *Campylobacter* diarrhea by antibodies in human milk. *J. Pediatr.* **116:**707–713.
35. **Siitonen, A., L. Kotola, H. Kyrönseppä, P. Oksanen, B. Naouri, A. Mechbal, and H. Peltola.** 1989. *Campylobacter* spp. is the leading cause of travelers' diarrhea among Finnish tourists to Morocco. *Program Abstr. 29th Intersci. Conf. Antimicrob. Agents Chemother.*, abstr. 44. American Society for Microbiology, Washington, D.C.
36. **Simor, A. E., and L. Wilcox.** 1987. Enteritis associated with *Campylobacter laridis*. *J. Clin. Microbiol.* **25:**10–12.
37. **Sjogren, E., G. Ruiz-Palacios, and B. Kaijser.** 1989. *Campylobacter jejuni* isolations from Mexican and Swedish patients, with repeated symptomatic and/or asymptomatic diarrhoea episodes. *Epidemiol. Infect.* **102:**47–57.
38. **Skirrow, M. B.** 1987. A demographic survey of *Campylobacter, Salmonella,* and *Shigella* infections in England. *Epidemiol. Infect.* **99:**647–657.
39. **Speelman, P., M. J. Struelens, and R. I. Glass.** 1983. Detection of *Campylobacter jejuni* and other potential pathogens in travellers' diarrhea in Bangladesh. *Scand. J. Gastroenterol.* **18**(Suppl. 84):19–23.
40. **Steele, T. W., and S. N. McDermott.** 1984. Technical note: the use of membrane filters applied directly to the surface of agar plates for the isolation of *Campylobacter jejuni* from feces. *Pathology* **16:**263–265.
41. **Steele, T. W., N. Sangster, and J. A. Lanser.** 1985. DNA relatedness and biochemical features of *Campylobacter* spp. isolated in Central and South Australia. *J. Clin. Microbiol.* **22:**71–74.
42. **Svedhem, A., and B. Kaijser.** 1980. *Campylobacter fetus* subspecies *jejuni:* a common cause of diarrhea in Sweden. *J. Infect. Dis.* **142:**353–359.
42a. **Taylor, D. N.** Unpublished data.
43. **Taylor, D. N., and M. J. Blaser.** 1991. *Campylobacter* infections, p. 151–172. *In* A. S. Evans and P. S. Brachman (ed.), *Bacterial Infections of Humans: Epidemiology and Control.* Plenum Publishing Corp., New York.
44. **Taylor, D. N., M. J. Blaser, P. Echeverria, C. Pitarangsi, L. Bodhidatta, and W. L. L. Wang.** 1987. Erythromycin-resistant *Campylobacter* infections in Thailand. *Antimicrob. Agents Chemother.* **31:**438–442.
45. **Taylor, D. N., and P. Echeverria.** 1986. The etiology and epidemiology of travelers' diarrhea in Asia. *Rev. Infect. Dis.* **8**(Suppl. 2):S136–S141.
46. **Taylor, D. N., P. Echeverria, M. Blaser, C. Pitarangsi, N. R. Blacklow, J. H. Cross, and B. Weniger.** 1985. The polymicrobial etiology of travelers' diarrhea. *Lancet* **i:**381–383.
47. **Taylor, D. N., P. Echeverria, C. Pitarangsi, J. Seriwatana, L. Bodhidatta, and M. Blaser.** 1988. Influence of strain characteristics and immunity on the epidemiology of *Campylobacter* infections in Thailand. *J. Clin. Microbiol.* **26:**863–868.
48. **Taylor, D. N., P. Echeverria, O. Sethabutr, C. Pitarangsi, U. Leksomboon, N. R. Blacklow, B. Rowe, R. Gross, and J. Cross.** 1988. Clinical and microbiologic features of *Shigella* and enteroinvasive *Escherichia coli* infections detected by DNA hybridization. *J. Clin. Microbiol.* **26:**1362–1366.
49. **Taylor, D. N., R. Houston, D. R. Shlim, P. Echeverria, M. Bhaibulaya, and B. L. P. Ungar.** 1988. Etiology of diarrheal disease among travelers and foreign residents in Nepal. *JAMA* **260:**1245–1248.
50. **Taylor, D. N., J. A. Kiehlbauch, W. Tee, C. Pitarangsi, and P. Echeverria.** 1991. Isolation of Group 2 aerotolerant *Campylobacter* species from Thai children with diarrhea. *J. Infect. Dis.* **163:**1062–1067.
51. **Taylor, D. N., C. Pitarangsi, P. Echeverria, and B. M. Diniega.** 1988. *Campylobacter* enteritis during doxycycline prophylaxis for malaria in Thailand. *Lancet* **ii:**578–579. (Letter.)
52. **Taylor, D. N., J. L. Sanchez, W. Candler, S. Thornton, C. McQueen, and P. Echeverria.** 1991. Treatment of travelers' diarrhea: ciprofloxacin plus loperamide compared with ciprofloxacin alone: a placebo-controlled, randomized trial. *Ann. Intern. Med.* **114:**731–734.

53. **Tee, W., B. N. Anderson, B. C. Ross, and B. Dwyer.** 1987. Atypical campylobacters associated with gastroenteritis. *J. Clin. Microbiol.* **25:**1248–1252.
54. **Zaki, A. M., H. L. DuPont, M. A. El Alamy, R. R. Arafat, K. Amin, M. M. Awad, L. Bassiouni, I. Z. Imam, G. S. El Malih, A. El Marsafie, M. S. Mohieldin, T. Naguib, M. A. Rakha, M. Sidaros, N. Wasef, C. E. Wright, and R. G. Wyatt.** 1986. The detection of enteropathogens in acute diarrhea in a family cohort population in rural Egypt. *Am. J. Trop. Med. Hyg.* **35:**1013–1022.

CHAPTER 4

Clinical and Epidemiologic Features of Non-*jejuni*, Non-*coli* *Campylobacter* Species

BAN MISHU, CHARLOTTE M. PATTON, AND ROBERT V. TAUXE

INTRODUCTION

Campylobacters have been long recognized as a cause of illness and abortion in animals. In the last two decades, awareness of the important role of *Campylobacter* species in human disease has been increasing. *Campylobacter jejuni* is now recognized as the most common bacterial cause of diarrhea in the world (5, 6, 11). More recently, there has been growing understanding that many *Campylobacter* species besides *C. jejuni* may also be human pathogens in immunocompromised persons, homosexual men, and the population at large. These are rarely recognized, and together represented only 1% of reported *Campylobacter* isolates in the United States from 1987 to 1989 (Table 1) (91). However, since most of these organisms are not likely to be detected or identified by standard clinical laboratory techniques for *C. jejuni*, they may be more common than current reports suggest. We will review the clinical, epidemiologic, and key biochemical characteristics of several *Campylobacter* species other than *C. jejuni* and *C. coli*, including *C. fetus* subsp. *fetus*, *C. hyointestinalis*, *C. lari*, *C. upsaliensis*, *C. cinaedi*, *C. fennelliae*, *C. concisus*, *C. jejuni* subsp. *doylei*, *C. sputorum*, and *C. butzleri*. *Helicobacter pylori*, formerly *C. pylori*, is not covered in this review.

C. FETUS SUBSP. *FETUS*

Campylobacters were recognized in the first decades of this century as causes of fetal infection and abortion in sheep; McFadyean and Stockman proposed the name *Vibrio fetus ovis* (53). In 1919, these organisms were also implicated as causes of abortions in cattle, and their name was shortened to *Vibrio fetus* (79). Although the strains were not preserved, evidence suggests they were *C. fetus* subsp. *fetus*, now established as a major cause of septic abortions in domestic animals (41). The other subspecies of *C. fetus*, *C. fetus* subsp. *venerealis*, is associated with infection of the reproductive tract in cattle (26) but is not an important human pathogen. In this report, *C. fetus* will refer to *C. fetus* subsp. *fetus* unless otherwise indicated. The first report of human infection with *C. fetus* was published in 1947; Vinzent et al. described a pregnant woman with *C. fetus* bacteremia who aborted at 6 months gestation (97). Since then, *C. fetus* has been recognized as a cause of bacteremic illness in immunocompromised persons and has been associated with a wide spectrum of extraintestinal infections as well. Between 1987 and 1989, 122 *C. fetus* isolates were reported to the Centers for Disease Control (CDC) *Campylobacter* Surveillance System (91). Many of these were blood isolates.

Campylobacters are microaerophilic, requiring 3 to 15% oxygen for growth. They do not ferment carbohydrates and are oxidase positive. Most species are catalase and nitrate positive. *C. fetus* is distinguished from the majority of other *Campylobacter* species by its ability to grow at 25 and 37°C, but most *C. fetus* strains do not grow at 42°C (19). *C. fetus* is susceptible to cephalothin and resistant to nalidixic acid, characteristics which often help to distinguish it from *C. jejuni* (40). Growth for 3 to 25 days may be

Ban Mishu, Division of Infectious Diseases, Department of Medicine, Vanderbilt University School of Medicine, Nashville, Tennessee 37232-2605. **Charlotte M. Patton and Robert V. Tauxe,** Enteric Diseases Branch, Division of Bacterial and Mycotic Diseases, National Center for Infectious Diseases, Centers for Disease Control, Atlanta, Georgia 30333.

TABLE 1. Number of isolates of *Campylobacter* strains other than *C. jejuni* and *C. coli* from 1982 to 1986 and 1987 to 1989 in the United States as reported to the CDC *Campylobacter* Surveillance System

Organism	No. of isolates in:	
	1982–1986	1987–1989
C. fetus	143	122
C. lari	7	21
C. sputorum	1	0
CLOs	1	0
C. upsaliensis	0	10
C. hyointestinalis	0	3

required for primary isolation from blood cultures (25). The best growth occurs in anaerobic BACTEC 7D blood culture bottles (101).

C. fetus infection typically causes bacteremia in elderly men with chronic underlying illness. More than three-fourths have underlying serious medical conditions such as cancer, alcoholism, cirrhosis or other liver disease, or diabetes or are receiving immunosuppressive therapy (34). *C. fetus* infection has also been associated with septic abortions, septic arthritis, abscesses, meningitis, intravascular infections, peritonitis, and salpingitis (10, 34, 49, 86). There have been three reports of *C. fetus* infection in persons with AIDS (72). Among adult patients, the ratio of affected males to females is 3:1 (34). The overall mortality rate among patients with *C. fetus* infection is approximately 20% (18, 72). The prognosis depends largely upon the severity of the underlying illness.

Only two outbreaks of *C. fetus* infection have been reported—both were related to eating contaminated food. In the first, 10 patients in California developed *C. fetus* sepsis after eating a nutritional supplement that contained raw calf's liver (14). In the second outbreak, patients in Wisconsin developed *C. jejuni*- and *C. fetus*-associated gastroenteritis that was epidemiologically linked to drinking unpasteurized milk (44). *C. fetus* was identified fortuitously because of the unusual thermotolerance of the strain; it was able to grow at 42°C.

The common modes of transmission of *C. fetus* infection in humans are not well understood. Because farm animals are a reservoir for *C. fetus* (Table 2), animal-to-human transmission seems plausible. However, more than two-thirds of patients with *C. fetus* infection are urban dwellers who report no occupational or environmental exposure to farm animals (73).

Recent studies suggest the intestinal tract may be the portal of entry of *C. fetus* into the bloodstream. *C. fetus* may be a quiet inhabitant of the gut, but in the setting of decreased host immunity, it can invade the mucosa and cause generalized infection. Although some early investigations indicated that *C. fetus* isolation from stools was rare, its natural habitat is the intestine, and as many as 40% of patients with *C. fetus* bacteremia have diarrhea preceding the onset of their other symptoms (34). *C. fetus* was capable of causing gastroenteritis in healthy persons who drank contaminated, unpasteurized milk; the unusual tolerance of the strain for the 42°C incubation temperature permitted its detection. Similarly, *C. fetus* has been detected in the stools of homosexual men with gastroenteritis; these isolates also grew at 42°C (17, 35).

The susceptibility of *C. fetus* to cephalothin and the fact that most strains do not grow at 42°C may explain why the organism is not isolated in stools more frequently. Assessment of the frequency of *C. fetus*-associated gastroenteritis is difficult because most clinical laboratories incubate samples at 42°C and use a medium that contains cephalothin (35). Also, many laboratories incubate blood cultures for only 1 week.

Sexual transmission may be another possible mode for the spread of *C. fetus* infection in humans. Venereal transmission of *C. fetus* subsp. *venerealis* is known to occur in cattle (26). The prepuce of the asymptomatic bull is the major habitat of *C. fetus* subsp. *venerealis;* the infection is transmitted to the cow, which develops chronic genital tract inflammation resulting in infertility (26). Sexual transmission of *C. fetus* subsp. *fetus* in humans has not been demonstrated, although there are isolated reports of infection occurring among homosexual males (34, 70). Finally, *C. fetus* infection can occur as a result of direct invasion of the bloodstream via a venipuncture or an intravenous line (34).

C. fetus accounts for more bacteremias in adults than any other *Campylobacter* species except *C. jejuni* (13). The bacteremia can be primary, or it can be secondary to infection of another site. Although the organism is rarely isolated from feces, diarrhea precedes or accompanies the bacteremia in nearly half of all patients (25, 34). Most patients experience high fever, but this is usually well tolerated. The prognosis depends upon the underlying illness; however, most patients recover fully with intravenous antibiotic therapy (19).

C. fetus was recognized as a cause of epidemic and sporadic abortion in animals more than 70 years ago. It also causes premature labor

TABLE 2. Animal reservoirs for *Campylobacter* species other than *C. jejuni* and *C. coli*

Organism	Animal reservoir
C. fetus	Cattle, sheep
C. hyointestinalis	Pigs, cattle, hamsters
C. lari	Gulls, dogs, cats, poultry, monkeys, fur seal
C. upsaliensis	Dogs, cats
H. cinaedi	Hamsters
H. fennelliae	None known
C. concisus	None known
C. sputorum subsp. *sputorum*	None known
C. sputorum subsp. *bubulus*	Cattle, sheep
C. (Arcobacter) butzleri	Pigs, cattle, ostrich, primates
C. jejuni subsp. *doylei*	None known

and perinatal sepsis in humans (15, 76). Fetal infection and abortion may follow maternal infection by several weeks. The pathogenesis of *C. fetus* infection of the placenta is not well understood, but the likely source of infection is the intestinal tract. In pregnant animals, ingestion of *C. fetus* leads to bacteremia and infection of the placenta and fetus (56). Intestinal infection followed by bacteremia and hematogenous spread to placental tissue is also the likely mechanism in humans; *C. fetus* has a tropism for placental tissue (51). Unlike maternal and fetal infection with *C. jejuni,* which can cause abortion early in pregnancy, infection with *C. fetus* usually occurs during the third trimester (76). The illness in the mother is generally mild and self-limited and precedes the onset of labor by several weeks. Fetal and neonatal mortality, however, is 80%. Infection of neonates may occur transplacentally or may occur during delivery (76). The incidence of neonatal mortality and morbidity secondary to this infection is unknown.

C. fetus exhibits a propensity to infect vascular endothelium; *C. fetus* infections have been associated with thrombophlebitis, mycotic aneurysms, and endocarditis (2, 12, 52, 58). It has been postulated that *C. fetus* has a receptor with an affinity for vascular endothelium (12).

C. fetus infection of the peritoneum has been reported in peritoneal dialysis patients; in this case it has been postulated that direct contamination of the catheter occurred (102). It has also occurred in patients with alcoholic cirrhosis; here the organism was believed to have been invasive from the bowel wall (86). *C. fetus*-associated salpingitis has been described in a nonpregnant young woman; however, the source of the infection was not known (10).

C. HYOINTESTINALIS

In 1983, a new *Campylobacter* species was identified and suggested as a possible cause of proliferative enteritis in pigs (Table 2); the name *C. hyointestinalis* was proposed (from the Latin word "hyo" meaning hog, and "intestinalis," pertaining to the intestines) (29). The organism described was most closely related to *C. fetus* but could be differentiated from *C. fetus* by its production of H_2S in triple sugar iron agar. Other investigators also identified the organism in pigs, cattle, hamsters, and deer (27, 36, 45, 92).

C. hyointestinalis is most closely related to *C. fetus* and, like *C. fetus,* is catalase positive, is susceptible to cephalothin, and is resistant to nalidixic acid. *C. hyointestinalis* differs from *C. fetus* mainly by its production of H_2S in triple sugar iron agar. The organism is considered thermotolerant rather than thermophilic because it tolerates 42°C but grows most abundantly at 37°C.

In 1986, *C. hyointestinalis* was isolated from the stool of a homosexual man with proctitis (21). Because no other enteric or sexually transmitted pathogens were isolated and because the organism disappeared and the patient's symptoms resolved after treatment with an antibiotic to which the strain was susceptible, *C. hyointestinalis* was thought to be the cause of illness. Edmonds et al. studied the genetic and epidemiologic characteristics of *C. hyointestinalis* strains isolated from the stools of four patients with watery, nonbloody diarrhea; this provided further evidence that *C. hyointestinalis* can be a human pathogen (20). For three of these patients, *C. hyointestinalis* was the only enteric pathogen isolated from the stools. The authors noted anecdotally that *C. hyointestinalis* was isolated from two other patients: a 72-year-old man with bloody diarrhea and a 3-year-old boy with watery diarrhea. *C. hyointestinalis* was also the presumed opportunistic pathogen in a case of diarrhea in a patient with chronic myeloid leukemia (57).

Among the eight patients reported with *C. hyointestinalis* infection, seven had diarrhea and one had proctitis. Of the seven patients with diarrhea, six had nonbloody diarrhea. Vomiting and abdominal pain were also occasionally seen. Three patients had fever of >38.5°C. The symptoms in most patients resolved in a few days and there were no deaths. Three of the eight patients were homosexual men, two patients were over 70 years old, and one was an infant. It is not yet known whether *C. hyointestinalis* is a potential pathogen only in immune compromised persons and homosexuals or whether it can affect other people as well.

C. hyointestinalis may be an important cause of diarrheal disease in homosexual men, compromised patients, and perhaps the population at large, but it is rarely identified by current laboratory practices. In the period from 1987 to 1989, there were only three isolates of *C. hyointestinalis* reported to the CDC *Campylobacter* Surveillance System (93). *C. hyointestinalis* strains can be susceptible to the concentration of cephalothin (15 μl/ml) used in selective media, and personnel in clinical laboratories may not be familiar with characteristics used to distinguish *C. hyointestinalis* from other *Campylobacter* species. Therefore, the true frequency of *C. hyointestinalis* in patients with enteritis is not known.

C. LARI

C. lari is a potential human pathogen that is only infrequently reported; 21 isolates were reported to the CDC *Campylobacter* Surveillance System from 1987 to 1989 (91). Most isolates are cultured from the stools of patients with diarrhea; however, there has been one report of fatal *C. lari* bacteremia in an immunocompromised patient and one report of *C. lari*-associated acute appendicitis. Typical symptoms of *C. lari* enteritis include nonbloody diarrhea and abdominal cramps with little or no fever.

C. lari was first described in 1980 by Skirrow and Benjamin as a thermophilic *Campylobacter* species that is distinct from *C. jejuni* and *C. coli* in several ways, most notably in its resistance to nalidixic acid (78). Other laboratory characteristics include a negative hippurate hydrolysis test and a negative indoxyl acetate hydrolysis (67), which are both positive for *C. jejuni*. Occasionally, urease-positive variants of *C. lari* are identified (55).

Because the strain was isolated most commonly in healthy gulls (25% of gulls, genus *Larus*, are infected), the name *C. laridis* was proposed (4). The name was revised to *C. lari* in 1990 (98). *C. lari* has been recovered from dogs, cats, chickens, and a monkey but not from cattle, pigs, or sheep (Table 2) (78). It has also been found in many other avian and mammalian species without causing any disease (50). Until 1984, only a few human isolates of *C. lari* had been reported, and these had no apparent association with illness (4).

The potential for human pathogenicity of this organism was first recognized in 1984, when Nachamkin et al. described a case of fatal *C. lari* bacteremia in a severely immunocompromised patient (59). Five additional patients with *C. lari* enteritis were described by Tauxe et al. in 1985 (87); all five isolates were cultured from the stools of immunocompetent individuals. One patient became infected and developed enteritis during the second trimester of pregnancy but experienced no complications; she recovered completely and delivered a healthy child. Four patients had diarrhea, four had abdominal pain, and one had fever. The illnesses were somewhat prolonged (range, 1 week to 4 months; median, 2 weeks), and two patients were hospitalized, but all recovered completely. Four patients had had contact with house pets and four had eaten chicken in the week before onset of symptoms. None had had contact with gulls (87). Simor and Wilcox described a patient with *C. lari* enteritis and were able to demonstrate specific serum bacteriocidal antibodies to the isolated strain, providing further evidence of an association between *C. lari* infection and enteritis (77). In 1988, Megraud et al. described two cases of enteritis in adults and one case of appendicitis in a child from whom urease-positive *C. lari* (i.e., urea-positive thermophilic *Campylobacter*) organisms were isolated (55). One diarrheal patient had abdominal pain, fever, and watery diarrhea; the second had pus and mucus in the stool.

One common-source outbreak of *C. lari* infection has been reported. In 1985, an outbreak of *C. lari* gastroenteritis occurred among construction workers who drank water accidentally contaminated by surface water from Lake Ontario, an area inhabited by gulls (9). A total of 162 symptomatic patients was identified; *C. lari* was cultured from the stools of seven patients. Diarrhea and abdominal pain were the most frequently reported symptoms, and only 20% of patients had fever. The low isolation rate was attributed to delayed specimen collection and absence of transport media.

The clinical and microbiologic features of *C. lari* may be difficult to distinguish from those of *C. jejuni.* The *C. lari*-related illnesses described, although somewhat prolonged, are within the clinical spectrum of infections caused by *C. jejuni.* Because many microbiology laboratories do not routinely test *Campylobacter* isolates for nalidixic acid susceptibility and indoxyl acetate hydrolysis, a number of isolates thought to be *C. jejuni* may in fact be *C. lari.* Furthermore, nalidixic acid-resistant strains of *C. jejuni* (1, 99) and nalidixic acid-susceptible *C. lari* strains have been described (7, 61), so distinguishing *C. jejuni* from *C. lari* may depend upon the hippurate hydrolysis test alone.

C. UPSALIENSIS

In 1983, Sandstedt et al. reported the isolation, from dogs with and without diarrhea, of thermotolerant *Campylobacter* species that were catalase negative or only weakly positive (75). The name *C. upsaliensis* was proposed, for the Swedish town where the dogs lived; the name has been recently validated (38). In 1989, Fox et al. reported the isolation of *C. upsaliensis* from asymptomatic cats used in biomedical research (Table 2) (24). *C. upsaliensis* is now a recognized human pathogen, causing diarrhea and bacteremia in both healthy and immunocompromised persons.

Several characteristics distinguish *C. upsaliensis* from other *Campylobacter* species (75). They have a negative or weakly positive catalase reaction. They grow well at 42°C but not at 25°C. They do not produce H_2S in triple sugar iron agar; the hippurate hydrolysis test result is negative; and they are susceptible to both cephalothin and nalidixic acid (74). Because cephalothin is commonly used in media for isolation of *C. jejuni,* the presence of *C. upsaliensis* may often go unrecognized. This organism may be a more common cause of gastroenteritis than indicated by current surveillance data. From 1987 to 1989, 10 isolates of *C. upsaliensis* were reported through the CDC *Campylobacter* Surveillance System (91). *C. upsaliensis* was isolated from 99 of 15,185 stool specimens that were cultured for "new" campylobacters (32).

The first report implicating a catalase-negative *Campylobacter* species (later determined to be *C. upsaliensis*) as a cause of human illness was in 1985; Steele et al. isolated *C. upsaliensis* from the feces of eight children less than 3 years old and one adult in Australia; all had diarrhea (82). Similarly, in France, *C. upsaliensis* was isolated from the stools of five small children with gastroenteritis (54). Taylor et al. investigated the clinical histories of seven patients with positive *C. upsaliensis* stool cultures; all the patients had diarrhea and five were less than 2 years old (88). Hirschl et al. described a patient with diarrhea who had *C. upsaliensis* isolated from her stools and who had a significant decrease in antibody titers against her own *C. upsaliensis* strain within 12 months of her illness (37), providing additional evidence of an association between *C. upsaliensis* infection and diarrhea. In a 3-year study of patients with diarrhea by Goossens et al., *C. upsaliensis* was isolated from 99 patients; of 83 patients for whom clinical information was available, 92% had an acute, self-limited diarrheal illness (32). Fecal isolation of *C. upsaliensis* from six children was described by Walmsley and Karmali (100). The clinical significance of these isolates was unknown; however, no other bacterial pathogens were isolated and three of the children had loose, watery stools, vomiting, and anorexia. The three other patients were asymptomatic.

Between 1980 and 1986, CDC received 11 human isolates of catalase-negative or weakly positive campylobacters that were identified as *C. upsaliensis* (66). The ages of the patients ranged from 6.5 months to 83 years. Eight of the isolates were from blood, and three were from stools. Of the three patients with positive stool cultures, two had a self-limited watery diarrhea and abdominal cramps. The third patient had acute leukemia and developed watery, blood-tinged diarrhea and spiking fevers that persisted until her death a short time later. Of the eight patients with positive blood cultures, six were adults. Five of these adults were immunocompromised but only one had AIDS; a sixth patient had a ruptured ectopic pregnancy. Indeed, four of the six adult patients with bacteremia had abdominal pathologic conditions, including two with recent abdominal surgery, suggesting a possible intestinal source of infection. Only two of the eight patients with positive blood cultures had diarrhea. The two children with *C. upsaliensis* bacteremia had acute respiratory illnesses, suggesting a possible upper airway source of infection. Of the 11 total patients described, 9 had fever, 9 required hospitalization, and 5 died within 3 months of their positive culture. *C. upsaliensis* has also been isolated from blood samples of 16 bacteremic pediatric patients in

South Africa (46). Of these 16 patients, 10 were less than 1 year old and all 16 had predisposing conditions.

Plasmid profile determination may become an epidemiologic typing tool for *C. upsaliensis. C. upsaliensis* is distinct from *C. jejuni* and other *Campylobacter* species in that a high proportion of *C. upsaliensis* strains contain plasmids. In one investigation, 89 of 99 strains contained plasmids (31). Similarly, in another investigation, plasmids were detected in 54 of 62 strains studied (63). In both studies, investigators found identical plasmids in strains of *C. upsaliensis* isolated from dogs and humans, suggesting a possible animal-to-human transmission as a common source.

Erythromycin is considered the treatment of choice for *Campylobacter* infections. However, in the investigation described above, Patton et al. found that 2 of the 11 *C. upsaliensis* isolates (1 from blood and 1 from stool) were resistant to erythromycin (66). Goossens et al. also found erythromycin resistance in 10 of 99 *C. upsaliensis* isolates (31). Preston et al. studied the antimicrobial susceptibility of 41 strains of *C. upsaliensis* and found them to be most susceptible to fluoroquinolones; all strains were resistant to trimethoprim (68). More studies may further define the range of antibiotic susceptibility of this organism and the clinical indications and efficacy of treatment with antimicrobial agents.

C. CINAEDI AND *C. FENNELLIAE*

During the late 1970s and early 1980s, there was increased recognition of the high rate of enteric infections among homosexual men (66). *Campylobacter* species and *Campylobacter*-like organisms (CLOs) were recognized as important rectal and intestinal pathogens in this population (69), a finding that was later corroborated by other investigators (48).

CLOs isolated from homosexual men were shown to belong to four genetic groups—CLO1A, CLO1B, CLO2, and CLO3—that were different from other known *Campylobacter* species (90). The CLO1A strains were called *C. cinaedi* (for the Latin word "cinaedi"; of a homosexual). CLO2 strains were called *C. fennelliae* for Cynthia Fennell, the technologist who first isolated the organisms from the rectal swabs of homosexual men. Both species were recently moved to the genus *Helicobacter* (96) and will henceforth be referred to as *Helicobacter cinaedi* and *H. fennelliae.* CLO1B strains are identical to *H. cinaedi.* Only one CLO3 strain has been identified, and its taxonomic structure needs further study (90, 96).

H. cinaedi and *H. fennelliae* require microaerobic conditions on cephalothin-free medium at 37°C for primary isolation. Growth is enhanced by an increased hydrogen atmosphere. In vitro susceptibilities of *H. cinaedi* and *H. fennelliae* to therapeutic antimicrobial agents are within the ranges characteristic of *C. jejuni* and *C. fetus.* However, they are distinguished from *C. jejuni* and *C. fetus* by their susceptibility to rifampin and are distinguished from *C. fetus* by their susceptibility to nalidixic acid (23). Ampicillin, gentamicin, spectinomycin, doxycycline, tetracycline, chloramphenicol, nalidixic acid, rifampin, and ceftriaxone were active against 43 *H. cinaedi* strains and 6 *H. fennelliae* strains studied (23).

Clinically and histopathologically, syndromes associated with *H. cinaedi, H. fennelliae,* and other CLO infections are similar to *C. jejuni* infections; they consist primarily of proctocolitis, enterocolitis, and diarrhea (22, 69). CLOs have also been isolated from asymptomatic men. In a study of 33 homosexual men with diarrhea and 35 with proctitis, *Campylobacter* species or CLOs were isolated from the stools of 23% of patients with diarrhea and 14% of patients with proctitis (47). *H. cinaedi* was recovered from two patients with acute diarrhea; CLO3 was recovered from the stools of a third patient. The gastroenteritis associated with these organisms has in most cases been mild and has resolved without use of antimicrobial agents, even in patients who are human immunodeficiency virus antibody positive (33). Abnormal findings on anoscopy and sigmoidoscopy, acute inflammation on rectal biopsy, and increased number of rectal leukocytes are seen in patients from whom CLOs are the only enteric organisms isolated (64).

Although CLOs appear to be important causes of acute enteric illness in homosexual men, they have not been shown to be a cause of chronic diarrheal disease in persons with symptomatic human immunodeficiency virus disease (103). Infection with these organisms is also not exclusive to homosexual men. Recently, there have been reports of *H. cinaedi* infections in women and children with acute diarrheal gastroenteritis, suggesting that *H. cinaedi* may be more widespread than previously thought (89, 95).

The invasive potential of CLOs in immunocompromised patients was established when Pasternak et al. reported that CLOs had been isolated from the blood of two homosexual patients with tuberculosis (65). Another report described bacteremia with a CLO (*H. cinaedi*) in a 29-year-old homosexual man with AIDS (16). Similarly, the potential for *H. fennelliae* bacteremia was recognized when Ng et al. reported successive *H. cinaedi* and *H. fennelliae* bacteremias in a 31-year-old bisexual patient with human immunodeficiency virus-related disease (60).

H. cinaedi has been isolated from only one nonhuman source; Gebhart et al. were able to isolate *H. cinaedi* from 75% of healthy hamsters obtained from two commercial sources (28). Initially, it was thought that hamsters were an animal reservoir from which the organism is introduced into humans (Table 2). However, additional studies are needed to corroborate the presence of this organism in hamsters.

In summary, *Campylobacter* species and CLOs have been isolated from homosexual men with gastroenteritis and proctitis. These CLOs were categorized into four groups; the names *C. cinaedi* and *C. fennelliae* were accepted for two of these, but the species were later moved to the genus *Helicobacter*. The clinical spectrum of disease associated with CLO infection ranges from asymptomatic colonization to bacteremia and death. *H. cinaedi* has also recently been identified in women and children, suggesting that the organism may be more widespread. Hamsters are the only known animal reservoir for *H. cinaedi*. Nonroutine laboratory techniques are required to culture these organisms.

C. CONCISUS

C. concisus has been associated with periodontal disease in humans, although a direct pathogenic role for this organism in gingival disease has not been proven. Gram-negative, anaerobic bacteria are commonly found in the oral lesions of persons with destructive periodontal disease. In 1981, Tanner et al. isolated 46 strains of gram-negative asaccharolytic bacteria from patients with periodontal disease and differentiated these into seven groups (84). One group fit the genus *Campylobacter*, and the name *C. concisus* (from the Latin word "concisus," meaning concise, brief) was proposed.

C. concisus could be differentiated from other gram-negative, asaccharolytic organisms (*Bacteroides gracilis*, *Wolinella recta*, recently placed in the *Campylobacter* genus as *C. recta* [96], and *Eikenella corrodens*) serologically by agglutination (3). Protein profiles obtained by sodium dodecyl sulfate-polyacrylamide gel electrophoresis further facilitated differentiation (83). *C. concisus* forms small, curved, unbranched cells. It is microaerophilic to anaerobic, and its growth is supported by formate or fumarate alone or with hydrogen.

In 1986, Paster and Gibbons demonstrated that *C. concisus* was not only supported by formate but was chemotactic to this substance as well; *C. concisus* was not chemotactic to a wide range of other substances tested (64). Interestingly, the formate concentration that gave the optimal chemotactic response was the mean concentration of formate in dental plaque (5×10^{-2} M). Thus, chemotaxis to formate may enable *C. concisus* to locate and colonize plaque-laden periodontal pockets. Treatment of periodontal disease with Widman flap surgery and tetracycline (1 g/day for 3 weeks) resulted in an increase in the proportion of *C. concisus* organisms at active sites of periodontal disease (85). Further studies of both the pathogenic role and possible therapeutic options for *C. concisus* infection of the oral cavity are needed.

Recently, reports have suggested that *C. concisus* may not be confined to the oral cavity in humans. In 1987, Johnson and Finegold isolated *C. concisus* from the foot ulcer of a diabetic patient with osteomyelitis (39). Vandamme et al. studied 14 strains of misidentified campylobacters and CLOs obtained from nonoral clinical sources: blood, esophagus, stomach, duodenum, and feces (94). All strains were unambiguously *C. concisus*. Although a direct pathogenic role for these organisms was not identified, the possibility remains open for a broader association between *C. concisus* infections and gastrointestinal illnesses.

C. SPUTORUM

Of the three biovars (subspecies) of *C. sputorum*, two have been associated with infections in humans. Two reports describe five patients with *C. sputorum* infection (8, 71). Two isolates were *C. sputorum* subsp. *sputorum*, and three were *C. sputorum* subsp. *bubulus*. All five isolates were from abscesses: one lung abscess, one axillary abscess, one scrotal abscess, and two groin abscesses.

C. BUTZLERI

C. butzleri was recently recognized as a species distinct from *C. cryaerophila* and is probably associated with diarrhea in humans (43). *C. cryaerophila* has been moved to the genus *Arcobacter* within the family *Campylobacteraceae,* and the species name has been corrected to *A. cryaerophila* (93, 96). *Campylobacter (Arcobacter) butzleri* does not grow at 42°C and cannot be isolated on media commonly used for primary isolation of *C. jejuni.* Further information on the pathogenic role of this organism is not currently available.

C. JEJUNI SUBSP. *DOYLEI*

In 1985, nitrate-negative strains that resembled *C. jejuni* were isolated from antral biopsies of adults with upper gastrointestinal symptoms (30, 42) and children with gastroenteritis (80, 81). The organisms were referred to as gastric CLOs (GLO-2). These nitrate-negative campylobacters were later determined to be a distinct subspecies of *C. jejuni* (62). In 1988, the name *C. jejuni* subsp. *doylei* was proposed after the veterinarian L. P. Doyle, who first isolated vibrios from the large bowels of pigs with dysentery (81).

C. jejuni subsp. *doylei* does not grow at 42°C and grows slowly at 37°C. The bacteria are characterized by a positive hippurate hydrolysis test result and an inability to reduce nitrate to nitrite and are more susceptible than *C. jejuni* to cephalothin and polymyxin (81). The role of *C. jejuni* subsp. *doylei* in causing human illness is unknown.

REFERENCES

1. **Altwegg, M., A. Burnens, J. Zollinger-Iten, and J. L. Penner.** 1987. Problems in identification of *Campylobacter jejuni* associated with acquisition of resistance to nalidixic acid. *J. Clin. Microbiol.* **25:**1807–1808.
2. **Anolik, J. R., D. Mildvan, J. W. Winter, D. Puttlitz, S. Rubenstein, and H. Lozman.** 1983. Mycotic aortic aneurysm: a complication of *Campylobacter fetus* septicemia. *Arch. Intern. Med.* **143:**609–610.
3. **Badger, S. J., and A. C. R. Tanner.** 1981. Serologic studies of *Bacteroides gracilis, Campylobacter concisus, Wolinella recta,* and *Eikenella corrodens,* all from humans with periodontal disease. *Int. J. Syst. Bacteriol.* **31:**446–451.
4. **Benjamin, J., S. Leaper, R. J. Owen, and M. B. Skirrow.** 1983. Description of *Campylobacter laridis,* a new species comprising the nalidixic acid resistant thermophilic *Campylobacter* (NARTC) group. *Curr. Microbiol.* **8:**231–238.
5. **Blaser, M. J., I. D. Berkowitz, M. LaForce, J. Cravens, L. B. Reller, and W. I. Wang.** 1979. *Campylobacter* enteritis: clinical and epidemiologic features. *Ann. Intern. Med.* **91:**179–185.
6. **Blaser, M. J., J. A. Hopkins, and M. L. Vasil.** 1984. *Campylobacter* enteritis. *N. Engl. J. Med.* **305:**1444–1452.
7. **Bolton, F. J., D. Coates, D. N. Hutchinson, and A. F. Godfree.** 1987. A study of thermophilic *Campylobacter* in a river system. *J. Appl. Bacteriol.* **62:**167–176.
8. **Borczyk, A., H. Lior, A. McKeown, and H. Svendsen.** 1987. Isolations of *Campylobacter sputorum* associated with human infections, abstr. 211. *In* B. Kaijser and E. Falsen (ed.) *Campylobacter IV.* University of Gothenburg, Gothenburg, Sweden.
9. **Borczyk, A., S. Thompson, D. Smith, and H. Lior.** 1987. Water-borne outbreak of *Campylobacter laridis*-associated gastroenteritis. *Lancet* **i:**164–165. (Letter.)
10. **Brown, W. J., and R. Sautter.** 1977. *Campylobacter fetus* septicemia with concurrent salpingitis. *J. Clin. Microbiol.* **6:**72–75.
11. **Butzler, J. P., and M. B. Skirrow.** 1979. Campylobacter enteritis. *Clin. Gastroenterol.* **8:**737–765.
12. **Carbone, K. M., M. C. Heinrich, and T. C. Quinn.** 1985. Thrombophlebitis and cellulitis due to *Campylobacter fetus* ssp. *fetus. Medicine* **64:**244–250.
13. **Centers for Disease Control.** 1981. *Campylobacter* sepsis associated with "nutritional therapy"—California. *Morbid. Mortal. Weekly Rep.* **30:**294–295.
14. **Centers for Disease Control.** 1984. Premature labor and neonatal sepsis caused by *Campylobacter fetus,* subsp. *fetus*—Ontario. *Morbid. Mortal. Weekly Rep.* 33:483–489.
15. **Centers for Disease Control.** 1988. *Campylobacter* isolates in the United States, 1982–1986. *Morbid. Mortal. Weekly Rep.* **37**(SS-2)**:**1–14.
16. **Cimolai, N., M. J. Gill, A. Jones, B. Flores, W. E. Stamm, W. Laurie, B. Madden, and M. S. Shahrabadi.** 1987. "*Campylobacter cinaedi*" bacteremia: case report and laboratory findings. *J. Clin. Microbiol.* **25:**942–943.
17. **Devlin, H. R., and L. McIntyre.** 1983. *Campylobacter fetus* subsp. *fetus* in homosexual males. *J. Clin. Microbiol.* **18:**999–1000.
18. **Dickgiesser, N., G. Kasper, and W. Kihm.** 1983. *Campylobacter fetus* ssp. *fetus* bacteremia: a patient with liver cirrhosis. *Infection* **5:**288.
19. **Edmonds, P., C. M. Patton, T. J. Barrett, G. K. Morris, A. G. Steigerwalt, and D. J. Brenner.** 1985. Biochemical and genetic characteristics of atypical *Campylobacter fetus* subsp. *fetus* strains isolated from humans in the United States. *J. Clin. Microbiol.* **21:**936–940.
20. **Edmonds, P., C. M. Patton, P. M. Griffin, T. J. Barrett, G. P. Schmid, C. N. Baker, M. A. Lambert, and D. J. Brenner.** 1987. *Campylobacter hyointestinalis* associated with human gastrointestinal disease in the United States. *J. Clin. Microbiol.* **25:**685–691.
21. **Fennell, C. L., A. M. Rompalo, P. A. Totten, K. L. Bruch, B. M. Flores, and W. E. Stamm.** 1986. Isolation of "*Campylobacter hyointestinalis*" from a human. *J. Clin. Microbiol.* **24:**146–148.

22. **Fennell, C. J., P. A. Totten, T. C. Quinn, C. L. Patton, K. K. Holmes, and W. E. Stamm.** 1984. Characterization of *Campylobacter*-like organisms isolated from homosexual men. *J. Infect. Dis.* **149:**58–66.
23. **Flores, B. M., C. L. Fennell, K. K. Holmes, and W. E. Stamm.** 1985. In vitro susceptibility of *Campylobacter*-like organisms to twenty antimicrobial agents. *Antimicrob Agents Chemother.* **28:**188–191.
24. **Fox, J. O., K. O. Maxwell, N. S. Taylor, C. D. Runsick, P. Edmonds, and D. J. Brenner.** 1989. "*Campylobacter upsaliensis*" isolated from cats as identified by DNA relatedness and biochemical features. *J. Clin. Microbiol.* **27:**2376–2378.
25. **Francioli, P., J. Herztein, J. P. Grob, J. J. Vallotton, G. Mombelli, and M. P. Glauser.** 1985. *Campylobacter fetus* subspecies *fetus* bacteremia. *Arch. Intern. Med.* **145:**289–292.
26. **Garcia, M. M., M. D. Eaglesome, and C. Rigby.** 1983. Campylobacters important in veterinary medicine. *Vet. Bull.* **53:**793–818.
27. **Gebhart, C. J., P. Edmonds, G. E. Ward, H. J. Kurtz, and D. J. Brenner.** 1985. "*Campylobacter hyointestinalis*" sp. nov.: a new species of *Campylobacter* found in the intestines of pigs and other animals. *J. Clin. Microbiol.* **44:**361–367.
28. **Gebhart, C. J., C. L. Fennell, M. P. Murtaugh, and W. E. Stamm.** 1989. *Campylobacter cinaedi* is the normal intestinal flora in hamsters. *J. Clin. Microbiol.* **27:**1692–1694.
29. **Gebhart C. J., G. E. Ward, K. Chang, and H. J. Kurtz.** 1983. *Campylobacter hyointestinalis* (new species) isolated from swine with lesions of proliferative ileitis. *Am. J. Vet. Res.* **44:**361–367.
30. **Goodwin, S., E. Blincow, J. Armstrong, and R. McCulloch.** 1985. *Campylobacter pyloridis* is unique: GCLO-2 is an ordinary *Campylobacter. Lancet* **ii:**38–39.
31. **Goossens, H., B. Pot, L. Vlaes, C. Van den Borre, C. Van den Abbeele, C. Van Naelten, J. Levy, H. Cogniau, P. Marbehant, J. Verhoef, K. Kersters, J. P. Butzler, and P. Vandamme.** 1990. Characterization and description of *Campylobacter upsaliensis* isolated from human feces. *J. Clin. Microbiol.* **28:**1039–1046.
32. **Goossens, H., L. Vlaes, M. De Bobck, B. Pot, K. Kersters, J. Levy, P. De Mol, J. P. Butzler, and P. Vandamme.** 1990. Is "*Campylobacter upsaliensis*" an unrecognized cause of human diarrhea? *Lancet* **336:**584–586.
33. **Grayson, M. L., W. Tee, and B. Dwyer.** 1989. Gastroenteritis associated with *Campylobacter cinaedi. Med. J. Aust.* **150:**214–215.
34. **Guerrant, R. L., R. G. Lahita, W. C. Winn, Jr., and R. B. Roberts.** 1976. Campylobacteriosis in man: pathogenic mechanisms and review of 91 bloodstream infections. *Am. J. Med.* **65:**584–592.
35. **Harvey, S. M., and J. R. Greenwood.** 1983. Probable *Campylobacter fetus* subsp. *fetus* gastroenteritis. *J. Clin. Microbiol.* **18:**1278–1279.
36. **Hill, B. D., R. J. Thomas, and A. R. Mackenzie.** 1987. *Campylobacter hyointestinalis*-associated enteritis in moluccan rusa deer. *J. Comp. Pathol.* **97:**687–694.
37. **Hirschl, A. M., M. Pletschette, D. Wolf, J. Berger, G. Diridl, and M. L. Rotter.** 1990. Frequency of occurrence and characterization of catalase negative *Campylobacter* isolated from human feces in Vienna. *Int. J. Med. Microbiol.* **272:**547–553.
38. **International Union of Microbiological Societies.** 1991. Validation of the publication of new names and new combinations previously effectively published outside the IJSB. *Int. J. Syst. Bacteriol.* **41:**331.
39. **Johnson, C. C., and S. M. Finegold.** 1987. Uncommonly encountered motile, anaerobic gram-negative bacilli associated with infection. *Rev. Infect. Dis.* **9:**1150–1162.
40. **Kaplan, R. L.** 1980. Campylobacter, p. 235–241. *In* E. H. Lennette, A. Balows, W. J. Hausler, Jr., and J. P. Truant (ed.), *Manual of Clinical Microbiology,* 3rd ed. American Society for Microbiology, Washington, D.C.
41. **Karmali, M. A., A. K. Allen, and P. C. Fleming.** 1981. Differentiation of catalase-positive campylobacters with special reference to morphology. *Int. J. Syst. Bacteriol.* **31:**64–71.
42. **Kasper, G., and N. Dickgiesser.** 1985. Isolation from gastric epithelium of *Campylobacter*-like bacteria that are distinct from *Campylobacter pyloridis. Lancet* **i:**111–112.
43. **Keihlbauch, J. A., D. J. Brenner, M. A. Nicholson, C. N. Baker, C. M. Patton, A. G. Steigerwalt, and I. K. Wachsmuth.** 1991. *Campylobacter butzleri* sp. nov. isolated from humans and animals with diarrheal illness. *J. Clin. Microbiol.* **29:**376–385.
44. **Klein, B. S., J. M. Vergeront, M. J. Blaser, P. Edmonds, D. J. Brenner, D. Janssen, and J. P. Davis.** 1986. *Campylobacter* infection associated with raw milk: an outbreak of gastroenteritis due to *Campylobacter jejuni* and thermotolerant *Campylobacter fetus* subsp. *fetus. JAMA* **255:**361–364.
45. **Lambert, M., J. M. W. Jones, and S. A. Lister.** 1984. Isolation of *Campylobacter hyointestinalis* from pigs in the United Kingdom. *Vet. Rec.* **115:**128–129.
46. **Lastovica, A. J., E. Le Roux, and J. L. Penner.** 1989. "*Campylobacter upsaliensis*" isolated from blood cultures of pediatric patients. *J. Clin. Microbiol.* **27:**657–659.
47. **Laughon, B. E., D. A. Druckman, A. Vernon, T. C. Quinn, B. F. Polk, J. F. Modlin, R. H. Yolken, and J. G. Bartlett.** 1988. Prevalence of enteric pathogens in homosexual men with and without acquired immunodeficiency syndrome. *Gastroenterology* **94:**984–993.
48. **Laughon, B. E., A. A. Vernon, D. A. Druckman, R. Fox, T. C. Quinn, B. F. Polk, and J. G. Bartlett.** 1988. Recovery of *Campylobacter* species from homosexual men. *J. Infect. Dis.* **158:**464–467.
49. **Lee, M. M., R. C. Welliver, and L. J. La Scolea.** 1985. *Campylobacter* meningitis in childhood. *Pediatr. Infect. Dis.* **4:**544–547.
50. **Lindblom, G. B., M. Jony, K. Khalil, K. Mazhar, G. M. Ruiz-Palacios, and B. Kaijser.** 1990. Enter-

otoxigenicity and frequency of *Campylobacter jejuni, C. coli,* and *C. laridis* in human and animal stool isolates from different countries. *Microbiol. Lett.* **66:**163–168.
51. **Lowrie, D. B., and J. H. Pearce.** 1970. The placental localisation of *Vibrio fetus. J. Med. Microbiol.* **3:**607–614.
52. **Marty, A. T., T. A. Webb, G. Stubbs, and R. R. Penkava.** 1983. Inflammatory abdominal aortic aneurysm infected by *Campylobacter fetus. JAMA* **249:**1190–1192.
53. **McFadyean, J., and S. Stockman.** 1913. Report of the department committee appointed by the Board of Agriculture and Fisheries to inquire into epizootic abortions. Appendix to part III. Abortion in sheep, p. 1–29. His Majesty's Stationery Office, London.
54. **Megraud, F., and F. Bonnet.** 1986. Unusual *Campylobacters* in human feces. *J. Infect.* **12:**275–276.
55. **Megraud, F., D. Chevrier, N. Desplaces, A. Sedallian, and J. L. Guesdon.** 1988. Urease-positive thermophilic Campylobacter (*Campylobacter laridis* variant) isolated from an appendix and from human feces. *J. Clin. Microbiol.* **26:**1050–1051.
56. **Miller, V. A., R. Jenson, and J. J. Gilroy.** 1959. Bacteremia in pregnant sheep following oral administration of *Vibrio fetus. Am. J. Vet. Res.* **20:**677–679.
57. **Minet, J., B. Grosbois, and F. Megraud.** 1988. *Campylobacter hyointestinalis:* an opportunistic enteropathogen? *J. Clin. Microbiol.* **26:**2659–2660.
58. **Morrison, V. A., B. K. Lloyd, J. K. S. Chia, and C. U. Tuazon.** 1990. Cardiovascular and bacteremic manifestations of *Campylobacter fetus* infection: case report and review. *Rev. Infect. Dis.* **12:**387–392.
59. **Nachamkin, I., C. Stowell, D. Skalina, A. M. Jones, R. M. Hoop, and R. M. Smibert.** 1984. *Campylobacter laridis* causing bacteremia in an immunosuppressed patient. *Ann. Intern. Med.* **101:**55–57.
60. **Ng, V. L., W. K. Hadley, C. L. Fennell, B. M. Flores, and W. E. Stamm.** 1987. Successive bacteremias with "*Campylobacter cianedi*" and "*Campylobacter fennelliae*" in a bisexual male. *J. Clin. Microbiol.* **25:**2008–2009.
61. **Owen, R. J., M. Costas, L. Sloss, and F. J. Bolton.** 1988. Numerical analysis of electrophoretic protein patterns of *Campylobacter laridis* and allied thermophilic campylobacters from the natural environment. *J. Appl. Bacteriol.* **65:**68–78.
62. **Owen, R. J., and C. Dawson.** 1986. DNA base compositions and base sequence relatedness of atypical *Campylobacter jejuni* strains from clinical material. *FEMS Microbiol. Lett.* **35:**283–287.
63. **Owen, R. J., and J. Hernandez.** 1990. Occurrence of plasmids in "*Campylobacter upsaliensis*" (catalase negative or weak group) from geographically diverse patients with gastroenteritis or bacteremia. *Eur. J. Epidemiol.* **6:**111–117.
64. **Paster, B. J., and R. J. Gibbons.** 1986. Chemotactic response to formate by *Campylobacter concisus* and its potential role in gingival colonization. *Infect. Immun.* **52:**378–383.
65. **Pasternak, J., R. Bolivar, R. L. Hopper, V. Fainstein, K. Mills, A. Rios, G. P. Bodey, C. L. Fennell, P. A. Totten, and W. E. Stamm.** 1984. Bacteremia caused by *Campylobacter*-like organisms in two male homosexuals. *Ann. Intern. Med.* **101:**339–341.
66. **Patton, C. M., N. Shaffer, P. Edmonds, T. J. Barrett, M. A. Lambert, C. Baker, D. M. Perlman, and D. J. Brenner.** 1989. Human disease associated with "*Campylobacter upsaliensis*" (catalase-negative or weakly positive *Campylobacter* species) in the United States. *J. Clin. Microbiol.* **27:**66–73.
67. **Popovic-Uroic, T., C. M. Patton, M. A. Nicholson, and J. A. Kiehlbauch.** 1990. Evaluation of indoxyl acetate hydrolysis test for rapid differentiation of *Campylobacter, Helicobacter,* and *Wolinella* species. *J. Clin. Microbiol.* **28:**2335–2339.
68. **Preston, M. A., A. E. Simor, S. L. Walmsey, S. A. Fuller, A. J. Lastovica, K. Sandstedt, and J. L. Penner.** 1990. In vitro susceptibility of *"Campylobacter upsaliensis"* to twenty-four antimicrobial agents. *Eur. J. Clin. Microbiol. Infect. Dis.* **9:**822–824.
69. **Quinn, T. C., S. E. Goodell, C. Fennell, S. P. Wang, M. D. Schuffler, K. K. Holmes, and W. E. Stamm.** 1984. Infections with *Campylobacter jejuni* and *Campylobacter*-like organisms in homosexual men. *Ann. Intern. Med.* **101:**187–192.
70. **Quinn, T. C., W. E. Stamm, S. E. Goodell, E. Mkrtichian, J. Benedetti, L. Corey, M. D. Schuffler, and K. K. Holmes.** 1983. The polymicrobial origin of intestinal infections in homosexual men. *N. Engl. J. Med.* **309:**576–582.
71. **Raffi, F., M. Derriennic, A. Michault, C. Arvin-Berod, M. Renouil, G. Durieux, D. Baron, and A. L. Courtieu.** 1985. Infections humaines a *Campylobacter sputorum:* a propos de deux observations. *Med. Mal. Infect.* **15:**65–67.
72. **Rao, G. G., Q. N. Karim, A. Maddocks, R. J. Hillman, J. R. W. Harris, and A. J. Pinching.** 1990. *Campylobacter fetus* infections in two patients with AIDS. *J. Infect.* **20:**170–172.
73. **Rettig, P. J.** 1979. Campylobacter infections in human beings. *J. Pediatr.* **94:**855–864.
74. **Sandstedt, K., and J. Ursing.** 1991. Description of *Campylobacter upsaliensis* sp. nov. previously known as the CNW group. *Syst. Appl. Microbiol.* **14:**39–45.
75. **Sandstedt, K., J. Ursing, and M. Walder.** 1983. Thermotolerant *Campylobacter* with no or weak catalase activity isolated from dogs. *Curr. Microbiol.* **8:**209–213.
76. **Simor, A. E., M. A. Karmali, T. Jadavji, and M. Roscoe.** 1986. Abortion and perinatal sepsis associated with campylobacter infection. *Rev. Infect. Dis.* **8:**397–402.
77. **Simor, A. E., and L. Wilcox.** 1987. Enteritis associated with *Campylobacter laridis. J. Clin. Microbiol.* **25:**10–12.
78. **Skirrow, M. B., and J. Benjamin.** 1980. "1001" campylobacters: cultural characteristics of intestinal campylobacters from man and animals. *J. Hyg.* **85:**427–442.

79. **Smith, T.** 1919. The etiological relationship of spirilla *(Vibrio fetus)* to bovine abortion. *J. Exp. Med.* **30:**313–322.
80. **Steele, T. W., J. A. Lanser, and N. Sangster.** 1985. Nitrate-negative *Campylobacter*-like organisms. *Lancet* **i:**394.
81. **Steele, T. W., and R. J. Owen.** 1988. *Campylobacter jejuni* subspecies *doylei* (subsp. nov.), a subspecies of nitrate-negative campylobacters isolated from human clinical specimens. *Int. J. Syst. Bacteriol.* **38:**316–318.
82. **Steele, T. W., N. Sangster, and J. A. Lanser.** 1985. DNA relatedness and biochemical features of *Campylobacter* spp. isolated in Central and South Australia. *J. Clin. Microbiol.* **22:**71–74.
83. **Tanner, A. C. R.** 1986. Characterization of *Wolinella* spp., *Campylobacter concisus, Bacteroides gracilis,* and *Eikenella corrodens* by polyacrylamide gel electrophoresis. *J. Clin. Microbiol.* **24:**562–565.
84. **Tanner, A. C. R., S. Badger, C. H. Lai, M. A. Listgarten, R. A. Visconti, and S. S. Socransky.** 1981. *Wolinella* gen. nov., *Wolinella succinogenes* (*Vibrio succinogenes* Wolin et al.) comb. nov., and description of *Bacteroides gracilis* sp. nov., *Wolinella recta* sp. nov., *Campylobacter concisus* sp. nov., and *Eikenella corrodens* from humans with periodontal disease. *Int. J. Syst. Bacteriol.* **31:**432–435.
85. **Tanner, A. C. R., J. L. Dzink, J. L. Ebersole, and S. S. Socransky.** 1987. *Wolinella recta, Campylobacter concisus, Bacteroides gracilis,* and *Eikenella corrodens* from periodontal lesions. *J. Periodont. Res.* **22:**327–330.
86. **Targan, S. R., A. W. Chow, and L. B. Guze.** 1976. Spontaneous peritonitis of cirrhosis due to *Campylobacter fetus. Gastroenterology* **71:**311–313.
87. **Tauxe, R. V., C. M. Patton, P. Edmonds, T. J. Barrett, D. J. Brenner, and P. A. Blake.** 1985. Illness associated with *Campylobacter laridis,* a newly recognized *Campylobacter* species. *J. Clin. Microbiol.* **21:**222–225.
88. **Taylor, D. E., K. Hiratsuks, and L. Mueller.** 1989. Isolation and characterization of catalase-negative and catalase-weak strains of *Campylobacter* species, including *"Campylobacter upsaliensis,"* from humans with gastroenteritis. *J. Clin. Microbiol.* **27:**2042–2045.
89. **Tee, W., B. N. Anderson, B. C. Ross, and B. Dwyer.** 1987. Atypical campylobacters associated with gastroenteritis. *J. Clin. Microbiol.* **25:**1248–1252.
90. **Totten, P. A., C. L. Fennell, F. C. Tenover, J. M. Wezenberg, P. L. Perine, W. E. Stamm, and K. K. Holmes.** 1985. *Campylobacter cinaedi* (sp. nov.) and *Campylobacter fennelliae* (sp. nov.): two new *Campylobacter* species associated with enteric disease in homosexual men. *J. Infect. Dis.* **151:**131–139.
91. **U.S. Department of Health and Human Services, Public Health Service.** 1990. *Centers for Disease Control Campylobacter Annual Tabulation 1987–1989.* U.S. Department of Health and Human Services, Washington, D.C.
92. **Ursing, J., K. Sandstedt, and E. Hansson.** 1984. Genetic and phenotypic characteristics of a new group of *Campylobacter* isolated from pigs and cattle. *Acta Pathol. Microbiol. Immunol. Scand. Sect. B* **92:**71–72.
93. **Vandamme, P., and J. De Ley.** 1991. Proposal for a new family, *Campylobacteraceae. Int. J. Syst. Bacteriol.* **41:**451–455.
94. **Vandamme, P., E. Falsen, B. Pot, B. Hoste, K. Kersters, and J. De Ley.** 1989. Identification of EF group 22 campylobacters from gastroenteritis cases as *Campylobacter concisus. J. Clin. Microbiol.* **27:**1775–1781.
95. **Vandamme, P., E. Falsen, B. Pot, K. Kersters, and J. De Ley.** 1990. Identification of *Campylobacter cinaedi* isolated from blood and feces of children and adult females. *J. Clin. Microbiol.* **28:**1016–1020.
96. **Vandamme, P., E. Falsen, R. Rossau, B. Hoste, R. Tytgat, and J. De Ley.** 1991. Revision of *Campylobacter, Helicobacter,* and *Wolinella* taxonomy: emendation of generic descriptions and proposal of *Arcobacter* gen. nov. *Int. J. Syst. Bacteriol.* **41:**88–103.
97. **Vinzent, R., J. Dumas, and N. Picard.** 1947. Septicemie grave au cours de la grossesse due a un vibrion. Avortement consecutif. *Bull. Acad. Natl. Med.* (Paris) **131:**90–92.
98. **Von Graevenitz, A.** 1990. Revised nomenclature of *Campylobacter laridis, Enterobacter intermedium,* and *"Flavobacterium branchophilia." Int. J. Syst. Bacteriol.* **40:**211.
99. **Walder, M., K. Sandstedt, and J. Ursing.** 1983. Phenotypic characteristics of thermotolerant *Campylobacter* from human and animal sources. *Curr. Microbiol.* **9:**291–296.
100. **Walmsley, S. L., and M. A. Karmali.** 1989. Direct isolation of thermophilic *Campylobacter* species from human feces on selective agar medium. *J. Clin. Microbiol.* **27:**668–670.
101. **Wang, W. L., and M. J. Blaser.** 1986. Detection of pathogenic *Campylobacter* species in blood culture systems. *J. Clin. Microbiol.* **23:**709–714.
102. **Wens, R., M. Dratwa, C. Potvliege, W. Hansen, C. Tielemans, and F. Collart.** 1985. *Campylobacter* fetus peritonitis followed by septicaemia in a patient on continuous ambulatory peritoneal dialysis. *J. Infect.* **10:**249–251.
103. **Wilcox, C. M., B. A. Byford, C. E. Forsmark, W. K. Hadley, J. P. Cello, and M. A. Jacobson.** 1990. *Campylobacter*-like organisms are uncommon pathogens in patients infected with the human immunodeficiency virus. *J. Clin. Microbiol.* **28:**2370–2371.

II. RESERVOIRS AND ANTIMICROBIAL RESISTANCE

CHAPTER 5

Food-Borne Transmission and Antibiotic Resistance of *Campylobacter jejuni*

MICHAEL P. DOYLE AND DENNIS M. JONES

FUTURE DIRECTIONS TO CONTROLLING FOOD-BORNE TRANSMISSION OF *CAMPYLOBACTER JEJUNI*

Campylobacter jejuni is carried in the intestinal tract of a wide variety of wild and domestic animals and, as a result of fecal contact during processing, frequently contaminates foods derived from animals (22, 24, 28). *C. jejuni* is often present on retail fresh poultry and is less frequently found on fresh beef, lamb, pork, and mushrooms and in raw milk (5, 6, 23). Shellfish, such as clams, may become contaminated by feeding in waters polluted by runoff from animal-raising farms.

Fortunately, *C. jejuni* does not grow or survive well outside the enteron of its host. The organism is not likely to grow in foods (that remain edible) or on food-processing surfaces because the bacterium (i) will not grow below 30°C, (ii) requires microaerobic (5% O_2 optimal) and capnophilic (3 to 5% CO_2) conditions for growth, (iii) grows slowly (even under optimal conditions its doubling time is about 1 h), and (iv) is not a good competitor with other bacteria (it will not utilize carbohydrates) (5). Furthermore, *C. jejuni* does not survive well in foods, being sensitive to drying, 21% oxygen, storage at 25°C, acidic conditions, and heat ($D_{55°C}$ in milk is ca. 1 min) (5, 10). However, refrigerating (4°C) foods will substantially promote survival (5), and keeping foods frozen may allow long-term survival of a small population of an originally large number of *C. jejuni* cells (5).

Although *C. jejuni* is not likely to grow or survive well in foods, foods of animal origin may be contaminated initially with large populations ($>10^3$/g) of the organism (16, 22). Often 45 to 85% of retail-ready poultry parts, carcasses, and giblets are *C. jejuni* positive (5). Furthermore, results of limited studies suggest that ingestion of only a small number (ca. 500 cells) of *C. jejuni* organisms will produce human illness (2, 19). The apparent high degree of virulence of the organism, as indicated by its apparent low infectious dose, coupled with its widespread prevalence in foods of animal origin, is important in explaining why this sensitive bacterium is a leading cause of gastroenteritis.

There is ample evidence to indicate that poultry and, to a lesser extent, pets (especially kittens and puppies) are important reservoirs of *C. jejuni* and are principal vehicles of *Campylobacter* enteritis (3, 4, 11). It is estimated that more than 50% of sporadic cases of *Campylobacter* enteritis are linked to eating or handling poultry (4, 11), and so reducing the carriage of *C. jejuni* by poultry should have a major impact on decreasing disease.

Stern (this volume) describes several well-conceived approaches to reducing the incidence of *C. jejuni* in poultry. However, an understanding of how the organism colonizes poultry is important for developing successful approaches to eliminating or reducing *C. jejuni* carriage. Studies by Beery et al. (1) have shown that the principal sites of *C. jejuni* colonization in chickens are mucus-filled cecal crypts. Within these crypts large populations of campylobacters appear to be freely suspended and unattached to mucosal surfaces. Hugdahl et al. (12) determined that *C. jejuni* is chemoattracted to the mucin component of mucus, specifically to L-fucose, which is

Michael P. Doyle, Department of Food Science and Technology, Georgia Experiment Station, University of Georgia, Griffin, Georgia 30223. **Dennis M. Jones,** Department of Clinical Bacteriology, Public Health Laboratory Service, Withington Hospital, Manchester M20 8LR, United Kingdom.

an exposed constituent of mucin. In addition, they found that the organism can utilize mucin as the sole substrate for growth. From these data, one could speculate that *C. jejuni* is chemoattracted to mucin within cecal crypts, where the organism thrives and multiplies on the ever-present supply of mucus being continuously secreted.

A practical approach to intervene in the colonization of poultry by *C. jejuni* is to expose newly hatched chickens to bacteria that can (i) colonize cecal crypts, (ii) utilize mucin as the sole substrate for growth, and (iii) produce metabolites that are bactericidal or antagonistic to *C. jejuni.* These bacteria theoretically should competitively prevent campylobacters from colonizing poultry. Hence, the poultry industry could use defined bacterial cultures to control *C. jejuni.*

Selecting and breeding chickens on the basis of their resistance to *C. jejuni* colonization also has the potential for success. However, substantial research is needed to elucidate the heritability factors that provide protection against colonization and to characterize the genome responsible for the resistance phenotype. A possible limitation of this approach is that the genome of interest may confer additional characteristics that are undesirable in broilers or laying hens.

Vaccination of poultry with noncolonizing *C. jejuni* or a "colonization antigen" of *C. jejuni* also has potential for protecting chickens. However, this approach, even if effective, may be limited by practical considerations such as cost and methods of application.

Although poultry is a leading vehicle of *Campylobacter* enteritis, the current philosophy of the U.S. Department of Agriculture (as described by Norcross et al. [this volume]) which regulates poultry processing in the United States is that *C. jejuni* is a normal inhabitant of the intestinal tract of poultry and may contaminate poultry carcasses during processing. It is the responsibility of the food handler to properly cook poultry and to use hygienic practices in handling cooked poultry to prevent recontamination with *C. jejuni.*

It is likely that improvements in the hygiene of chicken production could reduce the number of campylobacters entering the chicken-processing plants. Complete elimination may not be practically possible, but if fewer birds were colonized, the level of contamination of individual carcasses at point of sale would be reduced. This in itself might reduce the opportunities for infection of humans and cross-contamination of other foods to a significant degree. Attention to the quality of the water supply to chicken houses can significantly affect the colonization rates among poultry flocks, which in turn can result in reduction in human disease (17). Such effects can be maintained only if supported by continued good hygiene both within and outside the chicken houses. Perhaps not enough attention is given to the environmental contamination of groundwater that can occur in the vicinity of chicken houses. This can lead to increased numbers of campylobacters, whether culturable or not (20, 25), gaining access to the local water cycles and contributing to the *Campylobacter* colonization of a variety of animals, both wild and domesticated.

Irradiation has been documented to be an effective procedure for killing pathogens, including *C. jejuni,* on poultry (13, 26, 30). Irradiation of poultry at levels needed to kill *C. jejuni* has been sanctioned by the U.S. Food and Drug Administration; however, because it is believed that the consumer will not accept irradiated poultry, the industry will not readily adopt the practice. Consumer preference and marketing research are needed to determine whether such consumer attitudes exist and, if so, to develop strategies that will initiate consumer acceptance of irradiated poultry products. Perhaps a case-control study of diarrheal illness among individuals who eat irradiated versus nonirradiated poultry could be done and results could be used to educate consumers about the value of irradiation in reducing the incidence of food-borne disease. Additionally, research is needed to eliminate or reduce *C. jejuni* contamination during slaughter and processing operations. Present-day operations serve to disseminate *C. jejuni* on poultry carcasses and parts.

Besides poultry, other foods of concern include raw seafoods (especially oysters), fresh mushrooms, and raw milk, which have been shown to carry *C. jejuni* and have been implicated as vehicles of *Campylobacter* enteritis. Research is needed to develop practices to produce or process such foods to ensure that *C. jejuni*-free products would be available to consumers interested in eating these foods raw. An alternate consideration is to outlaw the sale of raw milk at retail and the sale of raw seafoods at restaurants. Novel approaches are needed to educate food handlers in proper hygienic practices in food preparations and to educate consumers to avoid eating uncooked foods of animal origin.

Although progress is being made to reduce the incidence of *C. jejuni* in poultry, relatively little research is being done to affect *C. jejuni* carriage by other animals, especially pets. Research is needed to develop treatments for animals, especially kittens and puppies, that may be in households of high-risk individuals, including infants, the elderly, and the immunocompromised. This may be of even greater concern in the future, because a large portion (estimated >20%) of the U.S. population will be ≥65 years of age by 2020.

ANTIBIOTIC RESISTANCE AMONG CAMPYLOBACTERS

The genetic aspects and the mechanisms of the resistance of *C. jejuni* and *C. coli* to tetracycline, chloramphenicol, kanamycin, and erythromycin are comprehensively covered by Taylor (chapter 9 of this volume) and Tenover et al. (this volume). Turning to the therapeutic aspects of resistance to antibiotics, erythromycin has long been regarded as the antibiotic of choice. Although the use of this antibiotic may reduce the severity of the symptoms in children (21) and curtail the convalescent carriage state, it generally does little to alter the natural course of the illness (14). Most cases of *Campylobacter* enteritis do not require treatment, being of short duration and self-limiting. Only if the symptoms are prolonged or unduly severe is treatment necessary. It has been suggested that very early treatment with erythromycin would exert some effect, but there are practical difficulties. One is the length of time taken by conventional methods to isolate the infecting organism, and progress in detection methods not involving culture would be welcome. Nevertheless, in a recent prospective survey of empirical treatment the patients had already had an average of 3 days of diarrhea before therapy (29).

The potential problem of antibiotic resistance was illustrated by a recent study in Thailand, where early erythromycin treatment, compared with untreated controls, had no observable clinical effect (27). In this study the prevalence of resistance was particularly high (53% for *C. jejuni* and 91% for *C. coli*) and could have been the reason for the observed results. In developed countries erythromycin resistance is commonly reported at about the 2% level for *C. jejuni* (about 10% for *C. coli*) although animal strains are more frequently resistant. The report of such high rates of erythromycin resistance in Thailand is disturbing and may indicate what could happen if antibiotics became widely used for treating *Campylobacter* infection in developed countries.

Thermophilic campylobacters are associated with a proportion of cases of traveler's diarrhea and are then likely to be treated with broad-spectrum antibiotics. It is in this context that resistance to trimethoprim-sulfamethoxazole and tetracycline becomes clinically important. Fluoroquinolones are now popular, and ciprofloxacin is frequently used for travel-associated diarrhea (7, 15). Ciprofloxacin is also effective in treating erythromycin-resistant *Campylobacter* infections. Infected patients with lymphoma, leukemia, hypogammaglobulinemia, and human immunodeficiency virus infection, and who therefore have some degree of immunosuppression, are likely to have severe and protracted symptoms with a tendency to relapse after treatment (18). These circumstances favor the development of antibiotic resistance, and strains resistant to erythromycin and ciprofloxacin have been encountered in the course of treating these patients (8). Perhaps more significantly, a sharp increase in the prevalence of quinolone resistance among campylobacters isolated from poultry seems to have followed the introduction of enrofloxacin for veterinary use in the Netherlands (9). The prevalence of resistance to ciprofloxacin in contemporary human isolates has risen to 11%. Once again, the use of antibiotics in animal husbandry could have serious consequences for the therapeutics of human infection. The concomitant appearance of resistance among human isolates provides additional evidence for the importance of poultry as a source of human *Campylobacter* infection.

In general, the occurrence of antibiotic resistance among campylobacters remains at a fairly low level, possibly because specific therapy is not widely indicated. In clinical situations in which effective therapy is required, problems of resistance to first-line antibiotics are emerging and determination of susceptibility to a range of antibiotics is required to manage some of these patients. The mechanics and genetics of the development of resistance are of great interest because of the general insight they afford to the genetics within the genus, but they also illuminate some of the possible future trends in antibiotic resistance.

REFERENCES

1. **Beery, J. T., M. B. Hugdahl, and M. P. Doyle.** 1988. Colonization of gastrointestinal tracts of chickens by *Campylobacter jejuni*. *Appl. Environ. Microbiol.* **54:**2365–2370.
2. **Black, R. E., M. M. Levine, M. L. Clements, T. P. Hughes, and M. J. Blaser.** 1988. Experimental

Campylobacter jejuni infection in humans. *J. Infect. Dis.* **157**:472–479.
3. **Blaser, M. J., F. M. LaForce, N. A. Wilson, and W.-L. L. Wang.** 1980. Reservoirs for human campylobacteriosis. *J. Infect. Dis.* **141**:665–669.
4. **Deming, M. S., R. V. Tauxe, P. A. Blake, S. E. Dixon, B. S. Fowler, T. S. Jones, E. A. Lockamy, C. M. Patton, and R. O. Sikes.** 1987. *Campylobacter* enteritis at a university: transmission from eating chicken and from cats. *Am. J. Epidemiol.* **126**:526–534.
5. **Doyle, M. P.** 1984. *Campylobacter* in foods, p. 164–180. *In* J.-P. Butzler (ed.), *Campylobacter Infection in Man and Animals.* CRC Press, Inc., Boca Raton, Fla.
6. **Doyle, M. P., and J. L. Schoeni.** 1986. Isolation of *Campylobacter jejuni* from retail mushrooms. *Appl. Environ. Microbiol.* **51**:449–450.
7. **DuPont, H. L., C. D. Ericsson, A. Robinson, and P. D. Johnson.** 1987. Current problems in antimicrobial therapy for bacterial enteric infection. *J. Med.* **82**:324–328.
8. **Endtz, P. H., J. W. M. van der Meer, and R. P. Mouton.** 1988. *Campylobacter jejuni* bacteraemia in hypogammaglobulinaemia: emergence of ciprofloxacin resistance and results of bactericidal assays, abstr. 50. *In* B. Kaijser and E. Falsen (ed.), *Campylobacter IV.* University of Gothenburg, Gothenburg, Sweden.
9. **Endtz, P. H., G. J. Ruijs, B. van Klingeren, W. H. Jansen, T. van der Reyden, and R. P. Mouton.** 1991. Quinolone resistance in campylobacter isolated from man and poultry following the introduction of fluoroquinolones in veterinary medicine. *J. Antimicrob. Chemother.* **27**:199–208.
10. **Griffiths, P. L., and R. W. A. Park.** 1990. Campylobacters associated with human diarrheal disease. *J. Appl. Bacteriol.* **69**:281–301.
11. **Harris, N. V., N. S. Weiss, and C. M. Nolan.** 1986. The role of poultry and meats in the etiology of *Campylobacter jejuni/coli* enteritis. *Am. J. Public Health* **76**:407–411.
12. **Hugdahl, M. B., J. T. Beery, and M. P. Doyle.** 1988. Chemotactic behavior of *Campylobacter jejuni. Infect. Immun.* **56**:1560–1566.
13. **Lambert, J. D., and R. B. Maxcy.** 1984. Effect of gamma radiation on *Campylobacter jejuni. J. Food Sci.* **49**:665–667, 674.
14. **Mandal, B. K., M. E. Ellis, E. M. Dunbar, and K. Whale.** 1984. Double-blind placebo-controlled trial of erythromycin in the treatment of clinical *Campylobacter* infection. *J. Antimicrob. Chemother.* **13**:619–623.
15. **Mikhail, I. A., A. L. Bourgeois, K. C. Hyams, J. K. Pogmore, C. R. Lissner, and S. Walz.** 1987. In-vitro activity of ciprofloxacin compared to trimethoprim-sulphamethoxazole against *Campylobacter* spp., *Shigella* spp., and enterotoxigenic *Escherichia coli* causing travellers diarrhea in Egypt. *Scand. J. Infect. Dis.* **19**:479–481.
16. **Oosterman, J., S. Notermans, H. Karman, and G. B. Engels.** 1983. Origin and prevalence of *Campylobacter jejuni* in poultry processing. *J. Food Prot.* **46**:339–344.
17. **Pearson, A. D., R. R. Colwell, D. Rollins, M. Watkin-Jones, T. Healing, M. Greenwood, M. Shahamat, E. Jump, M. Hood, and D. J. Jones.** 1988. Transmission of *C. jejuni* on a poultry farm, p. 281–284. *In* B. Kajser and E. Falsen (ed.) *Campylobacter IV.* University of Gothenburg, Gothenburg, Sweden.
18. **Perlman, D. M., N. M. Ampel, R. B. Shifman, D. L. Cohn, C. M. Patton, M. L. Aguirre, W. L. Wang, and M. Blaser.** 1988. Persistent *Campylobacter jejuni* infections in patients infected with human immunodeficiency virus (HIV). *Ann. Intern. Med.* **108**:540–546.
19. **Robinson, D. A.** 1981. Infective dose of *Campylobacter jejuni* in milk. *Br. Med. J.* **282**:1584.
20. **Rollins, D., and R. R. Colwell.** 1986. Viable but non-culturable stage of *Campylobacter jejuni* and its role in the natural aquatic environment. *Appl. Environ. Microbiol.* **52**:531–538.
21. **Salazar-Lindo, E., R. B. Sack, E. Chea-Woo, B. A. Kay, Z. A. Piscoya, R. Leon-Barua, and Y. August.** 1986. Early treatment with erythromycin of *Campylobacter jejuni*-associated dysentery in children. *J. Paediatr.* **109**:355–360.
22. **Skirrow, M. B.** 1991. Epidemiology of *Campylobacter* enteritis. *Int. J. Food Microbiol.* **12**:9–16.
23. **Stern, N. J., M. P. Hernandez, L. Blankenship, K. E. Deibel, S. Doores, M. P. Doyle, H. Ng, M. D. Pierson, J. N. Sofos, W. H. Sveum, and D. C. Westoff.** 1985. Prevalence and distribution of *Campylobacter jejuni* and *Campylobacter coli* in retail meats. *J. Food Prot.* **48**:595–599.
24. **Stern, N. J., and S. U. Kazmi.** 1989. *Campylobacter*, p. 71–110. *In* M. P. Doyle (ed.), *Foodborne Bacterial Pathogens.* Marcel Dekker, Inc., New York.
25. **Sutcliffe, E. M., D. M. Jones, and A. D. Pearson.** 1991. Use of latex agglutination for the detection of *Campylobacter* species in water. *Lett. Appl. Microbiol.* **12**:72–74.
26. **Tarján, V.** 1985. Investigation into the radio-sensitivity of *Campylobacter fetus* subspecies *jejuni* in ground chicken meat. *Int. J. Food Microbiol.* **1**:321–326.
27. **Taylor, D. N., M. J. Blaser, P. Echeverria, C. Pitarangsi, L. Bodhidatta, and W. W.-L. Wang.** 1987. Erythromycin-resistant *Campylobacter* infections in Thailand. *Antimicrob. Agents Chemother.* **31**:483–442.
28. **Wempe, J. M., C. A. Genigeorgis, T. B. Farver, and H. I. Yusufri.** 1983. Prevalence of *Campylobacter jejuni* in two California chicken-processing plants. *Appl. Environ. Microbiol.* **45**:355–359.
29. **Williams, D., J. Scharling, L. J. Barrett, I. Orgel, R. Koch, D. S. Shields, and R. L. Guerrant.** 1989. Early treatment of *Campylobacter jejuni* enteritis. *Antimicrob. Agents Chemother.* **33**:248–250.
30. **Yogasundram, K., S. M. Shane, R. M. Grodner, E. N. Lambremont, and R. E. Smith.** 1987. Decontamination of *Campylobacter jejuni* on chicken drumsticks using chemicals and radiation. *Vet. Res. Commun.* **11**:31–40.

CHAPTER 6

Reservoirs for *Campylobacter jejuni* and Approaches for Intervention in Poultry

NORMAN J. STERN

BACKGROUND

Campylobacter jejuni is acknowledged as the most common human enteropathogen in developed countries (113). This paper reviews literature describing the transmission of the organism from the environment, through the food chain, and, ultimately, to humans. The weight of the published information indicates that campylobacteriosis is a zoonotic disease. Pets, water, and contaminated foods are the main sources of sporadic infections in humans (40, 72, 112, 113). Cross-contamination and improper handling and cooking of foods of animal origin account for the majority of disease. If hygiene measures were universally applied, there would be no need for intervention in the carrier state of *C. jejuni* found in many livestock animals. Adherence to the fundamentals of hygienic food handling is all too often disregarded, which leads to numerous cases of campylobacteriosis.

No single animal food source can be excluded as a potential vehicle for infection of humans. However, the epidemiology and transmission of the organism have now been adequately determined, so that attention can be directed toward stopping the most significant flow of *C. jejuni* to humans. The literature indicates that 50 to 70% of cases of human campylobacteriosis are associated with poultry (24, 40). Certainly, development of intervention technology to control and prevent colonization of poultry by *C. jejuni* would help eliminate the disease and would substantially ameliorate this human food-borne health hazard. Pertinent literature which describes the reservoirs of *C. jejuni* are presented, and several areas of research which could affect the presence of the organism in poultry are discussed.

OUTBREAKS AND EPIDEMIOLOGICAL ASSOCIATIONS

Reservoirs

Waterborne outbreaks of campylobacteriosis have been associated with unchlorinated water and with unhygienic water sources. These outbreaks, with large numbers of stricken individuals, were easily traced back to the source of the disease (70, 90, 91, 96, 114). The requirements for adequate levels of chlorination and operating integrity in community water systems were not maintained in these incidents.

Outbreaks of *Campylobacter* enteritis have also been most prominently associated with consumption of unpasteurized milk. One of the first reports of the association between campylobacter enteritis and raw milk was provided by Blaser et al. (13). In that outbreak three members of one family became ill after consuming unpasteurized milk from a cow whose feces were infected with *C. jejuni.* The organism was also recovered from stool specimens of the patients. A larger outbreak of milk-borne *C. jejuni* infection in Scotland was reported by Porter and Reid (87). The organism was isolated from stools of 148 patients and from a milk filter. Taylor et al. (115) reported an outbreak in about 200 persons who consumed one brand of unpasteurized milk. The organism could not be detected in the milk or the milk filters.

In an even larger outbreak of *Campylobacter* enteritis, 2,500 children were infected (52). Although bacteriological proof could not be obtained, the source of the epidemic was almost certainly contaminated milk. Inspection of the milk-processing equipment indicated a malfunction of the bypass valve system, where un-

Norman J. Stern, U.S. Department of Agriculture–Agricultural Research Service, Richard Russell Research Center, Athens, Georgia 30613.

pasteurized bulk milk could have passed through the processing plant without undergoing the appropriate heat treatment.

Potter et al. (88) reported on an outbreak associated with certified raw milk. Fifty individuals developed campylobacteriosis; grade A milk was epidemiologically incriminated as the source of the organism, although the organism was not isolated from the milk. The authors noted that the only reasonable means available to ensure the safety of milk would be to properly pasteurize the product before its consumption. These conclusions were further underscored in reports by Hudson et al. (43) and Harris et al. (39). In the first report, *C. jejuni* was isolated from milk of one of the cows implicated in an outbreak. Both the human and the milk isolates of the organism were of the same serotype—Penner 2, Lior 4. The findings of Harris et al. demonstrated that raw milk was the cause of endemic *C. jejuni* enteritis and that infection of individuals drinking raw milk was more than four times as common as among the control subjects not drinking raw milk. Insistence on ignoring the health consequences of drinking raw milk continues. Birkhead et al. (12) reported that multiple strains of *C. jejuni* could be transmitted through nonpasteurized milk. Rather than treating the milk for the required 30 min at 145°F, they reported that milk was heated for only 25 min at 135°F to avoid a burnt taste. Whether this is an inalienable right or not, unpasteurized milk is clearly a source of *C. jejuni* for humans.

The sources of campylobacteriosis outbreaks are quite different from the sources of the far more numerous sporadic cases. In comparison with the estimated number of cases of *Campylobacter* enteritis in the United States, large outbreaks of the disease are relatively rare. This is a point of contrast when comparing the epidemiology of *Salmonella* spp. transmission with that of *Campylobacter* spp. The general rule of thumb is that *C. jejuni*-induced enteritis occurs in numerous, sporadic episodes. Tauxe and coworkers (113) indicate that the sources of sporadic cases of *Campylobacter* enteritis have been defined by several case-control investigations. They state that poultry is the predominant source of human infection. This strong assertion was supported in part by the studies of Harris et al. (40) and Deming et al. (24), which are discussed below.

One of the earliest episodes linking *C. jejuni* enteritis with chickens is described in a report by Brouwer et al. (18). In this colorful description, a survival exercise for 123 Dutch cadets was reviewed. Live chickens were provided to the cadets, who killed them and cooked them over a wood fire for their evening meal. During the following week, 89 of these individuals became ill with classical campylobacteriosis. The authors suggested that viable *C. jejuni* organisms had remained associated with the chickens because the carcasses were not thoroughly heated. It was also suggested that the hygiene exercised during food preparation may not have been optimal.

Another outbreak of *Campylobacter* enteritis occurred among 11 of 15 members and friends in an extended family gathering in Colorado (49). It was suggested that inadequate cooking of the barbecued chicken was responsible for this particular outbreak. In addition, using a brush to apply sauce to the chicken may have increased the risk of transmitting infection, since the brush itself could have been a vehicle for further contamination of the chicken with subsequent applications of sauce after cooking was finished.

Harris et al. (40) reported that when 218 individuals with *Campylobacter* enteritis were compared with 526 controls, consumption of chicken and Cornish game hens was associated with more than a twofold higher risk of infection. Consumption of raw or rare chicken was even more strongly associated with human disease. They concluded that ingestion of contaminated chicken was a primary source of *Campylobacter* enteritis, contributing to about half of the cases they analyzed.

In a similar case-control comparison, Deming et al. (24) found comparable results among students at the University of Georgia. In their study, they identified the following risk factors: eating chicken reported to be raw or undercooked, and having contact with a cat or kitten. In this study, 70% of the cases were accounted for by eating chicken. Other case-control studies have identified eating chicken as a risk factor for sporadic *Campylobacter* enteritis (58, 75, 79, 84). Especially noted among these reports is the implication that improperly barbecued chickens cause enteritis.

Another type of chicken-to-human transmission was found in a study by Grados et al. (37). They reported that direct contact with feces of *C. jejuni*-infected chickens in the Lima, Peru, household environment was largely responsible for transmission of the organism to susceptible infants. Studies involving combinations of serotyping and biotyping methods repeatedly indicate that serogroups of *C. jejuni* that are associated with human disease can be isolated from live and processed chickens (3, 8, 34, 53, 74, 82, 95).

Less prominently heralded are two outbreaks which implicate seafoods. These two incidents suggest that clams are associated with human disease (16, 51). It should be noted that other shellfish, e.g., oysters, are capable of concentrating *C. jejuni* from waters containing the organism and thus may serve as a vehicle of transmission (5).

Feral Animals and Insects

Several studies have been conducted to determine the reservoir of *C. jejuni* and *C. coli* in feral mammals and birds. Rosef et al. (93) isolated *C. jejuni* from 1 of 23 rabbits which they captured, but made no other isolations from three other species of rodents. Genigeorgis et al. (35) isolated *C. jejuni* from rodents around a poultry farm in California and concluded that this was an important reservoir for the domestic fowl.

Wild birds are an important reservoir of *C. jejuni*. Luechtefeld et al. (65) and Kapperud and Rosef (55) were some of the first researchers to document the isolation of the organism from wild birds. Kapperud and Rosef reported high isolation rates of *C. jejuni* from crows, gulls, and domestic pigeons. Luechtefeld et al. reported isolation of *Campylobacter* spp. from approximately one-third of the migratory birds from which they took samples. Ito et al. (50) reported that crows, blue magpies, gray starlings, domestic pigeons, and bulbuls yielded *C. jejuni* upon fecal culture in Japan. Yogasundram et al. (119) emphasized the importance of Galliformes as a reservoir for *C. jejuni* among wild birds in Louisiana, along with migratory waterfowl as carriers of the organism. At the other side of the spectrum, Hill and Grimes (41) documented the absence of *C. jejuni* from waterfowl on Lake Onalaska, Wis. They suggested that the distribution of the organism among migratory waterfowl was sporadic.

Flies are an additional source of *Campylobacter* spp. in the environment. Rosef and Kapperud (94) reported that about 51% of the flies from a chicken farm and 43% of the flies at a piggery yielded the organism. Wright (118) indicated that only 5 of 210 flies yielded the organism upon culture on selective media and that the hazard to health from the transmission from animals to human food by flies is small. Shane et al. (98) demonstrated that flies infected with *C. jejuni* transmitted the organism to specific-pathogen-free chickens. These data demonstrate the potential role of flies in the dissemination of *C. jejuni* among chickens.

Pets

Domestic pets, such as cats and dogs, have been implicated in transmission of *C. jejuni* to humans. Deming et al. (24) indicated that 30% of the cases which they studied were accounted for by contact with cats. They observed an association of sporadic cases of *Campylobacter* enteritis with handling kittens. Bruce et al. (19) found that up to 45% of clinically normal cats yielded *Campylobacter* spp.

Puppies may also serve as a reservoir for human infections (14). Variable frequencies of isolation from dogs have been reported: Nair et al. (77) recovered the organism from 21.7% of dogs with diarrhea and 3.1% of normal healthy dogs, and Bruce et al. (19) found that 49% of mostly healthy dogs yielded *C. jejuni*. Other, more exotic, pets such as the Syrian hamster may also harbor this human pathogen (32). Zoo animals and wild pigeons at zoological gardens have also been documented as carrying *Campylobacter* spp. (10, 59, 66), but these, and laboratory animals (31), are probably not significant sources of transmission to the general public. More significant potential health hazards are associated with infections transmitted by pets, especially dogs and cats.

Bovine and Porcine Carriage

Although bovines are an important source in milk-borne transmission of *C. jejuni*, cattle are not strongly implicated in transmission through meat products. Exceptions to this exist. A Dutch report indicated an outbreak affecting 28 military personnel living in one barrack (83). Steak tartare had been eaten by 93% of the affected individuals, whereas only half of the unaffected soldiers had eaten the food. Garcia et al. (34) reported that many of the serotypes of *C. jejuni* isolated from bovines are similar to those found in human disease. The implication is that a proportion of human campylobacteriosis could be traced back to beef products. This is further supported by Dilworth et al. (26), who identified cattle as the reservoir of infection in two unrelated cases of gastroenteritis. Biotyping and serotyping of isolates from both the humans and the suspected cattle provided documentation for this connection.

Garcia et al. described the distribution patterns of *Campylobacter* spp. from slaughter cattle (34). The organism was frequently carried by bovines and could be isolated from gallbladders, large intestines, small intestines, and livers. As noted above, the serogroups of the organism were similar for humans and cattle. Grau (38) characterized the presence of *Campylobacter* spp. in the intestinal tract and on carcasses of calves and cattle. He pointed out that calves carried the organism more frequently than did adult cattle, that feedlot cattle were more likely to have the organism in their intestines and on their carcasses than were pasture-fed cattle, and that chilling carcasses overnight significantly reduced the numbers of *Campylobacter* spp. associated with the carcass.

Several reports describe the association of *Campylobacter* spp. and beef products. One of the earliest reports was from England (116), describing a study in which the organism was isolated from 1.6% of more than 6,000 meat samples taken. Fukushima et al. (33) reported levels of *Campylobacter* spp. in raw beef, pork, and chicken similar to those found in the British study.

Stern et al. (108), using enrichment methodology, found that approximately 5% of all the red-meat samples from retail outlets throughout the United States yielded *Campylobacter* spp. Sampling and product handling is a critical consideration when attempting to isolate the organism from foods, or else the best culture methods are worthless. Because animal food products are frozen, the levels and detection rates of *Campylobacter* spp. are diminished (109). Indeed, when poultry livers were frozen, the *Campylobacter* levels detected were significantly diminished (107). Lammerding et al. (61) further characterized the high levels of *Campylobacter* spp. in a variety of foods of animal origin in Canada.

Unpasteurized milk can serve as a vehicle of infection in humans. Doyle and Roman (28) indicated that only 0.9% of grade A milk from bulk tanks on dairy farms yielded *Campylobacter* spp. They also indicated that the organism was inactivated over time in unpasteurized milk when held at 4°C. Humphrey and Beckett (46) found that *Campylobacter* spp. had colonized the dairy herds on five farms and were isolated from 10 to 72% of the animals tested by fecal culture. They indicated that *Campylobacter* spp. were detected at an incidence of 8.1% in the milk of animals from the five farms on which *Campylobacter* infection was found. In a continuation of these studies, Humphrey and Hart (47) reported that *Campylobacter* spp. were isolated from 6% of samples of unpasteurized cow's milk on sale to the public. In Canada, Davidson et al. (23) reported that 1.2% of the 256 milk samples taken from four dairies and 48 farms in Manitoba were contaminated with *Campylobacter* spp. Barrell (9) indicated that *Campylobacter* spp. were inactivated more rapidly in raw milk at 21°C than at ca. 5°C.

Campylobacter spp. are often isolated from feces of cows. Meanger and Marshall (68) reported that 22% of 273 rectal swabs from dairy cows yielded *Campylobacter* spp. Contamination of the milk can be of fecal origin or could occur through a mastitic infection. Lander and Gill (62) provided evidence by way of an experimental infection showing that such a mastitic condition could exist in cows. Raw milk from these cows could infect humans. Subsequently, Morgan et al. (72) reported the isolation of *C. jejuni* from a naturally occurring case of mastitis in association with human illness involving the same serotype. Raw milk is a known source of human campylobacteriosis, and pasteurization must be mandated by the regulatory authorities if this particular source of human disease is to be discontinued.

Rosef (92) described the presence of *Campylobacter* spp. in gallbladders and/or bile ducts of slaughter pigs in Norway. He found that 58% of the pigs sampled yielded the organism. In neighboring Sweden, Svedhem and Kaijser (112) reported that 95% of the pigs they sampled at slaughterhouses yielded *Campylobacter* spp. The biotypes and serotypes of *Campylobacter* spp. isolated from pigs and humans in Rotterdam were infrequently related to one another (8).

Several reports specifically considered the serology of isolates from pigs and compared the results with the serology of *C. jejuni* isolates from humans (8, 74, 86). Those reports, emanating from western Europe and Canada, concluded that isolates from pigs (mostly *C. coli*) belonged to serotypes uncommon among human isolates. Therefore, pigs do not appear to be a major source of human campylobacteriosis.

Several studies determining the presence of *Campylobacter* spp. associated with swine in North America have been conducted. In Georgia, 12.5% of slaughter pig carcasses yielded the organism, but after overnight chilling, no isolations were made (17). In Manitoba, Canada, 26% of the tissue and fecal samples from slaughter pigs yielded *Campylobacter* spp. (30). In a national surveillance program in Canada, *Campylobacter* spp. were isolated from 16.9% of the carcasses sampled (61). Additional farm animals such as sheep (25) and horses (6) have been shown to carry *Campylobacter* spp. In some instances a disease state exists in the animals, causing abortion or death. In most cases the farm animals exist in a more benign commensal state with the human pathogen.

Poultry Associations

C. jejuni exists within the intestinal tract of poultry in what must most frequently be considered a commensal association. Large numbers of the organism prevail there (up to 10^6 to 10^7 CFU/g [107]) without any apparent gross pathologic consequences for the chicken host (106). The organism resides in a comparatively rare niche within the intestinal tract, where competition for space and nutrients is minimal (11). This relationship is discussed below. Because of this symbiosis between the host and parasite, few pressures exist to dislodge the bacterium. When carriage of *C. jejuni* in chicken flocks is assessed, the organism is usually isolated in large numbers from the majority of birds sampled (89). However, there appears to be substantial variability in the colonization prevalence of different flocks and at different ages of the birds.

Grados et al. (37) indicated that free-range chickens were colonized by *C. jejuni.* These chickens would be allowed to forage in a back yard. Similarly, Adekeye et al. (1) found almost an identical frequency of the organism in intensive management and free-range management of chickens. The organism appears to be a member of the normal flora of chickens.

Aho and Hirn (2) reported finding very low levels of *C. jejuni* (1.7%) in the feces of broilers at 4 to 5 weeks of age. At slaughter (ca. 6 to 7 weeks of age), the ceca of these birds yielded a higher incidence of *C. jejuni* (24%). These ceca contained a mean $\log_{10}$ 7.2 CFU of *C. jejuni* per g. During processing of the chicken carcasses, the organism can be spread either from the large load of bacteria within the intestinal tract or from the load of *C. jejuni* on the feathers and skin of the birds. This enormous bacterial load results in substantial contamination of processed carcasses. Mean levels of $\log_{10}$ 4.5 CFU per *C. jejuni* per carcass have been reported (2). Neill et al. (78) monitored flocks of broiler chickens for colonization with *C. jejuni.* In 10 of 12 flocks, they could not isolate *C. jejuni* from chickens during the first 2 weeks of life. All the flocks but one became colonized during growth. These data could be interpreted to indicate that flock colonization is dependent mostly upon the introduction of *C. jejuni,* regardless of the source of the organism, after which most of the flock becomes colonized with *C. jejuni.*

Several reports indicate that the levels of *C. jejuni* found in chickens appear to diminish with age (27, 54). Kaino et al. (54) found that chickens ceased to excrete *C. jejuni* in their feces 3 months after challenge. Doyle (27) indicated that less than 25% of individually caged laying hens excreted detectable levels of *C. jejuni* in their feces over a 42-week period. Understanding the reasons for diminished carriage of the organism in chickens with increasing age could yield beneficial information and is considered below.

The earliest of numerous reports on the presence of *C. jejuni* associated with chicken carcasses was presented by Smith and Muldoon (101). They used less than optimal methodology and isolated the organism from fewer than 2% of the carcasses examined. Notermans et al. (80) reported that 16% of the chickens obtained from marketplaces in the Netherlands yielded *C. jejuni.* Fresh chicken obtained at retail outlets in Ontario, Canada, and Ohio yielded *C. jejuni* at a rate of 116 of 200 carcasses (85). In France, the rate of isolation of *Campylobacter* spp. from poultry was 44 of 45 carcasses sampled (67). In Canada, *Campylobacter* spp. were isolated from 74.7 and 38.2% of turkey and chicken carcasses, respectively (61). In Poland, the organisms were found on 80% of the chicken carcasses, 48% of the duck carcasses, 38% of the goose carcasses, and 3% of the turkey carcasses examined (60). In southern England, *C. jejuni* was isolated from 48% of the fresh carcasses sampled (42). Counts of a mean 1.5×10^6 CFU of *C. jejuni* per carcass were reported. A recent study in the southeastern United States was designed to assess a variety of enrichment methods and selective agar media (64). When such rigorous analyses were applied to retail market broilers, 98% of the 50 chicken carcasses yielded *C. jejuni.*

Strategies for intervention in the colonization of poultry by *C. jejuni* are dictated by the epidemiology of the organism in the flock. Consequently, it was important to understand whether the organism could be disseminated by eggs. Doyle (27) reported that although hens were excreting *C. jejuni* in their feces, the organism did not penetrate the eggshell to contaminate the contents of the eggs. The organism could, however, infrequently be isolated from shell surfaces. Continuing this line of research, Clark and Bueschkens (20) indicated that fertile chicken eggs could be infected with *C. jejuni* by using temperature or pressure differential methods of inoculation. They showed that up to 11% of the hatched chickens challenged in such a manner carried the organism within their intestinal tracts. In a continuation of this research

(21), it was demonstrated that the organism was susceptible to albumin and the conalbumin component of the egg white. Shane et al. (97) indicated that hens which were fecal shedders of *C. jejuni* (with 12 to 62% incidence) did not produce infected eggs.

Shanker et al. (99) reached a similar conclusion by providing data which argued against the vertical transmission of *C. jejuni* in commercial broiler production. Of a total of 524 eggs analyzed, only 2 were shown to contain the organism. Baker et al. (7) sampled 276 eggs from an egg farm in New York State and did not isolate *C. jejuni* from any of these samples.

POTENTIALS FOR INTERVENING IN POULTRY COLONIZATION

Production Intervention

Laboratory studies (22, 57, 100) have indicated that birds already colonized with *C. jejuni* (seeder birds) can rapidly spread the organism to a majority of hatch mates within less than 3 days. Because chickens are coprophagic, the fecal-oral spread among cohorts is plausible. However, the rapidity with which broiler chicken flocks shift from a noncolonized status to 100% colonization suggests that this route of transmission is not the only channel for flock infection. Montrose et al. (71) provide a potential explanation for the rapid spread of the organism through chicken flocks in a growout house. They observed a transient palatine colonization of *C. jejuni* in young chickens. Such a colonization could initially occur in a single chicken, perhaps exposed to rat feces contaminated with the organism. Subsequently, as palatine colonization occurs and as the chicken drinks from a communal water source, *C. jejuni* could be transmitted to a 20,000-bird flock in a logarithmic progression.

This hypothesis is supported by a number of studies. Smitherman et al. (102) monitored six chicken houses for *Campylobacter* colonization and found that one house had become positive within 2 weeks of bird placement, whereas the other five houses became positive after 6 to 7 weeks. When each house became positive, virtually all cloacal swabs and fecal droppings from that house became positive within 1 week. Engvall et al. (29) indicated that they could not isolate the organism from environmental or chicken samples from 16 flocks which they monitored during the first 2 weeks of growth, but subsequently the frequency of carriage rapidly increased. Pokamunski et al. (86) monitored five flocks of broiler chickens from hatch through slaughter. They never isolated the organism from hatchery chickens. Three of the flocks were 100% colonized at the 4-week sampling, one flock was positive at 8 weeks of age, and the fifth remained negative through the growout period. *C. jejuni* was not isolated from feed or water. Kasrazadeh and Genigeorgis (56) studied the origin of *C. jejuni* in ducks at the farm. They indicated that colonization of the birds did not come from the hatchery and that the organism was probably introduced by carrier rats, as rat feces frequently (87%) yielded the organism. Annan-Prah and Janc (4) monitored 10 broiler flocks but did not isolate the organism from their samples until the birds were 21 days old. They suggested that other farm animals and the farmer's boots could have been the source of contamination of the flocks. Lindblom et al. (63) indicated that once *C. jejuni* appeared in a flock, it spread rapidly to virtually all birds. They did, however, note that among laying hens at 42 weeks of age, only 20 to 46% of the birds remained colonized.

The fact that most chickens in commercial production remain free of *Campylobacter* spp. for several weeks is not due to an inherent resistance to the organism by the young chickens. Stern and colleagues (106) reported that the dose required to colonize 50% of orally challenged 24-h-old chickens (CD_{50}) was only 35 CFU. I suggest that the reason the organism is not typically isolated from the hatchery environment, or during early stages of production, is that the environmental fomite invades the production facility on sporadic occasions. As soon as this invasion does occur, the entire flock of chickens is at risk. The organism can remain viable in litter for some period (perhaps as long as 2 weeks), but becomes inactivated fairly rapidly (35, 71). The infrequent detection of *C. jejuni* in the first 2 weeks of chicken growout speaks against litter as a significant or consistent source for flock colonization.

Competitive exclusion (CE) is a concept introduced by Nurmi and Rantala (81) for the purpose of reducing the level of *Salmonella* spp. associated with poultry. The approach provides an undefined intestinal tract flora from pathogen-free adult chickens and uses this source to furnish a bacterial subculture for treatment of newly hatched chickens. One major concern with this process is that poultry pathogens could potentially also be transmitted through this undefined culture. Hudson et al. (44) indicated that *C. jejuni* will be killed during repeated subculture under anaerobic conditions. Another concern is that each CE culture is not equally effective in preventing colonization by *Salmonella* spp. Therefore, major, although as yet unsuccessful, efforts have been expended to provide an effective, defined CE culture for administration to commercially raised chickens. Similar goals and concerns have been considered to interfere with *Campylobacter* colonization in chickens. Humphrey et al. (48) found that cecal contents from chickens inhibited *C. jejuni* in vitro. Such an in vitro screen could be useful in a preliminary assessment of the efficacy of anti-*Campylobacter* CE cultures.

One of the first reports (104) indicating the applicability of such an approach involved the subculture of fecal droppings from *Campylobacter*-free chickens. In this study the authors reported that CE treatment reduced chicken colonization, as monitored by cloacal swabs. All 10 untreated chickens were colonized with *C. jejuni,* while only 5 of 10 birds from the treated group were colonized. In addition, the levels of the organism in feces were significantly reduced in the treated group as compared with the untreated group. The same research team reproduced analogous work in a separate study and reached similar conclusions (103). Stern et al. attempted to corroborate these findings, but failed to do so (106). In their work, four CE cultures, effective against *Salmonella* spp., did not elicit qualitative advantage in protecting chickens against cecal colonization by *C. jejuni.* CE material used in the study by Soerjadi-Liem et al. (104) was subsequently obtained to treat chickens. Again, no benefit was gained in preventing *C. jejuni* colonization when the birds were challenged with 10^5 CFU at 48 h of age. Shanker et al. (100) also indicated that treatment of 1-day-old chickens with adult cecal microbiota did not effect colonization.

Several research teams (11, 103, 117) indicated that the principal site of *C. jejuni* colonization in chicken is the cecum. Beery et al. (11) provided convincing data demonstrating that crypts within the ceca of chickens, where the organism is free swimming in the mucin layer, are the primary niche for *C. jejuni* colonization. Hugdahl et al. (45) noted that *C. jejuni* exhibited chemotactic movement toward substrates found in the mucin layer. If antagonistic members of the flora are to be effective, such organisms would probably be derived from the same niche where *C. jejuni* is found. Stern (105) obtained the cecum from an adult hen, inverted the organ onto a glass rod, washed the cecal material under anaerobic conditions from the lumen of the cecum, scraped the mucosal epithelial surface, and subcultured the scraping anaerobically three times. This mucosal CE (MCE) flora derivatization was effective against both *Salmonella* and *C. jejuni* colonization. The CD_{50} was increased approximately 100-fold in protecting against *C. jejuni* colonization. The mean $\log_{10}$ level of cecal carriage (colonization quotient) was similarly decreased by 100- to 1,000-fold. Not all of the trials were successful in increasing the CD_{50}, which indicates that all MCEs are not created equally.

More recently, Stern et al. (109a) conducted a field trial to study the applicability of using MCE to protect against *C. jejuni* colonization in chickens. Approximately 10,000 chickens were provided MCE by spraying eggs and chickens after one-half of the birds had pecked from their shells, and these chickens were MCE treated in their first drinking water after placement in the growout house on the farm. A control group of chickens in an untreated growout house was monitored for comparison. Cecal carriage, external contamination (of skin and feathers), and retail market-ready carcasses were monitored. At about 2.5 weeks of age the results were as follows: the ceca of 2 and 100% of the treated and untreated chickens, respectively, were colonized. At 6.5 weeks the ceca of almost all of the treated and untreated chickens were colonized; on the farm, 31 and 0% of the skin and feathers from the control and treated groups, respectively, were contaminated; at the processing plant, 56 and 18% of the control group and treated group, respectively, were externally contaminated with *C. jejuni;* finally, on the finished, retail-ready carcasses, 64 and 6% of the control and treated groups, respectively, yielded *C. jejuni.* These results indicate potential for intervening in the colonization of *C. jejuni* among broiler chickens. This large-scale field trial is being repeated.

Hygiene

Other potential approaches for intervention are being considered. Gondrosen (36) and Blaser et al. (15) noted that chlorinated tap water drastically reduce the survival of all *C. jejuni* strains tested. Application of chlorine to drinking water in broiler chicken houses might therefore diminish the presence of the organism if used in conjunction with nipple drinkers, which exclude fecal contact with the drinking water.

Heritability

Stern et al. (110) noted significant differences among chicken breeds in their *C. jejuni* colonization potential. On challenging 60 chickens from each of three breeds with *C. jejuni,* they found that the ceca of 3% of individuals from one breed were colonized whereas the ceca of 32% of chickens from another breed were colonized. Mulder et al. (73) also reported differences in resistance to *Campylobacter* colonization between experimental and commercial breeds of chickens. Work in this area of research has been continuing. Stern et al. have attempted to select chickens on the basis of colonization resistance or susceptibility from among a diverse gene pool. After selecting parental stock from the original group of 30 random-bred chicken families, they identified five resistant families and five susceptible families and bred them to produce offspring. These offspring were challenged with *C. jejuni,* and, from among approximately 400 chickens, 40 hens and roosters showing susceptibility to colonization and 40 hens and roosters showing resistance to colonization were bred. Stern et al. are currently gathering eggs from these pairings to test the F_1 generation for resistance and susceptibility. If inbred lines for resistance and susceptibility can be developed, it is hoped to identify the physiological differences between the breeds and, ultimately, to identify the genome responsible for the resistance phenotype. Gene insertion or Mendelian selection approaches to producing commercial chicken breeds are a long-term goal. Other studies, involving chickens with various chicken histocompatibility groups, have been initiated to determine whether such expressions are related to resistance against colonization.

Immunological Intervention

Meinersmann et al. (69) have been pursuing the long-term goal of immunologically neutralizing colonization factors expressed by *C. jejuni* in chickens. Myszewski and Stern (76) studied secretory and humoral immunoglobulin response of chickens to *C. jejuni* colonization. They observed that the chicken immunoglobulin response was only minimal and that this response did not diminish the level of colonization over 8 weeks. Stern et al. (111) demonstrated that passively administered antibody effectively increased the CD_{50} and decreased the CQ for chickens challenged with *C. jejuni.*

To further study colonization factors, Stern et al. (106) created a congenic pair of colonizing and noncolonizing *C. jejuni* organisms. Meinersmann et al. (69) described the antigenic differences expressed by this congenic pair. They are continuing the process of assessing the influence of antibody to these particular antigenic differences on the colonization of chickens by *C. jejuni.* Furthermore, they are cloning the genes which are responsible for expressing these pertinent antigenic differences. The goal of this research initiative is to identify colonization factor antigens which immunologically stimulate the chicken to resist colonization by *C. jejuni.*

Because *C. jejuni* is a highly significant bacterial enteropathogen transmitted through zoonotic infections, measures must be taken to identify critical control points. Not only must the consumer use appropriate hygiene and cooking procedures when handling foods of animal origin, but also the industries which produce these foods must take measures to intervene and reduce the presence of this bacterium. Government agencies and the food industry must begin to take note of this most important enteropathogen and respond to the needs of public health.

REFERENCES

1. **Adekeye, J. O., P. A. Abdu, and E. K. Bawa.** 1989. *Campylobacter fetus* subsp. *jejuni* in poultry reared under different management systems in Nigeria. *Avian Dis.* **33:**801–803.
2. **Aho, M., and J. Hirn.** 1988. Prevalence of campylobacteria in the Finnish broiler chicken chain from the producer to the consumer. *Acta Vet. Scand.* **29:**451–462.
3. **Annan-Prah, A., and M. Janc.** 1988. Chicken-to-human infection with *Campylobacter jejuni* and *Campylobacter coli:* biotype and serotype correlation. *J. Food Prot.* **51:**562–564.
4. **Annan-Prah, A., and M. Janc.** 1988. The mode of spread of *Campylobacter jejuni/coli* to broiler flocks. *J. Vet. Med.* **B35:**11–18.
5. **Arumugaswamy, R. K., R. W. Proudford, and M. J. Eyles.** 1988. The response of *Campylobacter jejuni* and *Campylobacter coli* in the Sydney rock oyster *(Crassostrea commercialis),* during depuration and storage. *Int. J. Food Microbiol.* **7:**173–183.
6. **Atherton, J. G., and S. W. Ricketts.** 1980. Campylobacter infection from foals. *Vet. Rec.* **107:**264. (Letter.)
7. **Baker, R. C., M. D. C. Paredes, and R. A. Qureshi.** 1987. Prevalence of *Campylobacter jejuni* in eggs and poultry meat in New York State. *Poult. Sci.* **66:**1766–1770.
8. **Banffer, J. R. J.** 1985. Biotypes and serotypes of *Campylobacter jejuni* and *Campylobacter coli* strains isolated from patients, pigs and chickens in the region of Rotterdam. *J. Infect.* **10:**277–281.
9. **Barrell, R. E.** 1981. The survival of *Campylobacter coli/jejuni* in unpasteurized milk. *J. Infect.* **3:**348–352.
10. **Bauwens, L., and W. de Meurichy.** 1981. The occurrence of thermophilic campylobacters in zoo animals. *Acta Zool. Pathol. Antverp.* **76:**181–189.

11. **Beery, J. T., M. B. Hugdahl, and M. P. Doyle.** 1988. Colonization of gastrointestinal tracts of chickens by *Campylobacter jejuni. Appl. Environ. Microbiol.* **54:**2365–2370.
12. **Birkhead, G., R. L. Vogt, E. Heun, C. M. Evelti, and C. M. Patton.** 1988. A multiple-strain outbreak of Campylobacter enteritis due to consumption of inadequately pasteurized milk. *J. Infect. Dis.* **157:**1095–1097. (Letter.)
13. **Blaser, M. J., J. Cravens, B. W. Powers, F. M. Laforce, and W.-L. L. Wang.** 1979. Campylobacter enteritis associated with unpasteurized milk. *Am. J. Med.* **67:**715–718.
14. **Blaser, M. J., F. M. LaForce, N. A. Wilson, and W.-L. L. Wang.** 1980. Reservoirs for human campylobacteriosis. *J. Infect. Dis.* **141:**665–669.
15. **Blaser, M. J., P. F. Smith, W.-L. L. Wang, and J. C. Hoff.** 1986. Inactivation of *Campylobacter jejuni* by chlorine and monochloramine. *Appl. Environ. Microbiol.* **51:**307–311.
16. **Blaser, M. J., D. N. Taylor, and R. A. Feldman.** 1984. Epidemiology of campylobacter infections, p. 143–161. *In* J. P. Butzler (ed.), *Campylobacter Infection in Man and Animals.* CRC Press, Inc., Boca Raton, Fla.
17. **Bracewell, A. J., J. O. Reagan, J. A. Carpenter, and L. C. Blankenship.** 1985. Incidence of *Campylobacter jejuni/coli* on pork carcasses in the northeast Georgia area. *J. Food Prot.* **48:**808–810.
18. **Brouwer, R., M. J. A. Mertens, T. H. Siem, and J. Katchaki.** 1979. An explosive outbreak of Campylobacter enteritis in soldiers. *Antonie Van Leeuwenhoek J. Microbiol.* **45:**517–519.
19. **Bruce, D., W. Zochowski, and G. A. Fleming.** 1980. Campylobacter infections in cats and dogs. *Vet. Rec.* **107:**200–201.
20. **Clark, A. G., and D. H. Bueschkens.** 1985. Laboratory infection of chicken eggs with *Campylobacter jejuni* by using temperature or pressure differentials. *Appl. Environ. Microbiol.* **49:**1467–1471.
21. **Clark, A. G., and D. H. Bueschkens.** 1986. Survival and growth of *Campylobacter jejuni* in egg yolk and albumen. *J. Food Prot.* **49:**135–141.
22. **Clark, A. G., and D. H. Bueschkens.** 1988. Horizontal spread of human and poultry-derived strains of *Campylobacter jejuni* among broiler chicks held in incubators and shipping boxes. *J. Food Prot.* **51:**438–441.
23. **Davidson, R. J., D. W. Sprung, C. E. Park, and M. K. Rayman.** 1989. Occurrence of *Listeria monocytogenes, Campylobacter* spp. and *Yersinia enterocolitica* in Manitoba raw milk. *Can. Inst. Food Sci. Technol. J.* **22:**70–74.
24. **Deming, M. S., R. V. Tauxe, P. A. Blake, S. E. Dixon, B. S. Fowler, T. S. Jones, E. A. Lockamy, C. M. Patton, and R. O. Sikes.** 1987. *Campylobacter* enteritis at a university: transmission from eating chicken and from cats. *Am. J. Epidemiol.* **126:**526–534.
25. **Diker, K. S., M. Sahal, and N. Aydin.** 1988. Ovine abortion associated with *Campylobacter coli. Vet. Rec.* **122:**87.
26. **Dilworth, C. R., H. Lior, and M. A. Belliveau.** 1988. Campylobacter enteritis acquired from cattle. *Can. J. Public Health.* **79:**60–62.
27. **Doyle, M. P.** 1984. Association of *Campylobacter jejuni* with laying hens and eggs. *Appl. Environ. Microbiol.* **47:**533–536.
28. **Doyle, M. P., and D. J. Roman.** 1982. Prevalence and survival of *Campylobacter jejuni* in unpasteurized milk. *Appl. Environ. Microbiol.* **44:**1154–1158.
29. **Engvall, A., Å. Bergqvist, K. Sandstedt, and M.-L. Danielsson-Tham.** 1986. Colonization of broilers with Campylobacter in conventional broiler-chicken flocks. *Acta Vet. Scand.* **27:**540–547.
30. **Finlay, R. C., E. D. Mann, and J. L. Horning.** 1986. Prevalence of *Salmonella* and *Campylobacter* contamination in Manitoba swine carcasses. *Can. Vet. J.* **27:**185–187.
31. **Fox, J. G.** 1982. Campylobacteriosis: a new disease in laboratory animals. *Lab. Anim. Sci.* **32:**625–637.
32. **Fox, J. G., S. Zanotti, and H. V. Jordan.** 1981. The hamster as a reservoir of *Campylobacter fetus* subsp. *jejuni. J. Infect. Dis.* **143:**856.
33. **Fukushima, H., K. Hoshina, R. Nakamura, and Y. Ito.** 1987. Raw beef, pork and chicken in Japan contaminated with *Salmonella* sp., *Campylobacter* sp., *Yersinia enterocolitica,* and *Clostridium perfringens:* a comparative study. *Zentralbl. Bakteriol. Mikrobiol. Hyg. Ser. B* **184:**60–70.
34. **Garcia, M. M., H. Lior, R. B. Stewart, G. M. Ruckerbauer, J. R. R. Trudel, and A. Skljarevski.** 1985. Isolation, characterization, and serotyping of *Campylobacter jejuni* and *Campylobacter coli* from slaughter cattle. *Appl. Environ. Microbiol.* **49:**667–672.
35. **Genigeorgis, C., M. Hassuneh, and P. Collins.** 1986. *Campylobacter jejuni* infection on poultry farms and its effect on poultry meat contamination during slaughtering. *J. Food Prot.* **49:**895–903.
36. **Gondrosen, B.** 1986. Survival of thermotolerant campylobacters in water. *Acta Vet. Scand.* **27:**1–10.
37. **Grados, O., N. Bravo, R. E. Black, and J. P. Butzler.** 1988. Paediatric campylobacter diarrhoea from household exposure to live chickens in Lima, Peru. *Bull. W.H.O.* **66:**369–374.
38. **Grau, F. H.** 1988. *Campylobacter jejuni* and *Campylobacter hyointestinalis* in the intestinal tract and on the carcasses of calves and cattle. *J. Food Prot.* **51:**857–861.
39. **Harris, N. V., T. Kimball, N. S. Weiss, and C. Nolan.** 1986. Dairy products, produce and other non-meat foods as possible sources of *Campylobacter jejuni* and *Campylobacter coli* enteritis. *J. Food Prot.* **49:**347–351.
40. **Harris, N. V., N. S. Weiss, and C. M. Nolan.** 1986. The role of poultry and meats in the etiology of *Campylobacter jejuni/coli* enteritis. *Am. J. Public Health* **76:**407–411.
41. **Hill, G. A., and D. J. Grimes.** 1984. Seasonal study of a freshwater lake and migratory waterfowl for *Campylobacter jejuni. Can. J. Microbiol.* **30:**845–849.

42. **Hood, A. M., A. D. Pearson, and M. Shahamat.** 1988. The extent of surface contamination of retailed chickens with *Campylobacter jejuni* serogroups. *Epidemiol. Infect.* **100:**17–25.
43. **Hudson, P. J., R. L. Vogt, J. Brondum, and C. M. Patton.** 1984. Isolation of *Campylobacter jejuni* from milk during an outbreak of campylobacteriosis. *J. Infect. Dis.* **150:**789. (Letter.)
44. **Hudson, W. R., C. S. Impey, and G. C. Mead.** 1987. 'Nurmi concept' and possible transmission of campylobacters to poultry. *Vet. Rec.* **120:**439.
45. **Hugdahl, M. B., J. T. Beery, and M. P. Doyle.** 1988. Chemotactic behavior of *Campylobacter jejuni. Infect. Immun.* **56:**1560–1566.
46. **Humphrey, T. J., and P. Beckett.** 1987. *Campylobacter jejuni* in dairy cows and raw milk. *Epidemiol. Infect.* **98:**263–269.
47. **Humphrey, T. J., and R. J. C. Hart.** 1988. Campylobacter and salmonella contamination of unpasteurized cows' milk on sale to the public. *J. Appl. Bacteriol.* **65:**463–467.
48. **Humphrey, T. J., D. G. Lanning, and G. C. Mead.** 1989. Inhibition of *Campylobacter jejuni* in vitro by broiler chicken cecal contents. *Vet. Rec.* **125:**272–273.
49. **Istre, G. R., M. J. Blaser, P. Shillam, and R. S. Hopkins.** 1984. *Campylobacter* enteritis associated with undercooked barbecued chicken. *Am. J. Public Health* **74:**1265–1267.
50. **Ito, K., Y. Kubokura, K. Kaneko, Y. Totake, and M. Ogawa.** 1988. Occurrence of *Campylobacter jejuni* in free-living wild birds from Japan. *J. Wildl. Dis.* **24:**467–470.
51. **Itoh, T., K. Saito, Y. Yanagawa, S. Sakai, and M. Ohashi.** 1982. Campylobacter enteritis in Tokyo, p. 5–12. *In* D. G. Newell (ed.), *Campylobacter: Epidemiology, Pathogenesis, and Biochemistry.* MTP Press, Lancaster, England.
52. **Jones, P. H., A. T. Willis, D. A. Robinson, M. B. Skirrow, and D. S. Josephs.** 1981. Campylobacter enteritis associated with the consumption of free school milk. *J. Hyg.* **87:**155–162.
53. **Juven, B. J., and M. Rogol.** 1986. Incidence of *Campylobacter jejuni* and *Campylobacter coli* serogroups in a chicken processing factory. *J. Food Prot.* **49:**290–292.
54. **Kaino, K., H. Hayashidani, K. Kaneko, and M. Ogawa.** 1988. Intestinal colonization of *Campylobacter jejuni* in chickens. *Jpn. J. Vet. Sci.* **50:**489–494.
55. **Kapperud, G., and O. Rosef.** 1983. Avian wildlife reservoir of *Campylobacter fetus* subsp. *jejuni, Yersinia* spp., and *Salmonella* spp. in Norway. *Appl. Environ. Microbiol.* **45:**375–380.
56. **Kasrazadeh, M., and C. Genigeorgis.** 1987. Origin and prevalence of *Campylobacter jejuni* in ducks and duck meat at the farm and processing plant level. *J. Food Prot.* **50:**321–326.
57. **Kazwala, R. R., J. D. Collins, J. Hannan, and R. A. P. Crinion.** 1990. The establishment and spread of *Campylobacter jejuni* in young chickens: experimental studies, p. 118–121. *In* R. W. A. W. Mulder (ed.), *Prevention and Control of Potentially Pathogenic Microorganisms in Poultry and Poultry Meat Processing.* Het Spelderholt, Ploufragan, France.
58. **Kist, M.** 1983. *Campylobacter* enteritis in an industrial country: epidemiologic features in urban and rural areas, p. 14–18. *In* M. Pearson (ed.), *Proceedings of the Second International Workshop on Campylobacter Infections.* Public Health Laboratory Service, London.
59. **Kuhn, T. A., J. C. Whitla, and R. J. Montali.** 1983. Isolation of (*Campylobacter fetus* subsp. *jejuni*) from wild pigeons at a zoo [sic]. *J. Zoo Anim. Med.* **14:**27–30.
60. **Kwiatek, K., B. Wojton, and N. J. Stern.** 1990. Prevalence and distribution of *Campylobacter* spp. on poultry and selected red meat carcasses in Poland. *J. Food Prot.* **53:**127–130.
61. **Lammerding, A. M., M. M. Garcia, E. D. Mann, Y. Robinson, W. J. Dorward, R. B. Truscott, and F. Tittiger.** 1988. Prevalence of *Salmonella* and thermophilic *Campylobacter* in fresh pork, beef, veal and poultry in Canada. *J. Food Prot.* **51:**47–52.
62. **Lander, K. P., and K. P. W. Gill.** 1980. Experimental infection of the bovine udder with *Campylobacter coli/jejuni. J. Hyg.* **84:**421–428.
63. **Lindblom, G.-B., E. Sjögren, and B. Kaijser.** 1986. Natural campylobacter colonization in chickens raised under different environmental conditions. *J. Hyg.* **96:**385–391.
64. **Line, E., and N. J. Stern.** 1991. Optimized enrichment methods and selective media for recovery of Campylobacter jejuni from chicken carcasses. *IAMFES Abstract* no. 56.
65. **Luechtefeld, N. A. W., M. J. Blaser, L. B. Reller, and W.-L. L. Wang.** 1980. Isolation of *Campylobacter fetus* subsp. *jejuni* from migratory waterfowl. *J. Clin. Microbiol.* **12:**406–408.
66. **Luechtefeld, N. W., R. C. Cambre, and W.-L. L. Wang.** 1981. Isolation of *Campylobacter fetus* subsp. *jejuni* from zoo animals. *J. Am. Vet. Med. Assoc.* **179:**1119–1122.
67. **Marinescu, M., B. Festy, R. Derimay, and F. Megraud.** 1987. High frequency of isolation of *Campylobacter coli* from poultry meat in France. *Eur. J. Clin. Microbiol.* **6:**693–695. (Letter.)
68. **Meanger, J. D., and R. B. Marshall.** 1989. Seasonal prevalence of thermophilic *Campylobacter* infections in dairy cattle and a study of infection of sheep. *N.Z. Vet. J.* **37:**18–20.
69. **Meinersmann, R. J., N. J. Stern, and L. C. Blankenship.** 1990. Antigenic differences in congenic chicken-colonizing and noncolonizing strains of *Campylobacter jejuni. Curr. Microbiol.* **21:**17–21.
70. **Mentzing, L. O.** 1981. Waterborne outbreaks of Campylobacter enteritis in Central Sweden. *Lancet* **ii:**352–353.
71. **Montrose, M. S., S. M. Shane, and K. S. Harrington.** 1985. Role of litter in the transmission of *Campylobacter jejuni. Avian Dis.* **29:**392–399.
72. **Morgan, G., P. Chadwick, K. P. Lander, and K. P. W. Gill.** 1985. *Campylobacter jejuni* mastitis in a cow: a zoonosis-related incident. *Vet. Rec.* **116:**111. (Letter.)

73. **Mulder, R. W. A. W., H. M. Bolder, and W. F. Jacobs.** 1990. Colonization of pathogenic microorganisms in different poultry breeds, p. 94–95. *In* R. W. A. W. Mulder (ed.), *Prevention and Control of Potentially Pathogenic Microorganisms in Poultry and Poultry Meat Processing.* Het Spelderholt, Ploufragan, France.
74. **Munroe, D. L., J. F. Prescott, and J. L. Penner.** 1983. *Campylobacter jejuni* and *Campylobacter coli* serotypes isolated from chickens, cattle, and pigs. *J. Clin. Microbiol.* **18:**877–881.
75. **Murray, B. J.** 1986. *Campylobacter*-enteritis—a college campus average incidence and a prospective study of the risk factors for exposure. *West. J. Med.* **145:**341–342.
76. **Myszewski, M. A., and N. J. Stern.** 1990. Cecal colonization by *Campylobacter jejuni* elicits limited immunoglobulin response in chicks. *Avian Dis.* **34:**588–594.
77. **Nair, G. B., R. K. Sarkar, S. Chowdhury, and S. C. Pal.** 1985. Campylobacter infection in domestic dogs. *Vet. Rec.* **116:**237–238.
78. **Neill, S. D., J. N. Campbell, and J. A. Greene.** 1984. *Campylobacter* species in broiler chickens. *Avian Pathol.* **13:**777–785.
79. **Norkrans, G., and A. Svedhem.** 1982 Epidemiological aspects of *Campylobacter jejuni* enteritis. *J. Hyg.* **89:**163–170.
80. **Notermans, S., E. H. W. Van Erne, H. J. Beckers, and J. Oosterom.** 1981. The assessment of the bacteriological condition of fresh poultry in shop and market places. *Fleischwirtschaft* **61:**101–104.
81. **Nurmi, E., and M. Rantala.** 1973. New aspects of Salmonella infection in broiler production. *Nature* (London) **214:**210–211.
82. **Oosterom, J., J. R. J. Banffer, S. Lauwers, and A. E. Busschbach.** 1985. Serotyping of and hippurate hydrolysis by *Campylobacter jejuni* isolates from human patients, poultry and pigs in the Netherlands. *Antonie van Leeuwenhoek J. Microbiol.* **51:**65–70.
83. **Oosterom, J., H. J. Beckers, L. M. van Noorle Jansen, and M. van Schothorst.** 1980. An outbreak of campylobacter in a barracks probably caused by eating raw hamburger. *Ned. Tijdschr. Geneeskd.* **124:**1631–1634.
84. **Oosterom, J., C. H. den Uyl, J. R. J. Banffer, et al.** 1984. Epidemiological investigations on *Campylobacter jejuni* in households with a primary infection. *J. Hyg.* **92:**325–332.
85. **Park, C. E., Z. K. Stankiewicz, and J. Lovett.** 1981. Incidence of *Campylobacter jejuni* in fresh eviscerated whole market chicken. *Can. J. Microbiol.* **27:**841–842.
86. **Pokamunski, S., N. Kass, E. Borochovich, B. Marantz, and M. Rogol.** 1986. Incidence of *Campylobacter* spp. in broiler flocks monitored from hatching to slaughter. *Avian Pathol.* **15:**83–92.
87. **Porter, I. A., and T. M. S. Reid.** 1980. A milk-borne outbreak of *Campylobacter* infection. *J. Hyg.* **84:**415–419.
88. **Potter, M. E., M. J. Blaser, R. K. Sikes, A. F. Kaufmann, and J. G. Wells.** 1983. Human *Campylobacter* infection associated with certified raw milk. *Am. J. Epidemiol.* **117:**475–483.
89. **Prescott, J. F., and O. S. Gellner.** 1984. Intestinal carriage of *Campylobacter jejuni* and *Salmonella* by chicken flocks at slaughter. *Can. J. Comp. Med.* **48:**329–331.
90. **Rautelin, H., K. Koota, R. Essen, M. Jahkola, A. Siitonen, and T. U. Kosunen.** 1990. Waterborne *Campylobacter jejuni* epidemic in a Finnish hospital for rheumatic diseases. *Scand. J. Infect. Dis.* **22:**321–326.
91. **Rogol, M., I. Sechter, H. Falk, Y. Shtark, S. Alfi, Z. Greenberg, and R. Mizrachi.** 1983. Waterborne outbreak of campylobacter enteritis. *Eur. J. Clin. Microbiol.* **2:**588–590.
92. **Rosef, O.** 1981. Isolation of *Campylobacter fetus* subsp. *jejuni* from the gallbladder of normal slaughter pigs, using an enrichment procedure. *Acta Vet. Scand.* **22:**149–151.
93. **Rosef, O., B. Gondrosen, G. Kapperud, and B. Underal.** 1983. Isolation and characterization of *Campylobacter jejuni* and *Campylobacter coli* from domestic and wild mammals in Norway. *Appl. Environ. Microbiol.* **46:**855–859.
94. **Rosef, O., and G. Kapperud.** 1983. House flies (*Musca domestica*) as possible vectors of *Campylobacter fetus* subsp. *jejuni. Appl. Environ. Microbiol.* **45:**381–383.
95. **Rosenfield, J. A., G. J. Arnold, G. R. Davey, R. S. Archer, and W. H. Woods.** 1985. Serotyping of *Campylobacter jejuni* from an outbreak of enteritis implicating chicken. *J. Infect.* **11:**159–165.
96. **Sacks, J. J., S. Lieb, L. M. Baldy, S. Berta, C. M. Patton, M. C. White, W. J. Bigler, and J. J. Witte.** 1986. Epidemic campylobacteriosis associated with a community water supply. *Am. J. Public Health* **76:**424–429.
97. **Shane, S. M., D. H. Gifford, and K. Yogasundram. 1986.** *Campylobacter jejuni* contamination of eggs. *Vet. Res. Commun.* **10:**487–492.
98. **Shane, S. M., M. S. Montrose, and K. S. Harrington.** 1985. Transmission of *Campylobacter jejuni* by the housefly (*Musca domestica*). *Avian Dis.* **29:**384–391.
99. **Shanker, S., A. Lee, and T. C. Sorrell.** 1986. *Campylobacter jejuni* in broilers: the role of vertical transmission. *J. Hyg.* **96:**153–159.
100. **Shanker, S., A. Lee, and T. C. Sorrell.** 1990. Horizontal transmission of *Campylobacter jejuni* amongst broiler chicks: experimental studies. *Epidemiol. Infect.* **104:**101–110.
101. **Smith, M. V., II, and P. J. Muldoon.** 1974. *Campylobacter fetus* subsp. *jejuni* (*Vibrio fetus*) from commercially processed poultry. *Appl. Microbiol.* **27:**995–996.
102. **Smitherman, R. E., C. A. Genigeorgis, and T. B. Farver.** 1984. Preliminary observations on the occurrence of *Campylobacter jejuni* at four California chicken ranches. *J. Food Prot.* **47:**293–298.
103. **Soerjadi, A. S., G. H. Snoeyenbos, and O. M. Weinack.** 1985. Comparative studies on competitive exclusion of three isolates of *Campylo-*

bacter fetus subsp. *jejuni* in chickens by native gut microflora. *Avian Dis.* **28**:139–146.
104. **Soerjadi-Liem, A. S., G. H. Snoeyenbos, and O. M. Weinack.** 1983. Intestinal colonization and competitive exclusion of *Campylobacter fetus* subsp. *jejuni* in young chicks. *Avian Dis.* **26**:520–524.
105. **Stern, N. J.** 1990. Influence of competitive exclusion on chicken cecal colonization by *Campylobacter jejuni. Poultry Sci.* **69**(Suppl. 1):130.
106. **Stern, N. J., J. S. Bailey, L. C. Blankenship, N. A. Cox, and F. McHan.** 1988. Colonization characteristics of *Campylobacter jejuni* in chick ceca. *Avian Dis.* **32**:330–334.
107. **Stern, N. J., S. S. Green, N. Thaker, D. J. Krout, and J. Chiu.** 1984. Recovery of *Campylobacter jejuni* from fresh and frozen meat and poultry collected at slaughter. *J. Food Prot.* **47**:372–374.
108. **Stern, N. J., M. P. Hernandez, L. Blankenship, K. E. Deibel, S. Doores, M. P. Doyle, H. Ng, M. D. Pierson, J. N. Sofos, W. H. Sveum, and D. C. Westhoff.** 1985. Prevalence and distribution of *Campylobacter jejuni* and *Campylobacter coli* in retail meats. *J. Food Prot.* **48**:595–599.
109. **Stern, N. J., and A. W. Kotula.** 1982. Survival of *Campylobacter jejuni* inoculated into ground beef. *Appl. Environ. Microbiol.* **44**:1150–1153.
109a. **Stern, N. J.** Unpublished data.
110. **Stern, N. J., R. J. Meinersmann, N. A. Cox, J. S. Bailey, and L. C. Blankenship.** 1990. Influence of host lineage on cecal colonization by *Campylobacter jejuni* in chickens. *Avian Dis.* **34**:602–606.
111. **Stern, N. J., R. J. Meinersmann, and H. W. Dickerson.** 1990. Influence of antibody treatment of *Campylobacter jejuni* on the dose required to colonize chicks. *Avian Dis.* **34**:595–601.
112. **Svedhem, Å., and B. Kaijser.** 1981. Isolation of *Campylobacter jejuni* from domestic animals and pets: probable origin of human infection. *J. Infect.* **3**:37–40.
113. **Tauxe, R. V., N. Hargrett-Bean, C. M. Patton, and I. K. Wachsmuth.** 1988. *Campylobacter* isolates in the United States, 1982–1986. *Morbid. Mortal. Weekly Rep.* **37**:1–13.
114. **Tauxe, R. V., R. L. Vogt, H. E. Sours, T. Barrett, R. A. Feldman, R. J. Dickinson, and L. Witherell.** 1982. Campylobacter enteritis associated with contaminated water. *Ann. Intern. Med.* **96**:292–296.
115. **Taylor, D. N., B. W. Porter, C. A. Williams, H. G. Miller, C. A. Bopp, and P. A. Blake.** 1982. *Campylobacter* enteritis: a large outbreak traced to commercial raw milk. *West. J. Med.* **137**:365–369.
116. **Turnbull, P. C. B., and P. Rose.** 1982. *Campylobacter jejuni* and salmonella in raw red meats. *J. Hyg.* **88**:29–37.
117. **Wempe, J. M., C. A. Genigeorgis, T. B. Farver, and H. I. Yusufu.** 1983. Prevalence of *Campylobacter jejuni* in two California chicken-processing plants. *Appl. Environ. Microbiol.* **45**:355–359.
118. **Wright, E. P.** 1983. The isolation of *Campylobacter jejuni* from flies. *J. Hyg.* **91**:223–226.
119. **Yogasundram, K., S. M. Shane, and K. S. Harrington.** 1989. Prevalence of *Campylobacter jejuni* in selected domestic and wild birds in Louisiana. *Avian Dis.* **33**:664–667.

CHAPTER 7

Importance of *Campylobacter* spp. to the Food Industry

MARVIN A. NORCROSS, RALPH W. JOHNSTON, AND JEFFREY L. BROWN

INTRODUCTION

The importance of *Campylobacter* spp. to the food industry is very difficult to assess because of the great diversity of food products consumed in the United States. The situation is further complicated by the many processes involved in preparing, shipping, marketing, and final use preparation of these products. Accordingly, this communication is limited to specific comments about meat and poultry products, which are regulated by the Food Safety and Inspection Service (FSIS). FSIS is responsible for ensuring that meat and poultry products are safe, wholesome, and accurately labeled. Although just a part of the overall food supply, meat and poultry present almost limitless areas for problems to occur and controls to be developed and applied.

Through the years, the food industry and public health regulators learned how to control food-borne pathogens to minimize their impact. Cooking procedures, proper cooling and sanitary handling, and public education were the keystones of control. It is widely recognized that even when the knowledge needed for control exists, compliance in all segments of the food industry from the farm to the table is a slow process. Nevertheless, progress has been made, and all of us have an active part in it. Technology and engineering have played a major role in the progress of food safety, as has our improved standard of living.

There are, however, some 250 million people in the United States, very few of whom produce food commercially. Most of the contemporary population exclusively consumes rather than produces food, and the practical wisdom of past generations is forgotten or inapplicable. Food production is now massive and regionalized. Shelf life has been extended by lowering storage temperatures and by the use of vacuum and modified-atmosphere packaging technologies (6). All of these changes are highly beneficial but at the same time have created discrete microcosms of risk, thus creating the need to tighten control systems to the maximum. Without appropriate and stringent controls, the effects can be widespread. Several years ago, both the food industry and regulatory officials were shocked by an outbreak of *Salmonella* infection caused by milk from a single dairy, which caused illness in approximately 18,000 individuals. The defective procedure suspected as the cause was not a major one, and the causative microorganism has been a food safety concern for a century. This clearly shows the need for advanced control systems, performed impeccably and designed to control all microbial pathogens whether they are the old chronic ones such as *Salmonella* spp. or the newly recognized ones such as *Campylobacter* spp.

CAMPYLOBACTER SPP. EMERGE

The principal food-borne pathogen has been, and remains, *Salmonella* spp., but, beginning in the 1970s, the food industry and the regulatory agencies became concerned about other food-borne pathogens, such as *Yersinia enterocolitica, Escherichia coli* serotype O157:H7, and *Listeria monocytogenes. Campylobacter* spp. emerged as a concern in the late 1970s and has presented a rather confusing picture. The association of *Campylobacter* spp. with human enteric illnesses is the direct result of recent advances in epidemiology and microbiology. It was apparent for decades that *Campylobacter* spp. are associated with warm-blooded animals,

Marvin A. Norcross, Ralph W. Johnston, and Jeffrey L. Brown, Science and Technology, Food Safety and Inspection Service, U.S. Department of Agriculture, Washington, D.C. 20250.

but their significance as human pathogens was not established because of the lack of adequate detection methods. Epidemiological studies indicate that *Campylobacter jejuni* causes acute diarrheal illness in humans (2, 3) and that isolations from such cases exceed those of *Salmonella* and *Shigella* spp. combined. The World Health Organization Surveillance Programme for Control of Foodborne Infections and Intoxications in Europe concludes that *C. jejuni* and *C. coli* cause *Campylobacter* enteritis, whereas the rarer *C. fetus* causes extraintestinal infections. Additional hazards associated with *Campylobacter* illnesses have been reported. Recently, *C. pylori* was associated with gastric ulcers. This bacterium was found to have subtle differences from other members of the genus and therefore has been reclassified as *Helicobacter pylori*. *C. jejuni* has been observed as the most common pathogen found in association with Guillain-Barré syndrome in adults (7). It has also been described in association with a severe case of Guillain-Barré syndrome in a child (4). There is some evidence, therefore, that *Campylobacter* spp. cause other diseases beyond gastroenteritis. These observations clearly make *Campylobacter* spp. a group of bacteria of concern to FSIS, particularly in view of their prevalence in uncooked meat and poultry. It is no longer of concern only to the food animal producer (5).

Much has been learned about *Campylobacter* spp. and their association with the environment and the food supply. From the voluminous data that exist to date, one can arrive at the following general conclusions. *Campylobacter* spp. are present in warm-blooded animals and their environment throughout most, if not all, parts of the world. They have been isolated from humans, food-producing animals, free-living birds, flies, pets, and other sources. Their incidence is generally higher in poultry, perhaps because of the higher body temperature of birds and the preference of *Campylobacter* spp. for high temperatures for optimum growth.

In addition to the issue of pervasiveness, work has been done that allows regulatory and public health officials to make some preliminary judgments on the relationship of the organism and food safety. *Campylobacter* spp. are similar to *Salmonella* spp. in that their primary reservoir is the enteric tract of warm-blooded animals.

Although conclusive enumeration studies for *Campylobacter* spp. have yet to be done, their numbers are estimated to be much larger than those of *Salmonella* spp. For survey or worst-case work, FSIS laboratories customarily rinse a whole bird and culture the rinse buffer for *Salmonella* spp. The test sample can exceed 1,000 g. Nonenrichment techniques used for many years for *Campylobacter* spp. have taken no more than 0.1 g as the test sample.

In contrast to *Salmonella* spp., *Campylobacter* spp. do not grow or compete well with other bacteria at common food abuse temperatures. They require a high temperature to grow but survive without growth at refrigeration temperatures. In general, when bacteria such as *Salmonella* spp. are given the opportunity to grow, as they are in recontaminated foods abused by being held at room temperatures, both the attack rate and the severity of illness increase. It appears that the level of *Campylobacter* spp. in contaminated foods is governed only by the extent of initial contamination and that temperature abuse is not a significant factor.

Although *Campylobacter* spp. occur in the enteric contents of poultry, they do not appear to cause any ill effects in these birds. In general, poultry scientists in the United States and Japan do not now consider *Campylobacter* spp. to be poultry pathogens. Limited feeding studies produce mixed findings. Studies under way at the Tokyo Metropolitan Institute of Health included oral feeding of high doses of *Campylobacter* spp. to primates. To date, only one strain has produced any untoward result, and that was soft stools. However, *Campylobacter* organisms were consistently found in the blood 1 h after the initial feeding dose. Other studies with other animals have produced enteric illnesses, but only inconsistently. For cooked products over which we have control, the risk of human disease is very low, probably because of the low heat resistance of the organism. *Campylobacter* species are easily destroyed by heat, and there has been no indication to date that drying increases heat resistance as it does with some *Salmonella* spp. Furthermore, *Campylobacter* species are susceptible to chlorine solutions which are commonly used in food-processing plants.

The events of the past two decades have made it evident to both the food industry and food regulatory officials that efforts to make all foods safe for all consumers cannot focus on one or even two pathogens. In the area of cooked food products, a completely new perspective is essential for food safety. There has been some progress in this regard, but documentation over time is not readily available.

As an example of such progress, the Centers for Disease Control report on food-borne illness outbreaks from known vehicle groups over several years (1) has been plotted in Fig. 1; these results in general show a downward trend for meat and poultry products.

With the information available to date, the current FSIS assessment of *Campylobacter* spp. in meat and poultry is as follows. (i) Significant contamination exists in uncooked meat and poultry (8), especially in poultry throughout the world. (ii) Uncooked meat and poultry are prepared without the benefit of a heating step. Consequently, no heat lethality exists to destroy external and internal contamination, which is unavoidable even in the best processing plants. The most common antimicrobial agent permitted in such processing is chlorine. Chlorine in the rinse water reduces the number of bacteria, including *Campylobacter* spp., but is not 100% effective. Some countries now prohibit the use of chlorine in meat and poultry processing because of the potential formation of halocarbons. Thus, the most common antimicrobial chemical agent approved for raw tissue and capable of reducing the number of *Salmonella* and *Campylobacter* organisms is being used less frequently by processors in the United States. (iii) *C. jejuni* is associated with human enteritis. The basic knowledge of strain differences in invasiveness and toxigenic components remains incomplete. (iv) *Campylobacter* contamination in uncooked meat and poultry will be very difficult to control. The economic impact of such control, given existing knowledge, may be prohibitive on a national and worldwide basis. (v) More research is necessary on farm and processing plant control methods.

The current position of FSIS in regard to the presence of *Campylobacter* spp. in food is essentially the same as that for *Salmonella* spp. In raw meat and poultry, *Campylobacter* spp. are considered unavoidable, although undesirable, contaminants. In ready-to-eat foods, the presence of *Campylobacter* spp. would indicate inadequate heat processing, recontamination, or both; the contaminated food would probably be subject to regulatory action. In general, this FSIS position is similar to that of most other countries and the World Health Organization.

EPIDEMIOLOGY AND CONTROL

One area of scientific endeavor that the food industry and regulatory officials must watch closely is the development of new scientific methods for epidemiological investigations. The results obtained from a retrospective epidemiological investigation conducted by using a questionnaire are not always conclusive. However, for the more subtle outbreaks of illnesses, in which only portions of the population are at risk, such investigations are capable of raising genuine concerns. The use of this technique showed very clearly that *L. monocytogenes* from one producer of Jalisco-type cheese caused illnesses and deaths. Although *L. monocytogenes* had been shown to be food borne a few years earlier,

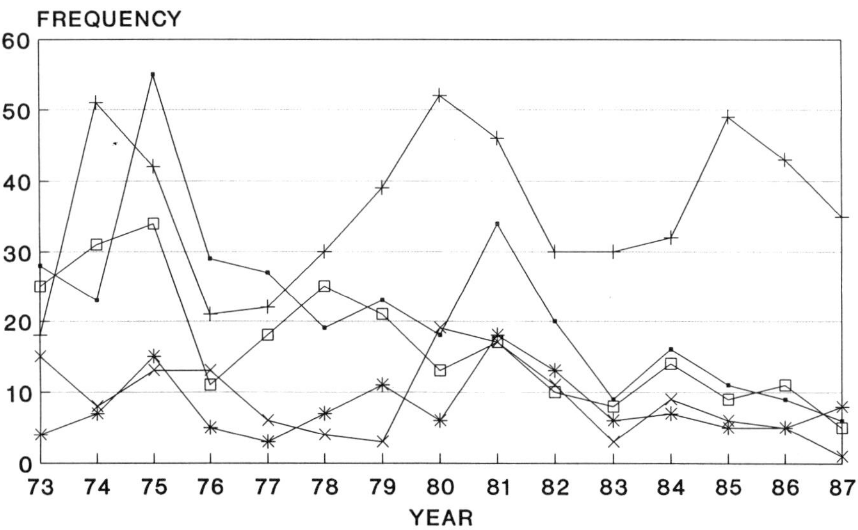

FIGURE 1. Food-borne illness outbreaks from known vehicle groups over several years. Data from the Centers for Disease Control (1). Symbols: ■, beef; +, fish; ✱, chicken, □, pork; ×, turkey.

its significance, particularly in causing deaths in the United States, was not fully appreciated. Food safety officials in both the food industry and government now take retrospective epidemiological investigations very seriously. More importantly, the number of additional genera of bacteria that must be addressed with standardized processing procedures has been greatly enlarged. In addition to our greater concerns regarding a larger number of bacteria, the newer knowledge of the heightened susceptibility of a small proportion of food consumers has made the task of control both more difficult and more important.

During fiscal year 1992, FSIS will initiate a monitoring program for *Campylobacter* spp. in cooked poultry and certain red meat items. No further work is planned for raw meat and poultry unless control breakthroughs develop or certain strains are shown to be more important than others. For both cooked and raw products, we will continue to emphasize sanitary controls.

CAMPYLOBACTER CONTROLS

For cooked products, FSIS is of the opinion that existing cooking and postprocessing sanitation procedures are adequate for *Campylobacter* control. There are, however, concerns regarding how FSIS can be sure that existing controls are applied at all facilities.

Control of *Campylobacter* spp. in uncooked meat and poultry products is clearly not being accomplished commercially. The most important source of *Campylobacter* spp. is the farm, and, regardless of the species of animal, farm controls are ineffective. Current farm controls are for general animal health and are not targeted specifically for *Campylobacter* spp. FSIS currently has no regulatory authority for farm control; thus, new concepts on how to attain the essential farm control of *Campylobacter* spp. are necessary. Farm losses due to *Campylobacter* spp. are economically negligible; this fact hinders both the development and implementation of controls.

Control in the processing plant is somewhat better than on the farm, but it is still a matter of reduction rather than elimination. Chlorine, organic acid sprays, hot-water rinses, and general good sanitation are the current weapons in the control arsenal. Irradiation is an effective control and has been recently approved for poultry. Although irradiation of poultry is deemed safe and efficacious by the Food and Drug Administration and FSIS, there remains a public acceptance barrier, and only time will tell whether the public will judge freedom from *Campylobacter* spp., *Salmonella* spp., *Listeria* spp., and other nonsporeforming bacteria to be a benefit that outweighs perceived irradiation concerns.

CURRENT RESEARCH AND RESEARCH NEEDS

FSIS has encouraged and contributed to the development of *Salmonella* controls for fresh meat and poultry. It is the philosophy of FSIS that any control developed for *Salmonella* spp. will probably have a similar effect on the emerging pathogens that are not adequately controlled today. Farm control methods must be economically feasible to be adopted commercially. Automation and regulatory flexibility to permit new processes and extension of shelf life are also important factors in the further development of microbiological controls.

In 1983 FSIS asked the Agricultural Research Service to conduct basic and applied research on *Campylobacter* spp., including studies on farm controls. Research now being conducted by the Agricultural Research Service, FSIS, and universities includes controlling *Salmonella* and *Campylobacter* spp. in animal feed; interventions in the growout area; novel studies on the effect of washing red-meat carcasses; poultry water filtration studies; a commercial poultry cage washer and sanitizer; improved methods to sanitize wood surfaces; improved *Salmonella* detection methods in poultry houses; and in-plant studies in Puerto Rico evaluating equipment design, processing operations and sanitation, and the addition of chlorine to the chiller tank.

In addition to the current research activities, FSIS perceives the following research needs. (i) The most important *C. jejuni* strains must be identified. It appears that some strains of *C. jejuni* are more important in human campylobacteriosis than others. These strains must be better defined so that, if necessary, they can be targeted in monitoring and control procedures by the food industry. (ii) Pet surveillance and control are necessary. Pets are important in transmission of campylobacteriosis since they carry *Campylobacter* spp. and are closely associated with people. Veterinary research into prevalence and sources of the organisms in pets and treatments to both eliminate and prevent infection is needed. (iii) Basic research must be carried out on the invasiveness and pathogenicity of *Campylobacter* spp. (iv) Basic research is needed to investigate the role and mechanisms of *Campylobacter* involvement in secondary pathogenicities such as Guillain-Barré syndrome. (v) Continued basic research is needed to find methods for economical control of *Campylobacter* spp. in food-producing animals, which appear to be the major reservoir.

HAZARD ANALYSIS AND CRITICAL CONTROL POINTS SYSTEM

A key FSIS initiative involving food safety control is the Hazard Analysis and Critical Control Points System (HACCP). In 1985, the National Academy of Sciences recommended that food-regulatory agencies initiate the HACCP procedure in their requirements. HACCP prevents food hazards, rather than remedying problems after they occur, by using scientific data to identify potential food hazards and putting a system into place to monitor and control those hazards. Implementing this recommendation would assure regulatory agencies that microbiological hazards would be better controlled and that such controls would probably be uniformly applied to all firms. FSIS is now planning and implementing HACCP pilot trials. Although HACCP will be applied to operations involving both cooked and raw products, knowledgeable scientists recognize that its success in controlling hazards in the cooked product will exceed its success with hazards at slaughter. HACCP will have the effect of increasing industry's accountability for controlling the food production process and preventing food hazards. At the same time, HACCP focuses FSIS inspection on the critical areas of food safety.

CONCLUSION

In summary, both FSIS and the food industry recognize *Campylobacter* spp. as a significant food safety concern. Steps have been taken to develop better controls. The two most critical areas for control efforts are animal rearing and food preparation. Both, unfortunately, are outside the jurisdiction of FSIS. Nevertheless, FSIS addresses these issues by producing public information materials for food handling and preparation and by encouraging research on methods to reduce *Campylobacter* levels on the farm. Should effective control procedures at the farm level be developed, academia, industry, and all levels of government will have to play a major, cooperative role in helping producers adopt such control procedures.

REFERENCES

1. **Bean, N. H., and P. Griffin.** 1990. Foodborne disease outbreaks in the United States, 1973–1987: pathogens, vehicles and trends. *J. Food Prot.* **53:**804–817.
2. **Blaser, M. J.** 1980. *Campylobacter fetus* subspecies *jejuni:* the need for surveillance. *J. Infect. Dis.* **141:**670.
3. **Blaser, M. J., and L. B. Reller.** 1981. *Campylobacter* enteritis. *N. Engl. J. Med.* **305:**444.
4. **DeBont, B., N. Mathews, K. Abbott, and G. P. Davidson.** 1986. Guillain-Barre syndrome associated with *Campylobacter* enteritis in a child. *J. Pediatr.* **109:**660–662.
5. **Doyle, M. P.** 1981. *Campylobacter fetus* subsp. *jejuni:* an old pathogen of new concern. *J. Food Prot.* **44:**480–488.
6. **Johnston, R. W., M. E. Harris, A. B. Moran, G. W. Krumm, and W. H. Lee.** 1982. A comparative study of the microbiology of commercial vacuum-packaged and hanging beef. *J. Food Prot.* **45:**223–228.
7. **Kaldor, J., and B. R. Speed.** 1984. Guillain-Barre syndrome and *Campylobacter jejuni:* a serological study. *Br. Med. J.* **288:**1867–1870.
8. **Stern, N. J., S. S. Green, N. Thaker, D. J. Krout, and J. Chiu.** 1984. Recovery of *Campylobacter jejuni* from fresh and frozen meat and poultry collected at slaughter. *J. Food Prot.* **47:**372–374.

CHAPTER 8

Antimicrobial Resistance in *Campylobacter* Species

FRED C. TENOVER, CAROLYN N. BAKER, CYNTHIA L. FENNELL, AND CAROLINE A. RYAN

INTRODUCTION

Studies of antimicrobial resistance in *Campylobacter* species range from surveys of resistance patterns of clinical isolates to studies characterizing the genetic determinants that encode the resistance phenotypes. Campylobacters can harbor a large array of resistance determinants, including several genes that are plasmid mediated (27). Unfortunately, few clinical laboratories routinely perform antimicrobial susceptibility testing on *Campylobacter* isolates. Thus, data that may indicate trends or changes in antimicrobial resistance patterns, or the introduction of novel resistance determinants from other organisms, are sparse. Nonetheless, a few laboratories throughout the world continue their surveillance of antimicrobial resistance in campylobacters and provide most of our new information on resistance in these organisms.

Most commercially available methods of antimicrobial susceptibility testing do not perform well with campylobacters. This necessitates the use of more tedious methods, such as agar dilution or broth microdilution. The development of simpler methods of susceptibility testing may entice more laboratories to test these organisms for resistance. However, because physicians infrequently request such information, microbiologists tend to view the undertaking of susceptibility testing as an unwarranted expense. Given the growing problem of resistance in these organisms (see below), the clinical need for such testing should become more apparent.

This chapter will focus on four aspects of antimicrobial resistance in *Campylobacter* species: (i) a review of traditional and novel methods of susceptibility testing, (ii) preliminary results of a survey of antimicrobial resistance among *Campylobacter jejuni* isolates from the United States, (iii) a review of the heterogeneity of kanamycin resistance determinants in *Campylobacter* species, and (iv) the movement of resistance determinants among species within the genus.

ANTIMICROBIAL SUSCEPTIBILITY TESTING

For many years, clinical laboratories have used the results of antimicrobial susceptibility testing of campylobacters to nalidixic acid and cephalothin as a tool for identifying various *Campylobacter* species (15). In fact, the pattern of resistance to these two antimicrobial agents is critical for differentiating *C. jejuni* from *C. lari* and *C. fetus*. Testing is done by the disk diffusion method, and any zone of inhibition around either the nalidixic acid disk or the cephalothin disk indicates susceptibility to the drug (15).

The testing of antimicrobial agents for guiding therapy, however, is not so clearly defined. No breakpoint values for resistance have been established for clinically useful drugs, nor has the effect of microaerobic incubation on the MICs of the antimicrobial agents been accurately quantitated. Vanhoof et al. reported that the disk diffusion test using Rosco Neosensitabs and Mueller-Hinton agar containing 5% lysed horse blood was an accurate means of determining the susceptibility of these organisms to several antimicrobial agents (39). However, they found an unacceptably high level of errors with

Fred C. Tenover and Carolyn N. Baker, Nosocomial Pathogens Laboratory Branch, Hospital Infections Program, National Center for Infectious Diseases, Centers for Disease Control, Atlanta, Georgia 30333. **Cynthia L. Fennell,** Department of Medicine, Harborview Medical Center, Seattle, Washington 98104. **Caroline A. Ryan,** Children's Hospital and Medical Center, Seattle, Washington 98105.

tetracycline and trimethoprim-sulfamethoxazole (cotrimoxazole). Although the breakpoints used for determining the MICs were those of the National Committee for Clinical Laboratory Standards, the concentrations of drugs used in the disk tests were not those commonly used by the National Committee for Clinical Laboratory Standards. Thus, the data are of limited utility.

Agar dilution and broth microdilution remain the standard methods of determining the susceptibility of campylobacters to antimicrobial agents. However, a review of the literature reveals that there is no consensus about the optimal medium, the requirement for blood supplementation, the temperature of incubation, or the duration of incubation. Temperature and time of incubation, for instance, vary from 42°C for 24 h (26) to 37°C for 48 h (40). For agar dilution testing, Mueller-Hinton agar containing 5% sheep blood, incubated in anaerobe jars with a gas mixture containing 5% O_2, 10% CO_2, and 85% N_2 for 48 h at 37°C, is the method most frequently used at the Centers for Disease Control (CDC) in the United States, whereas cation-adjusted Mueller-Hinton broth containing 5% lysed horse blood, incubated as described above, is used at the CDC for broth microdilution assays and specifically for testing trimethoprim-sulfamethoxazole. Other methods will produce acceptable results, but it is critical that quality control strains be tested in parallel to ensure the accuracy of the method.

Recently, a novel method of determining MICs, the E test (AB Biodisk, Solna, Sweden), was evaluated at the CDC for its accuracy in determining MICs for nonfastidious gram-negative and gram-positive organisms (2). The reagent for the E test consists of a nonporous carrier with a defined antibiotic gradient that is placed on an agar plate much like a disk diffusion test. The strip has 15 twofold dilutions of a single antibiotic. After overnight incubation, the MICs are read from a scale at the point where the zone of inhibition intersects the strip (Fig. 1).

A preliminary evaluation of the E test was performed in parallel with broth microdilution and agar dilution susceptibility testing on a group of 55 isolates of *C. jejuni*. Chloramphenicol, ciprofloxacin, erythromycin, gentamicin, and tetracycline MICs were determined (1a). For all the isolates, MICs of chloramphenicol and ciprofloxacin were ±1 dilution of the MICs determined by broth microdilution. The percent agreement for erythromycin, gentamicin, and tetracycline at ±1 dilution was 94, 80, and 66%, respectively. The percent agreement rose to 98.1% for all three drugs at ±2 dilutions. The

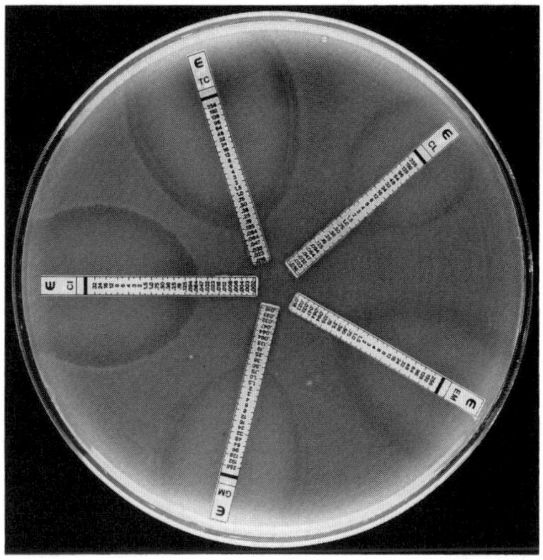

FIGURE 1. Zones of inhibition produced by five E test strips on a Mueller-Hinton agar plate containing 5% sheep blood inoculated with an isolate of *C. jejuni*. Each of the E test strips contains gradients of a single antibiotic. Abbreviations: CL, chloramphenicol; CI, ciprofloxacin; EM, erythromycin; GM, gentamicin; TC, tetracycline. The plate was incubated at 37°C for 24 h in an anaerobe jar containing an atmosphere of 5% CO_2, 10% O_2, and 85% N_2.

MICs of erythromycin and tetracycline were slightly higher with the E test than with broth microdilution, and the number of minor errors with erythromycin was due primarily to the use of National Committee for Clinical Laboratory Standards breakpoints that do not correspond to the doubling-dilution scheme used by the E test. The E test gave better agreement with the results of agar dilution than with the results of broth microdilution testing. The E test results could be interpreted easily after 24 h, whereas at least 25% of the agar dilution tests and 20% of the broth microdilution tests required a full 48 h of incubation before the endpoints were interpretable. Although the number of resistant organisms tested in this pilot study was relatively small, the preliminary results suggest that the E test is a simple, rapid, and accurate means of testing the susceptibility of *C. jejuni* isolates.

CDC NATIONAL *CAMPYLOBACTER* SURVEY

A national county-based survey of *Campylobacter* infections and isolates was undertaken in the Enteric Diseases Branch at the CDC.

The survey included approximately 700 isolates, the majority of which were *C. jejuni.* A variety of other campylobacters, including *C. coli, C. lari,* and several other species, were also represented. Preliminary analysis of the antimicrobial susceptibility patterns of 332 isolates of *C. jejuni* found that 144 (43%) were resistant to tetracycline, 25 (8%) were resistant to kanamycin, 8 (2%) were resistant to erythromycin, and 1 was resistant to ciprofloxacin. It was also found that 6% of the isolates were resistant to both tetracycline and kanamycin, 3% were resistant to tetracycline and erythromycin, and only one organism was resistant to all three of these antimicrobial agents. None of the isolates was resistant to chloramphenicol (MICs for all isolates were ≤ 8 μg/ml). β-Lactamase activity among the isolates was assayed by using the nitrocefin disk test; 55% of the isolates produced a strongly positive reaction, and an additional 22% were weakly positive. The majority of the isolates were susceptible to the β-lactamase inhibitor clavulanic acid (MIC, ≤ 2 μg/ml). This is unusual since clavulanic acid normally does not have antibacterial activity unless combined with a betalactam drug.

There are some interesting differences in these results and the results reported for the Food and Drug Administration-sponsored study of *Campylobacter* infections undertaken in the Seattle-King County, Wash., area in 1982 to 1983 (4). In the latter study, only 30% of the 276 human isolates examined were resistant to tetracycline and only 0.7% were resistant to erythromycin. Among the isolates that were tested for resistance to kanamycin, a resistance phenotype that is commonly plasmid mediated, only 10 human isolates showed resistance to the drug. No chloramphenicol resistance was noted among isolates in the Seattle-King County study, and ciprofloxacin resistance and β-lactamase production were not determined (4).

Only one ciprofloxacin-resistant isolate was found among the campylobacters tested at CDC. A larger number was expected since there have been reports of the development of ciprofloxacin resistance in campylobacters isolated from humans and animals in countries where quinolones are used frequently (6). As reported earlier by Taylor et al. (29), resistance to the 4-fluoroquinolones develops quickly in *C. jejuni* once the organism has been exposed to the agent. This can cause problems when identifying *Campylobacter* isolates to the species level since isolates may be classified as *C. lari* on the basis of resistance to cephalothin and nalidixic acid, when they are in fact ciprofloxacin- and nalidixic acid-resistant isolates of *C. jejuni* (1). Similar problems with the development of ciprofloxacin resistance in *C. jejuni* during therapy have been reported by Goodman et al. (8). Thus, surveys of *Campylobacter* infections may underestimate the level of ciprofloxacin resistance present nationwide since posttreatment cultures may be obtained infrequently.

KANAMYCIN RESISTANCE

The *aphA-3* Gene

Kanamycin resistance (Km^r) was first found in an isolate of *C. coli* by Lambert et al. in 1985 (11). In addition to kanamycin, this isolate was resistant to ampicillin, tetracycline, chloramphenicol, erythromycin, streptomycin, and spectinomycin. The gene responsible for Km^r was an *aphA-3* determinant, a gene previously detected only in gram-positive organisms. The nucleotide sequence of the *C. coli aphA-3* gene, which was encoded on a plasmid that also mediated tetracycline resistance, was determined by Trieu-Cuot et al. (38) and was shown to be highly related to the *aphA-3* genes from the staphylococcal plasmid pSH2 and the streptococcal plasmid pJH1. By cloning the *aphA-3* gene from *C. coli* onto two different shuttle vectors, these investigators also proved that the gene was capable of being expressed in both *Escherichia coli* and *Bacillus subtilis.* This was the first time that a "gram-positive" resistance determinant was documented in a gram-negative organism. DNA sequence analysis of the regions surrounding the *aphA-3* gene on the campylobacter, staphylococcal, and streptococcal plasmids suggests that the Km^r gene was the only determinant to survive entry into the *C. coli* cell from the donor source, which may have been a plasmid or transposon, such as Tn*1545* (3, 5). The remainder of this unknown replicon was lost when the Km^r gene integrated into a resident campylobacter plasmid by transposition or recombination. To date, no laboratory has been able to transfer a naturally occurring plasmid or transposon carrying the *aphA-3* gene from a streptococcal or staphylococcal donor to a campylobacter recipient.

Translocation of the *aphA-3* Gene

Data from Kotarski et al. (9) support the hypothesis that the *aphA-3* gene may have translocated from a replicon incapable of surviving in the campylobacter recipient to an indigenous plasmid. These investigators showed that the Km^r determinants present on plasmids from two different strains of *C. jejuni* were capable of translocating from a plasmid to the chromosome of the organism when exposed to ethidium bromide. Similarly, once the Km^r determinant was present in the *C. jejuni* chromosome, it could translocate back to a plasmid encoding a tetracycline resistance gene. When the Km^r determinant translocated from the chromosome to a plasmid, the plasmid increased in size by 4 kb. Similarly, when the Km^r phenotype was lost from a plasmid, the plasmid decreased in size, in most cases by 4 kb. In one instance, the loss of the Km^r gene from the plasmid was accompanied by an inversion of DNA adjacent to the region where the Km^r gene was previously mapped. The lack of recombination-deficient strains of *C. jejuni* prohibited these authors from ultimately proving the presence of a transposon in their strains. However, three findings suggest that the *aphA-3* gene can be located on a transposable element present on some campylobacter plasmids: (i) the Km^r gene could move between the plasmid and the chromosome of two isolates of *C. jejuni,* (ii) the unit had a predictable size of 4 kb, and (iii) rearrangements were noted in the plasmids in the area of the Km^r determinant (9).

Papadopoulou and Courvalin, who reported that the *aphA-3* gene was present in isolates of *C. jejuni* and *C. coli* from Thailand, Vietnam, and Spain (20), also noted that the Km^r determinant was present in the chromosome in one of the organisms investigated. This further supports the hypothesis that the *aphA-3* gene is capable of translocation since it is not always located on a plasmid yet has probably entered the cell from another organism.

Linkage of *aphA-3* to *tetO* and Other Genes

In campylobacters, Km^r genes frequently are located on plasmids that also encode tetracycline resistance (9, 23, 31). However, the relationship between the two resistance determinants, in terms of shared promoters or physical linkage, has not been explored in any detail. Preliminary restriction-mapping data from our laboratory suggest that Km^r determinants are located both upstream and downstream of *tetO* determinants on several campylobacter plasmids (29a). No hot spots of

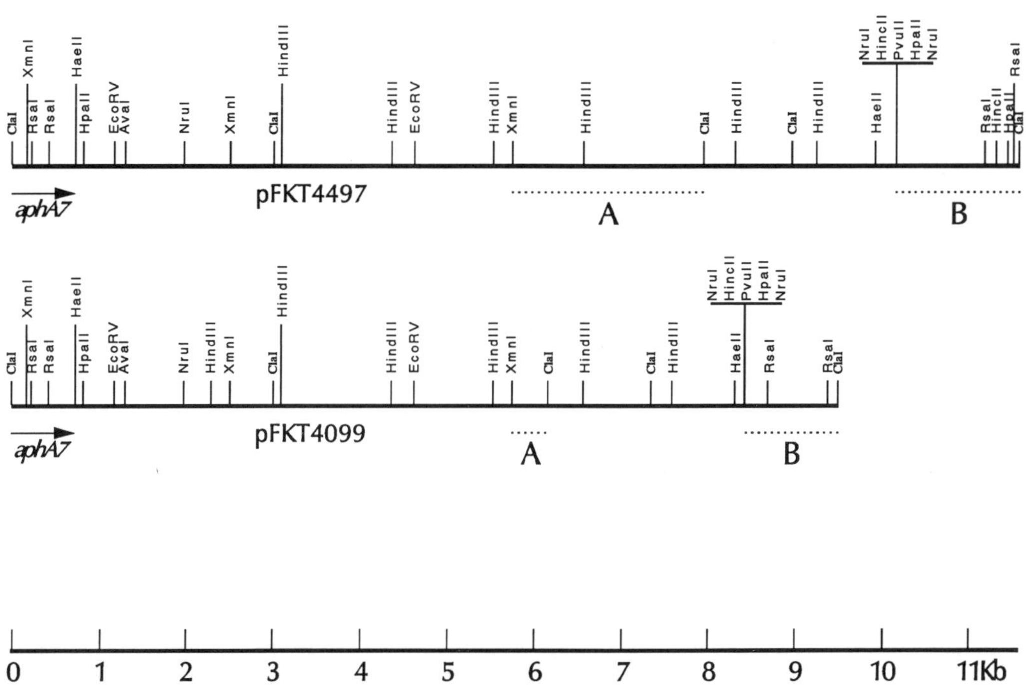

FIGURE 2. Restriction endonuclease maps of two *aphA-7*-encoding plasmids recovered from two different isolates of *C. jejuni.* The regions of diversity between the two maps are designated A and B. The size scale is in kilobases. Reprinted with permission from reference 32.

integration, as seen with Tn*21*-related elements (16), have been reported for the Km^r gene.

In addition to the frequent coupling of kanamycin and tetracycline resistance genes on campylobacter plasmids, Sagara et al. described an isolate of *C. coli* in which the Km^r determinant was located downstream from a chloramphenicol acetyltransferase gene on a plasmid that also mediated resistance to tetracycline (23). Although these investigators were not able to clone the *tet* gene and demonstrate its expression in *E. coli,* they were able to clone both the kanamycin and chloramphenicol resistance genes in *E. coli,* both of which expressed. Wang and Taylor (41), in continuing experiments with this isolate, demonstrated that the Km^r determinant was an *aphA-3* gene apparently under the control of the *cat* gene promoter. This makes this Km^r gene unique since most of the Km^r determinants seen in campylobacters appear to have functional promoters.

The *aphA-7* Kanamycin Phosphotransferase Gene

Tenover and Elvrum (31) were the first to report a Km^r gene other than the *aphA-3* gene in a *Campylobacter* species. [Although Ouellette et al. (17) described the presence of an *aphA-1* in a *Campylobacter*-like organism, this bacterium was never proven to be related to the other members of the genus *Campylobacter.* Similarly, the enzyme described as an APH(3′)-IV by Rivera et al. (21) fits the description of an *aphA-3* gene.] The novel gene, subsequently named *aphA-7,* was isolated initially from a *C. jejuni* isolate from a human infection in Seattle, Wash. When cloned and sequenced in *E. coli,* the gene was shown to share 55.4% nucleotide homology with the *aphA-3* gene (33). Unlike the *aphA-3* gene, however, the G+C ratio of the *aphA-7* gene was 32.8%, very similar to that of the *C. jejuni* chromosome (19) and unlike the 40% G+C of the *aphA-3* gene noted in *C. coli* by Trieu-Cuot et al. (36) and the 39% G+C ratio reported by Sougakoff et al. (24) and LeBlanc et al. (13) for the *tetO* determinant. The *aphA-7* gene also has a typical gram-negative promoter (7, 22) that is different from the promoters noted for the *aphA-3* and *tetO* genes, both of which are presumed to have been transferred into the genus from gram-positive organisms (37, 38). These data suggest that the *aphA-7* gene, unlike the *aphA-3* and *tetO* genes, may be indigenous to campylobacters. A recent survey of resistance determinants in 500 isolates of enterococci by Ounissi et al. (18), using both phosphocellulose paper-binding assays and gene probes, demonstrated a 100% correlation between enzyme assay results for kanamycin phosphotransferase activity and the presence of the *aphA-3* gene as detected by hybridization. This supports the hypothesis that the *aphA-7* gene present in *C. jejuni* was not scavenged from gram-positive cocci, or at least not from enterococci. It is possible that this gene is present only in other species of streptococci, but this, in our view, is unlikely since there seem to be few barriers to exchange of genes between enterococci and other streptococci (12).

The APH(3′)-VII Protein

The APH(3′)-VII protein mediates resistance to kanamycin, neomycin, and amikacin, but not to gentamicin or tobramycin (31). This protein also demonstrates the same amino acid motifs and domains found in other aminoglycoside-phosphorylating enzymes (33), suggesting that it probably evolved from the same ancestral gene as the other *aphA* phosphotransferases active on aminoglycosides (14). However, several deviations from the conserved amino acid sequences can be noted in the APH(3′)-VII protein in these domains, suggesting that the *aphA-7* gene may have diverged from the other determinants earlier, although this is speculative.

Plasmids Encoding the *aphA-7* Gene

The *aphA-7* gene has been found in only two isolates of *C. jejuni,* one from Seattle, Wash., and one from Athens, Ga. (32). Both genes were located on small mobilizable plasmids apparently devoid of other antimicrobial resistance determinants. Although the plasmids were obtained from isolates of *C. jejuni* that had different Lior and Penner serotypes and different auxotypes and were from different locations in the United States, the plasmids had very similar restriction endonuclease maps (32). Only two regions, which may represent either insertions or deletions, differentiated the two plasmids (Fig. 2).

The *aphA-7* gene was cloned in the plasmid pBR322 and expressed in *E. coli* (33). After deletion of several restriction fragments to reduce the size of the plasmid, the new chimeric plasmid was cloned into a streptococcal vector that, when introduced into *Streptococcus gordonii* Challis, expressed the Km^r phenotype (32). This demonstrated that *aphA-7* was capable of expression in a streptococcal host even though it is presumed to have originated in a campylobacter. This suggests that the promoter and regulatory functions for antimicrobial resistance determinants in campylobacters and streptococci are similar. Further support for this hypothesis is provided by Wang and Taylor, who were able to introduce the *tetM* streptococcal resistance determinant into a *C. coli* isolate and achieve expression (42). Thus, the similarity of the genetic regulatory systems of campylobacters and streptococci bears further investigation.

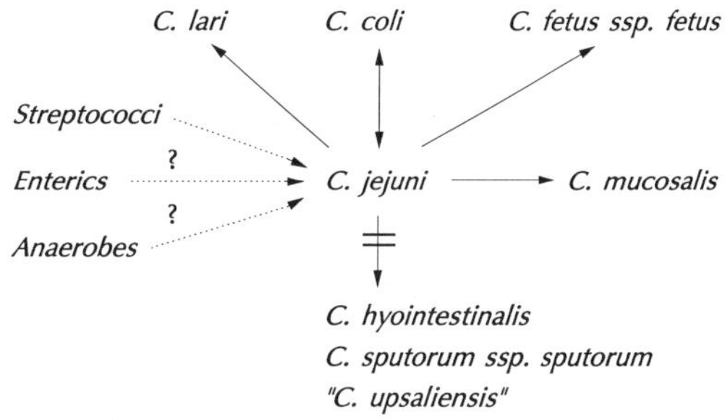

FIGURE 3. Pathways of genetic exchange among campylobacters determined by mating a donor strain of *C. jejuni* containing the 48-kb *tetO*-encoding R factor pFKT1025 and the 9.5-kb *aphA-7*-encoding plasmid pFKT4099 with various recipients under microaerobic conditions. Dotted lines indicate potential pathways of exchange that have yet to be documented in vitro.

CONJUGATION AMONG *CAMPYLOBACTER* SPECIES

In 1981, Taylor et al. (28) reported that tetracycline-encoding plasmids in *C. jejuni* could be transferred to *C. fetus* subsp. *fetus* by conjugation. Following that report, Tenover et al. noted that a 57-kb plasmid mediating resistance to tetracycline from an isolate of *C. jejuni* taken from a simian could transfer itself as well as a small cryptic plasmid to a recipient strain of *C. jejuni* during conjugal matings (30). Since then, many studies have reported conjugal transfer of tetracycline-encoding plasmids between *C. jejuni* and *C. coli* and various campylobacter recipients (9, 11, 23, 31, 34). However, there are no reports of transmission of plasmids to other genera, although many investigators have attempted matings with gram-negative enteric and anaerobic bacilli.

In recent experiments, Tenover et al. have shown that a strain of *C. jejuni* harboring the tetracycline R factor pFKT1025 and the Km^r plasmid pFKT4099 could transfer both R plasmids in filter matings to *C. coli, C. fetus* subsp. *fetus,* and *C. lari.* However, only the tetracycline R factor was recovered in matings with *C. mucosalis* (Fig. 3). No transconjugants manifesting either tetracycline or kanamycin resistance were recovered from matings with *C. jejuni, C. coli,* or *C. lari* donors and *C. hyointestinalis, C. sputorum* subsp. *sputorum,* or *C. upsaliensis* recipients even when the mating pairs were incubated under various atmospheric conditions (31a). Plasmids could be transferred to *C. mucosalis* but not to *C. upsaliensis,* another thermophilic *Campylobacter* species that has been recovered from human infections, but this may relate more to the particular strains tested rather than to species barriers. However, this remains an open question. The transfer of the tetracycline R factor to *C. mucosalis* was surprising given the lack of DNA homology between these two organisms and the fact that they occupy quite different ecological niches (15). This genetic pathway between commensal and thermophilic campylobacters may prove to be important in linking campylobacters with other genera, in that plasmids may be introduced into *C. mucosalis* and transferred to *C. jejuni* rather than being introduced from streptococci or other donors directly into *C. jejuni* or *C. coli.* Mating experiments in which streptococcal donors are paired with *C. mucosalis* recipients are in progress.

Although conjugation with other genera by using naturally occurring plasmids or transposons has not been reported, shuttle vectors allowing conjugation between *E. coli* and *C. jejuni* have been described (10). Labigne-Roussel et al. constructed a vector for gene cloning consisting of an *aphA-3* Km^r determinant, the replication functions from a cryptic plasmid of *C. coli,* and the *oriT* of plasmid pEYDG1 cloned into the vector pBR322 (10). This allowed cloning of *Campylobacter* genes in *E. coli* and their subsequent mobilization back into *C. jejuni* via conjugation by using the helper plasmid pRK212.1. This suggests that the machinery for genetic exchange between the family *Enterobacteriaceae* and the genus *Campylobacter* does exist, but that the failure of plasmids to replicate in the recipient organism is the critical factor prohibiting the introduction of a variety of enteric genes into *Campylobacter* recipients. Trieu-Cuot et al. have hypothesized that a genetic pathway between *E. coli* and streptococci exists based on the discovery of erythromycin resistance genes common to streptococci in some isolates of *E. coli* (35). If the maintenance and transfer machinery for plasmids is indeed similar in campylobacters and streptococci, there might be a common pathway for genetic exchange between *E. coli* and campylobacters as well, even though enteric plasmids cannot replicate in a campylobacter host. If a recombination event resulting in placement of a campylobacter *oriV* on an enteric plasmid occurred, similar to what Labigne-Roussel et al. (10) constructed in vitro, it is possible that the entry of enteric genes into campylobacters would be observed.

In summary, it is possible that the major pathway of entry of resistance genes into the genus *Campylobacter* is through species of this organism infrequently associated with human infections. As a precedent for this, it is worth recalling that the TEM-type β-lactamase gene that entered into strains of *Neisseria gonorrhoeae* in 1976 probably was introduced on DNA through either transformation or conjugation from *Haemophilus influenzae* (25). We must not forget to look for alternate pathways of genetic exchange if the obvious pathways do not prove fruitful.

REFERENCES

1. **Altwegg, M., A. Burnens, J. Zollinger-Iten, and J. L. Penner.** 1987. Problems in identification of *Campylobacter jejuni* associated with acquisition of resistance to nalidixic acid. *J. Clin. Microbiol.* **25:**1807–1808.

1a. **Baker, C. N., and M. A. Nicholson.** 1990. The PDM Epsilometer: an improved method for antimicrobial susceptibility testing of *Campylobacter jejuni,* abstr. 216, p. 132. *Sixth Int. Congr. Rapid Methods Automation Microbiol. Immunol.* Helsinki-Espoo, Finland.

2. **Baker, C. N., S. A. Stocker, D. H. Culver, and C. Thornsberry.** 1991. Comparison of the E test to agar dilution, broth microdilution, and agar diffusion susceptibility testing techniques by using a special challenge set of bacteria. *J. Clin. Microbiol.* **29:**533–538.

3. **Caillaud, F., P. Trieu-Cuot, C. Carlier, and P. Courvalin.** 1987. Nucleotide sequence of the kanamycin resistance determinant of the pneumococcal transposon Tn*1545:* evolutionary relationships and transcriptional analysis of *aphA*-3 genes. *Mol. Gen. Genet.* **207:**509–513.

4. **Communicable Disease Control Section Seattle-King County Public Health Department.** 1984. *Surveillance of the Flow of Salmonella and Campylobacter in a Community.* Seattle-King County Department of Public Health, Seattle.

5. **Courvalin, P., and C. Carlier.** 1987. Tn*1545:* a conjugative shuttle transposon. *Mol. Gen. Genet.* **206:**259–264.

6. **Endtz, H. P., G. J. Ruijs, B. van Klingeren, W. H. Jansen, T. van der Reyden, and R. P. Mouton.** 1991. Quinolone resistance in campylobacter isolated from man and poultry following the introduction of fluoroquinolones in veterinary medicine. *J. Antimicrob. Chemother.* **27:**199–208.

7. **Gold, L., D. Pribnow, T. Schneider, S. Shinedling, B. S. Singer, and G. Stormo.** 1981. Translational initiation in prokaryotes. *Annu. Rev. Microbiol.* **35:**365–403.

8. **Goodman, L. J., G. M. Trenholme, R. L. Kaplan, J. Segreti, D. Hines, R. Petrak, J. A. Nelson, K. W. Mayer, W. Landau, G. W. Parkhurst, and S. Levin.** 1990. Empiric antimicrobial therapy of domestically acquired acute diarrhea in urban adults. *Arch. Intern. Med.* **150:**541–546.

9. **Kotarski, S. K., T. L. Merriwether, G. T. Tkalcevic, and P. Gemski.** 1986. Genetic studies of kanamycin resistance in *Campylobacter jejuni. Antimicrob. Agents Chemother.* **30:**225–230.

10. **Labigne-Roussel, A., J. Harel, and L. Tompkins.** 1987. Gene transfer from *Escherichia coli* to *Campylobacter* species: development of shuttle vectors for genetic analysis of *Campylobacter jejuni. J. Bacteriol.* **169:**5320–5323.

11. **Lambert, T., G. Gerbaud, P. Trieu-Cuot, and P. Courvalin.** 1985. Structural relationship between the genes encoding 3′-aminoglycoside phosphotransferases in *Campylobacter* and gram positive cocci. *Ann. Inst. Pasteur* (Paris) **136B:**135–150.

12. **LeBlanc, D. J., L. N. Lee, M. Banai, L. D. Rollins, and J. M. Inamine.** 1987. Dissemination of streptococcal antibiotic resistance determinants in the natural environment, p. 42–57. *In* J. J. Ferretti and R. Curtiss III (ed.), *Streptococcal Genetics.* American Society for Microbiology, Washington, D.C.

13. **LeBlanc, D., L. N. Lee, B. M. Titmas, C. J. Smith, and F. C. Tenover.** 1988. Nucleotide sequence analysis of tetracycline resistance gene *tetO* from *Streptococcus mutans* DL5. *J. Bacteriol.* **170:** 3618–3626.

14. **Martin, P., E. Julien, and P. Courvalin.** 1988. Nucleotide sequence of *Acinetobacter baumannii aphA*-6 gene: evolutionary and functional implications of sequence homologies with nucleotide binding proteins, kinases and other aminoglycoside modifying enzymes. *Mol. Microbiol.* **2:**615–625.

15. **Morris, G. K., and C. M. Patton.** 1985. *Campylobacter,* p. 302–308. *In* E. H. Lennette, A. Balows, W. J. Hausler, Jr., and H. J. Shadomy (ed.), *Manual of Clinical Microbiology,* 4th ed. American Society for Microbiology, Washington, D.C.

16. **Ouellette, M., L. Bissonnette, and P. H. Roy.** 1987. Precise insertion of antibiotic resistance determinants into Tn*21*-like transposons: nucleotide sequence of the OXA-1 β-lactamase gene. *Proc. Natl. Acad. Sci. USA* **84:**7378–7382.

17. **Ouellette, M., G. Gerbaud, T. Lambert, and P. Courvalin.** 1987. Acquisition by a *Campylobacter*-like strain of *aphA-1,* a kanamycin resistance determinant from members of the family *Enterobacteriaceae. Antimicrob. Agents Chemother.* **31:**1021–1026.

18. **Ounissi, H., E. Derlot, C. Carlier, and P. Courvalin.** 1990. Gene homogeneity for aminoglycoside-modifying enzymes in gram-positive cocci. *Antimicrob. Agents Chemother.* **34:**2164–2168.

19. **Owen, R. J.** 1983. Nucleic acids in the classification of campylobacters. *Eur. J. Clin. Microbiol.* **2**:367–377.
20. **Papadopoulou, B., and P. Courvalin.** 1988. Dispersal in *Campylobacter* spp. of *aphA-3,* a kanamycin resistance determinant from gram-positive cocci. *Antimicrob. Agents Chemother.* **32**:945–948.
21. **Rivera, M. J., J. Castillo, C. Martin, M. Navarro, and R. Gomez-Lus.** 1986. Aminoglycoside-phosphotransferases APH (3′)-IV and APH (3″) synthesized by a strain of *Campylobacter coli. J. Antimicrob. Chemother.* **18**:153–158.
22. **Rosenberg, M., and D. Court.** 1979. Regulatory sequences involved in the promotion and termination of transcriptions. *Annu. Rev. Genet.* **13**:319–353.
23. **Sagara, H., A. Mochizuki, N. Okamura, and R. Nakaya.** 1987. Antimicrobial resistance of *Campylobacter jejuni* and *Campylobacter coli* with special reference to plasmid profiles of Japanese clinical isolates. *Antimicrob. Agents Chemother.* **31**:713–719.
24. **Sougakoff, W., B. Papadopoulou, P. Nordmann, and P. Courvalin.** 1987. Nucleotide sequence and distribution of gene *tetO* encoding tetracycline resistance in *Campylobacter coli. FEMS Microbiol. Lett.* **44**:153–159.
25. **Sparling, P. F., T. E. Sox, W. Mohammed, and L. F. Guymon.** 1978. Antibiotic resistance in the gonococcus: diverse mechanisms of coping with a hostile environment, p. 44–52. *In* G. F. Brooks, E. C. Gotschlich, K. K. Holmes, W. D. Sawyer, and F. E. Young (ed.), *Immunobiology of Neisseria gonorrhoeae.* American Society for Microbiology, Washington, D.C.
26. **Svedham, A., B. Kaiser, and E. Sjogren.** 1981. Antimicrobial susceptibility of *Campylobacter jejuni* isolated from humans with diarrhea and healthy chickens. *J. Antimicrob. Chemother.* **7**:301–305.
27. **Taylor, D. E., and P. Courvalin.** 1988. Mechanisms of antibiotic resistance in *Campylobacter* species. *Antimicrob. Agents Chemother.* **32**:1107–1112.
28. **Taylor, D. E., S. A. DeGrandis, M. A. Karmali, and P. C. Fleming.** 1981. Transmissible plasmids from *Campylobacter jejuni. Antimicrob. Agents Chemother.* **19**:831–835.
29. **Taylor, D. E., L.-K. Ng, and H. Lior.** 1985. Susceptibility of *Campylobacter* species to nalidixic acid, enoxacin, and other DNA gyrase inhibitors. *Antimicrob. Agents Chemother.* **28**:708–710.
29a. **Tenover, F. C.** Unpublished data.
30. **Tenover, F. C., M. A. Bronsdon, K. P. Gordon, and J. J. Plorde.** 1983. Isolation of plasmids encoding tetracycline resistance from *Campylobacter jejuni* strains isolated from simians. *Antimicrob. Agents Chemother.* **23**:320–322.
31. **Tenover, F. C., and P. M. Elvrum.** 1988. Detection of two different kanamycin resistance genes in naturally occurring isolates of *Campylobacter jejuni* and *Campylobacter coli. Antimicrob. Agents Chemother.* **32**:1170–1173.
31a. **Tenover, F. C., and C. L. Fennell.** Unpublished data.
32. **Tenover, F. C., C. L. Fennell, L. Lee, and D. N. LeBlanc.** Characterization of two plasmids from *Campylobacter jejuni* isolates that carry the *aphA-7* kanamycin resistance determinant. *Antimicrob. Agents Chemother.,* in press.
33. **Tenover, F. C., T. Gilbert, and P. O'Hara.** 1989. Nucleotide sequence of a novel kanamycin resistance gene, *aphA-7,* from *Campylobacter jejuni* and comparison to other kanamycin phosphotransferase genes. *Plasmid* **22**:52–58.
34. **Tenover, F. C., S. Williams, K. P. Gordon, C. Nolan, and J. J. Plorde.** 1985. Survey of plasmids and resistance factors in *Campylobacter jejuni* and *Campylobacter coli. Antimicrob. Agents Chemother.* **27**:37–41.
35. **Trieu-Cuot, P., C. Carlier, P. Martin, and P. Courvalin.** 1987. Plasmid transfer by conjugation from *Escherichia coli* to gram positive bacteria. *FEMS Microbiol. Lett.* **48**:289–294.
36. **Trieu-Cuot, P., and P. Courvalin.** 1983. Nucleotide sequence of the *Streptococcus faecalis* plasmid gene encoding the 3′5″-aminoglycoside phosphotransferase type III. *Gene* **23**:331–334.
37. **Trieu-Cuot, P., and P. Courvalin.** 1986. Evolution and transfer of aminoglycoside resistance genes under natural conditions. *J. Antimicrob. Chemother.* **18**(Suppl. C):93–102.
38. **Trieu-Cuot, P., G. Gerbaud, T. Lambert, and P. Courvalin.** 1985. In vivo transfer of genetic information between Gram-positive and Gram-negative bacteria. *EMBO J.* **4**:3583–3587.
39. **Vanhoof, R., R. Dierickx, H. Coignau, J. M. H. Hubreachts, L. Kaufman, and J. P. Butzler.** 1984. Disk sensitivity testing for *Campylobacter jejuni. Eur. J. Clin. Microbiol.* **3**:160–162.
40. **Wang, W.-L., L. B. Reller, and M. J. Blaser.** 1984. Comparison of antimicrobial susceptibility patterns of *Campylobacter jejuni* and *Campylobacter coli. Antimicrob. Agents Chemother.* **26**:351–353.
41. **Wang, Y., and D. E. Taylor.** 1990. Chloramphenicol resistance in *Campylobacter coli:* nucleotide sequence, expression, and cloning vector construction. *Gene* **94**:23–28.
42. **Wang, Y., and D. E. Taylor.** 1990. Natural transformation in *Campylobacter* species. *J. Bacteriol.* **172**:949–955.

CHAPTER 9

Antimicrobial Resistance of *Campylobacter jejuni* and *Campylobacter coli* to Tetracycline, Chloramphenicol, and Erythromycin

DIANE E. TAYLOR

INTRODUCTION

In 1988 Taylor and Courvalin (57) reviewed what was known about the antibiotic resistance mechanisms found in *Campylobacter* species. It is not my intention here to describe work already covered in our previous review. However, since that time we have gained a better understanding of two plasmid-mediated resistance mechanisms, namely those encoding tetracycline and chloramphenicol resistance. Consequently I will discuss these studies in detail. Recently progress has been made in understanding the genetic and biochemical basis of erythromycin resistance, which I will also describe in this chapter. The attention of the reader is drawn to the previous chapter (Tenover et al., this volume), which describes a recent survey of the incidence of antimicrobial resistance in *Campylobacter jejuni* and *C. coli* and reviews the mechanism of kanamycin resistance in these species.

TETRACYCLINE RESISTANCE

Incidence of Tetracycline Resistance

The incidence of tetracycline resistance (Tc^r) varies widely depending on the geographic location of the strains surveyed (57). In Canadian surveys completed in the early 1980s, Tc^r incidence ranged from 8% (56) to 12% (23). Wang et al. (68) in 1984 reported widespread resistance (86%) among *Campylobacter* species from hogs (therefore mostly *C. coli*) and considerable resistance (30%) among human isolates (mostly *C. jejuni*) in the United States. In the recent Centers for Disease Control survey of campylobacters performed on strains isolated from 1987 to 1989, 43% of strains were found to be resistant to tetracycline (MICs, >16 μg/ml; see Tenover et al., this volume). Therefore the incidence of Tc^r among clinical *Campylobacter* isolates in the United States is considerable and may be increasing.

Genetics of Tetracycline Resistance

All Tc^r strains of *C. jejuni* and *C. coli* investigated to date encode resistance to high levels of the antibiotic (MICs, ≥ 64 μg of tetracycline per ml and ≤ 32 μg of minocycline per ml) (57). Resistance in both *C. jejuni* and *C. coli* is frequently mediated by self-transmissible plasmids (56–58). The host range of these plasmids is narrow, because they can transfer to and be maintained in only closely related *Campylobacter* species, such as *C. lari, C. fetus* subsp. *fetus,* and *C. fetus* subsp. *venerealis* (58). We found that most Tc^r plasmids are about 45 to 50 kb in size (54, 56, 62). Restriction maps of several plasmids were constructed (54, 56, 60, 62), and the position of the Tc^r determinant on the *C. jejuni* plasmid pUA466 has been mapped by deletion mutant analysis (54, 60).

Tc^r determinants from a *C. jejuni* plasmid (pUA466) and a *C. coli* plasmid (pIP1433) have been cloned and expressed in *Escherichia coli,* and the DNA sequences have been determined (31, 51, 54, 60). These two determinants are highly homologous at the nucleotide level (57) and have been given the designation TetO to conform to the currently accepted designation

Diane E. Taylor, Department of Medical Microbiology and Infectious Diseases and Canadian Bacterial Diseases Network, University of Alberta, Edmonton, Alberta, Canada T6G 2H7.

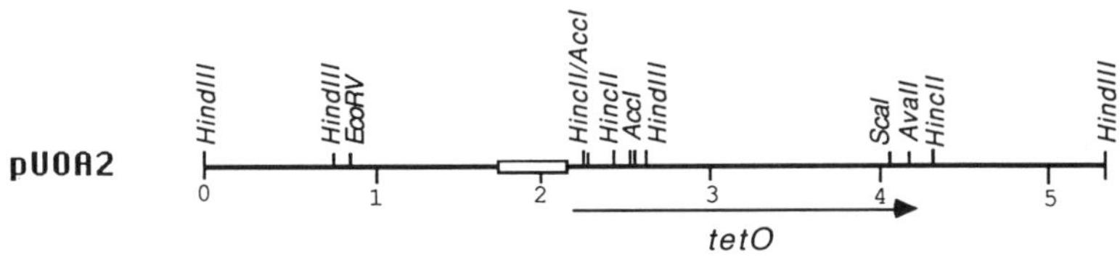

FIGURE 1. Restriction map of pUOA2, which contains the *tetO* gene cloned from *C. jejuni* plasmid pUOA466 cloned into pUC8 (60). The position of the *tetO* ORF and the 300-kb A+T-rich upstream region (open box) are shown. Sizes are in kilobase pairs.

for Tc^r^ determinants from gram-negative and gram-positive organisms (29).

Although Tc^r^ is usually plasmid mediated, we have identified one strain of *C. coli,* UA703, in which the TetO determinant has integrated into the chromosome (35). This finding suggests that the TetO determinant could be carried on a transposable element. The process of natural transformation which has recently been found in *Campylobacter* species (see chapter 29, this volume) was used to test for transposition of TetO into *C. coli* UA585. Chromosomal DNA from *C. coli* UA703 was isolated and used to transform *C. coli* UA585 by natural transformation, using the biphasic growth system described previously (69). After a period of expression in nonselective medium, transformed cells of UA585 were plated on Mueller-Hinton agar containing 8 μg of tetracycline per ml. The frequency of transformation of tetracycline resistance was approximately 10^{-4} transformant per viable cell (61). Four independent Tc^r^ transformants of *C. coli* UA585 were examined by pulsed-field gel electrophoresis to separate chromosomal fragments of UA585 which had been digested by *Sma*I (10). Southern blots, which were prepared from agarose gels containing *Sma*I fragments of UA585 DNA, were hybridized to a ^{32}P-labeled 1.8-kb *Hin*cII fragment of plasmid UA466 DNA, which has proven to be a useful probe for the TetO determinant (35). All four tetracycline-resistant transformants of UA585 contained the TetO determinant in the same *Sma*I fragment (61). The fact that TetO is located in an apparently identical position in the UA585 genome of the four transformants rather than in a number of different positions strongly suggests, but does not prove, that TetO is incorporated via the general recombination processes of the host cell rather than by a transposition mechanism. However, there are transposons, such as Tn*7* in *E. coli,* which frequently integrate into the same chromosomal site (13). Therefore, additional studies are required before the possibility of TetO transposition in *Campylobacter* spp. can be entirely ruled out.

The TetO determinant consists of the *tetO* gene, which has an open reading frame (ORF) of 1,911 bp and could encode a polypeptide with a maximum of 637 amino acid residues and a calculated molecular weight of 72,297 (31, 51). This value is consistent with an observed protein of 68 kDa in an *E. coli* in vitro transcription-translation system and in *E. coli* minicells (31, 60), as well as in maxicell analysis of the cloned *tetO* fragment from the *C. jejuni* plasmid pKFT1025 (66). A restriction map of the TetO determinant of pUA466 which was cloned into pUC8 is shown in Fig. 1. Upstream of the TetO determinant lies a sequence of about 300 bp which is relatively A+T rich (74%) compared with the *tetO* ORF (60%) or *C. jejuni* chromosomal DNA (68%). No potential ORF encoding more than 20 amino acids was found in either direction within this sequence (71). This stretch of 300 nucleotides contains a number of potential promoter sequences. Primer extension analysis suggested that in *C. jejuni* transcription initiates at an A residue 42 nucleotides upstream of the ATG start codon (Fig. 2). Only a possible −10 region located at 73 to 78 nucleotides upstream of the *tetO* ORF was identified, but no obvious −35 region was present. In *E. coli,* primer extension analysis indicated that transcription initiates at an A residue 272 nucleotides upstream of the ATG start codon and both −10 and −35 regions were identified as shown in Fig. 2. Sougakoff et al. (51) identified the TetO promoter sequence for *C. coli* plasmid pIP1433 at 282 to 288 nucleotides (−10 region) and 306 to 311 nucleotides (−35 region) upstream of the ATG codon. Within the 5′-flanking region of *tetO,* 41 nucleotides upstream of *tetO* are two inverted repeats followed by a string of T residues (Fig. 2), which resembles a classical *E. coli* transcription terminator (41).

Although all cloned TetO determinants contain the upstream region (57), transposon mutation analysis of TetO with Tn*1000* dem-

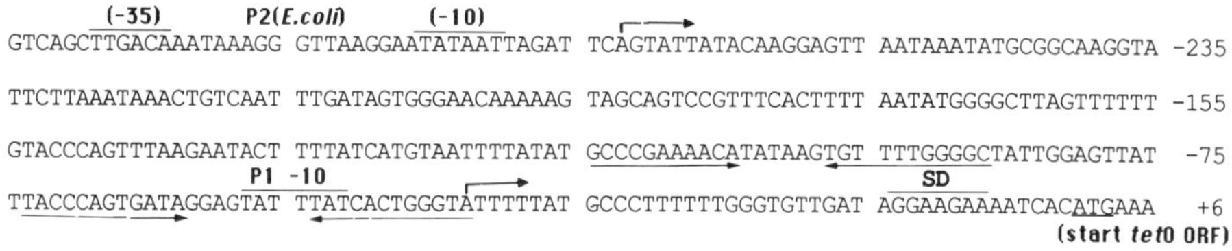

FIGURE 2. Nucleotide sequence of the DNA fragment upstream of the *tetO* ORF. Inverted repeats are depicted by arrows below the sequence. Transcription initiation sites are depicted by arrows above the sequence. The promoter sites (−10 and −35) are indicated, as is the ribosome-binding sequence identified by Shine and Dalgarno (SD).

onstrated that only insertions within the TetO ORF gene gave rise to tetracycline-susceptible (Tc^s) mutants (31, 60). We constructed a mutant plasmid (pUOA2E2) which lacked the upstream region and in which the wild-type promoter was replaced by a LacZ promoter. In *E. coli* the mutant specified an MIC of 16 μg of tetracycline per ml, compared with 64 μg of tetracycline per ml specified by the wild-type plasmid containing the upstream sequence (71). Therefore the upstream region appears to contribute in some way to the TetO phenotype, either by its effect on transcription and/or translation of the TetO protein or in some as yet unrecognized way.

Mechanism of TetO Resistance

Amino acid sequence comparisons of the TetO protein with other known Tc^r proteins revealed that it is completely unrelated to Tc^r determinants from members of the family *Enterobacteriaceae* but is highly related to the TetM determinant originally discovered in *Streptococcus* spp. (8). Tc^r mechanisms have been reviewed recently (44). Briefly, three different types have been reported. In members of the *Enterobacteriaceae*, Tc^r is usually mediated by an efflux mechanism (classes A to E) in which a cytoplasmic membrane protein actively pumps tetracycline out of cells (28). In *Bacteroides fragilis* the class F determinant involves inactivation of tetracycline in *E. coli* but not in the original host species (52). TetM and TetO specify a completely different mechanism which was initially shown by Burdett, for the streptococcal TetM, to act at the level of protein synthesis (7).

Tetracycline is believed to inhibit protein synthesis by binding to a single high-affinity site on the 30S subunit within the 70S ribosome. It may, however, also bind to a large number of low-affinity sites. The major inhibitory effect of tetracycline on protein synthesis is believed to result from blocking of the entry of aminoacyl-tRNA into the ribosomal A site. Goldman et al. (16) showed that tetracycline binds mainly to ribosomal protein S7, but more recent studies have demonstrated that S14 and S19 are also involved in binding (11). These proteins are located within the head of the 30S particle, including the 3′ major domain of 16S rRNA, from bases 920 to 1396, with which tetracycline is also known to interact (33).

Effect of TetO on protein synthesis

We investigated the mechanism by which TetO mediates resistance to tetracycline at the molecular level (30). *E. coli* K-12 containing plasmid pUOA2 (60), a derivative of pUC8 which carries the TetO determinant (Fig. 1), was used in all studies. Both in vivo and in vitro protein syntheses were resistant to the inhibitory action of tetracycline when the TetO plasmid was present in *E. coli* cells. In ^{35}S-labeling experiments with *E. coli* JM107 and JM107(pUOA2), 56 μM tetracycline (equivalent to 25 μg of tetracycline per ml) completely inhibited the incorporation of [^{35}S]methionine into cellular proteins in strain JM107. In JM107(pUOA2) a fourfold increase in the concentration of tetracycline was necessary before in vivo protein synthesis was reduced. Poly(U)-directed polyphenylalanine synthesis in S-30 fractions was used to study in vitro protein synthesis. Whereas 56 μM tetracycline (25 μg/ml) inhibited poly(U)-directed polyphenylalanine incorporation by 75% in an S-30 fraction prepared from JM107, 450 μM tetracycline (200 μg/ml) was required to obtain the same level of inhibition in JM107(pUOA2). Therefore, results show that the TetO mechanism, like that of TetM, acts at the level of protein synthesis.

Ribosome-binding studies

We also tested the ability of 70S ribosomes from Tc^r and Tc^s *E. coli* cells to bind to [^{3}H]tetracycline (30). Ribosomes isolated from

JM107 and from JM107(pUOA2) bound almost identical amounts of [^{3}H]tetracycline. These results suggest that interference in the binding of tetracycline to the 30S subunit is not the primary mechanism by which TetO mediates tetracycline resistance.

Protective effect of TetO on ribosomes

A hydrophilicity profile analysis of the TetO protein suggested that it is moderately hydrophilic in nature (30) and is probably associated with the soluble fraction in tetracycline-resistant cells. We were able to use an S-100 fraction prepared from Tc^r cells to convert Tc^s ribosomes to Tc^r ones as measured by incorporation of poly(U)-directed polyphenylalanine (30). When ribosomes were obtained from Tc^r cells they also provided similar protection when mixed with an S-100 fraction from Tc^s cells. The nature of the protective effect of the S-100 fraction on susceptible ribosomes is not yet understood but depends on the continued presence of the S-100 fraction, since pretreatment of ribosomes with S-100 fractions followed by washing failed to protect the ribosomes from the inhibitory effect of tetracycline.

The available evidence suggests that the TetO protein modifies some component of the ribosome so that tetracycline is no longer inhibitory. The [^{3}H]tetracycline-binding experiments (discussed above) suggest that tetracycline still binds to ribosomes even in the presence of TetO. However, this binding may represent low-affinity binding which occurs at numerous sites. The specific binding which blocks the attachment of aminoacyl-tRNA may be prevented by TetO. Further work is required to analyze high- and low-affinity binding in the presence of TetO.

Homology of TetO with GTP-binding proteins

The amino acid sequence of the TetO protein was compared with known sequences of various proteins of the protein synthetic machinery. TetO showed no homology to any ribosomal subunit proteins (30). The amino-terminal portion of the TetO protein is, however, highly homologous to the amino-terminal regions of several GTP-binding proteins involved in protein synthesis, especially elongation factors Tu (EF-Tu) and G (EF-G) (30). This homology extends to the first 250 amino acids of TetO and the first 200 amino acids of EF-Tu (Fig. 3). X-ray crystallographic studies have revealed that the regions of EF-Tu that show similarity with TetO are involved in the binding of GTP and GDP (22). Amino acids 19 to 28 in EF-Tu, HXXXGKTTXX (single-letter code for amino acids), constitute the phosphate-binding loop (P-loop). Many ATP- and GTP-binding proteins contain the characteristic P-loop, whose primary structure typically consists of a glycine-rich sequence followed by a conserved lysine and a serine or threonine (47).

A Tc^r determinant from *Streptomyces rimosus,* the organism which produces tetracycline, was cloned (37) and, more recently, sequenced (21). The amino-terminal region of the predicted amino acid sequence of the OtrA

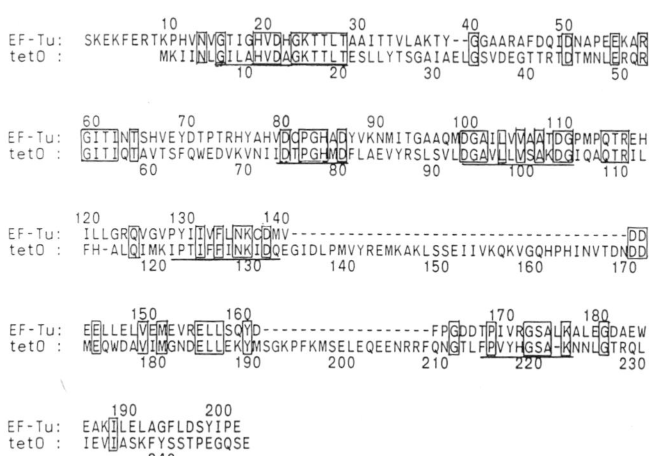

FIGURE 3. Amino acid alignment of TetO (31) and the trypsin-modified form of EF-Tu (22). Regions of complete identity are boxed, and regions of major similarity are underlined.

ORF from *S. rimosus* was also found to be highly homologous with TetM and TetO, although the rest of the protein sequences show little similarity with one another.

How does TetO function?

It seems likely that TetM, TetO, and OtrA bind GDP and GTP and act as GTPases and that this function is critical to their activity. There is no evidence yet to support the suggestion (46) that these proteins mimic the function of EF-Tu or EF-G. Neither of these elongation factors has been shown to be inhibited by tetracycline.

TetO is present only in small amounts in the cell. Attempts to overproduce the TetO protein by cloning the *tetO* gene in expression vectors in bacterial systems have failed (30, 71a). It may be that overproduction of the TetO protein is toxic to bacterial cells. We believe, therefore, that TetO is likely to function in a catalytic fashion. Evidence consistent with this includes the small amount of TetO protein produced in Tc^r cells, the ability of S-100 fractions prepared from Tc^r cells to convert Tc^s ribosomes to tetracycline resistance during protein biosynthesis, and the fact that Tc^r ribosomes are resistant to the inhibitory action of tetracycline even in the presence of a Tc^s S-100 fraction.

Reversed-phase high-performance liquid chromatography (RP-HPLC) as well as sodium dodecyl sulfate-polyacrylamide gel electrophoresis (SDS-PAGE) analyses of ribosomal proteins failed to detect the presence of TetO either associated with the ribosomes or in the S-100 fraction (30). Therefore, although TetO appears to be acting in a catalytic fashion, its precise function remains a matter of speculation. TetO may modify one or more ribosomal proteins or the 16S rRNA. Subtle changes, such as acetylation, methylation, or phosphorylation of protein(s) or methylation of rRNA, would probably not be detected by RP-HPLC or SDS-PAGE. Further experiments are required to determine whether and how the TetO protein can bring about such changes.

Origin of the TetO Determinant

It has been suggested that TetO arose in gram-positive bacteria and subsequently spread to *Campylobacter* spp. (47, 51). Three pieces of evidence support this hypothesis. First, the TetO determinant has been found in both *Enterococcus* and *Streptococcus* spp. (26, 77). Second, the G+C content of *tetO* is 40%, which is close to that of *tetM* (32) but significantly higher than those of *C. jejuni* and *C. coli* chromosomal DNA (32.5 mol%) and plasmid DNA (31 to 33 mol%) (31, 59). Third, the presumed Shine-Dalgarno sequence in TetO closely resembles a gram-positive ribosome-binding site (51). Homology noted among TetO, TetM, and OtrA from *S. rimosus* at the amino terminus of the proteins could mean that the TetM and TetO determinants were acquired from a streptomycete and were developed to protect that organism from its metabolic product, tetracycline. The lack of homology in the rest of the OtrA protein sequence suggests that a considerable amount of time has elapsed since the separation of TetM and TetO from OtrA.

CHLORAMPHENICOL RESISTANCE

Incidence of Chloramphenicol Resistance

Plasmid-mediated resistance to Chloramphenicol (Cm^r) is very rare among *Campylobacter* isolates. In the study by Wang et al. (68), MICs ranged from 4 to 16 μg/ml, with 90% of strains susceptible to 8 μg of chloramphenicol per ml. Similarly, in the Centers for Disease Control study (chapter 8, this volume), no strains were found with chloramphenicol MICs of more than 8 μg/ml. In Japan, however, Sagara et al. (43) identified a Cm^r strain of *C. coli*, for which the MIC was 100 μg/ml.

Genetic and Molecular Studies of Chloramphenicol Resistance

Sagara et al. cloned and expressed high-level chloramphenicol resistance from the *C. coli* plasmid in *E. coli* (43). Using the cloned fragment from this *C. coli* plasmid, kindly supplied to us by R. Nakaya as plasmid pNR9013, we sequenced the Cm^r determinant (70). The MIC of chloramphenicol for *E. coli* K-12(pUOA18), which contains the cloned fragment, is 128 μg/ml (71a). The Cm^r determinant contained an ORF of 621 bp, which could code for a polypeptide of 207 amino acids with a calculated molecular weight of 24,294.

The *C. coli cat* gene exhibited significant sequence homology with chloramphenicol acetyltransferase *(cat)* genes isolated from other bacteria (70). It shares about 57% nucleotide sequence homology with other known *cat* genes such as the *E. coli* Tn*9* sequence (49), but it is most closely related to *cat* sequences from both *Clostridium perfringens* (53) and

```
C. coli          1    MQFTKIDI-------NNWTRKEYFDHYFGNTPCTYSMTVKLDIS----KLKKDGKKLYPT
C. perfringens   1    MVFEKIDK-------NSWNRKEYFDHYFASVPCTYSMSLKVDIT----QIKEKGMKIYPA
C. difficile     1    MVFEKIDK-------NSWNRKEYFDHYFASVPCTYSMTVKVDIT----QIKEKGMKIYPA
E. coli Tn9      1    MEKKI--TGYTTVDISQWHRKEHFEAFQSVAQCTYNQTVQLDITAFLKTVKKNKHKFYPA

consensus             M F KID        N W RKEYFDLYF   PCTYSM  K DI     K    G K YP


C. coli          50   LLYGVTTIINRHEEFRTALD-ENGQVGVFSEMLPCYTVFHKETETFSSIWTEFTADYTEF
C. perfringens   50   MLYYIAMIVNRHSEFRTAIN-QDGELGIYDEMIPSYTIFHNDTETFSSLWTECKSDFKSF
C. difficile     50   MLYYIAMIVNRHSEFRTAIN-QDGELGIYDEMIPSYTIFHNDTETFSSLWTECKSDFKSF
E. coli Tn9      59   FIHIIARIMNAHPEFRMAMK-D-GELVIWDSVHPCYTVFHEQTETFSSLWSEYHDDFROF

consensus              LY     I NRH EFRTA     G      EM P YT FH  TETFSS WTE   D   F


C. coli          109  LQNYQKDIDAFGERMGMSAKPNPPENTFPVSMIPWISFEGFNLNLKKGYDYLLPIFTFGK
C. perfringens   109  LADYESDTQRYGNNHRMEGKPNAPENIFNVSMIPWSTFDGFNLNLQKGYDYLIPIFTMGK
C. difficile     109  LADYESDTQRYGNNHRMEGKPNAPENIFNVSMIPWSTFDGFNLNLQKGYDYLIPIFTMGK
E. coli Tn9      117  LHIYSQDVACYGENLAYFPKGFI-ENMFFVSANPWVSFTSFDLNVANMDNFFAPVFTMGK

consensus             L  Y  D    G     M  KPN  PEN F VSMIPW   F GFNLNL KGYDYL PIFT GK


C. coli          168  YYEEGGKYYIPLSIQVHHAVCDGFHVCRFLDELQDLL-NK
C. perfringens   168  IIKKDNKIILPLAIQVHHAVCDGFHICRFVNELQELI-IV--TQVC-L
C. difficile     168  IIKKDNKIILNLAIQVHHAVCDGFHICRFVNELQELI-IV--TQVC-L
E. coli Tn9      175  YYTQGDKVLMPLAIQVHHAVCDGFHVGRMLNELQQYC-DEWQGG---A

consensus                   K   L IQVHHAVCDGFH RF  ELQ L
```

FIGURE 4. Amino acid alignment of the *C. coli* CAT monomer with CAT monomers from *Clostridium perfringens, Clostridium difficile,* and *E. coli* Tn*9*. The consensus sequence of the *C. coli* and clostridial determinants is shown below the main sequences. Underlining indicates that the identity extends to the *E. coli* Tn*9* CAT. The sequence consisting of PLAIQVHHAVCDGFH, close to the C terminus (shaded), is highly conserved and is believed to be part of the active center of the enzyme.

Clostridium difficile (73), with which it shares about 67% identity. Similarly, at the amino acid level, the *C. coli* chloramphenicol acetyltransferase (CAT) shared 44% identity with all other CAT amino acid sequences except the *C. perfringens* and *C. difficile* CAT sequences which showed 57% homology. If amino acids of similar chemical structure are considered, the *C. coli* CAT also exhibited greatest homology with the clostridial CAT enzymes (73%). The sequence consisting of PLSIQVHHAVCDGFH close to the C terminus (Fig. 4) is highly conserved and is believed to be part of the active center of the enzyme (27, 49).

Plasmid pYW69, which consists of pUC13 into which was cloned a portion of pNR9013 containing the *cat* gene (70), was introduced into *E. coli* CSR603 for maxicell analysis (45). Labeled proteins were examined by SDS-PAGE. The *cat* gene encodes a protein of 23.5 kDa identified as CAT, which is produced constitutively in fairly large amounts. Directly downstream of the *cat* gene is an *aphA-3* gene which specifies a type 3 aminoglycoside phosphotransferase observed as a 31.5-kDa polypeptide in maxicells (70). It appears that in this plasmid the *aphA-3* gene is transcribed from the *cat* promoter, since the *aphA-3* gene in pNR9013 does not have the promoter sequence found in the *aphA-3* gene in the *C. coli* plasmid pIP1433 (67).

There are two pairs of 12-bp direct repeats upstream of the *cat* gene and another similar 11-bp direct repeat downstream of the *aphA-3* gene. Although these structures suggest that the Cm^r and Km^r determinants could be located on a transposable element, we have found no evidence of transposition of these determinants in either *E. coli* or *C. coli* (61).

Origin of Chloramphenicol Resistance in *Campylobacter* spp.

Studies of evolutionary relationships among *cat* genes from different bacteria by using evolutionary parsimony analysis (18) indicate that the plasmid-encoded *cat* genes from *C. coli, C. perfringens,* and *C. difficile* have evolved from a common ancestor (4). Perhaps *C. coli* has acquired the *cat* gene from the clostridia.

STREPTOMYCIN RESISTANCE

The incidence of resistance to streptomycin is rarely reported in surveys of susceptibility patterns. Therefore it is not possible to comment on the incidence of streptomycin resistance in campylobacters. Resistance to streptomycin in three strains of *C. jejuni* and three strains of *C. coli* was clearly shown to be due to an acetyltransferase [AAD(6)] which confers resistance to streptomycin but not spectinomycin (39). A DNA probe for the *aadE* gene from gram-positive cocci, which encodes a 6-aminoglycoside adenylyltransferase, hybridized with all six streptomycin-resistant (Str^r) strains. Another *Campylobacter*-like strain resistant to both streptomycin and spectinomycin hybridized to a DNA probe for the *aadA* probe (3″,9-aminoglycoside adenylyltransferase) commonly found in gram-negative bacteria (19). Therefore campylobacters seem to have acquired genes specifying enzymes that inactivate these aminoglycosides from both gram-negative and gram-positive organisms.

Besides the acquisition of genes encoding inactivating enzymes, *Campylobacter* spp. can also mutate to streptomycin resistance. Spontaneous mutants of *C. coli* UA417, designated UA417R, which are Str^r, were isolated by plating fresh cells onto Mueller-Hinton agar containing 10 μg of streptomycin per ml. The mutation frequency for Str^r in UA417 was $<10^{-9}$ per viable cell plated (69).

The Str^r marker from UA417R can be transformed by the process of natural transformation to *C. coli* UA417 at frequencies of approximately 4×10^{-4} transformant per viable cell (69). The position of the Str^r marker on the genome of UA417R was mapped by combining pulsed-field gel electrophoresis of UA417R DNA with natural transformation. DNA fragments of the UA417R genome were extracted from low-melting-point agarose and used to transform *C. coli* UA417. Analysis of Str^r transformants enabled us to map the approximate position of the Str^r determinant on the *C. coli* UA417 genome (Fig. 5).

Mutational resistance to streptomycin in *E. coli* is usually due to a change in the L12 ribosomal protein, which prevents the binding of the antibiotic to its target site (15). The StrA mutation maps to the *rpsL* gene at 73 min on the *E. coli* genetic map (3). A DNA probe containing the *E. coli rpsL* gene (pNO2005) (40) did not hybridize to the DNA fragment in the genome of *C. coli* UA417R which was associated with Str^r, but to another DNA fragment (63). Therefore the mutation in *C. coli* which results in Str^r appears to be in a different ribosomal protein gene from that of the StrA mutation in *E. coli.*

ERYTHROMYCIN RESISTANCE

Incidence of Erythromycin Resistance

In the recent CDC survey of *Campylobacter* isolates, 2.4% of strains were found to be resistant to erythromycin (MIC, $\geq$16 μg/ml) (Tenover et al., this volume). This value is comparable with findings of $\leq$1% erythromycin-resistant (Ery^r) strains from Canadian sources (23, 56) and with 3% Ery^r strains of *C. jejuni* from the United States (68). In the latter study Wang et al. noted a greater incidence of erythromycin resistance among *C. coli* isolates, with 70% of isolates from hogs found to be resistant (MIC, $>$32 μg/ml). Several studies have also demonstrated that erythromycin resistance is more usually associated with *C. coli* than with *C. jejuni* (9, 24, 64).

We recently tested 15 Ery^r *Campylobacter* strains from Canadian and European sources. Only 2 of 15 were identified as *C. jejuni,* whereas the rest were *C. coli* (55). The MICs for all strains were $\geq$1,024 μg of erythromycin per ml. As reported previously, these strains show cross-resistance to spiramycin, lincomycin, and clindamycin (9, 23, 74). They are also resistant to azithromycin (Pfizer Inc.), a 15-member macrolide (MIC, $\geq$1,024 μg/ml) (55).

Genetics of Erythromycin Resistance

Erythromycin resistance in both *C. jejuni* and *C. coli* strains was unrelated to the presence of plasmid DNA and is therefore considered to be chromosomally mediated (57). However, unlike streptomycin resistance, it has not been pos-

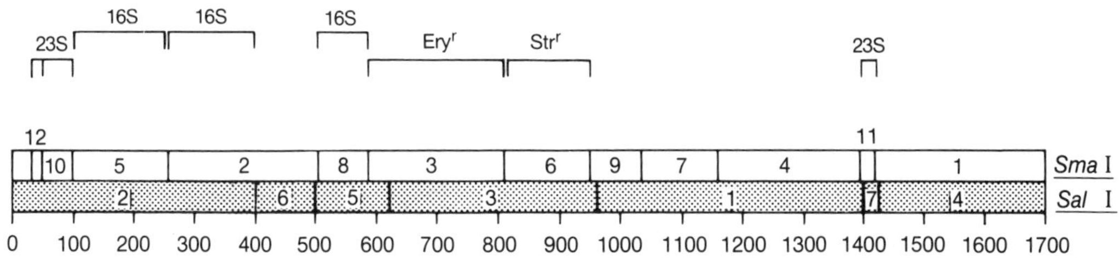

FIGURE 5. Genome map of *C. coli* UA417. The *Sal*I and *Sma*I restriction sites are as shown. Sizes are in kilobase pairs. Positions of 16S and 23S rRNA genes were determined by hybridization with DNA probes, whereas positions of the streptomycin resistance marker (Str^r) and erythromycin resistance marker (Ery^r) were determined by natural transformation (76).

sible to select spontaneous Ery^r mutants of either *C. coli* or *C. jejuni* by plating on medium containing low concentrations of erythromycin (74).

We have been able to identify the location of the chromosomal Ery^r marker on the genome of *C. coli* UA417 by pulsed-field gel electrophoresis followed by natural transformation (76). Ery^r is associated with transformation of the 240-kb *Sma*I fragment 3 from UA585 to UA417 (Fig. 5). Uptake of this fragment from UA585 and recombination between a portion of this DNA fragment and the *C. coli* UA417 genome resulted in the acquisition by UA417 of erythromycin resistance.

Mechanism of Erythromycin Resistance in *Campylobacter* spp.

Ery^r Campylobacter strains have been examined for the presence of the various mechanisms known to result in erythromycin resistance in other species, namely, for RNA methylase genes, for erythromycin-activating enzymes, for efflux of erythromycin, and for evidence of mutations in RNA or ribosomal protein genes. Work was carried out on a pair of isogenic *C. coli* strains, UA585 (MIC, >1,024 μg of erythromycin per ml) and its erythromycin-susceptible (Ery^s) derivative UA586 (MIC, 2 μg of erythromycin per ml). The strain UA586 is a laboratory-derived isolated of UA585 and both strains are plasmid free. Two strains of *C. jejuni*, UA709 (MIC, >1,024 μg of erythromycin per ml) and UA736 (MIC, 4 μg of erythromycin per ml), which were originally obtained from the same patient in the Netherlands, were also studied. These two strains, however, differ in serotype and biotype and in pulsed-field gel electrophoresis patterns of genomic DNA (75).

DNA probes and cloning studies

DNA probes for *ermA, ermAM, ermB,* and *ermC* methylases from *Staphylococcus* and *Streptococcus* spp. (34) and for the *ermE* methylase from *Streptomyces erythraeus* (6), which is also homologous to *ermD* (from *Bacillus* spp.), did not hybridize with DNA from Ery^r campylobacters (12, 65, 74, 76a). These RNA methylases produce an N^6,N^6-dimethylation of specific adenine residues within the 23S rRNA (25) which reduces the affinity of the antibiotics for the target site, the 50S ribosome. The genes for erythromycin resistance are presumed to have evolved from the erythromycin-producing organism *S. erythraeus* (6). This is the so-called MLS mechanism of resistance, where MLS refers to resistance to macrolides, lincosamides, and streptogramin B. The *erm* genes have been cloned from various species and have been expressed without difficulty in *E. coli* (2, 5, 34). In contrast, the *Campylobacter* Ery^r determinant has never been successfully cloned in *E. coli,* despite extensive efforts in three different laboratories (12, 65, 74). Failure to clone the *Campylobacter* Ery^r determinant suggests that the determinant has a recessive phenotype, more reminiscent of a direct change in the target (50S ribosome) than in the acquisition of a RNA methylase.

Induction studies

The ability of macrolides to induce erythromycin resistance was tested in Ery^r *C. jejuni* and *C. coli* strains (74, 76a). Strains were preincubated with subinhibitory levels of erythromycin prior to the addition of high concentration of erythromycin, and growth rates of the cultures were monitored over a 72-h period. No significant difference in growth rate between induced and uninduced cultures was detected. Identical results were also obtained for strains preincubated with lincomycin or oleandomycin. Therefore, erythromycin resistance in *C. jejuni* and *C. coli* is constitutive.

In *S. erythraeus* the *erm* gene is transcribed constitutively; however, in many other organisms erythromycin resistance is inducible (6, 34). In the absence of erythromycin the mRNA for methylase is inactive and the 23S rRNA remains unmethylated. In the presence of subinhibitory concentrations of the antibiotic the mRNA for the methylase is subjected to an attenuation mechanism during translation and active methylase is made (20, 34). This attenuation mechanism is characteristic of MLS resistance.

Thus evidence from DNA hybridization, cloning, and induction experiments with Ery^r *Campylobacter* strains is not consistent with production of an RNA methylase.

Absence of erythromycin-modifying enzymes

High-level resistance to erythromycin in members of the *Enterobacteriaceae* has been shown to be due to macrolide-inactivating enzymes of two types: erythromycin esterases and macrolide 2′-phosphotransferases (1, 2, 36). Therefore, campylobacters were examined for erythromycin-modifying activity. Biological assays were performed on Ery^r and Ery^s strains of *C. jejuni* and *C. coli*, with *E. coli* BM2571-(pIP1527), which specifies an erythromycin esterase, as the positive control. *Staphylococcus aureus* ATCC 25923 was used as the indicator (1). None of the *Campylobacter* strains were able to modify erythromycin and did not allow the growth of the *S. aureus* indicator (74, 76a). Therefore, erythromycin resistance in *C. jejuni* and *C. coli* is not due to the production of extracellular enzymes capable of modifying erythromycin.

In vivo uptake and accumulation of [^{14}C]erythromycin

Resistance to macrolides and streptogramin B (MS resistance) was identified in *Staphylococcus* spp. (42). The protein MsrA, which is the product of the *msrA* gene, was found to contain two ATP-binding domains and to confer resistance by a mechanism of active efflux (42). Resistance in *S. epidermidis* mediated by plasmid pNE24 was also found to result from energy-dependent efflux of macrolides (17). Therefore the ability of *C. coli* UA585 and UA586 to take up and accumulate [^{14}C]erythromycin was assessed (74, 76a). Both strains took up and accumulated [^{14}C]erythromycin, with optimal uptake reached by 60 min followed by a slight decrease over the next 120 min. There was no significant difference between the two strains in [^{14}C]erythromycin uptake activity. Similar results were observed with *C. jejuni* UA736 and UA709. Therefore, the mechanism of erythromycin resistance in *Campylobacter* spp. does not appear to be due to decreased uptake of the antibiotic into resistant cells, such as would be expected to occur if an efflux mechanism were responsible.

Protein synthesis in Ery^r strains

Erythromycin binds to the 50S ribosomal subunit and inhibits protein synthesis (38). We studied the amount of [^{35}S]methionine incorporation into *Campylobacter* cells as a measure of in vivo protein synthesis (74, 76a). Addition of 5 μg of erythromycin per ml to *C. coli* UA586 almost completely inhibited [^{35}S]methionine incorporation, whereas in *C. coli* UA585 [^{35}S]methionine incorporation was unaffected by 100 μg of erythromycin per ml. Similar results were obtained with *C. jejuni* UA736 and UA709. Thus, as expected, the mechanism of erythromycin resistance in *C. jejuni* and *C. coli* is at the level of protein synthesis.

Ribosome-binding studies

Erythromycin resistance in *C. jejuni* and *C. coli* has been studied directly at the level of the ribosome. Binding of [^{14}C]erythromycin to both 70S and 50S ribosomal subunits of Ery^r and Ery^s strains of *C. jejuni* and *C. coli* was investigated (74, 76a). Both 70S and 50S ribosomal subunits isolated from *C. coli* UA585 (Ery^r) bound significantly less [^{14}C]erythromycin than did those from UA586 (Ery^s). Similar results were found with the Ery^r *C. jejuni* UA709, in which both 50S and 70S ribosomal subunits bound much lower levels of [^{14}]erythromycin than did those from UA736, which is Ery^s. As expected [^{14}C]erythromycin did not bind to 30S ribosomal subunits from any of the strains tested.

Does Ery^r depend on changes in rRNA or ribosomal proteins?

The experiments discussed above rule out both inactivation and active efflux of the antibiotic. They also suggest that production of an RNA methylase is not the primary mechanism of resistance. Alternative mechanisms could involve mutations in either rRNA genes or ribosomal protein genes. Studies in *E. coli* have demonstrated that Ery^r can result from a mutation in the 23S rRNA gene when one of the seven rRNA (*rrn*) operons (*rrnH*) was cloned on a multicopy plasmid (14, 50). *C. jejuni* and *C. coli* contain three copies of 23S rRNA genes which have been located on the *C. coli* UA417 map (Fig. 5). None of the 23S rRNA genes correspond to the location of the Ery^r marker in UA417 (74, 76a). Therefore, the Ery^r determinant is unlikely to be due to a change in 23S rRNA gene(s) resulting in decreased erythromycin-binding to 50S ribosomal subunits.

In *E. coli* and *Bacillus stearothermophilus*, mutations in the gene for the L4 protein, which is a component of the 50S ribosomal subunit, can result in erythromycin resistance (48, 72). Ery^r mutants of *E. coli* (*rplD* or *eryA*) map at 73 min on the *E. coli* genetic map (40). Two-dimensional PAGE of ribosomal proteins from the 50S subunit has been used to demonstrate alterations in the L4 proteins in both *E. coli* and *B. stearothermophilus* (48, 72).

Experiments are in progress in our laboratory to search for differences between 50S ribosomal subunit proteins from Ery^r and Ery^s *Campylobacter* strains by using two-dimensional gel electrophoresis. We are also continuing to map ribosomal protein genes on the *C. jejuni* and *C. coli* maps to determine whether any of these are associated with the Ery^r marker. These experiments should enable us to determine whether Ery^r in *Campylobacter* strains results from a mutation in a gene encoding a ribosomal protein.

Is erythromycin resistance in Campylobacter spp. likely to increase?

Erythromycin resistance occurs fairly infrequently in human *Campylobacter* clinical isolates and is not able to be selected at high frequency in the laboratory. This is comforting news for the clinician since erythromycin is the treatment of choice for serious *Campylobacter* infections. However, the much higher incidence of erythromycin resistance in *C. coli* from animal sources and the varied nature of the mechanisms mediating erythromycin resistance in other species makes one wonder whether the incidence of resistance of *C. jejuni* strains to erythromycin will continue to remain low and whether other Ery^r mechanisms will subsequently be acquired by campylobacters.

ACKNOWLEDGMENTS. I thank E. K. Manavathu, S. Salama, M. Eaton, Y. Wang, and W. Yan for their contribution to understanding antibiotic resistance in *Campylobacter* spp. and D. Maher for reading the manuscript. I am grateful to R. K. Read for providing Fig. 3, J. I. Rood for providing data prior to publication, and Heather Mitchell for superb secretarial assistance. Work in my laboratory described in this chapter has been supported by the Natural Sciences and Engineering Research Council of Canada.

REFERENCES

1. **Andremont, A., G. Gerbaud, and P. Courvalin.** 1986. Plasmid-mediated high-level resistance to erythromycin in *Escherichia coli. Antimicrob. Agents Chemother.* **29:**515–518.
2. **Arthur, M., A. Andremont, and P. Courvalin.** 1987. Distribution of erythromycin esterase and rRNA methylase genes in members of the family *Enterobacteriaceae* highly resistant to erythromycin. *Antimicrob. Agents Chemother.* **30:**694–700.
3. **Bachmann, B. J.** 1987. Linkage map of *Escherichia coli* K-12, edition 7, p. 807–876. *In* F. C. Neidhardt, J. L. Ingraham, K. B. Low, B. Magasanik, M. Schaechter, and H. E. Umbarger (ed.), *Escherichia coli and Salmonella typhimurium: Cellular and Molecular Biology.* American Society for Microbiology, Washington, D.C.
4. **Bannam, T. L., and J. I. Rood.** 1991. Relationship between the *Clostridium perfringens catQ* gene product and chloramphenicol acetyltransferases from other bacteria. *Antimicrob. Agents Chemother.* **35:**471–476.
5. **Berryman, D. I., and J. I. Rood.** 1989. Cloning and hybridization analysis of *ermP,* a macrolide-lincosamide-streptogramin B resistance determinant from *Clostridium perfringens. Antimicrob. Agents Chemother.* **33:**1346–1353.
6. **Bibb, M. J., G. R. Janssen, and J. M. Ward.** 1985. Cloning and analysis of the promotor region of the erythromycin resistance gene (*ermE*) of *Streptomyces erythreus. Gene* **38:**215–226.
7. **Burdett, V.** 1986. Streptococcal tetracycline resistance mediated at the level of protein synthesis. *J. Bacteriol.* **165:**564–569.
8. **Burdett, V., J. Inamine, and S. Rajagopalan.** 1982. Heterogeneity of tetracycline resistance determinants in *Streptococcus. J. Bacteriol.* **149:**995–1004.
9. **Burridge, R., C. Warren, and I. Phillips.** 1986. Macrolide, lincosamide and streptogramin resistance in *Campylobacter jejuni/coli. J. Antimicrob. Chemother.* **17:**315–321.
10. **Chang, N., and D. E. Taylor.** 1990. Use of pulsed-field agarose gel electrophoresis to size *Campylobacter* spp. genomes and to construct a *Sal*I map of *Campylobacter jejuni* UA580. *J. Bacteriol.* **172:**5211–5217.
11. **Cooperman, B. S., M. A. Buck, C. L. Fernandez, C. J. Weitzmann, and B. F. D. Ghrist.** 1989. Antibiotic photoaffinity labeling probes of *Escherichia coli* ribosomal structure and function, p. 123–139. *In* P. E. Nielsen (ed.), *NATO Series,* vol. 272: *Photochemical Probes in Biochemistry.* Kluwer Academic Publishers, Inc., Boston.
12. **Courvalin, P. (Institut Pasteur, Paris).** Personal communication.
13. **Craig, N. L.** 1989. Transposon Tn*7,* p. 211–225. *In* D. E. Berg and M. M. Howe (ed.), *Mobile DNA.*

American Society for Microbiology, Washington, D.C.
14. **Ettayebi, M., S. M. Prasad, and E. A. Morgan.** 1985. Chloramphenicol-erythromycin resistance mutations in a 23S rRNA gene of *Escherichia coli. J. Bacteriol.* **162:**551–557.
15. **Funatsu, G., and H. G. Wittman.** 1972. Ribosomal proteins. XXIII. Location of amino-acid replacement in protein L12 isolated from *Escherichia coli* mutants resistant to streptomycin. *J. Mol. Biol.* **68:**547–550.
16. **Goldman, R. A., T. Hasan, C. C. Hall, W. A. Strycharz, and B. S. Cooperman.** 1983. Photoincorporation of tetracycline into *Escherichia coli* ribosomes. Identification of the major proteins photolabelled by native tetracycline and tetracycline photoproducts and implications for the inhibitory action of tetracycline on protein synthesis. *Biochemistry* **22:**359–368.
17. **Goldman, R. C., and J. O. Capobianco.** 1990. Role of an energy-dependent efflux pump in plasmid pNE24-mediated resistance to 14- and 15-membered macrolides in *Staphylococcus epidermidis. Antimicrob. Agents Chemother.* **34:**1973–1980.
18. **Hein, J. 1990.** Unified approach to alignment and phylogenies. *Methods Enzymol.* **183:**626–645.
19. **Hollingshead, S., and D. Vapnek.** 1985. Nucleotide sequence analysis of a gene encoding a streptomycin/spectinomycin adenyltransferase. *Plasmid* **13:**17–30.
20. **Horinouchi, S., and B. Weisblum.** 1980. Post-transcriptional modification of mRNA conformation: mechanism that regulates erythromycin-induced resistance. *Proc. Natl. Acad. Sci. USA* **77:**7079–7083.
21. **Hunter, I. (University of Glasgow).** Personal communication.
22. **Jurnak, F.** 1985. Structure of the GDP domain of Ef-Tu and location of the amino acids homologous to *ras* oncogene proteins. *Science* **230:**32–36.
23. **Karmali, M. A., S. DeGrandis, and P. C. Fleming.** 1981. Antimicrobial susceptibility of *Campylobacter jejuni* with special reference to resistance patterns of Canadian isolates. *Antimicrob. Agents Chemother.* **19:**593–597.
24. **Karmali, M. A., S. A. DeGrandis, D. E. Taylor, and P. C. Fleming.** 1982. On the association between erythromycin resistance and failure to hydrolyze hippurate in *Campylobacter jejuni*, p. 218–220. *In* D. G. Newell (ed.), *Campylobacter. Epidemiology, Pathogenesis and Biochemistry.* MTP Press, Lancaster, United Kingdom.
25. **Lai, C. J., and B. Weisblum.** 1971. Altered methylation of ribosomal RNA in an erythromycin-resistant strain of *Staphylococcus aureus. Proc. Natl. Acad. Sci. USA* **68:**856–860.
26. **LeBlanc, D. J. L., L. N. Lee, B. M. Titimas, C. J. Smith, and F. C. Tenover.** 1988. Nucleotide sequence analysis of tetracycline resistance gene *tetO* from *Streptococcus mutans* DL5. *J. Bacteriol.* **170:**3618–3626.
27. **Leslie, A. G. M., P. C. E. Moody, and W. V. Shaw.** 1988. Structure of chloramphenicol acetyltransferase at 1.75-Å resolution. *Proc. Natl. Acad. Sci. USA* **85:**4133–4137.
28. **Levy, S. B.** 1988. Tetracycline resistance determinants are widespread. *ASM News* **54:**418–421.
29. **Levy, S. B., L. M. McMurry, V. Burdett, P. Courvalin, W. Hillen, M. C. Roberts, and D. E. Taylor.** 1989. Nomenclature for tetracycline resistance determinants. *Antimicrob. Agents Chemother.* **33:**1373–1374.
30. **Manavathu, E. K., C. L. Fernandez, B. S. Cooperman, and D. E. Taylor.** 1990. Molecular studies on the mechanism of tetracycline resistance mediated by Tet(O). *Antimicrob. Agents Chemother.* **34:**71–77.
31. **Manavathu, E. K., K. Hiratsuka, and D. E. Taylor.** 1988. Nucleotide sequence analysis and expression of a tetracycline resistance gene from *Campylobacter jejuni. Gene* **62:**17–26.
32. **Martin, P., P. Trieu-Cuot, and P. Courvalin.** 1986. Nucleotide sequence of the *tetM* tetracycline resistance determinant of the streptococcal conjugative shuttle transposon Tn*1545. Nucleic Acids Res.* **14:**7047–7058.
33. **Moazed, D., and H. F. Noller.** 1987. Interaction of antibiotics with functional sites in 16S ribosomal RNA. *Nature* (London) **327:**389–394.
34. **Murphy, E. 1985. Nucleotide sequence of** *ermA*, a macrolide-lincosamide-streptogramin B determinant in *Staphylococcus aureus. J. Bacteriol.* **162:**633–640.
35. **Ng, L.-K., M. E. Stiles, and D. E. Taylor.** 1987. DNA probes for identification of tetracycline resistance genes in *Campylobacter* species isolated from swine and cattle. *Antimicrob. Agents Chemother.* **31:**1669–1674.
36. **O'Hara, K., T. Kanda, K. Ohmiya, T. Ebisu, and M. Kono.** 1989. Purification and characterization of macrolide 2′-phosphotransferase from a strain of *Escherichia coli* that is highly resistant to erythromycin. *Antimicrob. Agents Chemother.* **33:**1354–1357.
37. **Ohnuki, T., T. Katoh, T. Imanaka, and S. Aiba.** 1985. Molecular cloning of tetracycline resistance gene from *Streptomyces rimosus* in *Streptomyces griseus* and characterization of the cloned gene. *J. Bacteriol.* **161:**1010–1016.
38. **Peska, S.** 1977. Inhibitors of protein synthesis, p. 468–553. *In* H. Weissbach and S. Peska (ed.), *Molecular Mechanisms of Protein Biosynthesis.* Academic Press, Inc., New York.
39. **Pinto-Alphandary, H., C. Mabilat, and P. Courvalin.** 1990. Emergence of aminoglycoside resistance genes *aadA* and *aadE* in the genus *Campylobacter. Antimicrob. Agents Chemother.* **34:**1294–1296.
40. **Post, L. E., and M. Nomura.** 1980. DNA sequences from the *str* operon of *Escherichia coli. J. Biol. Chem.* **255:**4660–4666.
41. **Rosenberg, M., and D. Court.** 1979. Regulatory sequences involved in the promotion and termination of RNA transcription. *Annu. Rev. Genet.* **13:**319–353.
42. **Ross, J. I., E. A. Eady, J. H. Cove, W. J. Cundliffe, S. Baumberg, and J. C. Wootton.** 1990. Inducible

erythromycin resistance in staphylococci is encoded by a member of the ATP-binding transport super-gene family. *Mol. Microbiol.* **7**:1207–1214.

43. **Sagara, K., A. Mochizuki, N. Okamura, and R. Nakaya.** 1987. Antimicrobial resistance of *Campylobacter jejuni* and *Campylobacter coli* with special reference to plasmid profiles of Japanese clinical isolates. *Antimicrob. Agents Chemother.* **31**:713–719.
44. **Salyers, A. A., B. S. Speer, and N. B. Shoemaker.** 1990. New perspectives in tetracycline resistance. *Mol. Microbiol.* **4**:151–156.
45. **Sancar, A., A. M. Hack, and W. D. Rupp.** 1979. Simple method for identification of plasmid-coded proteins. *J. Bacteriol.* **137**:692–693.
46. **Sanchez-Pescador, R., J. T. Brown, M. Roberts, and M. S. Urdea.** 1988. Homology of the TetM with translational elongation factors: implication for potential modes of tetM conferred tetracycline resistance. *Nucleic Acids Res.* **16**:1218.
47. **Saraste, M., P. R. Sibbald, and A. Wittinghofer.** 1990. The P-loop—a common motif in ATP- and GTP-binding proteins. *Trends Biochem. Sci.* **15**:430–434.
48. **Schnier, J., H.-S. Gewitz, S.-E. Behrens, A. Lee, C. Ginther, and T. Leighton.** 1990. Isolation and characterization of *Bacillus stearothermophilus* 30S and 50S ribosomal protein mutations. *J. Bacteriol.* **172**:7306–7309.
49. **Shaw, W. V.** 1983. Chloramphenicol acetyltransferase: enzymology and molecular biology. *Crit. Rev. Biochem.* **14**:1–47.
50. **Sigmund, C. D., and E. A. Morgan.** 1982. Erythromycin resistance due to a mutation in a ribosomal RNA operon of *Escherichia coli. Proc. Natl. Acad. Sci. U.S.A.* **79**:5602–5606.
51. **Sougakoff, W., B. Papadopoulou, P. Nordmann, and P. Courvalin.** 1987. Nucleotide sequence and distribution of gene *tetO* encoding tetracycline resistance in *Campylobacter coli. FEMS Microbiol. Lett.* **44**:153–159.
52. **Speer, B. S., and A. A. Salyers.** 1989. Novel aerobic tetracycline resistance gene that clinically modifies tetracycline. *J. Bacteriol.* **171**:148–153.
53. **Steffen, C., and H. Matzura.** 1989. Nucleotide sequence analysis of a chloramphenicol-acetyltransferase gene from *Clostridium perfringens. Gene* **75**:349–354.
54. **Taylor, D. E.** 1986. Plasmid-mediated tetracycline resistance in *Campylobacter jejuni:* expression in *Escherichia coli* and identification of homology with streptococcal class M determinant. *J. Bacteriol.* **165**:1037–1039.
55. **Taylor, D. E., and N. Chang.** 1991. In vitro susceptibilities of *Campylobacter jejuni* and *Campylobacter coli* to azithromycin and erythromycin. *Antimicrob. Agents Chemother.* **35**:1917–1918.
56. **Taylor, D. E., N. Chang, R. S. Garner, R. Sherburne, and L. Mueller.** 1986. Incidence and antibiotic resistance and characterization of plasmids in *Campylobacter jejuni* isolated from clinical sources in Alberta, Canada. *Can. J. Microbiol.* **32**:28–32.
57. **Taylor, D. E., and P. Courvalin.** 1988. Mechanisms of antibiotic resistance in *Campylobacter* species. *Antimicrob. Agents Chemother.* **32**:1107–1112.
58. **Taylor, D. E., S. A. DeGrandis, M. A. Karmali, and P. C. Fleming.** 1981. Transmissible plasmids from *Campylobacter jejuni. Antimicrob. Agents Chemother.* **19**:831–835.
59. **Taylor, D. E., R. S. Garner, and B. J. Allan.** 1983. Characterization of tetracycline resistance plasmids from *Campylobacter jejuni* and *Campylobacter coli. Antimicrob. Agents Chemother.* **24**:930–935.
60. **Taylor, D. E., K. Hiratsuka, H. Ray, and E. K. Manavathu.** 1987. Characterization and expression of a cloned tetracycline resistance determinant from *Campylobacter jejuni* plasmid pUA466. *J. Bacteriol.* **169**:2984–2989.
61. **Taylor, D. E., S. Salama, and Y. Wang.** Unpublished data.
62. **Taylor, D. E., W. Yan, L.-K. Ng, E. K. Manavathu, and P. Courvalin.** 1988. Genetic characterization of kanamycin resistance in *Campylobacter coli. Ann. Inst. Pasteur Microbiol.* **139**:665–676.
63. **Taylor, D. E., W. Yan, and M. Eaton.** Unpublished data.
64. **Taylor, D. N., M. J. Blaser, P. E. Echeverria, C. Pitarangsi, L. Bodhidatta, and W.-L. L. Wang.** 1987. Erythromycin-resistant *Campylobacter* infections in Thailand. *Antimicrob. Agents Chemother.* **31**:438–442.
65. **Tenover, F. C. (Centers for Disease Control, Atlanta, Ga.).** Personal communication.
66. **Tenover, F. C., D. J. LeBlanc, and P. Elvrum.** 1987. Cloning and expression of a tetracycline resistance determinant from *Campylobacter jejuni* and *Escherichia coli. Antimicrob. Agents Chemother.* **31**:1301–1306.
67. **Trieu-Cuot, P., G. Gerbaud, T. Lambert, and P. Courvalin.** 1985. In vivo transfer of genetic information between gram-positive and gram-negative bacteria. *EMBO J.* **4**:3583–3587.
68. **Wang, W.-L. L., L. B. Reller, and M. J. Blaser.** 1984. Comparison of antimicrobial susceptibility patterns of *Campylobacter jejuni* and *Campylobacter coli. Antimicrob. Agents Chemother.* **26**:351–353.
69. **Wang, Y., and D. E. Taylor.** 1990. Natural transformation of *Campylobacter* species. *J. Bacteriol.* **172**:949–955.
70. **Wang, Y., and D. E. Taylor.** 1990. Chloramphenicol resistance in *Campylobacter coli:* nucleotide sequence, expression, and cloning vector construction. *Gene* **94**:23–28.
71. **Wang, Y., and D. E. Taylor.** 1991. A DNA sequence upstream of the *tet* (O) gene is required for full expression of tetracycline resistance. *Antimicrob. Agents Chemother.* **35**:2020–2025.

71a. **Wang, Y., and D. E. Taylor.** Unpublished data.

72. **Wittman, H. G., G. Stoffler, D. Apirion, L. Rosen, K. Tanaka, M. Tamaki, R. Takata, S. Dekio, E. Otaka, and S. Osawa.** 1973. Biochemical and genetic studies on two different types of erythromycin resistant mutants of *Escherichia coli* with

altered ribosomal proteins. *Mol. Gen. Genet.* **127**:175–189.

73. **Wren, B. W., P. Mullany, C. Clayton, and S. Tabaqchali.** 1989. Nucleotide sequence of a chloramphenicol acetyltransferase gene from *Clostridium difficile. Nucleic Acids Res.* **17**: 4877.
74. **Yan, W.** 1990. Characterization of erythromycin resistance in *Campylobacter* spp. Ph.D. thesis, University of Alberta, Edmonton, Alberta, Canada.
75. **Yan, W., N. Chang, and D. E. Taylor.** Pulsed-field gel electrophoresis of *Campylobacter jejuni* and *Campylobacter coli* genomic DNA and its epidemiological application. *J. Infect. Dis.* **163**:1068–1072.
76. **Yan, W., and D. E. Taylor.** 1991. Sizing and mapping of the genome of *Campylobacter coli* strain UA417R using pulsed-field gel electrophoresis. *Gene* **101**:117–120.

76a. **Yan, W., and D. E. Taylor.** 1991. Characterization of erythromycin resistance in *Campylobacter jejuni* and *Campylobacter coli. Antimicrob. Agents Chemother.* **35**:1989–1996.

77. **Zilhao, R., B. Papadopoulou, and P. Courvalin.** 1988. Occurrence of the *Campylobacter* resistance gene *tetO* in *Enterococcus* and *Streptococcus* spp. *Antimicrob. Agents Chemother.* **32**:1793–1796.

III. CLINICAL MICROBIOLOGY

Chapter 10

Diagnosis of *Campylobacter* Infections

Bertil Kaijser and Francis Mégraud

ISOLATION

Isolation of *Campylobacter* species from clinical specimens is considered to be the gold standard for diagnosis despite other means of detection. Several parameters are important for culture isolation: (i) culture medium, including growth and selective supplements; (ii) temperature; and (iii) atmosphere of incubation.

Many protocols have been proposed since the first isolation from stool samples by Dekeyser et al. (5). The main question for the clinical microbiologists is that of which technique should be used. This depends upon the goal that one wishes to achieve. Considering that *Campylobacter jejuni* subsp. *jejuni* causes the majority of enteric infections due to *Campylobacter* spp., several selective media incubated at 42°C could be used. The medium of choice should be a blood-free charcoal-based medium such as that proposed by Karmali et al. (13) and Bolton and Coates (1), an alternative being the semisolid medium developed by Goossens et al. (8). In a recent study comparing six media for the isolation of *Campylobacter* spp. from stool specimens, Endtz et al. (6) obtained the best detection rate with two charcoal-based media (87 and 83%). Antimicrobial agents such as rifampin, polymyxin, and cephalothin should be avoided because of the susceptibility of some isolates, which can lead to false-negative results.

If the goal is to isolate most of the known *Campylobacter* spp. in addition to *C. jejuni* subsp. *jejuni,* a selective medium alone is not sufficient. In this case, as discussed by Goossens and Butzler (this volume), the technique of choice is filtration (19, 22, 36), but because of its low sensitivity, it cannot be used alone. False-negative results will be obtained with stool samples containing fewer than 10^4 organisms per g of stool. Specimens processed by filtration should be incubated at 37°C because some of the unusual *Campylobacter* spp. are not thermophilic. The cost-effectiveness of culture methods must also be considered. Even though it is possible to decrease the cost by testing several specimens on the same plate, filters can be expensive.

In addition to primary plating, some investigators have suggested the use of enrichment broth cultures. We have compared enrichment by the two techniques mentioned above. In our experience, enrichment broth culture was less effective than selective plate culture (Karmali's medium). However, when enrichment was combined with the selective medium, it improved the efficiency and was helpful in detecting small numbers of *Campylobacter* cells (35).

In summary, a selective medium is sufficient for routine diagnosis, but it is important that in some settings a filtration method should also be included to detect species other than *C. jejuni* subsp. *jejuni* and *C. coli.* Enrichment may be useful when the sample has not been transported under optimal conditions or when very few bacteria are expected in the original fecal sample (35).

Molecular biologic approaches to direct detection of *Campylobacter* cells in stool samples may play a role in the future and displace culture techniques. The main problem with assays described so far is test sensitivity. Direct detection systems seem to have a sensitivity in the range of 10^5 organisms per g of stool (39, 41). DNA extraction is also time-consuming and/or expensive when using columns. In two published studies involving a synthetic nucleic acid probe, the sensitivity was 66 and 82% with 6 and 23 culture-positive stool samples, respectively (24, 40). However, when detecting *C. jejuni* and *C. coli,*

Bertil Kaijser, Department of Clinical Bacteriology, University of Göteborg, Göteborg, Sweden. **Francis Mégraud,** Laboratoire de Bactériologie, Hôpital des Enfants, and University of Bordeaux II, Bordeaux, France.

the tests had specificities close to 100%. Similar sensitivity problems have been described for immunologic detection as well. An intermediate solution may be a short enrichment period beforehand. In the future, the polymerase chain reaction may be an important test for detecting enteric pathogens.

IDENTIFICATION

Some changes have occurred recently concerning the nomenclature of spiral bacteria following extensive taxonomic studies of *Campylobacter* spp. and related bacteria. Two former *Campylobacter* spp., *C. cryaerophila* and *C. nitrofigilis,* have been transferred to the genus *Arcobacter* (43) within the proposed family *Campylobacteraceae* (42). In addition, a group of *Arcobacter cryaerophila*-like organisms has been transferred to a new species, *"Campylobacter (Arcobacter) butzleri"* (14). *Campylobacter* is easily identified at the genus level. Presumptive identification can be made on the basis of the observation of gram-negative spiral bacteria, motility, and positive oxidase reaction. Immunologic tests for culture confirmation have also been described (23).

Phenotypic Approach

Identification at the species level can include the tests listed in Table 1 of Goossens and Butzler (this volume), including that for indoxyl acetate hydrolysis (10). Three groups of campylobacters that are also different genotypically can be differentiated. Within the thermophilic group, identification of *C. jejuni* subsp. *jejuni* can be confirmed by using hippurate hydrolysis. Some hippurate-negative strains do exist (see Patton and Wachsmuth, this volume) and must be differentiated from *C. coli.* Because some strains of *C. coli* may also be nalidixic acid resistant (5% in France, for example), several characteristics may be used to differentiate *C. coli* from *C. fetus,* such as a lack of growth at 25°C, resistance to cephalothin, and rapid coccoid formation. *C. lari* can be differentiated on the basis of anaerobic growth in trimethylamine oxide; however, we have not found this test to be reproducible. Recently some urease-positive variants of *C. lari* with different phenotypic characteristics have been described (21). Another related subspecies, *C. jejuni* subsp. *doylei,* is cephalothin sensitive and may exhibit a weak or negative catalase test. In contrast to other *Campylobacter* spp., *C. jejuni* subsp. *doylei* is nitrate reductase negative. This species usually grows slowly at 37°C and not at 42°C but hydrolyzes hippurate (37). *C. upsaliensis,* formerly called CNW strain (32), has emerged as an enteric pathogen in recent years (7, 27, 38). Its poor phenotypic characteristics makes its identification difficult without the help of probes. *C. fetus* subsp. *fetus,* which is increasingly isolated from feces, can be differentiated from *C. hyointestinalis* by its lack of production of H_2S in triple sugar iron medium. Identification of *Campylobacter* spp. by using detection of preformed enzymes and carbon substrate utilization has been successful in our laboratories (20). A strip using such tests is commercially available.

Genotypic Approach

Because of the small number of phenotypic characteristics that can be studied in *Campylobacter* spp., the variability of antimicrobial susceptibility, and the unreliability of other tests such as tolerance tests, it is sometimes difficult to identify organisms to the species level. On the other hand, nucleic acid probes should provide a useful alternative for species identification since there is little genetic relatedness between the different *Campylobacter* spp. We have developed a battery of nonisotopic labeled probes with acetylaminofluorene as a marker to identify all *Campylobacter* spp. and related bacteria (4), with the goal of identifying in particular *C. lari, C. upsaliensis,* and uncommon species. This approach has also been used to identify other bacterial species (39). In the future, nonisotopic probes should become available for routine identification of *Campylobacter* spp.

TYPING

Since the role of *Campylobacter* spp. as major causes of bacterial gastrointestinal disease was accepted almost 15 years ago, different typing schemes have been established, similar to techniques used for typing of *Salmonella* spp., *Shigella* spp., *Escherichia coli,* and other bacterial pathogens. Several typing schemes have been published (9, 12, 16–18, 25, 26, 29–31, 33, 34), and these systems can be categorized into phenotypic and genotypic methods with various degrees of simplicity and ability to discriminate between strains as discussed by Patton et al. (28).

Because *Campylobacter* spp. are among the most common causes of bacterial diarrhea worldwide (11), often causing epidemic outbreaks, there is a need for simple typing methods. Good marker systems for widespread use in reference laboratories are lacking. Typing is limited to a small number of reference laboratories, even though there are, in theory, a great number of published typing methods. The genotypic methods seem to be the most sensitive markers and have the advantage over phenotypic methods that they measure stable chromosomal differences. Genotypic results are potentially more consistent and can be applied to all species. Plasmid analysis, however, has the drawback that the incidence of plasmids in *Campylobacter* spp. is fairly low (2, 3, 15). Genotypic methods, although specific, are cumbersome and complex and require specialized equipment and training. They appear to be more applicable for research purposes. In clinical laboratories, phenotypic methods seem to be preferred. Biotyping is simple and easily available (17). The ability of biotyping to discriminate among strains is limited when used alone, and this test should be combined with another method such as serotyping (17). Phage typing can provide additional discrimination among strains; however, typability is usually low and the availability of phages is limited thus far (9).

The serotyping methods, based on heat-stabile (29, 30) or heat-labile (17, 18) antigens, are the most sensitive and discriminative phenotypic procedures. They are true epidemiologic markers and offer a rapid and simple method. Furthermore, they have gained international acceptance as a reference method for typing *Campylobacter* spp. The present disadvantage is the fairly large number of antisera for the whole setup of the system and their lack of commercial availability. On the other hand, 10 to 20 antisera from each system could type 70 to 90% of *C. jejuni* and *C. coli* strains (12). The battery of this limited number of antisera could be used in many laboratories, while the total typing system should be limited to a few reference laboratories.

REFERENCES

1. **Bolton, F. J., and D. Coates.** 1983. Development of a blood-free *Campylobacter* medium: screening tests on basal media and supplements, and the ability of selected supplements to facilitate aerotolerance. *J. Appl. Bacteriol.* **54:**115–125.
2. **Bopp, C. A., K. A. Birkness, I. K. Wachsmuth, and T. J. Barrett.** 1985. In vitro antimicrobial susceptibility, plasmid analysis and serotyping of epidemic-associated *Campylobacter jejuni. J. Clin. Microbiol.* **21:**4–7.
3. **Bradbury, W. C., M. A. Marko, J. N. Hennessy, and J. P. Penner.** 1983. Occurrence of plasmid DNA in serologically defined strains of *Campylobacter jejuni* and *Campylobacter coli. Infect. Immun.* **40:**460–463.
4. **Chevrier, D., D. Larzul, F. Mégraud, and L. Guesdon.** 1989. Identification and classification of *Campylobacter* strains by using nonradioactive DNA probes. *J. Clin. Microbiol.* **27:**321–326.
5. **Dekeyser, P., M. Gossuin-Detrain, J. P. Butzler, and J. Sternon.** 1972. Acute enteritis due to related *Vibrio:* first positive stool culture. *J. Infect. Dis.* **125:**390.
6. **Endtz, H. P., G. J. H. M. Ruijs, A. H. Zwinderman, T. van der Reijden, M. Biever, and R. V. Mouton.** 1991. Comparison of six media, including a semisolid agar, for the isolation of various *Campylobacter* species from stool specimens. *J. Clin. Microbiol.* **29:**1007–1010.
7. **Goossens, H., B. Pot, L. Vlaes, C. Van den Borre, R. Van den Abbeele, C. Van Naelten, J. Levy, H. Cogniau, P. Marbehant, J. Verhoef, K. Kersters, J.-P. Butzler, and P. Vandamme.** 1990. Characterization and description of *"Campylobacter upsaliensis"* isolated from human feces. *J. Clin. Microbiol.* **28:**1039–1046.
8. **Goossens, H., L. Vlaes, I. Galande, C. van den Borre, and J. P. Butzler.** 1989. Semisolid blood-free selective-motility medium for the isolation of campylobacters from stool specimens. *J. Clin. Microbiol.* **27:**1077–1080.
9. **Grajewski, B. A., J. W. Kusek, and H. M. Gelfand.** 1985. Development of bacteriophage typing system for *Campylobacter jejuni* and *Campylobacter coli. J. Clin. Microbiol.* **22:**13–18.
10. **Hodge, D. S., A. Borczyk, and L. L. Wat.** 1990. Evaluation of the indoxyl acetate hydrolysis test for the differentiation of campylobacters. *J. Clin. Microbiol.* **28:**1482–1483.
11. **Kaijser, B.** 1988. *Campylobacter jejuni/coli*—a review. *APMIS* **96:**283–288.
12. **Kaijser, B., and E. Sjögren.** 1985. Campylobacter strains in Sweden. Serotyping and correlation to clinical symptoms. *Acta Pathol. Immunol. Microbiol. Scand. Sect. B* **93:**315–322.
13. **Karmali, M. A., A. E. Simor, M. Roscoe, P. C. Fleming, S. S. Smith, and J. Lane.** 1986. Evaluation of a blood-free, charcoal-based, selective medium for the isolation of *Campylobacter* organisms from feces. *J. Clin. Microbiol.* **23:**456–459.
14. **Kiehlauch, J. A., D. J. Brenner, M. A. Nicholson, C. N. Baker, C. M. Patton, A. G. Steigerwalt, and I. K. Wachsmuth.** 1991. *Campylobacter butzleri* sp. nov. isolated from humans and animals with diarrheal illness. *J. Clin. Microbiol.* **29:**376–385.
15. **Lind, L., E. Sjögren, C. Welinder-Olsson, and B. Kaijser.** 1989. Plasmids and serogroups in Campylobacter jejuni. *APMIS* **97:**1097–1102.
16. **Lindblom, G.-B., L.-E. Cervantes, E. Sjögren, B. Kaijser, and G. M. Ruiz-Palacios.** 1990. Adherence, enterotoxigenicity, invasiveness and serogroups in Campylobacter jejuni and C. coli from adult patients with acute enterocolitis. *APMIS* **98:**179–184.
17. **Lior, H.** 1984. New, extended biotyping scheme for *Campylobacter jejuni, Campylobacter coli,* and

"*Campylobacter laridis.*" *J. Clin. Microbiol.* **20**:636–640.
18. **Lior, H., D. L. Woodward, J. A. Edgar, L. J. Laroche, and P. Gill.** 1982. Serotyping of *Campylobacter jejuni* by slide agglutination based on heat-labile antigenic factors. *J. Clin. Microbiol.* **15**:761–768.
19. **Mégraud, F.** 1987. Isolation of *Campylobacter* from pigeon feces by a combined enrichment-filtration technique. *Appl. Environ. Microbiol.* **53**:1394–1395.
20. **Mégraud, F., A. Belbouri, D. Monget, and J. P. Gayral.** 1989. A micromethod to identify *Campylobacter* species. Preliminary results, p. 72–73. *In* B. Kaijser and E. Falsen (ed.), *Campylobacter IV.* University of Göteborg, Göteborg, Sweden.
21. **Mégraud, F., D. Chevrier, N. Desplaces, A. Sedallian, and J. L. Guesdon.** 1988. Urease-positive thermophilic *Campylobacter* (*Campylobacter laridis* variant) isolated from appendix and human feces. *J. Clin. Microbiol.* **26**:1050–1051.
22. **Mégraud, F., and Z. Elharrif.** 1985. Isolation of *Campylobacter* by filtration. *Eur. J. Clin. Microbiol.* **4**:437–438.
23. **Nachamkin, I., and S. Barbagallo.** 1990. Culture confirmation of *Campylobacter* spp. by latex agglutination. *J. Clin. Microbiol.* **28**:817–818.
24. **Olive, D. M., M. Johny, and S. K. Sethi.** 1990. Use of an alkaline phosphatase-labeled synthetic oligonucleotide probe for detection of *Campylobacter jejuni* and *Campylobacter coli. J. Clin. Microbiol.* **28**:1565–1569.
25. **O'Sullivan, N., J. Benjamin, and M. B. Skirrow.** 1987. Lectin typing of clinical *Campylobacter* isolates, p. 102. *In* B. Kaijser and E. Falsen (ed.), *Campylobacter IV.* University of Göteborg, Göteborg, Sweden.
26. **Patton, C. M., T. J. Barrett, and G. K. Morris.** 1985. Comparison of the Penner and Lior methods for serotyping *Campylobacter* spp. *J. Clin. Microbiol.* **22**:558–565.
27. **Patton, C. M., N. Shaffer, P. Edmonds, T. J. Barrett, M. A. Lambert, C. Baker, D. M. Perlman, and D. J. Brenner.** 1989. Human disease associated with "*Campylobacter upsaliensis*" (catalase-negative or weakly positive *Campylobacter* species) in the United States. *J. Clin. Microbiol.* **27**:66–73.
28. **Patton, C. M., I. K. Wachsmuth, G. M. Evins, J. A. Kiehlbauch, B. D. Plikaytis, N. Troup, L. Tompkins, and H. Lior.** 1991. Evaluation of 10 methods to distinguish epidemic-associated *Campylobacter* strains. *J. Clin. Microbiol.* **29**:680–688.
29. **Penner, J. L., and J. N. Hennessy.** 1980. Passive hemagglutination technique for serotyping *Campylobacter fetus* subsp. *jejuni* on the basis of soluble heat-stable antigens. *J. Clin. Microbiol.* **12**:732–737.
30. **Penner, J. L., J. N. Hennessy, and R. V. Congi.** 1983. Serotyping of Campylobacter jejuni and Campylobacter coli on the basis of thermostable antigens. *Eur. J. Clin. Microbiol.* **2**:378–383.
31. **Rogol, M., I. Sechter, I. Braunstein, and C. B. Gerichter.** 1983. Extended scheme for serotyping *Campylobacter jejuni.* Results obtained in Israel from 1980 to 1981. *J. Clin. Microbiol.* **18**:283–286.
32. **Sandstedt, K., and J. Ursing.** 1991. Description of *Campylobacter upsaliensis* sp. nov. previously known as the CNW group. *Syst. Appl. Microbiol.* **14**:39–45.
33. **Sjögren, E., K. Alestig, and B. Kaijser.** 1989. Campylobacter strains from Swedish patients with diarrhoea. Distribution of serotypes over a five year period. *APMIS* **97**:221–226.
34. **Sjögren, E., M. Johny, and B. Kaijser.** 1989. The serotype distribution of Campylobacter in patients with diarrhoea in Kuwait. *FEMS Microbiol. Lett.* **57**:237–240.
35. **Sjögren, E., G.-B. Lindblom, and B. Kaijser.** 1987. Comparison of different procedures, transportation media and enrichment media for the isolation of *Campylobacter* from healthy hens and humans with diarrhea. *J. Clin. Microbiol.* **25**:1966–1968.
36. **Steele, T. W., and N. McDermott.** 1984. The use of membrane filters applied directly to the surface of agar plates for the isolation of *Campylobacter jejuni* from feces. *Pathology* **16**:263–265.
37. **Steele, T. W., and R. J. Owen.** 1988. *Campylobacter jejuni* subsp. *doylei* subsp. nov., a subspecies of nitrate-negative campylobacters isolated from human clinical specimens. *Int. J. Syst. Bacteriol.* **38**:316–318.
38. **Taylor, D. C., K. Hiratsuka, and L. Mueller.** 1989. Isolation and characterization of catalase-negative and catalase-weak strains of *Campylobacter* species including "*Campylobacter upsaliensis*" from humans with gastroenteritis. *J. Clin. Microbiol.* **27**:2042–2045.
39. **Tenover, F. C.** 1988. Diagnostic deoxyribonucleic acid probes for infectious diseases. *Clin. Microbiol. Rev.* **1**:82–101.
40. **Thorne, G. M., A. Macone, and D. A. Goldman.** 1990. Enzymatically labelled nucleic acid probe assays for detection of *Campylobacter* spp. in human fecal specimens and in culture. *Mol. Cell. Probes* **4**:133–142.
41. **Tompkins, L. S., and M. Krajden.** 1986. Approaches to the detection of enteric pathogens, including *Campylobacter,* using nucleic acid hybridization. *Diagn. Microbiol. Infect. Dis.* **4**:71S–78S.
42. **Vandamme, P., and J. Deley.** 1991. Proposal for a new family, *Campylobacteraceae. Int. J. Syst. Bacteriol.* **41**:451–455.
43. **Vandamme, P., E. Falsen, R. Rossau, B. Hoste, P. Segers, R. Tytgat, and J. Deley.** 1991. Revision of *Campylobacter, Helicobacter,* and *Wolinella* taxonomy: emendation of generic descriptions and proposal of *Arcobacter* gen. nov. *Int. J. Syst. Bacteriol.* **41**:88–103.

CHAPTER 11

Isolation and Identification of *Campylobacter* spp.

HERMAN GOOSSENS AND JEAN-PAUL BUTZLER

INTRODUCTION

Campylobacter enteritis has emerged as one of the most common forms of human diarrheal illness. Reports of enteritis caused by *Campylobacter jejuni* and the very similar organism *Campylobacter coli* have risen dramatically in developed countries (105).

Campylobacter enteritis was first reported at the end of the nineteenth century by Theodor Escherich. In several articles (reviewed by Kist [76]) he described finding, in the feces of children with diarrhea, spiral organisms that could not be cultured on solid media. Unfortunately, these articles were published in German in journals such as *Medizinische Wochenschrift* and hence went unrecognized for many decades. King, in 1957 (75), was the first to recognize that these organisms could be associated with enteric disease. Her work was corroborated in Belgium in the early 1970s, when Butzler et al. (21) successfully used a veterinary bacteriological method to isolate these organisms from the feces of children suffering from acute diarrhea. This technique consisted of differential filtration of fecal suspensions through 0.65-μm-pore-size filters which allowed *Campylobacter* organisms to pass through (21, 30). The filtrate was then inoculated onto a selective medium. This, however, proved too time-consuming for the routine investigation of large numbers of specimens. Skirrow, in 1977 (124), published a more simple technique for culturing *C. jejuni* and *C. coli* from stool specimens, which allowed widespread isolation of these organisms. During the 1980s, major advances included the development of improved isolation techniques. Following this progress, it became obvious that the incidence of *C. jejuni* usually exceeds that of better-known human enteric pathogens such as *Salmonella* spp. and that the economic effects of *Campylobacter* infections are considerable.

In this chapter we will discuss various aspects of isolation and identification techniques for campylobacters known to cause human enteritis, i.e., *C. jejuni* and *C. coli.* We will also focus on atypical or "new" campylobacters which have been isolated from human feces by means of a nonselective isolation system and which have been associated with enteritis. It will become obvious that the isolation techniques have a number of disadvantages. Therefore, we will also discuss alternative diagnostic methods, such as immunological methods, and the more recently described molecular diagnostic systems.

The review will not include the recently described *Arcobacter* and *Helicobacter* spp. (140).

COLLECTION AND TRANSPORT

The demonstration of *C. jejuni* in a sample depends on the initial number of organisms, the sampling technique, and the efficiency of the culturing technique. The ability of *C. jejuni* to survive in samples is difficult to assess from the literature. Survival for a particular time depends on the inherent resistance of the strains, the number of organisms initially inoculated into a particular sample, and the size of the sample examined. Very often, details of the procedure are not given, and the reports on the survival of organism are sometimes based on "presence or absence" tests. The reports on the existence of viable but nonculturable forms of campylobacters have further complicated the situation (112).

Many factors should be taken into consideration when preparing to transport campylobacters, as follows. (i) They die slowly at temperatures between 10 and 30°C (1, 9, 32, 45,

Herman Goossens and Jean-Paul Butzler, WHO Collaborating Centre for Enteric Campylobacter, St. Pieters University Hospital, 1000 Brussels, Belgium.

132). Blaser et al. (9) reported that, from feces containing 6×10^6 to 9×10^9 organisms, campylobacters could be recovered after 3 weeks at 4°C, but that when the same samples were stored at 25°C, no viable organisms could be recovered after 1 week; however, Ladron de Guevara et al. (79) reported that they lost approximately 16% of their positive samples after storage for only 24 h at 4°C. (ii) They are sensitive to drying, except under refrigeration (33, 84, 122). (iii) Concentrations of NaCl exceeding 2% are inhibitory (33, 57). (iv) Acidic environments (lower than pH 5.0), such as yogurt, are inhibitory; organic acids are more inhibitory than inorganic ones (26, 29, 45). Finally, (v) they are sensitive to atmospheric oxygen (39, 43, 61, 62, 127).

Thus, if a transport medium is used, it should be possible to maintain all viable campylobacters but at the same time prevent the growth of irrelevant bacteria present in the sample. A transport medium might be advantageous (i) for stool samples when campylobacters are present in small numbers in follow-up studies, when the patient has been treated with antibiotics, or when the stool samples cannot be processed within 24 h, and (ii) for food products and environmental samples (102). A transport medium is also necessary when rectal swabs are being used, not only because of the small number of bacteria but also because of their increased exposure to oxygen (71).

Several transport media have been developed for fecal samples. Wang et al. (144) recommended a semisolid brucella agar with 10% ovine blood without antibiotics. Rosef et al. (116) recommended a SIFF medium for transport of pure *Campylobacter* cultures; SIFF medium is a modification of Stuart medium, with increased osmotic pressure and added starch (119). Luechtefeld et al. (84) transported turkey cecal contents in a Cary-Blair medium with decreased agar concentration (23). This medium was found to be the best of six transport media for the preservation of *C. jejuni* and *C. coli* in turkey cecal specimens held at 35°C; a commercial modified Stuart medium and buffered glycerol saline performed poorly (84).

Wang et al. (145) evaluated many media and concluded that the best transport medium for human feces at 25°C is alkaline peptone water with thioglycolate and cystine (RAPW medium). Sjögren et al. (123) recommended the use of a semisolid motility test medium (24) for transport of human fecal samples. All these experiments were carried out with either pure cultures or samples with a high *Campylobacter* concentration.

Aho et al. (3) evaluated the stability of small numbers of campylobacters at room temperature in four different transport media (SIFF, Cary-Blair, RAPW, and brucella broth with charcoal and ferrous sulfate-sodium metabisulfite-sodium pyruvate [FBP]). They found that SIFF medium was the best for samples with low *Campylobacter* concentrations, although Cary-Blair medium was almost equally efficient.

Storage and transport of *Campylobacter* organisms have also been studied by Monhort et al. (91), who found that the organism survives in animal feces for at least 3 h at 4°C but for less than 2 h at 25°C; the holding atmosphere had no effect on isolation rates. The organism may be killed by toxic metabolites, and transport at ambient temperature may also be the real problem according to these authors.

In conclusion, when stool samples are collected for culture of *C. jejuni,* they should be sent to the laboratory without any delay and stored at 4°C. For stool samples that cannot be processed within 24 h or for specimens with small numbers of campylobacters, such as food and water, a transport medium should be used.

PREENRICHMENT AND ENRICHMENT

The advantage of combining a direct method with an enrichment procedure has been shown by many researchers (24, 34, 59, 70, 85), whereas others have found direct culture to be at least as effective as enrichment procedures (2, 6, 44).

What was said regarding transportation can also be extrapolated for the enrichment of samples: enrichment is seldom required when large numbers of organisms are present, but is essential for isolation from samples with a small number of viable cells (31). Since *C. jejuni* may have a low infective dose (111), it is important that sensitive and specific techniques be developed for its isolation from food, milk, and environmental samples.

The use of a preenrichment period at 37°C, sometimes called resuscitation, may be important in the development of such techniques. Indeed, cells of *C. jejuni* damaged by heating or freezing show increased sensitivity to antibiotics (68) and to hydrogen and oxygen radicals (64, 65) and seem to be less able to tolerate elevated growth temperatures compared with undamaged cells. A significant proportion of a population of injured cells die when they are inoculated into culture broth or selective media, and this loss of viability is greater at 43°C than at 37°C (63).

This may explain why preenrichment at 37°C for 2 h before exposure to selective agents significantly increases the isolation of *C. jejuni* from naturally contaminated samples of river water and pasteurized cow's milk (63).

Humphrey and Lanning (69) showed, however, that if heavily contaminated samples such as sewage or chicken skin are processed, preenrichment has no effect on isolation rates, probably because of competition from contaminants. If preenrichment is used for such specimens, a selective preenrichment broth should be used. Indeed, Humphrey (66) showed that preenrichment of the sample in a selective enrichment broth for 4 h at 37°C prior to incubation for 4 h at 43°C gave improved isolation rates of the organism from chicken skin, presumably by allowing repair of sublethally damaged cells prior to exposure to stress temperatures. Aho et al. (4) showed that when a preenrichment step in 1% buffered peptone water under a microaerophilic atmosphere for 5 h at 43°C was added to the isolation method, it was possible to detect fewer than 100 CFU of campylobacters in SIFF medium to which thawing drip from deep-frozen broiler carcasses had been added.

Several enrichment systems have been developed: alkaline peptone water (134), Bruce-Zochowski medium (19), *Campylobacter* enrichment broth (85), Campy-thio broth (8), Gifu anaerobe-modified semisolid medium (121), Preston medium (17), a semisolid medium (24), etc. There are many conflicting data on the efficiency of these enrichment media; this is probably due to the differences in methods rather than to the performance of the media. In fact, there are nearly as many articles on this subject as there are enrichment media, which makes it difficult to make recommendations about the type of enrichment medium to be used.

Isolation of *C. jejuni* from water may have some specific problems. Rollins and Colwell (112) showed that campylobacters assume a nonculturable state within 3 weeks in aquatic environments at 25 and 37°C. The nonculturable state of campylobacters has serious epidemiological implications because the cells are still viable. It is not clear whether preenrichment or enrichment procedures would allow the isolation of such forms.

Humphrey (63) has shown that for the isolation of damaged *C. jejuni* cells from water by using the membrane filtration technique, the plating medium should contain oxygen-quenching agents, even if blood is added to the selective plating medium; the plates should also be preincubated at 37°C for up to 4 h. In a study on the comparison of three different enrichment broths on two selective growth media for isolating thermophilic campylobacters by combined membrane filtrations and enrichment procedures from surface waters, Korhonen and Martikainen (77) showed that the enrichment time (24 or 48 h) did not affect the isolation frequency of campylobacters but that a longer enrichment time increased the growth of contaminants.

In conclusion, there is an increasing amount of evidence supporting the value of preenrichment and enrichment culture for the isolation of *C. jejuni* from food, water, and other environmental sources. However, we believe that for the isolation of *C. jejuni* from human feces collected from patients with diarrhea, direct culture onto a good selective medium should be adequate provided that the specimens are sent immediately to the laboratory or stored at 4°C until use.

ISOLATION

Solid Selective Media

Effective plating media should have several characteristics. They must support the growth of a very wide range of strains of the particular type required and should, whenever possible, inhibit the growth of other bacteria which are able to form colonies on the same medium. Differential appearence not only increases the chances of successful isolation, but also decreases the number of colonies that must be screened by biochemical methods to confirm the isolation of the organism. The selective media used for campylobacters all rely on antibiotics to inhibit unwanted organisms.

The first selective medium for campylobacters which gained widespread acceptance was that described by Skirrow (124). It consists of a nutrient base, lysed blood, trimethoprim, polymyxin B, and vancomycin. Although campylobacters can grow on media not containing blood, its presence promotes growth. Skirrow's supplement proved successful in his isolation of *C. jejuni* from human feces and is still widely used. However, it has a weaker inhibitory effect on the fecal flora (7), and plates are frequently overgrown by competing organisms, including swarming *Proteus* spp., making identification and subculturing difficult. Subsequently other antibiotic combinations were proposed as selective supplements for basal media (8, 17, 22, 48, 49, 72).

Gram-negative bacteria present in fecal flora are inhibited by including cephalosporins such as cephazolin or cefoperazone, polymyxins such as polymyxin B and colistin, or trimethoprim. Several studies have shown that suppression of *Pseudomonas* spp., as well as of other gram-negative organisms, was almost certainly due to the action of cefoperazone (49, 72). Therefore, it is our opinion that higher selectivity is obtained with media containing cefoperazone than with those containing other cephalosporins.

Skirrow medium and Campy-BAP, containing blood agar base and brucella agar, respectively, contain nutritionally rich ingredients and are therefore likely to contain sufficiently high levels of thymidine to reverse the inhibitory effect of trimethoprim. Skirrow added 7% lysed horse blood to his medium to remove thymidine, but Campy-BAP contains 10% sheep blood, which is low in thymidine phosphorylase. However, at the concentration of blood used, thymidine phosphorylase is likely to have little effect in this respect. Bopp et al. (18) showed that trimethoprim was inactive in both blood agar base and brucella agar even when lysed horse blood or thymidine phosphorylase was added. Trimethoprim had activity when used in combination with the other antimicrobial agents normally included in Skirrow medium and Campy-BAP, probably indicating synergism between trimethoprim and one or more of the antimicrobial agents. Bopp et al. also showed that sheep blood could be substituted for lysed horse blood in Skirrow medium without compromising the activity of trimethoprim.

The inhibitory effect of colistin on the growth of some strains of *C. jejuni* has been shown to be temperature dependent; therefore, incubation of plates at 42°C has been recommended (44). We have studied the effect of colistin on detection of *C. jejuni* and *C. coli* in stool specimens. We modified our selective medium (49) by omitting colistin, and since we were expecting heavier growth of contaminating fecal flora, we doubled the concentration of cefoperazone to 30 mg/liter. We found that the growth of *C. coli* was reduced on the medium with colistin in comparison with the medium without colistin. This reduction did not result in a lower isolation rate of *C. coli* on the medium with colistin, although investigators with little experience may fail to recognize *Campylobacter* colonies if only a few have grown on the primary plate. MIC determinations were performed for all *C. coli* and *C. jejuni* strains isolated during the study, and it was found that *C. coli* was more susceptible to polymyxin B and colistin than was *C. jejuni*. These results concur with the findings of Ng et al. (94). These authors also showed that *C. coli* was more susceptible to antibiotics than *C. jejuni* and that the addition of blood or growth supplements reduced but did not eliminate the inhibitory effect. Primary isolation media should not be excessively inhibitory. When using water and foods, in which *Campylobacter* spp. are likely to be present in small numbers, care should be taken in choosing an appropriate selective medium, particularly if polymyxin B or colistin is included.

For inhibition of gram-positive organisms, vancomycin and rifampin have been used most frequently. Both are showing satisfactory results. Fricker (41) demonstrated that media containing rifampin, even if blood was also present, became toxic to *C. jejuni* and other *Campylobacter* species during storage. Presumably this was due to the accumulation of hydrogen peroxide. Humphrey (67) showed that this could be overcome by the addition of FBP and confirmed that the presence of blood alone is insufficient to protect *C. jejuni* from hydrogen peroxide. Lee et al. (83) found that some components of FBP deteriorated during storage of both dehydrated and hydrated media. Therefore, for maximal isolation of *C. jejuni*, particularly when using media containing rifampin, it is essential to use plates that have been stored for a short time and/or that contain freshly prepared solutions of FBP because this can oxidize during storage.

For inhibition of yeasts, either cycloheximide or amphotericin B is included in selective media. Although we do not believe that either has an advantage over the other, Karmali et al. (72) suggested that cycloheximide at 100 mg/liter was more active than amphotericin B at 2 mg/liter in the charcoal medium.

Bolton et al. (10, 11) discovered that charcoal can effectively replace blood in media for growing campylobacters. Indeed, the requirement for blood in selective media may be a problem for some laboratories, and so Bolton's medium was a promising development pertinent to *Campylobacter*-selective media. Several investigators (36, 49, 72) have shown that charcoal-based media are as effective as blood-containing ones for growing *Campylobacter* spp. and that swarming and effuse colonies are found on these media as well as on blood-based media. Charcoal used in selective media may also be able to neutralize toxic oxygen products (10).

Comparison of the different antibiotic supplements is difficult because, besides differences in their concentrations, there are also differences in the basal media used with the antibiotics. Indeed, Ng et al. (95) compared the quantitative growth of *Campylobacter* cells on blood agar base no. 2 (Oxoid), brucella agar (BBL Microbiology Systems and Difco Laboratories), *Campylobacter* agar base (Difco), Columbia agar base (Difco and Oxoid), and Mueller-Hinton agar (Difco and Oxoid). They were able to show that Columbia agar base and blood agar base no. 2 were inhibitory to most of the strains tested; however, the inhibitory effect of these media could be eliminated by the addition of 7% defibrinated sheep blood. The most consistent and best results were obtained with the Mueller-Hinton agar, and they concluded that Mueller-Hinton agar should be the basal medium of choice for growth of *C. jejuni,* especially when antibiotics are included in the medium. It has also been shown that, besides the basal media used for the composition of these selective media, the agar concentration may play a major role in the results of isolation of *Campylobacter* spp. from fecal specimens. Indeed, Patton et al. (103) increased the amount of agar in *Campylobacter* media to 30 g/liter, which reduces swarming of the organisms.

Martin et al. (85), Ng et al. (95), and Goossens et al. (48) indicated that the increased agar concentration results in reduced colony size; this may explain why Patton et al. (103) reported in the same study that the percentage of *Campylobacter*-positive specimens was increased by 9% when the primary isolation plates were incubated for 72 h instead of the generally recommended 48 h. However, variation in colony morphology (from round, convex, smooth colonies to flat, grayish, watery colonies) may be a result not only of the agar concentration, but also of the moisture content of the medium. Buck and Kelly (20) were able to show that fresh medium produced flat, grayish, spreading colonies but that plates which had been incubated at 30°C for 48 h produced round, convex, butyroid colonies.

Fricker (41) also showed that freshly poured media were able to recover more campylobacters than were media stored under aerobic or anaerobic conditions at room temperature or at 4°C and that the growth of *C. lari* was particularly reduced by storage of media.

Addition of FBP supplement to solid media as described by George et al. (43) was shown to enhance the growth of campylobacters, and a final concentration of 0.05% of each of the constituents has been suggested for routine use (62). The mechanism of action of this supplement is not clear, although it has been suggested that it quenches superoxide anions, which are thought to be generated in the medium and to which campylobacters are said to be more sensitive than are aerobic bacteria (61). Similarly, the role of blood in *Campylobacter* selective media is unclear. It is known, however, that blood contains enzymes such as catalase, peroxidase, and superoxide dismutase (11) which decompose toxic oxygen derivatives. Clearly, if toxic oxygen derivatives are generated within the media, the duration and conditions of storage of such media may affect their ability to recover campylobacters.

Therefore, we believe that freshly prepared media should be used immediately but that if storage is necessary, these plates should be held at 4°C, preferably under anaerobic conditions. These precautions appear to be essential for the optimum isolation of *C. lari.*

A number of studies (36, 103) have shown that extending the incubation time from 48 to 72 h led to an increase in the isolation rate regardless of the medium used. We believe that the incubation time of selective media depends to some extent on the experience of the investigator in the isolation of campylobacters. Skilled microbiologists may be able to recognize small *Campylobacter* colonies present after 48 h of growth on a selective medium, whereas others may need another 24 h of incubation to be able to recognize these colonies. Moreover, if plates are checked after 24, 48, and 72 h, investigators may prefer to proceed to staining after 72 h rather than after 48 h; therefore, we should be cautious about studies comparing the isolation rate after 24, 48, and 72 h.

Semisolid Selective Medium

Recognition of *Campylobacter* colonies on the selective solid isolation media can be difficult for several reasons: first, contaminating fecal flora may overgrow campylobacters; second, the fecal flora may mimic *Campylobacter* colonies; and third, *Campylobacter* colonies may not always appear as swarming flat colonies. Therefore, recovery of campylobacters from stool specimens can be time-consuming; very often suspected colonies will have to be stained to confirm the typical campylobacter morphology. Finally, developing countries are having trouble in isolating campylobacters because supplies of sterile blood are not readily available and because the blood-free basal medium is expensive.

For these reasons we developed a new isolation method based on swarming through a semisolid blood-free selective medium (SSM medium) (53). This SSM medium is composed of Mueller-Hinton broth containing 0.28 to 0.4% agar, cefoperazone (30 mg/liter), and trimethoprim (50 mg/liter). It was found to be a good medium for the isolation of campylobacters from stool specimens at 42°C but not at 37°C, and it performed equally well whether it was incubated in a special incubator (with 6% CO_2, 4% H_2, 6% O_2, and 84% N_2) or in a candle jar.

The SSM medium has several advantages. First, it is very cheap; Mueller-Hinton broth and agar are the only basal ingredients. The use of small petri dishes (diameter, 5 cm) further reduces the cost of the medium, and these dishes are very easily placed in a candle jar (two plates can be put next to each other in a 2.5-liter jar). Only two antibiotics have to be incorporated (inhibition of gram-positive organisms and yeasts is no longer necessary). Second, the cultures on this medium are easy to interpret; plates are read only for swarming, not for organisms. Third, the typical spiral forms of campylobacters were observed exclusively with the SSM medium. Indeed, coccoid transformation, as can be seen with campylobacters on solid media, was never seen in the semisolid medium. Fourth, contamination with members of the fecal flora is much lower than in any other selective medium which has been developed so far. Indeed, only 4.1% of the SSM plates were contaminated with members of the fecal flora versus 29.3% for our new modified selective medium (49), 42.6% for Karmali medium (72), 65.3% for Skirrow medium (72), 59.7% for Preston medium, and 37.6% for the blood-free medium. As a consequence, the time saved with the SSM medium is considerable. Fifth, SSM medium is highly sensitive. Sixth, the antibiotic supplement in the SSM medium did not inhibit the growth of *C. coli* as has been shown for other supplements (49, 72). Indeed, inhibition of *C. coli* is mainly due to the presence of polymyxins, which were omitted from the SSM medium. Seventh, the SSM medium does not require the addition of blood. Commercially available blood is expensive, and the addition of blood can cause variable and misleading results (94).

A disadvantage of the SSM medium is that nonmotile campylobacters might not be identified. Another disadvantage is that it cannot be used for incubation at 37°C in a candle jar. Also, for obtaining single colonies, campylobacters which have swarmed through the medium must be subcultured on a solid medium.

Only one study, published by Endtz et al. (36), has compared the SSM medium with two charcoal-based selective media, two blood-based selective media, and a passive 0.65-μm pore size cellulose triacetate membrane filter technique for the recovery of campylobacters from stools of patients with diarrhea. The authors reported a sensitivity of only 72% after 72 h of incubation in the SSM medium. However, we believe that the results may have to be interpreted with caution because a change in the brand of agar or lot number, as well as is the basal broth, markedly affects the performance of the SSM medium. We obtained the best results with Difco Bacto-Agar and Mueller-Hinton broth (47).

Filtration Method

The filtration method was first used to isolate campylobacters when *Vibrio fetus* (*C. fetus*) was isolated from semen and preputial samples from bulls (107). Similar techniques were used by Smibert (126), Seamon (120), and Morris and Park (92) for the isolation of campylobacters from animal feces. The first reported isolation from human feces was made by using this technique (30). However, with the development of selective media for the isolation of campylobacters, the filtration technique has been set aside until recently.

Steele and McDermott (128) described a filtration method which no longer involves filtration of fecal material through a syringe. With this method the fecal suspension was placed onto 47-μm pore size membrane filters which had been placed on a base medium with blood. Six to 8 drops of suspension were placed on the surface of the filter with a Pasteur pipette. The filter was removed and discarded 30 min after the suspension had been applied. Steele and McDermott (128) used a Gelman cellulose triacetate membrane filter. However, other investigators have successfully used other filters from Millipore (88, 136) and Sartorius (16, 49); cellulose nitrate and acetate are both suitable. Bolton et al. (16) showed that more strains of *C. jejuni* and *C. coli* were isolated by using 0.65-μm than 0.45-μm filters. However, the major drawback of the large pore size is the increase in the growth of other organisms that passed through the membrane (37% of culture plates from the membrane with large pores versus only 4% of the plates from the 0.45-μm membranes grew contaminants). The plates should be incubated for at least 3 days. *C. concisus* needs 4 days for sufficient growth. Although most *C. upsaliensis* strains will grow at 42°C, we advise incubation at 37°C. Indeed, some campylobacters, such as *C. fetus* and *C. concisus,* may fail to grow at 42°C on selective media.

In our department, we introduced this filtration method on 1 July 1986 and have compared it, for the isolation of campylobacters from 15,185 stool specimens, with our previously described solid and SSM media, as well as with the blood-free charcoal medium supplemented with cefoperazone (31). A total of 99 catalase-negative or weakly reacting strains were isolated: these were subsequently found to belong to the *C. upsaliensis* group (51). Ninety-five strains were isolated by the filtration method only. None of the presently available selective isolation media was found satisfactory for the isolation of these strains. Walmsley and Karmali (143) have reported successful isolation of *C. upsaliensis* with their previously described CSM medium, which consists of Columbia agar base, activated charcoal, cefoperazone (32 mg/liter), vancomycin (20 mg/liter), and cycloheximide (100 mg/liter). However, they may have been dealing with an outbreak strain, exceptionally resistant to cefoperazone, vancomycin, and cycloheximide (46). Unfortunately, bacterial contamination of less than 10^5 CFU/g of feces cannot be detected by the filter method. Steele and McDermott (128) suggested that less than 10% of the campylobacters present in fecal suspensions pass through the membrane. Therefore, a disadvantage of filtration might be that it is relatively insensitive (49, 88), so that positive samples with small numbers of viable campylobacters may be missed. Many authors advocate both direct inoculation onto a selective agar and filtration onto a nonselective medium for maximum isolation of campylobacters (15, 89). This, however, is rather inconvenient for the average diagnostic laboratory, and most laboratories continue to work only with selective agar methods.

ATMOSPHERE

All members of the genus *Campylobacter* are microaerophilic, generally requiring oxygen at lower tensions than in air for growth, but tolerance to oxygen varies greatly depending on the species and strain.

The growth supplement FBP improves the aerotolerance of campylobacters (43). Various methods are available for producing the microaerophilic atmosphere; these include the evacuation-replacement technique, microaerobic gas sachets, a candle placed within a gas jar, and even a microaerobic station and incubator for processing a large number of samples. Usually, the replacement mixture contains 10% CO_2, 8% N_2, and 10% H_2. The presence of H_2 has been shown to be beneficial for some strains: Skirrow et al. (125) have shown that the final gas atmosphere should contain at least 7% H_2.

Subculture in liquid medium can be best initiated by using a large inoculum as a lump. Indeed, slow-growing organisms that are dispersed with a low inoculum in a medium are vulnerable to oxygen. Workers new to campylobacter isolation sometimes lose their strains on subculturing because the inoculum for the liquid medium is not dense enough.

TEMPERATURE

Campylobacters differ with respect to their critical and optimum temperature requirements. *C. jejuni* and *C. coli* grew well at 42 to 43°C and hence are often referred to as the thermophilic campylobacters. *C. lari* and *C. upsaliensis* strains also grow at these temperatures and therefore also belong to the thermophilic group. However, *C. jejuni* subsp. *doylei* does not grow well at 42°C, and therefore plates should be incubated at 37°C for optimal isolation of these organisms. All four species mentioned grow well at 37°C and do not grow below 30°C. *C. fetus* grows at both 25 and 37°C. *C. concisus* and *C. rectus* grow poorly at 42°C, but well at 37°C (see Table 1).

DIRECT DETECTION IN STOOL SPECIMENS

Escherich in the 1890s (76) was able to use only microscopic examination to detect campylobacters in stools. Indeed, direct microscopy of stool specimens allows the detection of campylobacters on the basis of their typical morphological characteristics. Campylobacters appear as slender, gram-negative organisms that are comma, S, or spiral shaped; they can be readily observed by using stained preparations of stool specimens, such as the Gram stain, provided that the stools are fresh.

A direct dark-field microscopy technique for the typical darting motility of campylobacters was described by Paisley et al. (101), but its sensitivity was very low compared with that of culture. This was surpassed by fluorescent-antibody technique methods (58, 109), which rely very heavily on microscopic interpretation.

An immunological latex agglutination assay (55, 56), Microscreen Campylobacter (Mercia Diagnostics), allows approximately 60% of positive samples to be detected within approximately 3 min of receipt of the sample. This latex agglutination test is based on the coating of specific polyclonal antibodies on the surface of latex

TABLE 1. Differentiation between *Campylobacter* species[a]

Species	Catalase	Nitrate reduction	Nitrite reduction	H_2 requirement[b]	Urease production	H_2S production (TSI)[c]	Hippurate hydrolysis
C. fetus subsp. *fetus*	+[f]	+	−[f]	−	−	−	−
C. fetus subsp. *venerealis*	+	+	−	−	−	−	−
C. hyointestinalis	+	+	−	V[f]	−	+	−
C. sputorum bv. sputorum	−	+	+	−	−	+	−
C. sputorum bv. bubulus	−	+	+	−	−	+	−
C. sputorum bv. fecalis	+	+	+	−	−	+	−
C. jejuni subsp. *jejuni*	+	+	−	−	−	−	+
C. jejuni subsp. *doylei*	V	−	−	−	−	−	V
C. coli	+	+	−	−	−	−	−
C. lari	+	+	−	−	V	−	−
C. upsaliensis	W[f]	+	−	−	−	−	−
C. mucosalis	−	+	+	+	−	+	−
C. concisus	−	+	+	+	−	+	−
C. curvus	−	+	+	+	−	+	−
C. rectus	−	+	+	+	−	+	−

[a] Data from reference 140.
[b] For microaerophilic growth.
[c] TSI, triple sugar iron agar.
[d] Susceptibility to antibiotics was determined by using 30-μg disks. Abbreviations: S, susceptible; R, resistant.
[e] TMAO, trimethylamine-*N*-oxide hydrochloride.
[f] +, positive reaction; −, negative reaction; W, weak reaction; V, variable reaction.
[g] ND, not determined.

particles. The advantages of latex tests are that they are rapid and simple to perform and do not require laborious microscopy. Sutcliffe (131) evaluated this latex test for the detection of *Campylobacter* species in water. The latex test gave negative results with water samples that were culture positive for *C. coli.* Latex-positive, culture-negative water samples were found for a number of samples from chicken houses. This finding provided no evidence for the presence of viable nonculturable campylobacters in water but is consistent with this possibility.

We evaluated the Microscreen for the direct detection of campylobacters in stool specimens and found the test unsatisfactory. We tested 42 stool specimens, all positive for *C. jejuni* and *C. coli* by culture. We obtained a negative latex agglutination test with seven stool samples and a weak reaction with four stool samples. Moreover, agglutination reactions were also observed with stool samples negative for campylobacters by culture.

As technology progressed, several methods involving the use of DNA probes to detect campylobacters were developed. The first diagnostic campylobacter probe was specific for *C. jejuni* and *C. coli* (27). Subsequently, probes containing radioactive labels for *C. jejuni* were developed (78, 106, 110). The development of nonradioactive probes will further allow laboratories to use this technology for rapid diagnosis. The radiolabeled probes have several disadvantages: the possible danger to health, the short half-life of probes, complicated protocols, and requirement for specialized equipment.

Molecular Biosystems prepared an alkaline phosphate-labeled synthetic oligonucleotide probe in kit form for detection of *C. jejuni* and *C. coli* in stool specimens. Although this kit had excellent sensitivity and specificity for isolated bacterial colony isolates, its main limitation may be the sensitivity limit on direct isolation of campylobacters in stools (96).

Zhou and Wang (147) showed a sensitivity and specificity of 92 and 89.5%, respectively, with a biotin-labeled DNA probe for the detection of *C. jejuni* in 100 chicken feces specimens. However, the whole procedure included an overnight hybridization; furthermore, a limited number of specimens were tested, and no human fecal specimens were included in their evaluation. Other nonradioactive probes have been

TABLE 1. *Continued*

Species	Indoxyl acetate hydrolysis	Growth at: 15°C	25°C	42°C	Growth in the presence of: 3.5% NaCl	1% Glycine	0.1% TMAO (anaerobic)[e]	Susceptibility to[d]: Nalidixic acid	Cephalothin
C. fetus subsp. *fetus*	−	−	+	−	−	+	−	R	S
C. fetus subsp. *veneralis*	−	−	+	−	−	−	−	R	S
C. hyointestinalis	−	−	+	+	−	+	+	R	S
C. sputorum bv. sputorum	−	−	−	+	−	+	V	S	S
C. sputorum bv. bubulus	−	−	−	+	+	+	+	R	S
C. sputorum bv. fecalis	−	−	−	+	−	+	+	R	S
C. jejuni subsp. *jejuni*	+	−	−	+	−	+	−	S	R
C. jejuni subsp. *doylei*	+	−	−	−	−	+	−	S	S
C. coli	+	−	−	+	−	+	−	S	R
C. lari	−	−	−	+	−	+	+	R	R
C. upsaliensis	+	−	−	+	−	V	−	S	S
C. mucosalis	−	−	−	+	−	+	−	R	S
C. concisus	−	−	−	+	−	+	−	R	R
C. curvus	+	−	−	+	−	+	ND[g]	S	ND
C. rectus	+	−	−	W	−	+	ND	S	ND

commercialized; these include the Du Pont probe, which is claimed to detect *C. jejuni, C. coli, C. lari,* and *C. upsaliensis* directly in stools within 4 h of receipt by the laboratory.

DETECTION OF OTHER CAMPYLOBACTERS IN STOOL SPECIMENS

The use of nonselective isolation techniques, such as the filtration method, has made us aware that several species will not grow on selective media designed specifically for isolation of *C. jejuni.* In particular, *C. upsaliensis* has emerged as a new pathogen.

C. upsaliensis has been isolated in humans by several investigators. Mégraud and Bonnet (86) isolated five strains by a filter method in France; these were probably *C. upsaliensis* strains, although DNA hybridization was not performed. They were all isolated from children with diarrhea, either from gypsy families or African immigrants. Three of them yielded significant *Campylobacter* antibody titers in complement fixation tests with a commercial preparation of a *C. jejuni* antigen (Virion). Steele and McDermott (128) isolated eight *C. upsaliensis* strains by the filter technique from children aged 3 years or younger with gastroenteritis in Australia. Patton et al. (104) reported 11 clinical isolates of *C. upsaliensis* that were received at the Centers for Disease Control, Atlanta, Ga., from 1983 to 1986. Three stool and eight blood isolates were obtained from 11 ill persons. Five persons had diarrhea: three had positive stool cultures and two had positive blood cultures. Of the three persons with positive stool cultures, two had acute, nonbloody diarrhea, cramping abdominal pain, and fever; they were treated with erythromycin and recovered rapidly. The third patient had bloody diarrhea. Of the eight persons with positive blood cultures, only two had diarrhea; the others had fever or respiratory infection. However, six of these blood isolates were obtained from patients who had underlying disease and who were immunocompromised (one person had AIDS).

Taylor et al. (135) isolated seven *C. upsaliensis* strains in Canada by using the CCDA medium (14). All the strains were isolated from patients with diarrhea (five were children aged

2 years or younger, and two were adults). Walmsley and Karmali (143) isolated *C. upsaliensis* strains from six children aged 3 years or younger in Canada. Three of the five children had signs and symptoms compatible with gastroenteritis (loose watery stools, vomiting, and anorexia). These investigators have isolated the *C. upsaliensis* strains by using the charcoal-based selective medium (CSM) (72). Lastovica et al. (81) isolated 16 *C. upsaliensis* strains from the blood of ill persons in South Africa by using the automatic BACTEC system. Ten of the patients were younger than 1 year old, and all 16 patients were afflicted with a debilitating illness. Eight patients had gastroenteritis, indicating the possibility that *C. upsaliensis* bacteremias were secondary to intestinal infections with the same organisms. However, stools were not cultured for *C. upsaliensis* in this study. Grayson et al. (54) isolated *C. upsaliensis* strains in six patients in Australia. However, no further information was given for these strains.

We isolated *C. upsaliensis* in 99 patients during a 3-year period (46, 50, 51). There are several reasons why we believe that *C. upsaliensis* can cause diarrhea in humans: (i) it was the only organism detected in 83 patients; (ii) it was present in large numbers (more than 10^5 CFU/g of feces); (iii) diarrhea was present in 71 of 77 patients in whom *C. upsaliensis* was the only organism isolated; and (iv) the diarrheal symptom disappeared when the organism was eradicated by antibiotic therapy in all 13 patients treated.

Recently, we isolated *C. upsaliensis* from a person with bloody diarrhea and from his dog, also presenting with diarrhea. The strains were identical, suggesting that *C. upsaliensis* infection may be a zoonosis. Simultaneously, we isolated *C. upsaliensis* from dogs with diarrhea (52). Several investigators had reported the isolation of *C. upsaliensis* in animals. Sandstedt et al. (118) isolated 63 *C. upsaliensis* strains from asymptomatic and diarrhetic dogs; Fox et al. (40) isolated three *C. upsaliensis* strains from asymptomatic cats.

Steele et al. (130) isolated a number of *Campylobacter*-like organisms, referred to as atypical *C. jejuni* in their paper, from children younger than 5 years who had been admitted to hospital in central Australia with diarrhea. Similar strains were isolated by Kasper and Dickgiesser (73) from gastric biopsies of adults in the Federal Republic of Germany; these strains were referred to as GCLO-2. One similar gastric strain was isolated in the United Kingdom (99). Lastovica and Ambrosio (80) reported on such strains isolated from children with diarrhea in South Africa. The name *C. jejuni* subsp. *doylei* was proposed by Steele and Owen (129). We isolated *C. jejuni* subsp. *doylei* as the sole organism from four children, all with diarrhea; this suggests that these organisms might also be pathogenic in humans. All strains were isolated by the filtration method alone because of their sensitivity to cephalothin.

In 1983, strains of a new species, *C. hyointestinalis,* were isolated from pigs with proliferative enteritis (42). In 1986, isolation of *C. hyointestinalis* from a human was reported for the first time by Fennell et al. (38). They isolated *C. hyointestinalis* from the rectal culture of a homosexual man with proctitis. In 1987, Edmonds et al. (35) reported the isolation of this organism from the stool specimens of four persons, all of whom were experiencing nonbloody watery diarrhea (one child aged 8 months and three adults). In 1988, Minet et al. (90) reported a new case of *C. hyointestinalis*-associated diarrhea in a patient suffering from an evolutive chronic myeloid leukemia. We isolated *C. hyointestinalis* in two patients: in our first case the organism was isolated from a child with typhoid fever, and in our second case it was isolated from an adult with duodenal ulcer. Therefore, we have no strong arguments to suggest that *C. hyointestinalis* is pathogenic in humans. Although we were able to isolate these organisms from our selective medium as well as by filtration, it would appear that susceptibility to cephalothin may be a variable characteristic. Therefore, the use of a cephalothin-free medium for primary isolation of *C. hyointestinalis* would provide for the recovery of strains that exhibit susceptibility to cephalothin.

C. concisus was described in 1979 by Tanner et al. (133), who discovered these organisms in the human oral cavity. Vandamme et al. (139) identified *C. concisus* strains isolated from various nonoral human clinical specimens and showed that these campylobacters were associated with gastrointestinal disorders. Lauwers et al. (82), using the filtration method (i.e., Columbia blood agar incubated at 37°C for 4 days in an atmosphere of 7% CO_2, 4.5% O_2, 7% H_2, and 81.5% N_2), have isolated 148 *C. concisus* strains from stool specimens; none of the strains was detected on the selective medium composed of Columbia blood agar with colistin, cefoperazone, rifampin, and amphotericin B. Most *C. concisus*-positive patients presented with diarrhea, suggesting that this species may be pathogenic in humans.

Other atypical thermophilic campylobacters were detected by Bolton et al. (12, 13) and Mégraud et al. (87), who isolated them from various sources: feces of humans with diarrhea, an appendix of a child with appendicitis, river water, seawater, mussels, and cockles. These organisms resembled *C. lari* most closely. They were named the UPTC group (urease-positive thermophilic campylobacters) and the NASC group (nalidixic acid-sensitive campylobacters). Using sodium dodecyl sulfate-polyacrylamide gel electrophoresis, Owen et al. (100) and Vandamme et al. (139) identified the UPTC and NASC groups as atypical *C. lari* strains. They were referred to as *C. lari* variants. For isolation of these organisms from stool specimens, an isolation technique similar to that used for *C. lari* should be appropriate.

IDENTIFICATION

Conventional Methods

Campylobacter spp. represent a taxonomically heterogeneous group. Table 1 illustrates the characteristics of all *Campylobacter* species based on biochemical tests, resistance patterns, and growth temperatures. The identification of these campylobacters can be difficult since strains have relatively fastidious growth requirements and are asaccharolytic, and since only a limited number of biochcmical tests give adequate discrimination. For example, separation of *C. coli* from *C. jejuni* subsp. *jejuni* relies almost solely on hippurate hydrolysis. However, for both of these taxa, strains that do not give the expected result in this test have been reported (114). The development of reproducible tests that provide good discrimination for such taxa, and indeed for the group as a whole, would therefore be of considerable value.

Resistance to various agents, temperature tolerances, and growth requirements are among the phenotypic tests used in characterizing campylobacters. However, no standard methods for the performance of such tests have been published, and therefore most workers use methods peculiar to their own laboratories. Differences in methods may lead to differences in the outcome of, nominally, the same test. Certainly, such discrepancies have been published for campylobacters. For example, the proportion of *C. fetus* subsp. *fetus* strains able to grow at 42°C varies from 0% (142) to 59% (5). Furthermore, *C. mucosalis* was first described as being tolerant to salt (82a), but the species description was later emended since salt tolerance was found to vary with the test method used (115).

It is well established in antimicrobial susceptibility testing that several factors may influence the outcome (146). These factors include the size of the inoculum and the composition of the basal medium. However, On and Holmes (97) showed recently that the reproducibility of certain tests for certain taxa is questionable, even when the inoculum is standardized in terms of culturable age, optical density, and size and the tests are standardized in terms of atmospheric conditions and formulation. Indeed, test reproducibility proved to be dependent on the basal medium used. In general, the media giving the most favorable results for growth also yielded the most reproducible results overall (blood agar followed by nutrient agar followed by brucella agar).

In their study, On and Holmes (98) suggested that blood agar should be the medium of choice for most tolerance tests used in the identification of campylobacters, provided that important factors (such as the size of the inoculum and atmospheric conditions) are also considered. However, their study was carried out on a limited number of strains, and further work involving a large number of strains is required before recommendations for a particular basal medium can be made.

Finally, we would recommend the following tests for identification of *Campylobacter* species: oxidase; catalase; nitrate and nitrite reduction; urease; H_2S production; hippurate hydrolysis; indoxyl acetate hydrolysis; growth at 15, 25, and 42°C; and testing for susceptibility to nalidixic acid and cephalothin. The least reproducible tests in our hands are the growth in the presence of 1% glycine, 3.5% NaCl, and 0.1% trimethylamine-*N*-oxide hydrochloride. However, most clinical laboratories identify strains only as far as "*Campylobacter* species," which is sufficient information in most cases for the physicians involved. This diagnosis is based on typical colony and cell morphology and a positive oxidase reaction.

Latex Agglutination

Latex agglutination tests have been developed for confirmation of a variety of microorganisms including campylobacters (55, 60, 74, 93, 117). Three products, Campy-Slide (BBL Microbiology Systems), Microscreen Campylobacter, and Meritec-Campy (Meridian Diagnostics), are commercially available latex agglutination kits for culture confirmation. Like all latex agglutination tests, a specific antibody, in this case one that reacts with all *C. jejuni* and *C. coli* strains, is coated onto the surface of latex particles. In the presence of *Campylobacter* cells, these antibodies agglutinate to give a visible reaction. A 30-min extraction step prior to testing is required for the BBL test (60) but not for the Microscreen Campylobacter test (55) or the Meritec-Campy test (93). All three tests have an excellent sensitivity and specificity for the identification of *C. jejuni* and *C. coli.*

DNA Probes

DNA-DNA hybridization has been a successful reference method in taxonomic studies of *Campylobacter* species (140). Several groups have developed probes that recognize *Campylobacter* species. Totten et al. (138) have developed probes that differentiate *C. coli* isolates from hippurate-negative *C. jejuni* isolates. Romaniuk and Trust (113) have developed DNA probes to rRNA targets that can differentiate *C. jejuni* and *C. lari* from other *Campylobacter* species. In addition, Chevrier et al. (25), Cudjoe et al. (28), Ezaki et al. (37), Korolik et al. (78), and Picken et al. (106) have all developed probes for culture confirmation of *C. jejuni.* Fox et al. (40) and Patton et al. (104) have used probes for the identification of *C. upsaliensis.*

The problems associated with radioactive labels have encouraged the development of nonradioactive detection systems. Chevrier et al. (25) have reported on a nonradioactive probe based on labeling the probe with *N*-acetoxy-*N*-2-acetylaminofluoride (AAAF) and detection by using a monoclonal antibody to AAAF. Tenover et al. (137) and Popovic-Urovic et al. (108) have evaluated a Gen-Probe nonradioactive DNA probe, labeled with acridinium esters, that hybridized to an rRNA target. The assay is based on the selective chemical degradation of the label. During the selection step, acridinium ester covalently attached to nonhybridized probe is rapidly hydrolyzed, while the label associated with probe hybridized to the target rRNA is protected. After this differential hydrolysis, the remaining acridinium ester, which is associated only with DNA-rRNA hybrids, is activated with hydrogen peroxide. Under alkaline conditions, light is emitted upon relaxation to the ground state. Emitted light is captured by a photomultiplier and converted to a digital signal.

In both studies, all *C. jejuni, C. coli,* and *C. lari* isolates were correctly identified. The probe did not react with *C. upsaliensis, C. concisus, C. fetus, C. sputorum, C. mucosalis, C. curvus, C. rectus,* or most *C. hyointestinalis* strains.

CONCLUSION

The isolation of strains belonging to the genus *Campylobacter* and its relatives such as *Arcobacter* and *Helicobacter* is often troublesome, particularly because they require incubation in a microaerophilic atmosphere at 42°C and are rather slow growers. The use of selective media has greatly improved the isolation procedure, which has permitted more accurate studies of the epidemiology of *C. jejuni.* These isolation procedures allow growth of most of the *C. jejuni* and *C. coli* strains, but are too inhibitory for the isolation of several other *Campylobacter* species, such as *C. jejuni* subsp. *doylei* (31, 32), *C. upsaliensis* (31, 32), *C. concisus* (139), *C. curvus* (140), *C. hyointestinalis* (38), and *C. fetus* (105). These campylobacters can be isolated successfully only by means of the differential filtration technique. It is necessary to inoculate samples onto a nonselective agar base at 37°C in a microaerophilic atmosphere containing hydrogen.

The identification of these campylobacters is often difficult but is not strictly necessary for treatment of the patients. However, correct identification is important for the study of the antibiotic susceptibility, epidemiology, and pathogenicity of these organisms. At present, the relationship between the various *Campylobacter* species is well known (140, 141). This knowledge should function as a reference for identification. New diagnostic tools, such as latex agglutination and DNA probes, have been introduced into the clinical laboratory with limited success.

REFERENCES

1. **Abram, D. D., and N. N. Potter.** 1984. Survival of Campylobacter jejuni at different temperatures in broth, beef, chicken and cod supplemented with sodium chloride. *J. Food Prot.* **47:**795–800.
2. **Aguila, A., F. J. Merino, P. A. Villasante, A. Diaz, and A. C. Velasco.** 1987. Evaluation of four enrichment media for isolation of *Campylobacter jejuni. J. Clin. Microbiol.* **25:**174–175.
3. **Aho, M., M. Kauppi, and J. Hvin.** 1988. The stability of small number of campylobacteria in from different transport media. *Acta Vet. Scand.* **29:**437–442.
4. **Aho, M., M. Kauppi, and J. Hvin.** 1988. Pre-enrichment and enrichment methods for isolating small number of Campylobacteria from contaminating flora. *Acta Vet. Scand.* **29:**443–449.
5. **Barrett, T. J., C. M. Patton, and G. K. Morris.** 1988. Differentiation of Campylobacter species using phenotypic characterisation. *Lab. Med.* **19:**96–102.
6. **Beuchat, L. R.** 1985. Efficacy of media and methods for detecting and enumerating *Campylobacter*

jejuni in refrigerated chicken meat. *Appl. Environ. Microbiol.* **50**:934–939.

7. **Billingham, J. D.** 1980. A comparison of two media for the isolation of Campylobacter in the tropics. *Trans. R. Soc. Trop. Med. Hyg.* **75**: 645–646.
8. **Blaser, M. J., I. D. Berkowitz, F. M. Laforce, J. Cravens, B. Reller, and W.-L. L. Wang.** 1979. Campylobacter enteritis: clinical and epidemiological features. *Ann. Intern. Med.* **91**:179–185.
9. **Blaser, M. J., H. L. Hardesty, B. Powers, and W-L. L. Wang.** 1980. Survival of *Campylobacter fetus* subsp. *jejuni* in biological milieus. *J. Clin. Microbiol.* **11**:309–313.
10. **Bolton, F. J., and D. Coates.** 1983. Development of a blood-free Campylobacter medium: screening tests on basal media and supplements, and the ability of selected supplements to facilate aerotolerance. *J. Appl. Bacteriol.* **54**:115–125.
11. **Bolton, F. J., D. Coates, and D. N. Hutchinson.** 1984. The ability of campylobacter media supplements to neutralise photochemically induced toxicity and hydrogen peroxide. *J. Appl. Bacteriol.* **56**:151–157.
12. **Bolton, F. J., D. Coates, D. N. Hutchinson, and A. L. Godfree.** 1987. A study of thermophilic campylobacter in a river system. *J. Appl. Bacteriol.* **62**:167–176.
13. **Bolton, F. J., A. V. Holt, and D. N. Hutchinson.** 1985. Urease positive thermophilic campylobacters. *Lancet* **i**:1217–1218.
14. **Bolton, F. J., D. N. Hutchinson, and D. Coates.** 1984. Blood-free selective medium for the isolation of *Campylobacter jejuni* from feces. *J. Clin. Microbiol.* **19**:169–171.
15. **Bolton, F. J., D. N. Hutchinson, and G. Parker.** 1987. Isolation of Campylobacter. What are we missing? *J. Clin. Pathol.* **40**:702–703.
16. **Bolton, F. J., D. N. Hutchinson, and G. Parker.** 1988. Reassessment of selective agar and filtration techniques for isolation of Campylobacter species from faeces. *Eur. J. Clin. Microbiol.* **7**:155–160.
17. **Bolton, F. J., and L. Robertson.** 1982. A selective medium for isolating Campylobacter jejuni/coli. *J. Clin. Pathol.* **35**:462–467.
18. **Bopp, C. A., J. G. Wells, and T. J. Barrett.** 1982. Trimethoprim activity in media selective for *Campylobacter jejuni. J. Clin. Microbiol.* **16**:808–812.
19. **Bruce, D., W. Zochowski, and G. A. Fleming.** 1980. Campylobacter infections in cats and dogs. *Vet. Rec.* **107**:200–201.
20. **Buck, G. E., and M. T. Kelly.** 1981. Effect of moisture content of the medium on colony morphology of *Campylobacter fetus* subsp. *jejuni. J. Clin. Microbiol.* **14**:585–586.
21. **Butzler, J. P., P. Dekeyser, M. Detrain, and F. Dehaen.** 1973. Related vibrio in stools. *J. Pediatr.* **82**:493–495.
22. **Butzler, J. P., and M. B. Skirrow.** 1979. Campylobacter enteritis. *Clin. Gastroenterol.* **8**:737–765.
23. **Cary, S. G., and E. B. Blair.** 1964. New transport medium for shipment of clinical specimens. I. Fecal specimens. *J. Bacteriol.* **88**:96–98.
24. **Chan, F. T. H., and A. M. R. Mackenzie.** 1982. Enrichment medium and control system for isolation of *Campylobacter fetus* subsp. *jejuni* from stools. *J. Clin. Microbiol.* **15**:12–15.
25. **Chevrier, D., D. Larzul, F. Megraud, and J.-L. Guesdon.** 1989. Identification and classification of *Campylobacter* strains by using nonradioactive DNA probes. *J. Clin. Microbiol.* **27**:321–326.
26. **Christopher, F. M., G. C. Smith, and C. Vanderzant.** 1982. Effect of temperature and pH on the survival of Campylobacter fetus. *J. Food Prot.* **45**:253–259.
27. **Claus, P., S. L. Moseley, and S. Falkow.** 1983. The use of gene-specific DNA probes for the identification of enteric pathogens. *Prog. Food Nutr. Sci.* **7**:139–142.
28. **Cudjoe, K. S., G. Kupperud, and O. Olsvik.** 1991. Identification of thermotolerant Campylobacter species from poultry using enzyme-labelled oligonucleotide DNA probe. *Int. J. Food. Microbiol.* **12**:271–274.
29. **Cuk, Z., A. Annan-Prak, M. Janc, and J. Zajc-Salter.** 1987. Yoghurt an unlikely source of Campylobacter jejuni/coli. *J. Appl. Bacteriol.* **63**:201–205.
30. **Dekeyser, P., M. Detrain-Gossuin, J. P. Butzler, and J. Sternon.** 1972. Acute enteritis due to related vibrio: first positive stool cultures. *J. Infect. Dis.* **125**:390–392.
31. **Doyle, M. P.** 1984. Campylobacter in foods, p. 163–180. *In* J. P. Butzler (ed.), *Campylobacter Infection in Man and Animals.* CRC Press, Inc., Boca Raton, Fla.
32. **Doyle, M. P., and D. J. Roman.** 1981. Growth and survival of Campylobacter fetus subsp. jejuni as a function of temperature and pH. *J. Food Prot.* **44**:596–601.
33. **Doyle, M. P., and D. J. Roman.** 1982. Sensitivity of Campylobacter jejuni to drying. *J. Food Prot.* **45**:507–510.
34. **Doyle, M. P., and D. J. Roman.** 1982. Response of *Campylobacter jejuni* to sodium chloride. *Appl. Environ. Microbiol.* **43**:561–565.
35. **Edmonds, P., C. M. Patton, P. M. Griffin, T. J. Barrett, G. P. Schmid, C. N. Baker, M. A. Lambert, and D. J. Brenner.** 1987. *Campylobacter hyointestinalis* associated with human gastrointestinal disease in the United States. *J. Clin. Microbiol.* **25**:685–691.
36. **Endtz, H. P., G. J. H. M. Ruijs, A. H. Zwinderman, T. Van Der Reijden, M. Biever, and R. P. Mouton.** 1991. Comparison of six media, including a semisolid agar, for the isolation of various *Campylobacter* species from stool specimens. *J. Clin. Microbiol.* **29**:1007–1010.
37. **Ezaki, T., N. Takeuchi, S. L. Liu, and A. Kai.** 1988. Small-scale DNA preparation for rapid genetic identification of Campylobacter species without radioisotope. *Microbiol. Immunol.* **32**:141–150.
38. **Fennell, C. L., A. M. Rompalo, P. A. Totten, K. L. Bruch, B. M. Flores, and W. E. Stamm.** 1986. Isolation of "*Campylobacter hyointestinalis*" from a human. *J. Clin. Microbiol.* **24**:146–148.

39. **Fletcher, R. D., and W. N. Plastridge.** 1964. Gaseous environment and growth of microaerophilic vibrios. *J. Bacteriol.* **87**:352–355.
40. **Fox, J. G., K. O. Maxwell, N. S. Taylor, C. D. Runsick, P. Edmonds, and D. J. Brenner.** 1989. *Campylobacter upsaliensis* isolated from cats as identified by DNA relatedness and biochemical features. *J. Clin. Microbiol.* **27**:2376–2378.
41. **Fricker, C. R.** 1985. A note on the effect of different storage procedures on the ability of Preston medium to recover campylobacters. *J. Appl. Bacteriol.* **58**:57–62.
42. **Gebhart, C. J., G. E. Ward, K. Chang, and H. J. Kurtz.** 1983. Campylobacter hyointestinalis (new species) isolated from swine with lesions of proliferative ileitis. *Am. J. Vet. Res.* **44**:361–367.
43. **George, H. A., P. S. Hoffman, R. M. Smibert, and N. R. Krieg.** 1978. Improved media for growth and aerotolerance of *Campylobacter fetus*. *J. Clin. Microbiol.* **8**:36–41.
44. **Gilchrist, M. J. R., C. M. Grewell, and J. A. Washington.** 1981. Evaluation of media for isolation of *Campylobacter fetus* subsp. *jejuni* from fecal specimens. *J. Clin. Microbiol.* **14**:393–395.
45. **Gill, C. O., and L. M. Harris.** 1983. Limiting conditions of temperatures and pH for growth of "thermophilic" campylobacters on solid media. *J. Food Prot.* **46**:767–768.
46. **Goossens, H., and J. P. Butzler.** 1989. Isolation of *Campylobacter upsaliensis* from stool specimens. *J. Clin. Microbiol.* **27**:2143–2144.
47. **Goossens, H., and J. P. Butzler.** 1991. Isolation of *Campylobacter* spp. from stool specimens with a semisolid medium. *J. Clin. Microbiol.* **29**:2681–2682.
48. **Goossens, H., M. De Boeck, and J. P. Butzler.** 1983. A new selective medium for the isolation of *Campylobacter jejuni* from human faeces. *Eur. J. Clin. Microbiol.* **2**:389–394.
49. **Goossens, H., M. De Boeck, H. Coignau, L. Vlaes, C. Van den Boore, and J. P. Butzler.** 1986. Modified selective medium for isolation of *Campylobacter* spp. from feces: comparison with Preston medium, a blood-free medium, and a filtration system. *J. Clin. Microbiol.* **24**:840–843.
50. **Goossens, H., B. Pot, L. Vlaes, M. De Boeck, K. Kersters, J. Levy, P. Demol, J. P. Butzler, and P. Vandamme.** 1990. Is "C. upsaliensis" an unrecognised cause of human diarrhoea? *Lancet* **335**:584–586.
51. **Goossens, H., B. Pot, L. Vlaes, C. Van den Borre, R. Van den Abbeele, C. Van Naelten, H. Coignau, P. Marbehant, J. Verhoef, K. Kersters, J. P. Butzler, and P. Vandamme.** 1990. Characterization and description of "Campylobacter upsaliensis" isolated from human feces. *J. Clin. Microbiol.* **28**:1039–1046.
52. **Goossens, H., L. Vlaes, J. P. Butzler, A. Adnet, P. Hanicq, D. Massart, G. De Schrijver, and W. Blomme.** 1991. Campylobacter upsaliensis enteritis associated with canine infections. *Lancet* **i**:1486–1487.
53. **Goossens, H., L. Vlaes, I. Galand, C. Van den Borre, and J. P. Butzler.** 1989. Semisolid blood-free selective-motility medium for the isolation of campylobacters from stool specimens. *J. Clin. Microbiol.* **27**:1077–1080.
54. **Grayson, M. L., W. Tee, and B. Dwyer.** 1989. Gastroenteritis associated with Campylobacter cinaedi. *Med. J. Aust.* **150**:214–215.
55. **Griffiths, P. L., I. Hooper, C. R. Fricker, and R. W. A. Park.** 1991. Rapid serological detection of Campylobacters in stool cultures using a latex agglutination test, abstr. J3-89, p. 125–126. *In* G. M. Ruiz-Palacios, E. Calva, and B. R. Ruiz-Palacios (ed.), *Vth Int. Workshop on Campylobacter Infections.* Instituto Nacional de la Nutricion, Mexico City, Mexico.
56. **Griffiths, P. L., K. S. Walter, G. S. Morenco, and C. Tonkin.** 1989. Experience with using the "Microscreen" Campylobacter latex diagnostic kit on enrichment broth cultures for the detection of campylobacters. *J. Appl. Bacteriol.* **67**:36–37.
57. **Hänninen, M.-L.** 1981. Effect of NaCl in Campylobacter jejuni/coli. *Acta Vet. Scand.* **22**:578–588.
58. **Hodge, D. S., J. F. Prescott, and P. E. Shewen.** 1986. Direct immunofluorescence microscopy for rapid screening of *Campylobacter* enteritis. *J. Clin. Microbiol.* **24**:863–865.
59. **Hodge, D. S., and R. Terro.** 1984. Comparative efficacy of liquid enrichment medium for isolation of *Campylobacter jejuni*. *J. Clin. Microbiol.* **19**:434.
60. **Hodinka, R. L., and P. H. Gilligan.** 1988. Evaluation of the Campyslide agglutination test for confirmatory identification of selected *Campylobacter* species. *J. Clin. Microbiol.* **26**:47–49.
61. **Hoffman, P. S., H. A. George, N. R. Krieg, and R. M. Smibert.** 1979. Studies of the microaerophilic nature of Campylobacter fetus subsp. jejuni. II. Role of exogenous superoxide anions and hydrogen peroxide. *Can. J. Microbiol.* **25**:8–16.
62. **Hoffman, P. S., N. R. Krieg, and R. M. Smibert.** 1979. Studies of the microaerophilic nature of Campylobacter fetus subsp. jejuni. I. Physiological aspects of enhanced aerotolerance. *Can. J. Microbiol.* **25**:1–7.
63. **Humphrey, T. J.** 1986. Techniques for the optimum recovery of cold injured Campylobacter jejuni from milk or water. *J. Appl. Bacteriol.* **61**:125–132.
64. **Humphrey, T. J.** 1986. Injury and recovery in freeze- or heat-damaged Campylobacter jejuni. *Lett. Appl. Microbiol.* **3**:81–84.
65. **Humphrey, T. J.** 1988. Peroxide sensitivity and catalase activity in Campylobacter jejuni following injury and during recovery. *J. Appl. Bacteriol.* **64**:337–343.
66. **Humphrey, T. J.** 1989. An appraisal of the efficacy of preenrichment for the isolation of Campylobacter jejuni from water and food. *J. Appl. Bacteriol.* **66**:119–126.
67. **Humphrey, T. J.** 1990. The synergistic inhibition of Campylobacter jejuni by rifampicin and hydrogen peroxide. *Lett. Appl. Microbiol.* **10**:97–100.
68. **Humphrey, T. J., and J. G. Cruickshank.** 1985. Antibiotic and deoxycholate resistance in Cam-

pylobacter jejuni following freezing or heating. *J. Appl. Bacteriol.* **59**:65–71.

69. **Humphrey, T. J., and D. G. Lanning.** 1987. Salmonella and campylobacter contamination of broiler chicken carcasses and scald tank water: the influence of water pH. *J. Appl. Bacteriol.* **63**:21–25.
70. **Hutchinson, D. N., and F. J. Bolton.** 1983. Is enrichment culture necessary for the isolation of Campylobacter jejuni from faeces? *J. Clin. Pathol.* **36**:1350–1352.
71. **Kaplan, R. L., L. J. Goodman, J. E. Barrett, G. M. Trenholme, and W. Landau.** 1982. Comparison of rectal swabs and stool cultures in detecting *Campylobacter fetus* subsp. *jejuni. J. Clin. Microbiol.* **15**:959–960.
72. **Karmali, M. A., A. E. Simor, M. Roscoe, P. C. Fleming, S. S. Smith, and J. Lane.** 1986. Evaluation of a blood-free, charcoal based, selective medium for the isolation of *Campylobacter* organisms from feces. *J. Clin. Microbiol.* **23**:456–459.
73. **Kasper, G., and N. Dickgiesser.** 1985. Isolation from gastric epithelium of Campylobacter-like bacteria that are distinct from "Campylobacter pyloridis." *Lancet* **i**:111–112.
74. **Kimura, F., N. Koizumi, K. Yoshida, S. Nakajima, T. Itoh, M. Takahashi, A. Kal, and Y. Yangawa.** 1991. Rapid identification of *Campylobacter jejuni/coli* in a latex agglutination test using monoclonal antibody, abstr. 13–88. *In* G. M. Ruiz-Palacios, E. Calva, and B.R. Ruiz-Palacios (ed.), *Vth Int. Workshop on Campylobacter Infections.* Instituto Nacional de la Nutricion, Mexico City, Mexico.
75. **King, E. O.** 1957. Human infections with Vibro fetus and a closely related vibrio. *J. Infect. Dis.* **101**:119–128.
76. **Klst, M.** 1986. Wir entdeckte Campylobacter jejuni/coli. Eine Zusammen-volume sassing lishen unberucksichtiger Literaturquelles. *Zentralbl. Bakteriol. Hyg. A* **261**:177–186.
77. **Korhonen, L. K., and P. J. Martikainen.** 1990. Comparison of some enrichment broths and growth media for the isolation of thermophilic campylobacters from surface water samples. *J. Appl. Bacteriol.* **68**:593–599.
78. **Korolik, V., P. J. Coloe, and V. Krishnapillai.** 1988. A specific DNA probe for the identification of Campylobacter jejuni. *J. Gen. Microbiol.* **134**:521–529.
79. **Ladron De Guevara, C., M. T. Perez-Pomata, A. Aguila, F. J. Merino, P. A. Villasante, and A. C. Velasco.** 1989. Recovery of campylobacter from human faeces stored at 4°C. *Epidemiol. Infect.* **102**:281–285.
80. **Lastovica, A. J., and R. E. Ambrosio.** 1986. Plasmid profiles of clinical isolates of Campylobacter with weak or no catalase activity. *S. Afr. Med. J.* **70**:337–338.
81. **Lastovica, A. J., E. Le Roux, and J. L. Penner.** 1989. *Campylobacter upsaliensis* isolated from blood cultures of pediatric patients. *J. Clin. Microbiol.* **27**:657–659.
82. **Lauwers, S., T. Devreker, P. Van Etteryck, J. Breynaert, A. Van Zeebroeck, L. Smekens, K. Kersters, and P. Vandamme.** 1991. Isolation of Campylobacter concisus from human faeces. *Microb. Ecol. Health Dis.* **4**:591.

82a. **Lawson, G. H. K., J. L. Leaver, G. W. Pettigrew, and A. C. Rowland.** 1987. Some features of *Campylobacter sputorum* subsp. *mucosalis* subsp. nov., nom. rev., and their taxonomic significance. *Int. J. Syst. Bacteriol.* **31**:385–391.

83. **Lee, M. H. T., R. M. Smibert, and N. R. Krieg.** 1988. Effects of incubation temperature, ageing, and bisulfite content of unsupplemented Brucella agar on aerotolerance of Campylobacter jejuni. *Am. J. Microbiol.* **34**:1069–1074.
84. **Luechtefeld, N. W., W.-L. L. Wang, M. J. Blaser, and L. B. Reller.** 1981. Evaluation of transport and storage techniques for isolation of *Campylobacter fetus* subsp. *jejuni* from turkey cecal specimens. *J. Clin. Microbiol.* **13**:438–443.
85. **Martin, W. Y., C. M. Patton, G. K. Morris, M. E. Potter, and N. D. Puhr.** 1983. Selective enrichment broth medium for isolation of *Campylobacter jejuni. J. Clin. Microbiol.* **17**:853–855.
86. **Mégraud, F., and F. Bonnet.** 1986. Unusual campylobacters in human faeces. *J. Infect.* **12**:275–276.
87. **Mégraud, F., D. Chevrier, N. Desplaces, A. Sedallian, and J. L. Guesdon.** 1988. Urease-positive thermophilic campylobacter (*Campylobacter laridis* variant) isolated from an appendix and from human feces. *J. Clin. Microbiol.* **26**:1050–1051.
88. **Mégraud, F., and Z. Elhariff.** 1985. Isolation of Campylobacter species by filtration. *Eur. J. Clin. Microbiol.* **4**:437–438.
89. **Mégraud, F., and A. M. Gavinet.** 1988. Comparison of three protocols to isolate Campylobacter species from human species, p. 90–91. *In* B. Kaijser and E. Falsen (ed.), *Campylobacter IV.* University of Göteborg, Göteborg, Sweden.
90. **Minet, J., B. Grosbois, and F. Mégraud.** 1988. *Campylobacter hyointestinalis*: an opportunistic enteropathogen? *J. Clin. Microbiol.* **26**:2659–2660.
91. **Monhort, J. D., H. F. Stills, and S. Bech-Nulsen.** 1989. Effects of sample holding time, temperature and atmosphere on the isolation of *Campylobacter jejuni* from dogs. *J. Clin. Microbiol.* **27**:1419–1420.
92. **Morris, J. A., and R. W. A. Park.** 1971. The isolation of microaerophilic vibrios. *Soc. Appl. Bacteriol. Tech. Ser.* **5**:207–217.
93. **Nachamkin, I., and S. Barbagallo.** 1990. Culture confirmation of *Campylobacter* spp. by latex agglutination. *J. Clin. Microbiol.* **28**:817–818.
94. **Ng, L. K., M. E. Stiles, and D. E. Taylor.** 1985. Inhibition of *Campylobacter jejuni* and *Campylobacter coli* by antibiotics used in selective growth media. *J. Clin. Microbiol.* **22**:510–514.
95. **Ng, L. K., M. E. Stiles, and D. E. Taylor.** 1985. Comparison of basal media for culturing *Campylobacter jejuni* and *Campylobacter coli. J. Clin. Microbiol.* **21**:226–230.
96. **Olive, D. M., M. Johny, and S. K. Sethi.** 1990. Use of an alkaline phosphatase-labeled synthetic

oligonucleotide probe for detection of *Campylobacter jejuni* and *Campylobacter coli*. *J. Clin. Microbiol.* **28:**1565–1569.

97. **On, S. L. W., and B. Holmes.** 1991. Effect of inoculum size on the phenotypic characterization of *Campylobacter* species. *J. Clin. Microbiol.* **29:**923–926.
98. **On, S. L. W., and B. Holmes.** 1991. Reproducibility of tolerance tests that are useful in the identification of campylobacteria. *J. Clin. Microbiol.* **29:**1785–1788.
99. **Owen, R. J., A. Beck, and P. Borman.** 1985. Restriction endonuclease digest patterns of chromosomal DNA from nitrate-negative Campylobacter jejuni-like organisms. *Eur. J. Epidemiol.* **1:**281–287.
100. **Owen, R. J., M. Costas, L. L. Sloss, and F. J. Bolton.** 1988. Numerical analysis of electrophoretic protein patterns of Campylobacter laridis and allied thermophilic campylobacters from the natural environment. *J. Appl. Bacteriol.* **65:**69–78.
101. **Paisley, J. W., S. Mirretts, B. A. Lauer, M. Roe, and L. B. Reller.** 1982. Dark-field microscopy of human feces for presumptive diagnosis of *Campylobacter fetus* subsp. *jejuni* enteritis. *J. Clin. Microbiol.* **15:**61–63.
102. **Palumbo, S. A.** 1986. Campylobacter jejuni in foods: its occurrence, isolation from foods and injury. *J. Food Prot.* **49:**161–166.
103. **Patton, C. M., S. W. Mitchell, M. E. Potter, and A. F. Kaufman.** 1981. Comparison of selective media for primary isolation of *Campylobacter fetus* subsp. *jejuni*. *J. Clin. Microbiol.* **13:**326–330.
104. **Patton, C. M., N. Shaffer, P. Edmonds, T. Barrett, M. A. Lambert, C. Baker, M. Pellman, and D. J. Brenner.** 1989. Human disease associated with "*Campylobacter upsaliensis*" (catalase negative or weakly positive campylobacter species) in the United States. *J. Clin. Microbiol.* **27:**66–73.
105. **Penner, J. L.** 1988. The genus *Campylobacter*: a decade of progress. *Clin. Microbiol. Rev.* **1:**157–172.
106. **Picken, R. N., Z. Wang, and H. L. Yang.** 1987. Molecular cloning of a species-specific DNA probe for Campylobacter jejuni. *Mol. Cell. Probes* **1:**245–259.
107. **Plumer, G. L., W. C. Duvall, and V. M. Shepler.** 1962. A preliminary report on a new technic for isolation of Vibrio fetus from carrier bulls. *Gen. Vet.* **52:**110–122.
108. **Popovic-Uroic, T., C. M. Patton, K. Wachsmuth, and P. Roeder.** 1991. Evaluation of an oligonucleotide probe for identification of Campylobacter species. *Lab. Med.* **22:**533–539.
109. **Price, A. B., J. M. Dolby, P. R. Dunscombe, and J. Stirling.** 1984. Detection of campylobacter by immunofluorescence in stools and rectal biopsies of patients with diarrhoea. *J. Clin. Pathol.* **37:**1007–1013.
110. **Rashtchian, A., M. Abbott, D. H. Lovern, G. A. Mock, and M. M. Shaffer.** 1986. Use of synthetic oligonucleotides complementary to rRNA for detection of *Campylobacter*, abstr. C-90, p. 343. *In Abstr. Annu. Meet. Am. Soc. Microbiol. 1986.* American Society for Microbiology, Washington, D.C.
111. **Robinson, D. A.** 1981. Infective dose of Campylobacter jejuni in milk. *Br. Med. J.* **282:**1584.
112. **Rollins, D. M., and R. R. Colwell.** 1986. Viable but nonculturable stage of *Campylobacter jejuni* and its role in survival in the natural aquatic environment. *Appl. Environ. Microbiol.* **52:**531–538.
113. **Romaniuk, P. J., and T. J. Trust.** 1987. Identification of Campylobacter species by southern hybridization of genomic DNA using oligonucleotide probe for 16S rRNA genes. *FEMS Microbiol. Lett.* **43:**331–335.
114. **Roop, R. M., II, R. M. Smibert, J. L. Johnson, and N. R. Krieg.** 1984. Differential characteristics of catalase-positive campylobacters correlated with DNA homology groups. *Can. J. Microbiol.* **30:**938–951.
115. **Roop, R. M., II, R. M. Smibert, J. L. Johnson, and N. R. Krieg.** 1985. *Campylobacter mucosalis* (Lawson, Leaver, Pettigrew and Rowland 1981) comb. nov.: emended description. *Int. J. Syst. Bacteriol.* **35:**189–192.
116. **Rosef, O., B. Gondrosen, G. Kapperud, and B. Underdal.** 1983. Isolation and characterization of *Campylobacter jejuni* and *Campylobacter coli* from domestic and wild mammals in Norway. *Appl. Environ. Microbiol.* **46:**855–859.
117. **Samel, C., and I. Nachamkin.** 1988. Presumptive culture identification of Campylobacter spp. using latex agglutination, p. 70. *In* B. Kaijser and E. Falsen (ed.), *Campylobacter IV.* University of Göteborg, Göteborg, Sweden.
118. **Sandstedt, K., J. Ursing, and M. Walder.** 1983. Thermotolerant Campylobacter with no or weak catalase activity isolated from dogs. *Curr. Microbiol.* **8:**209–213.
119. **Sandven, P., O. Solberg, K. Odegaard, and G. Myhre.** 1982. Improved medium for the transportation of gonococcal specimens. *Acta Pathol. Microbiol. Immunol. Scand. Sect. B* **90:**73–77.
120. **Seamon, P. J.** 1968. A membrane filtration technique for the isolation of Vibrio species from contaminated material. *J. Med. Lab. Technol.* **25:**25–26.
121. **Shimada, K., and H. Tsuji.** 1986. Enrichment for detection of *Campylobacter jejuni*. *J. Clin. Microbiol.* **23:**887–890.
122. **Simmons, N. A., and F. J. Gibbs.** 1979. Campylobacter spp. in oven-ready poultry. *J. Infect.* **1:**159–162.
123. **Sjögren, E., G-B. Lindblom, and B. Kaijser.** 1985. Optimal transport and enrichment methods for the isolation of Campylobacter jejuni, p. 62–63. *In* A. D. Pearson, M. B. Skirrow, H. Lior, and B. Rowe (ed.), *Campylobacter III.* Public Health Laboratory Service, London.
124. **Skirrow, M. B.** 1977. Campylobacter enteritis: a "new" disease. *Br. Med. J.* **2:**9–11.

125. **Skirrow, M. B., T. J. Merry, and C. R. Vickery.** 1991. Hydrogen facilitates the isolation of *Campylobacter jejuni,* abstr. J3-82. *In* G. M. Ruiz-Palacios, E. Calva, and B. R. Ruiz-Palacios (ed.), *Vth Int. Workshop on Campylobacter Infections.* Instituto Nacional de la Nutricion, Mexico City, Mexico.
126. **Smibert, R. M.** 1965. Vibrio fetus var. intestinalis isolated from fecal and intestinal contents of clinically normal sheep: biochemical and cultural characteristics of microaerophilic vibrios isolated from the intestinal contents of sheep. *Am. J. Vet. Res.* **20:**320–327.
127. **Smibert, R. M.** 1978. The genus *Campylobacter. Annu. Rev. Microbiol.* **32:**673–709.
128. **Steele, T. W., and S. N. McDermott.** 1984. The use of membrane filters applied directly to the surface of agar plates for the isolation of Campylobacter jejuni from feces. *Pathology* **16:**263–265.
129. **Steele, T. W., and R. J. Owen.** 1988. *Campylobacter jejuni* subsp. *doylei* subsp. nov., a subspecies of nitrate-negative campylobacters isolated from human clinical specimens. *Int. J. Syst. Bacteriol.* **38:**316–318.
130. **Steele, T. W., N. Sangster, and J. A. Lanser.** 1985. DNA relatedness and biochemical features of *Campylobacter* spp. isolated in central and South Australia. *J. Clin. Microbiol.* **22:**71–74.
131. **Sutcliffe, E. M.** 1991. Latex agglutination for the detection of Campylobacter species in water. *Lett. Appl. Microbiol.* **12:**72–74.
132. **Svedhem, A., B. Kayser, and E. Sjögren.** 1981. The occurrence of Campylobacter jejuni in fresh food and survival under different conditions. *J. Hyg.* **87:**421–425.
133. **Tanner, A. C. R., C. Haffer, G. T. Bratthall, R. A. Visconti, and S. S. Sokransky.** 1979. A study of bacteria associated with advancing periodontitis in man. *J. Clin. Periodontol.* **6:**278–307.
134. **Tanner, E. I., and C. H. Bullin.** 1977. Campylobacter enteritis. *Br. Med. J.* **ii:**579.
135. **Taylor, D. E., K. Hiratsuka, and L. Muller.** 1989. Isolation and characterization of catalase-negative and catalase-weak strains of *Campylobacter* species, including "*Campylobacter upsaliensis*" from humans with gastroenteritis. *J. Clin. Microbiol.* **27:**2042–2045.
136. **Taylor, D. N., J. A. Kiehlbauch, W. Tee, C. Pitarargsi, and P. Echeverria.** 1991. Isolation of group 2 aerotolerant campylobacter species from Thai children with diarrhea. *J. Infect. Dis.* **163:**1062–1067.
137. **Tenover, F. C., L. Carlson, S. Barbagallo, and I. Nachamkin.** 1990. DNA probe culture confirmation assay for identification of thermophilic *Campylobacter* species. *J. Clin. Microbiol.* **28:**1284–1287.
138. **Totten, P. A., C. M. Patton, F. C. Tenover, T. J. Barrett, W. E. Stamm, A. G. Steigerwalt, J. Y. Lin, J. K. Holmes, and D. J. Brenner.** 1987. Prevalence and characterization of hippurate-negative *Campylobacter jejuni* in King County, Washington. *J. Clin. Microbiol.* **25:**1747–1752.
139. **Vandamme, P., E. Falsen, B. Pot, B. Hoste, K. Kersters, and J. De Ley.** 1989. Identification of EF group 22 campylobacters from gastroenteritis cases as *Campylobacter concisus. J. Clin. Microbiol.* **27:**1775–1781.
140. **Vandamme, P., and H. Goossens.** Taxonomy of Campylobacter, Arcobacter and Helicobacter. A review. *Zentralbl. Bakteriol.,* in press.
141. **Vandamme, P., B. Pot, and K. Kersters.** 1991. Differentiation of campylobacters and Campylobacter-like organisms by numerical analysis of one-dimensional electrophoretic protein patterns. *Syst. Appl. Microbiol.* **14:**57–66.
142. **Véron, M., and R. Chatelain.** 1973. Taxonomic study of the genus *Campylobacter* Sebald and Véron and designation of the neotype strain for the type species *Campylobacter fetus* (Smith and Taylor) Sebald and Véron. *Int. J. Syst. Bacteriol.* **23:**122–134.
143. **Walmsley, S. L., and M. A. Karmali.** 1989. Direct isolation of atypical thermophilic *Campylobacter* species from human feces on selective agar medium. *J. Clin. Microbiol.* **27:**668–670.
144. **Wang, W.-L. L., N. W. Luechtefeld, L. B. Reller, and M. J. Blaser.** 1980. Enriched brucella medium for storage and transport of cultures of *Campylobacter fetus* subsp. *jejuni. J. Clin. Microbiol.* **12:**479–480.
145. **Wang, W.-L. L., L. B. Reller, B. Smallwood, N. W. Luechtefeld, and M. J. Blaser.** 1983. Evaluation of transport media for *Campylobacter jejuni* in human fecal specimens. *J. Clin. Microbiol.* **18:**803–807.
146. **Waterworth, P. M.** 1973. Laboratory methods, p. 490–531. *In* L. P. Garrod, H. P. Lambert, and F. O'Grady (ed.), *Antibiotic and chemotherapy,* 4th ed. Churchill Livingstone, Edinburgh.
147. **Zhou, Y.-T., and S.-Q. Wang.** 1989. Application of a biotin-labeled DNA probe to detect Campylobacter. *Zentralbl. Bakteriol.* **272:**186–190.

CHAPTER 12

Typing Schemes: Are Current Methods Useful?

CHARLOTTE M. PATTON AND I. KAYE WACHSMUTH

INTRODUCTION

Since the introduction of appropriate isolation procedures approximately 15 years ago, campylobacters have been recognized as a major cause of morbidity throughout the world, with enteritis the most common clinical manifestation. In the United States, an estimated 2 million cases of *Campylobacter* enteritis occur per year, making *C. jejuni* and *C. coli* the most frequently isolated enterobacterial pathogens. *Campylobacter* sporadic disease outnumbers *Salmonella* sporadic disease at least 2:1, as shown in hospital-based and prevalence studies (17, 64, 133, 139). To identify common-source outbreaks of disease or to track individual strains in a community, it was necessary to develop methods to subtype *C. jejuni* and *C. coli* strains within the high background of sporadic disease and asymptomatic carriage. Also, a variety of animals have been identified as reservoirs, and subtyping is necessary to compare these isolates with human isolates to address the role of these animals in human illness.

The various subspecies typing systems reviewed in this chapter have shown a tremendous diversity within *Campylobacter* species, particularly *C. jejuni* and *C. coli.* By distinguishing individual strains, these systems have been essential in epidemiologic studies of the genus, providing information on relationships between isolates, determining the extent of disease outbreaks, and identifying sources of the organism and modes of transmission. It may even be possible to use typing systems in the future to differentiate between pathogenic and nonpathogenic *Campylobacter* strains.

In this chapter we present a broad overview of the typing methods that have been applied to *C. jejuni* and, where appropriate, discuss briefly the strong and weak points of each. We also present a critical review of typing methods most frequently used today and discuss future needs. Perhaps the best known and most widely used typing methods today are the heat-stable (HS) antigenic scheme described by Penner and Hennessy (114) and the heat-labile (HL) antigenic scheme described by Lior et al. (90).

OVERVIEW

Since 1980 approximately 35 methods or modifications of methods for subtyping *C. jejuni, C. coli,* and *C. lari* have been developed. To review the usefulness of these methods, we have separated them into two categories: (i) methods that are infrequently used either because they do not discriminate well or because they are too complex, and (ii) methods that are frequently used because they are relatively simple to perform and discriminate to a high degree. This distinction can be seen in Table 1, which lists the methods discussed below.

One desirable feature of any typing system is its ability to quantitate data which can then be compared among laboratories. For example, a *Campylobacter* serotype HS2:HL4 would be the same in any laboratory, whereas an outer membrane protein (OMP) pattern A profile may differ from laboratory to laboratory. Table 1 indicates whether the system has a quantitative means for comparing results and whether the system can be applied outside *Campylobacter* to other genera. Since the epidemiologic usefulness of any method might best be evaluated in an outbreak setting, those appropriate references are also listed in a separate column.

Charlotte M. Patton and I. Kaye Wachsmuth, Enteric Diseases Branch, Division of Bacterial and Mycotic Diseases, National Center for Infectious Diseases, Centers for Disease Control, Atlanta, Georgia 30333.

METHODS INFREQUENTLY USED

Method Simple; Discrimination Low or None

Bacteriocin typing

Bacteriocin typing and sensitivity to rod-type (R-type) pyocins of *Pseudomonas aeruginosa,* which are used for typing *Neisseria gonorrhoeae,* are simple, economical procedures but have little or no value in typing *Campylobacter* strains. Blackwell et al. (12) found that none of 50 thermophilic *Campylobacter* strains, tested one against the other for bacteriocin activity, inhibited the growth of any other strain. In the same study only four distinct patterns of sensitivity to R-type pyocins were identified among 13 of 80 thermophilic *Campylobacter* organisms sensitive to R-type pyocins.

Preformed enzymes

An identification method involving a rapid commercial strip for detecting 67 enzymes of thermophilic campylobacters showed diversity of enzyme production within species (36). The epidemiologic or subtyping importance has not been evaluated.

Method Simple; Discrimination Moderate

Auxotyping

Auxotyping uses the nutritional requirements of bacteria as markers to distinguish strains. In 1985, investigators in the United States and the Federal Republic of Germany independently developed different chemically defined media for auxotyping *Campylobacter* strains (33, 148). Twelve auxotrophic patterns were identified among approximately 500 isolates from the United States (149). Fewer than one-half of the *C. jejuni* strains and none of the *C. coli* strains showed auxotrophic requirements. Similar results were observed in the German study with the medium described by Dickgiesser and Czylwik (33), in which 42% of 52 *C. jejuni* strains were found to be auxotrophic. Auxotyping requires no special equipment, and large numbers of isolates can be tested at one time. *Campylobacter* auxotypes are the same from laboratory to laboratory, and the system is applicable to other organisms (132, 147); however, components of the auxotyping medium must be modified to accommodate the nutritional requirements of the genera under study.

Antimicrobial susceptibility patterns

The usefulness of antimicrobial susceptibility testing as a typing method is dependent upon resistance to antimicrobial agents. Most *Campylobacter* strains are sensitive to antimicrobial agents suggested for use in routine susceptibility assays, thereby limiting the diversity of patterns. Antimicrobial susceptibility testing by agar MIC and by MBC procedures is time-consuming, especially for *C. jejuni,* and MBC procedures are not standardized. Studies show that determination of the antimicrobial susceptibility pattern correlates with other marker systems and identifies the epidemic strain in approximately two-thirds of outbreaks (22, 49). Antimicrobial susceptibility testing is a quantitative means of comparing results and is applicable to other organisms by using a set of antimicrobial agents suitable for those genera.

Lectin typing

Lectins are proteins or glycoproteins that are derived mainly from plants (141). They bind specifically with carbohydrates, and reactions with bacteria result in specific agglutination. Lectins are used to determine strain variation in epidemic studies of a wide variety of bacterial species (141). Using five commercially available lectins, Wong et al. placed 98% of 155 *C. jejuni* and *C. coli* strains into 12 lectin agglutination patterns (159). No correlation was found between the lectin pattern and the serotype of one or more strains of 57 HS serotypes. Similarly, Corbel and Gill, using 11 lectins, found no relationship between lectin agglutination and HS serotype (30). Using the same five lectins as Wong et al., O'Sullivan et al. (105) applied lectin agglutination to 376 *Campylobacter* clinical isolates and identified 23 patterns. Discrimination with these five lectins was somewhat limited since 42% of *C. jejuni* and 35% of *C. coli* strains were lectin type 4. With further investigation, lectin typing may be a suitable typing system. Lectin agglutination testing by slide or microtiter procedure requires minute amounts of reagent and no special equipment. *Campylobacter* lectin agglutination patterns are analogous from laboratory to laboratory.

Method Moderate; Discrimination Moderate

Plasmid profiles

The usefulness of plasmid analysis for subtyping depends on the presence of plasmid DNA in isolates. Plasmids have been identified in 19

TABLE 1. Application, evaluation, and bibliography of typing methods for *C. jejuni*, *C. coli*, and *C. lari*

Method	Difficulty of performance	Discrimination	Comments	Quantitative comparison	Applicable to other genera	References for discrimination within: Genus	References for discrimination within: Outbreaks
Infrequently used							
Bacteriocin	Simple	None				12	
R-type pyocin	Simple	Low	4 patterns	Yes	Yes	12	
Auxotyping	Simple	Moderate	12 patterns	Yes	Yes	33, 148, 149	148
Antimicrobial susceptibility	Simple	Moderate	Dependent on resistance	Yes	Yes		22, 49
Lectin agglutination	Simple	Moderate	23 patterns	Yes	Yes	30, 159	
Plasmid profile	Moderate	Moderate	Dependent on presence of plasmid DNA	No	Yes	7, 23, 24, 86, 130, 151	22, 113, 150
Phage typing							
Lior	Moderate	Moderate	24 phages typed 78% of *C. jejuni*	Yes	No	50, 76	76
Preston	Moderate	Moderate	16 phages	Yes	No		109, 131
Total protein profile	Complex	Moderate	Species, strain, serotype discrimination	No	Yes	5, 37, 128	
Outer membrane protein	Complex	Low	9 subtypes, *C. jejuni*	No	Yes	14, 32, 92, 95	14, 49
REA	Complex	High	Dependent on RE[a]	No	Yes	27, 41, 71, 100, 106, 107, 117	25, 109, 113, 154
Ribotyping	Complex	High	Dependent on RE and probe				
			16S rDNA probe (*C. jejuni*)	No	Yes		113
			16S + 23S rRNA probe (*E. coli*)	No	Yes		109, 113, 154
			Oligonucleotide (unique to *Campylobacter* 16S rRNA)	No	No	100, 124	
MEE	Complex	High	Dependent on number of enzymes assayed	No	Yes	3	113
			Determines genetic relatedness				
PFGE	Complex	High	Dependent on RE	No	No	161	161

(Continued)

TABLE 1. *(Continued)*

Method	Difficulty of performance	Discrimination	Comments	Quantitative comparison	Applicable to other genera	References for discrimination within: Genus	Outbreaks
Frequently used							
Biotyping							
Skirrow	Simple	Low	2 *C. jejuni* types	Yes	No	140	Numerous
Lior	Simple	Low	4 *C. jejuni*, 2 *C. coli*, 2 *C. lari* types	Yes	No	87, 89	Numerous
Preston	Simple	Moderate	55 *C. jejuni* types	Yes	No	21	60, 61, 98, 109
Serotyping							
HS	Simple[b]	High	42 *C. jejuni*, 18 *C. coli*	Yes	No	85, 115	Numerous[c]
HL	Simple[b]	High	63 *C. jejuni*, 37 *C. coli*, 8 *C. lari*	Yes	No	63, 68, 90, 123	Numerous[c]

[a] RE, restriction endonuclease.
[b] Simple when reagents are available.
[c] See text.

to 53% of *C. jejuni* and *C. coli* strains (7, 23, 24, 86, 130, 151). The highest carriage rate in human isolates was identified in strains from Japan (130), and the highest carriage rate in animal isolates was identified in strains from Canada (23). Carriage rates of approximately 30% were found in strains from the United States and Sweden and in the Penner serotype reference strains (24, 86, 151). A different plasmid profile was seen for each of the 19 Penner reference strains that carried plasmids. The technique requires special equipment, but once established, it can be applied to other genera. Plasmid analysis has no quantitative means for comparing results from laboratory to laboratory.

Phage typing

Several investigators have isolated phages of *C. jejuni* and *C. coli,* and individual or small sets of *C. jejuni* and *C. coli* phages have been used to study lytic activity in isolates from humans and animals (18, 28, 39, 122). In 1985 Grajewski et al. (50) developed a phage-typing system for *C. jejuni* and *C. coli* strains by using a set of 14 phages selected from poultry feces. The system typed 94.5% of 255 human isolates from Illinois and 88.1% of 51 isolates from outside Illinois. All or only certain phages from this system are included, as indicated below, in the two current phage typing systems.

The Lior phage-typing system, composed of the above 14 phages plus 10 others, typed 78% of 301 *C. jejuni* strains from worldwide sources, including isolates from 34 outbreaks (76). Lior phage typing is suggested for use with HL serotyping and Lior biotyping to provide additional strain discrimination. There are now 29 Lior phages. The Preston phage-typing scheme contains 6 Grajewski phages and 10 phages from a variety of sources in the United Kingdom and is recommended for use with other typing methods (131).

Method Complex; Discrimination Moderate or Low

Protein profiles

Total protein profile and OMP profile analyses are complex research tools that have been valuable in studies of specific campylobacter proteins such as porins and flagella. However, these two methods demonstrate only low to moderate discrimination of campylobacters. The methods require specialized reagents and equipment but, once established, can be used with other organisms. Neither method has a quantitative means of interlaboratory comparison of profiles.

Total protein profile analysis by polyacrylamide gel electrophoresis (PAGE) with or without sodium dodecyl sulfate (SDS) of a limited number of strains distinguished *Campylobacter* species, including *C. jejuni* and *C. coli* (37), strains within the same species (108, 128), and strains of the same serotype (5).

The use of OMP profile analyses with SDS-PAGE could not discriminate between strains of *C. jejuni* and *C. coli* in two separate studies (14, 92). However, nine subtypes of *C. jejuni* could be distinguished on the basis of migration of the major bands. Two profiles accounted for 76% of strains studied (14). In contrast, other studies have shown that *Campylobacter* species, including *C. jejuni* and *C. coli* strains, could be distinguished by their OMP SDS-PAGE profiles (32, 95). With strains identified by a quantitative filter DNA hybridization technique, OMP results showed that *C. jejuni* and *C. coli* were distinct; discrepant results were attributed to differences in methodology (32). Although the second set of studies could differentiate *C. jejuni* and *C. coli* by OMP profile, strains within a species could not be distinguished for typing purposes.

Method Complex, Immunologic; Discrimination High

Antibodies

Monoclonal antibodies directed against flagellar antigens (103) or clones reacting with the polysaccharides (79) have been produced and suggested as a possible basis for a serotyping system. This approach should result in a very precise typing schema; recent data discussed elsewhere in this volume indicate that *C. jejuni* flagellar antigens have both conserved and type-specific epitopes, but to date few monoclonal antibody reagents have been characterized and documented as suitable for typing.

Method Complex, Genetic; Discrimination High

DNA analysis

Methods that examine the chromosomal DNA and detect minor changes in nucleotide sequences have been applied to campylobacters. Restriction endonuclease analysis (REA), Southern blot and hybridization of DNA fragments produced by REA with rRNA or rDNA (ribotyping), electrophoretic typing by multilocus enzyme electrophoresis (MEE), and pulsed-field gel electrophoresis (PFGE) measure relatively stable chromosomal differences and do not depend on phenotypic expression of bacterial cell products; therefore, they should provide consistent and reproducible results. All four methods are complex, require specialized reagents and equipment, and lack a quantitative means of comparing results. However, they can be applied to other genera and do offer the greatest discrimination among strains. Additionally, MEE can determine the genetic relatedness of strains.

The sensitivity of the REA, ribotyping, and PFGE depends on the choice of restriction enzyme. Numerous enzymes have been used in REA experiments to distinguish between *Campylobacter* species and subspecies and strains within the thermophilic species (25, 27, 41, 70, 71, 106, 107, 113, 117, 154). REA with *Hin*dIII distinguished strains of the closely related HS serotype complex 4,13,16,43,50 and strains of the closely related 8,17 antigens in studies of a milk-borne outbreak and a laboratory-acquired infection of campylobacteriosis (25, 117). PFGE with *Sma*I confirmed REA results again in the milk-borne outbreak associated with the HS serotype complex 4,13,16,43,50 (161). In other outbreak studies, REA with the enzymes *Bgl*III, *Xho*I, *Pvu*II, and *Pst*I correctly identified all strains epidemiologically implicated in four outbreaks and further distinguished strains of the same serotype (113).

Ribotyping

Ribotype discrimination is dependent on the choice of both enzyme and specific probe for hybridization (100, 107, 109, 113, 124, 154). The pattern of three to six restriction fragments or bands, produced in most ribotyping experiments, is much easier to interpret than are REA patterns containing 100 or more bands. Of the two probes used in one study of outbreak strains, the *Escherichia coli* 16S+23S rRNA probe was more sensitive than the *C. jejuni* 16S rDNA probe (113). In a study of strains from five outbreaks caused by serotype HS2:HL4, ribotyping of *Pst*I, *Pvu*II, and *Cla*I digests showed considerable heterogeneity among strains of this commonly occurring serotype (154). The greatest discrimination among strains was found in the *Pst*I digests (Fig. 1).

Multilocus enzyme electrophoresis

MEE has been used for many years in eucaryotic population genetics to estimate genetic diversity; more recently it has been applied to bacterial populations (134). MEE is based on the electrophoretic migration distance of enzymes present in most bacteria. In the statistical analysis of the electrophoresis data, enzyme mobility differences are assumed to relate directly to allelic variation in the structural gene locus for each enzyme. From this analysis, an estimate of the genetic relatedness among strains and the electrophoretic type can be determined (134). In a recent application of MEE to *Campylobacter* strains, 50 and 14 electrophoretic types were identified among 104 *C. jejuni* and 21 *C. coli* strains, respectively, thus demonstrating a high degree of genetic diversity within these two species (3). MEE was also one of the most sensitive of 10 techniques for distinguishing epidemic-associated strains (113).

MEE is highly complex and depends on the number of enzymes analyzed and the use of appropriate electrophoretic parameters. Also, in comparison with other genetic methods, it is relatively time-consuming. The technique might best be used to study the population genetics of a large group of strains or of epidemic-associated strains when background data already exist.

Application to Outbreaks

The above methods have been used to a limited extent in *Campylobacter* outbreak investigations (references are given in Table 1). Although some appear to be epidemiologically useful, none appears to be suitable for routine typing: either the system did not discriminate related and unrelated strains or the method was too complex for routine use in microbiology laboratories. The complex molecular techniques appear to be the most promising and discriminating of the infrequently used methods. The other methods, when applied to outbreaks, were most useful primarily in conjunction with other typing methods.

METHODS FREQUENTLY USED

Biotyping and serotyping have been used more often than the above methods to type *C. jejuni* and *C. coli.* The schemes are relatively simple and were developed for worldwide application to distinguish *Campylobacter* strains. Each system has a quantitative means for comparing results, but the systems are applicable to *Campylobacter* species only.

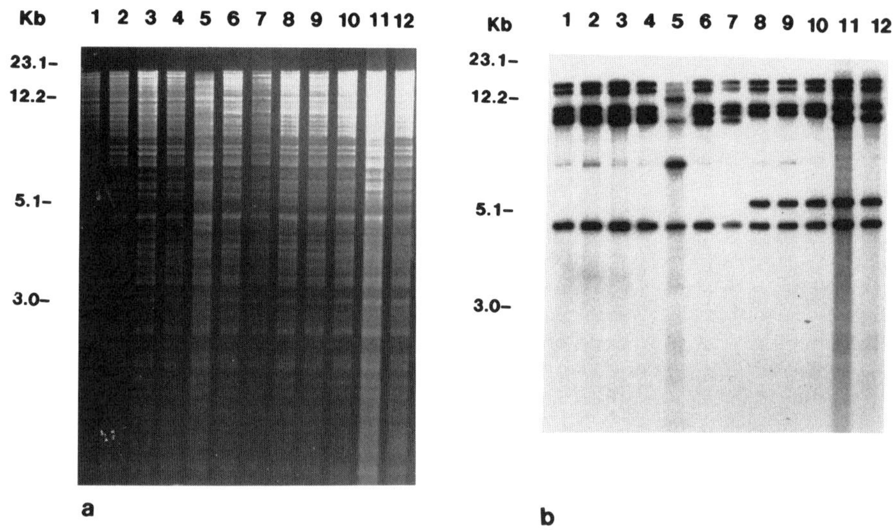

FIGURE 1. Ribotyping with *PstI* of *C. jejuni* strains, serotype Penner 2, Lior 4, causing outbreaks of diarrheal disease in the United States. (a) Restriction endonuclease patterns following 6-h *PstI* digestion. (b) Ribotyping pattern following hybridization with *E. coli* 16+23S rRNA. Lanes 1 and 2 correspond to the human and source isolate of the Vermont 1982 outbreak; lanes 3 to 5 correspond to the human and source isolate (milk) of the Vermont 1983 outbreak, followed by the isolate (fecal) of a different serotype from the source animal; lanes 6 and 7 represent human and source isolates from the Vermont 1986 outbreak; lanes 8 to 10 represent the human and two source isolates from the Kansas 1988 outbreak; and lanes 11 and 12 represent the human isolate and the isolate from a suspected human food handler source. Lanes 1 to 4 represent pattern A, lane 5 represents pattern B, lanes 6 and 7 represent pattern C, lanes 8 to 10 represent pattern D, and lanes 11 and 12 represent pattern E. (Reprinted from reference 154 with permission.)

Method Simple; Discrimination Low or Moderate

Biotyping

Of the six biotyping schemes proposed for distinguishing campylobacters, those of Skirrow and Benjamin (140), Lior and Patel (87, 89), and Bolton et al. (21) (Preston biotyping) are used most commonly. Skirrow and Benjamin described a means for distinguishing the species *C. jejuni, C. coli,* and *C. lari* by using the tests for hippurate hydrolysis, rapid H_2S production, and resistance to nalidixic acid. Additionally, two biotypes of *C. jejuni* are identified by the rapid H_2S test. Lior's biotyping scheme, using hippurate hydrolysis, rapid H_2S production, and DNase activity, can separate *C. jejuni* into four biotypes and *C. coli* and *C. lari* into two biotypes each and was developed to separate strains of the same HL serotype. The Preston scheme uses 12 tests, including 10 resistotyping tests that determine resistance to antibiotics, dyes, and chemicals, for biotyping four *Campylobacter* species. It differentiates 55 types of *C. jejuni.* The Preston scheme can also identify campylobacters to the species level. On the basis of test arrangement and results, a four-figure code, generated for each strain, indicates both the *Campylobacter* species and biotype. Lior's biotyping scheme is the most widely used for distinguishing epidemiologically related strains.

The schemes of Hebert et al. (52), Hollander (56), and Roop et al. (125) are no longer used in most laboratories. *C. jejuni* and *C. coli* strains are not distinguished by the schemes of Hebert et al. and Hollander, and inconclusive results with the test for alkaline phosphatase activity, used in the schemes of Roop et al. and Hollander, have made these biotyping schemes ineffective.

Method Simple; Discrimination High

Serotyping

The antigens of the *C. jejuni-C. coli* group are heterogeneous and complex, and their characteristics are discussed in detail in other chapters. Serotyping methods for *Campylobacter* species are somewhat analogous to those for members of the family *Enterobacteriaceae,* which use tolerance to heat as a means to separate somatic, flagellar, and capsular antigens. Comprehensive reviews of the historical developments leading to the methods in current use are outlined by Lauwers and Penner (84) and Lior (88). Both HS and HL antigens have been demonstrated by a variety of procedures (1, 29, 53, 63, 80, 81, 85, 90, 114, 123). Two groups in Canada and Belgium independently developed passive hemagglutination techniques by using unabsorbed antisera to detect thermostable antigens (85, 114). Another serotyping scheme involving specific antisera to detect HL antigens by slide agglutination was developed by other investigators in Canada and Israel (90, 123). The antisera are made specific by absorption of the homologous HS antibody and removal of heterologous cross-reacting HL antibody. A slightly different slide agglutination method, involving Formalin-treated cells instead of live cells, and the corresponding unabsorbed antisera to Formalin-treated cells to detect HL antigens, was also developed by workers in Japan (63).

In Czechoslovakia, a serotyping scheme involving live cells and unabsorbed antiserum to live cells in a slide test is used to serotype isolates from sporadic cases and outbreaks (67, 68). Cross-reactions are eliminated by diluting the unabsorbed antisera 1:8. A set of 25 antisera typed 312 strains, with 11 antisera accounting for 74.6% of typable isolates. Comparative studies with other systems have not been performed.

To standardize serotyping on an international basis, the International Committee on Serotyping *Campylobacter* recommended in 1985 that the systems of Penner and Lior, which are based on two sets of standardized strains from geographically diverse areas, be adopted and referred to as the HS and HL systems, respectively. The strains defined by the investigators in Belgium (8, 73, 104, 126) have been integrated into the HS system. The official serotyping system for Japan is now the HL system, and the Committee is working to incorporate the other HL schemes into that of the HL system.

The HS scheme identifies 60 serotypes (42 *C. jejuni* and 18 *C. coli*) (Table 1). Antisera are specific for each species, and species can be serotyped separately; however, isolates that do not type in antisera of one species may type in antisera of the other species (115). The HS antigen extract, instead of the viable subculture, can be shipped for serotyping (42, 83).

The HL scheme identifies 108 serotypes (88a), including 8 among *C. lari* strains (Table 1). The scheme types live cells, first with polyvalent, pooled, unabsorbed antisera, then with single unabsorbed serum, and then with single absorbed antiserum.

CRITICAL REVIEW OF SEROTYPING METHODS

Because the HS and HL serotyping schemes have been used extensively and globally, these systems, their utility, problems, and possible solutions to problems are discussed in detail here. Other methods, as they compare with serotyping, will also be included.

Worldwide Usefulness

The serotype distribution has been determined for *C. jejuni* and *C. coli* isolated from humans and animals from around the world. The effectiveness of the HS system in serotyping strains from 12 countries is shown in Table 2, with references included in the table. From 69 to 100% of human strains and 24 to 95% of animal strains were typable. The sources of the animal strains included strains from poultry, pets, farm animals, laboratory animals, wild birds, and seafood. The smallest number of typable *C. jejuni* and *C. coli* strains was found among isolates from wild birds by using 29 antisera (156). Although the number of antisera used to type the strains varied by country, many studies revealed that as many as 75% of isolates were typable with as few as 10 to 12 antisera (44, 66, 75, 94, 101, 119, 135, 136, 155).

Similarly, the HL system was capable of serotyping 65 to 100% of human strains and 59 to 100% of animal strains from 14 countries (Table 3). Poultry, pets, farm animals, and wild birds were the sources of these strains. As with the HS system, 10 to 12 antisera typed as many as three-fourths of the strains (2, 38, 46, 55, 69, 96, 111, 136, 138).

The distribution of the common serotypes in various geographic locations varied somewhat. Except for isolates from certain developing countries, most were the same as those found to be common serotypes in HS and HL schemes (Table 4). Differences are highlighted in boldface type in Table 4. The three most common HS serotypes in human isolates in 11 countries were types 1, 2, and 4. HL serotypes 1, 2, 4, and 36 occurred most commonly among human strains in 12 countries.

The serotypes common in domestic animals in each country (20, 57, 137; see also references

TABLE 2. Effectiveness of HS system for serotyping human and animal *C. jejuni* and *C. coli* strains from 12 countries

Country	Human isolates: No. of antisera	No. of strains tested	% Typable	Animal isolates: No. of antisera	No. of strains tested	% Typable	References
Bangladesh	42	102	74	42	26	65	102
Canada	55	285	97	16	83[a]	87	75, 119
	55	168	100	20	316	76	94, 101
Central African Republic	56	185	74				47
England	26	310	83	26	595	82	65
	28[b]	921	NI[c]	28	824[d]	76	44
	39	431	94	50	56	55	66, 158
Kuwait	20	51	78				136
Mexico	23	136	69				138
Nigeria				36	181	87	35
Norway	42	79	84				97
Scotland	29	650	76	29[e]	NI	24	156
South Africa	76[f]	258	79				82
Sweden	19	253	76				69
	19	105	76				135
United States	57	645	98	57	445	95	110
	55	99	94	55	195	94	155[g]
				20	36	58	40[h]
				20	119	51	146
				16	45	91	162

[a] Chicken isolates only.
[b] Coagglutination/passive hemagglutination.
[c] NI, not indicated.
[d] Food samples from poultry, beef, pork, lamb, offal (liver, kidney, heart), and seafood.
[e] Wild-bird (*Larus* sp.) isolates only.
[f] Includes 60 standard and 16 provisional antisera.
[g] Strains primarily from Iowa.
[h] Beagle isolates only.

in Tables 2 and 3) generally correspond to common serotypes in human strains (Table 4), except for isolates from swine in developed countries, e.g., Canada, United States, and the Federal Republic of Germany (101, 155, 157).

Epidemic investigations and other epidemiologic studies in numerous countries have shown that each system is also effective in separating related isolates from unrelated isolates, thereby identifying sources and modes of transmission of *Campylobacter* species. This has been shown with cow and goat milk (11, 16, 34, 51, 58, 59, 66, 78, 99, 111, 133, 153); poultry (66, 110); water (16, 26, 110, 111, 118, 121, 129, 144), including mountain streams (145) and untreated surface water (4); foods (13, 15, 127); pets (16, 31, 98, 111); and occasionally person-to-person spread, including neonate infection during delivery (16, 54, 74). Serotypes commonly isolated from humans and animals are also frequently found in river water (19, 44, 143) and sewage (6, 142), implicating these and consumable products contaminated with river water or sewage as possible sources of infection for humans and animals. The most common serotype in nine milk-borne outbreaks and one food-borne outbreak in the United States was HS2:HL4, and multiple serotypes were found in humans in two of four waterborne outbreaks (110a, 111).

Three laboratories have compared the HS and HL systems and have found them to be complementary (66, 69, 111). Strains of the same serotype in one system comprise multiple serotypes in the other system, resulting in a variety of HS-HL combinations. The combination of the two systems obviously gives greater discrimination.

At the Centers for Disease Control we have worked with both systems for the past 9 years, and both systems have proven effective. In the

TABLE 3. Effectiveness of HL system for serotyping human and animal *C. jejuni* and *C. coli* strains from 14 countries

	Human isolates			Animal isolates			
Country	No. of antisera	No. of strains tested	% Typable	No. of antisera	No. of strains tested	% Typable	References
Austria	NI[a]	121	98				55
Canada				21	105[b]	80	46
Central African Republic	20	209	71				48
Chile	96	76	100	96	25	100	38
England	10	431	65				66
France	17	226	82				96
Germany	62	109	92				157
India	73	30	83	73	25	88	10
Japan				60	76[c]	59	72
Kuwait	23	51	96				136
Mexico	20	136	93				138
Nigeria	NI	101	100	NI	99	100	2
Sweden	19	253	90				69
	19	105	98				135
United States	55	645	92	55	445	90	111

[a] NI, antisera provided by H. Lior. Number of antisera not indicated.
[b] Cattle isolates only.
[c] *C. jejuni*, *C. coli*, and *C. lari* strains from gulls.

following paragraphs, we discuss some of the problems encountered and simplifications of the HS and HL schemes which offer potential solutions to those problems.

HS Serotyping System

Although preparation of antisera is straightforward, the actual passive hemagglutination procedure is labor- and time-intensive, requiring several washes of the erythrocytes before and after sensitization and several incubation periods. In our experience, one person can serotype approximately 30 to 40 strains in 1 week. Over a 5-year period, 20% of frozen antisera had declined to minimal titer; replacement would require more than 6 months.

We and others occasionally observe high-titer, transient antigens, apparently unrelated to other antigens on the cell (111). These do not seem to be associated with a certain serotype, but certain antigens are transient more frequently than others. The factors that affect their presence or detection have not been determined. One strain may also react in several antisera, resulting in a serotype complex such as 4,13,16,43,50; the presence and titer of these antigens may vary from test to test. These problems usually result in repeated antigenic extraction and retesting, adding to the time and labor problems.

HL Serotyping System

Although the time required for the actual HL assay of 30 to 40 strains is only 3 days, a tremendous time and labor investment is required to produce and maintain antisera. Additionally, test strains may require as many as 10 subcultures for antigen expression (38, 55, 111, 157). Of the 108 serotypes in the system, the Centers for Disease Control maintain antisera to 60 strains, requiring the preparation and quality control of a total of 129 absorbed and unabsorbed antisera. In our laboratory, the growth from 40 to 60 plates (15 by 150 mm) is required to absorb 2 ml of serum, making incubator space a limiting factor. HL antisera prepared in other laboratories may require less growth for absorption (90). In some cases, the specific HL antibody is lost during multiple absorptions, or the resulting titer is extremely low. As with HS antisera, titers have declined to unacceptable levels during storage. To replace these sera and replenish other antisera would require more than 2.5 years.

TABLE 4. Common serotypes in HS and HL systems and in human isolates from several countries

Country	Common serotypes[a]	Reference
HS system	1; 2; 3; 4; 5; 6,7; 8; 11; 13,16; 23,26	Penner[b]
Bangladesh	5; **10;** 13; **15; 21; 22;** 23; **33; 41; 53**	102
Central African Republic	1,3; 3; 5; **24; 30; 34; 37,56; 49; 49,53**	47
South Africa	1; 2; 4; 5; **5,31; 12;** 13,16,50; **19;** 23,36	82
Kuwait	1; 3; 4; 5; 8; 11; 13; 23; **25**	136
Mexico	1; 4; 5; 8; 11; 13; **15; 21; 37**	138
Canada	1; 2; 3; 4; 5; 8; 13,16; **18; 21;** 23,36	94
England	1,44; 2; 3; 4; 6,7; 8; **9,37; 21;** 23	65
Scotland	1; 2; 4; 5; 6; 8; 11; 13; 23; **31**	156
Sweden	1; 2; 4; 5; 6; 8; 13; 16; **18; 37**	69
Norway	1; 4; 6; 7; **12,40;** 13,16; 23,36	97
United States	1; 2; 3; 4; 5; 6,7; 8; **15; 16,50; 19**	Patton[c]
HL system	1; 2; 4; 5; 6; 7; 8; 9; 11; 17; 36	Lior[b]
Central African Republic	1; 2; 4; 7; **21; 28; 29;** 36; **44; 46**	48
India	2; **29; 46; 54; 55**	10
Nigeria	2; 4; 5; 9; **18; 29;** 36; **46; 53**	2
Kuwait	1; 2; 4; 6; 9; **10;** 11; **21;** 36	136
Mexico	2; 4; 9; 11; **13; 20; 21;** 36	138
Chile	2; 4; 7; 8; 9; **13; 21; 29,55; 79**	38
Austria	1; 2; 4; 6; 11; **13; 21; 28; 29;** 36	55
England	1; 2; 4; 5; 6; 7; 8; 9; 11; 17	46
France	1; 4; 5; 6; 9; 11; **29; 45; 46**	96
Germany	1; 4; 5; 6; 7; 8; **10; 16;** 36	157
Sweden	1; 2; 4; 6; 7; 8; 9; **13;** 17	69
United States	1; 2; 4; 6; 7; 9; 11; **16;** 17; 36	Patton[c]

[a] Differences from common serotypes in HS and HL systems highlighted in boldface type.
[b] Personal communications from J. Penner (HS system) and H. Lior (HL system).
[c] Preliminary data, C. Patton.

Solving Problems of HS-HL Systems

Serotyping using referenced methodology is beyond the scope of many public health and clinical laboratories. As a result, other methods or modifications of the current serotyping procedures have been proposed.

Combined HS-HL systems

A coagglutination system to simultaneously type HS and HS antigens of *C. jejuni* and *C. coli* has been devised (160). Although HS and HL antisera were produced as described for the HS and HL schemes (90, 114), sera (antibodies) were subsequently absorbed to *Staphylococcus aureus* (protein A) cells and reacted with *Campylobacter* cells in a slide agglutination test. Antisera reacted specifically with serotype reference strains (160), but discrepancies were noted when wild-type strains were assayed (112). With further refinement in reagents and technique, coagglutination procedure could become a practical method for public health and clinical laboratories.

Simplified HS system

Several modifications of the passive hemagglutination procedure have been described. The Penner microtiter passive hemagglutination method was converted to a slide format by using pooled antisera followed by testing in individual sera (116). Results correlated with the microtiter procedure for 88% of 197 isolates tested. Most differences were attributed to isolates with low levels of somatic antigen or cross-reacting antigens. With the availability of antisera, the simplified procedure may be an alternative means of serotyping for epidemic investigations.

Investigators in Great Britain developed a more rapid microtiter passive hemagglutination test and subsequently combined the modifications with a slide format (43). By reducing the time for antigen extraction and erythrocyte sensitization and using nucleated avian erythrocytes that agglutinate more rapidly than sheep erythrocytes, the test could be done in 1 day.

These investigators then combined the chicken erythrocyte passive hemagglutination slide test with coagglutination of *S. aureus* antibody-coated cells (45, 62). The combined passive hemagglutination-coagglutination slide test is considered presumptive, and the serotype was confirmed by the modified microtiter technique (44). With the availability of antisera and appropriate reagents, these modifications may allow routine application of serotyping in clinical laboratories.

Simplified HL system

For a short period, a commercial kit with absorbed and unabsorbed antisera to the 25 most common serotypes was available for the HL serotyping system. In one study (9), the kit typed approximately 50% of thermophilic campylobacters. The kit was relatively expensive because of antiserum production and quality control requirements and is no longer manufactured.

A mathematical, computer-based method to simplify *Campylobacter* serotyping by using the Lior data set of 21 antisera has been proposed (152). Seven key sera, selected according to criteria that include cross-reaction information, would be expected to identify approximately 60% of cases (strains). For the remaining cases (strains), screening in "intersecting pools" is needed. Since selection of key sera depends on the cross-reactions, and antisera produced in different rabbits to the same antigen preparation may have different major and minor cross-reactions, each laboratory must analyze its own serum collection to determine the key sera and pools.

Use of a limited number of antisera

To simplify serotyping, some investigators have limited the number of antisera and use either a combination of both serotyping schemes (66, 69), or one serotyping system with a combination of biotyping (61) or phage typing (131), or all three (91).

Because of the time and effort required to maintain each system and the significant decline in epidemic support requests, the Centers for Disease Control will maintain a limited number of typing antisera. To select those sera, the most common serotypes in a collection of 646 isolates from 19 laboratories in 14 states across the United States will be determined. In a preliminary analysis, the common serotypes appear similar to the common types in the HS and HL schemes (110a). A set of approximately 20 antisera in each system should serotype 90% of isolates from sporadic cases and outbreaks.

In future outbreak studies, common serotype, nontypable, or problematic isolates will be ribotyped. This decision is based on a recent collaborative study of strains from four well-defined outbreaks evaluating 10 methods for sensitivity and specificity (113). The methods in this study included HS and HL serotyping, Lior biotyping, Lior phage typing, plasmid profile analysis, electrophoretic typing by MEE, REA with various enzymes, and ribotyping with various enzymes and probes.

When data from this study were analyzed for maximal discrimination or sensitivity, MEE, REA, and ribotyping with the *E. coli* 16S+23S rRNA identified nine types among the 22 strains. These methods were further capable of distinguishing strains of the same serotype.

Although the HS and HL serotypes could be further discriminated, serotyping methods were as successful as other procedures for distinguishing strains within each epidemic. For this reason, and because serotypes are internationally recognized, serotyping seems to be the initial typing method of choice for epidemic investigations, if high-quality antisera are available.

FUTURE NEEDS

Although molecular approaches to subtyping *Campylobacter* spp. are promising, they are not quantifiable and the methods remain complex. One future direction of research should be the generation of quantitative data for these methods. The use of digoxygenin in place of ^{32}P for ribotyping and the addition of a statistical analysis to determine strain relationships by using ribotyping data are very promising (77, 154).

A future direction of research for serotyping might be to prepare specific antisera to purified antigens (93, 120) and to make those reagents widely available.

The Centers for Disease Control will continue serotyping since we have made the initial investment to establish the systems; also, our needs for typing have changed from outbreak support to surveillance activities, which require a quantitative, comparative system such as serotyping. The epidemiologic study of 646 sporadic cases of strains from across the United States will provide invaluable epidemiologic information; it will take approximately 6 months to determine the HS and HL serotypes of 300 strains from this collection, but this would be virtually impossible to accomplish by ribotyping. Future public health studies will require the further application of subtyping methods to the study of *Campylobacter* sporadic disease, which occurs far more frequently than outbreak disease.

In answer to the question posed in the title of this chapter, current methods are useful but are not easily adapted to routine use in microbiology or clinical laboratories.

ACKNOWLEDGMENTS. We are grateful to Mable Ann Nicholson, Dan Cameron, Nancy Puhr, and Ramona Walters, who kindly provided help and support for both the oral presentation of these data and the preparation of the manuscript.

REFERENCES

1. **Abbott, J. D., B. Dale, J. Eldridge, D. M. Jones, and E. M. Sutcliffe.** 1980. Serotyping of *Campylobacter jejuni/coli. J. Clin. Pathol.* **33**:762–766.
2. **Adegbola, R. A., S. A. Alabi, F. O. Akinkuade, A. O. Coker, and T. Odugbemi.** 1990. Correlation between human and animal bio-serogroups of *Campylobacter* isolates in Nigeria. *J. Trop. Med. Hyg.* **93**:280–283.
3. **Aeschbacher, M., and J. Piffaretti.** 1989. Population genetics of human and animal enteric *Campylobacter* strains. *Infect. Immun.* **57**:1432–1437.
4. **Aho, M., M. Kurki, H. Rautelin, and T. U. Kosunen.** 1989. Waterborne outbreak of campylobacter enteritis after outdoors infantry drill in Utti, Finland. *Epidemiol. Infect.* **103**:133–141.
5. **Altwegg, M., A. Burnens, J. Zollinger-Iten, and J. L. Penner.** 1987. Problems in identification of *Campylobacter jejuni* associated with acquisition of resistance to nalidixic acid. *J. Clin. Microbiol.* **25**:1807–1808.
6. **Arimi, S. M., C. R. Fricker, and R. W. A. Park.** 1988. Occurrence of "thermophilic" campylobacters in sewage and their removal by treatment processes. *Epidemiol. Infect.* **101**:279–286.
7. **Austen, R. A., and T. J. Trust.** 1980. Detection of plasmids in the related group of the genus *Campylobacter. FEMS Microbiol. Lett.* **8**:201–204.
8. **Banffer, J. R.** 1985. Biotypes and serotypes of *Campylobacter jejuni* and *Campylobacter coli* strains isolated from patients, pigs and chickens in the region of Rotterdam. *J. Infect.* **10**:277–288.
9. **Bar, W., G. Fricke, and H. Goossens.** 1989. Distribution of serotypes and biotypes of thermophilic campylobacters in the Federal Republic of Germany: a comparison with other countries. *Zentralbl. Bakteriol.* **271**:127–134.
10. **Bhadra, R. K., H. Lior, S. K. Misra, S. C. Pal, and G. B. Nair.** 1989. Serotypes and biotypes of *Campylobacter jejuni* and *C. coli* from diverse sources in Calcutta. *Indian J. Med. Res.* **89**:225–228.
11. **Birkhead, G., R. L. Vogt, E. Heun, C. M. Evelti, and C. M. Patton.** 1988. A multiple-strain outbreak of Campylobacter enteritis due to consumption of inadequately pasteurized milk. *J. Infect. Dis.* **157**:1095–1097.
12. **Blackwell, C. C., F. P. Winstanley, and W. A. T. Brunton.** 1982. Sensitivity of thermophilic campylobacters to R-type pyocines of *Pseudomonas aeruginosa. J. Med. Microbiol.* **15**:247–251.
13. **Blaser, M. J., P. Checko, C. Bopp, A. Bruce, and J. M. Hughes.** 1982. *Campylobacter* enteritis associated with foodborne transmission. *Am. J. Epidemiol.* **116**:886–894.
14. **Blaser, M. J., J. A. Hopkins, R. M. Berka, M. L. Vasid, and W. L. Wang.** 1983. Identification and characterization of *Campylobacter jejuni* outer membrane proteins. *Infect. Immun.* **42**:276–284.
15. **Blaser, M. J., and C. M. Patton.** 1985. *Campylobacter* enteritis associated with foodborne transmission: new serotyping data. *Am. J. Epidemiol.* **121**:625–626.
16. **Blaser, M. J., J. L. Penner, and J. G. Wells.** 1982. Diversity of serotypes in outbreaks of enteritis due to *Campylobacter jejuni. J. Infect. Dis.* **146**:826.
17. **Blaser, M. J., J. G. Wells, R. A. Feldman, R. A. Pollard, J. R. Allen, and The Collaborative Diarrheal Disease Study Group.** 1983. Campylobacter enteritis in the United States: a multicenter study. *Ann. Intern. Med.* **98**:360–365.
18. **Bokkenheuser, V. D., N. J. Richardson, J. H. Bryner, D. J. Roux, A. B. Schutte, H. J. Koornhof, I. Freiman, and E. Hartman.** 1979. Detection of enteric campylobacteriosis in children. *J. Clin. Microbiol.* **9**:227–232.
19. **Bolton, F. J., D. Coates, D. N. Hutchinson, and A. F. Godfree.** 1987. A study of thermophilic campylobacters in a river system. *J. Appl. Bacteriol.* **62**:167–176.
20. **Bolton, F. J., H. C. Dawkins, and D. N. Hutchinson.** 1985. Biotypes and serotypes of thermophilic campylobacters isolated from cattle, sheep and pig offal and other red meats. *J. Hyg.* (Cambridge) **95**:1–6.
21. **Bolton, F. J., A. V. Holt, and D. N. Hutchinson.** 1984. Campylobacter biotyping scheme of epidemiological value. *J. Clin. Pathol.* **37**:677–681.
22. **Bopp, C. A., K. A. Birkness, I. K. Wachsmuth, and T. J. Barrett.** 1985. In vitro antimicrobial susceptibility, plasmid analysis, and serotyping of epidemic-associated *Campylobacter jejuni. J. Clin. Microbiol.* **21**:4–7.
23. **Bradbury, W. C., and D. L. G. Munroe.** 1985. Occurrence of plasmid and antibiotic resistance among *Campylobacter jejuni* and *Campylobacter coli* isolated from healthy and diarrheic animals. *J. Clin. Microbiol.* **22**:339–346.
24. **Bradbury, W. C., A. M. Murray, J. N. Hennessy, and J. L. Penner.** 1983. Occurrence of plasmid DNA in serologically defined strains of *Campylobacter jejuni* and *Campylobacter coli. Infect. Immun.* **40**:460–463.

25. **Bradbury, W. C., A. D. Pearson, M. A. Marko, R. V. Congi, and J. L. Penner.** 1984. Investigation of a *Campylobacter jejuni* outbreak by serotyping and chromosomal restriction endonuclease analysis. *J. Clin. Microbiol.* **19:**342–346.
26. **Broczyk, A., S. Thompson, D. Smith, and H. Lior.** 1987. Water-borne outbreak of *Campylobacter laridis*-associated gastroenteritis. *Lancet* **i:**164–165.
27. **Bruce, D., J. V. Hookey, and S. A. Waitkins.** 1988. Numerical classification of campylobacters by DNA-restriction endonuclease analysis. *Zentralbl. Bakteriol. Mikrobiol. Hyg. Ser. A* **269:**284–297.
28. **Bryner, J. H., A. E. Ritchie, and J. W. Foley.** 1982. Techniques for phage typing *Campylobacter jejuni,* abstr. 18, p. 52–56. *In* D. G. Newell (ed.), *Campylobacter: Epidemiology, Pathogenesis and Biochemistry.* MTP Press, Lancaster, United Kingdom.
29. **Butzler, J. P., and M. B. Skirrow.** 1979. Campylobacter enteritis. *Clin. Gastroenterol.* **8:**737–765.
30. **Corbel, M. J., and K. P. W. Gill.** 1987. Lectin agglutination of thermophilic *Campylobacter* species. *Vet. Microbiol.* **15:**163–173.
31. **Deming, M. S., R. V. Tauxe, P. A. Blake, S. E. Dixon, B. S. Fowler, T. S. Jones, E. A. Lockamy, C. M. Patton, and R. K. Sikes.** 1987. *Campylobacter* enteritis at a university: transmission from eating chicken and from cats. *Am. J. Epidemiol.* **126:**526–534.
32. **Derclaye, I., I. Delor, M. Van Bouchaute, P. Moureau, G. Wauters, and G. R. Cornelis.** 1989. Identification of *Campylobacter jejuni* and *C. coli* by gel electrophoresis of the outer membrane proteins. *J. Clin. Microbiol.* **27:**1072–1076.
33. **Dickgiesser, N., and D. Czylwik.** 1985. Chemically defined media for auxotyping of *C. jejuni. Zentralbl. Bakteriol. Mikrobiol. Hyg. Ser. A* **260:**57–64.
34. **Dilworth, C. R., H. Lior, and M. A. Belliveau.** 1988. *Campylobacter* enteritis acquired from cattle. *Can. J. Public Health* **79:**60–62.
35. **Elegbe, I. A., A. Juba, and J. O. Adebayo.** 1987. Species and serotypes of *Campylobacter* from domestic animals in Nigeria. *J. Diarrhoeal Dis. Res.* **2:**97–101.
36. **Elharrif, Z., and F. Megraud.** 1986. Characterization of thermophilic *Campylobacter.* II. Enzymatic profiles. *Curr. Microbiol.* **13:**317–322.
37. **Ferguson, D. A., Jr., and D. W. Lambe, Jr.** 1984. Differentiation of *Campylobacter* species by protein-banding patterns in polyacrylamide slab gels. *J. Clin. Microbiol.* **20:**453–460.
38. **Figueroa, G., M. Troncoso, H. Galeno, V. Soto, and M. S. Toledo.** 1990. Biotypes, serogroups and antibiotic susceptibility of *Campylobacter jejuni* and *Campylobacter coli* in Chile. *J. Infect. Dis.* **20:**123–127.
39. **Fletcher, R. D.** 1965. Activity and morphology of *Vibrio coli* phage. *Am. J. Vet. Res.* **26:**361–364.
40. **Fox, J. G., M. C. Claps, N. S. Taylor, K. O. Maxwell, J. I. Ackerman, and S. B. Hoffman.** 1988. *Campylobacter jejuni/coli* in commercially reared beagles: prevalence and serotypes. *Lab. Anim. Sci.* **38:**262–265.
41. **Fox, J. G., N. S. Taylor, J. L. Penner, B. Shames, R. V. Gurgis, and F. N. Tomson.** 1989. Investigation of zoonotically acquired *Campylobacter jejuni* enteritis with serotyping and restriction endonuclease DNA analysis. *J. Clin. Microbiol.* **27:**2423–2425.
42. **Fricker, C. R.** 1986. Campylobacter serotyping on shipped antigen extracts. *Lancet* **i:**554.
43. **Fricker, C. R., M. M. Alemohammad, and R. W. A. Park.** 1987. A study of factors affecting the sensitivity of the passive hemagglutination method for serotyping *Campylobacter jejuni* and *Campylobacter coli* and recommendations for a more rapid procedure. *Can. J. Microbiol.* **33:**33–39.
44. **Fricker, C. R., and R. W. A. Park.** 1989. A two-year study of the distribution of "thermophilic" campylobacters in human, environmental and food samples from the Reading area with particular reference to toxin production and heat-stable serotype. *J. Appl. Bacteriol.* **66:**477–490.
45. **Fricker, C. R., J. Uradzinske, M. M. Alemohammad, R. W. A. Park, C. Whelan, and R. W. A. Girdwood.** 1986. Serotyping of campylobacters by co-agglutination on the basis of heat-stable antigens. *J. Med. Microbiol.* **21:**83–86.
46. **Garcia, M. M., H. Lior, R. B. Stewart, G. M. Ruckerbauer, J. R. Trudel, and A. Skljarevski.** 1985. Isolation, characterization, and serotyping of *Campylobacter jejuni* and *Campylobacter coli* from slaughter cattle. *Appl. Environ. Microbiol.* **49:**667–672.
47. **Georges-Courbot, M. C., C. Baya, A. M. Beraud, D. M. Y. Meunier, and A. J. Georges.** 1986. Distribution and serotypes of *C. jejuni* and *C. coli* in enteric *Campylobacter* strains isolated from children in the Central African Republic. *J. Clin. Microbiol.* **23:**592–594.
48. **Georges-Courbot, M. C., I. Gouandjika, P. M. V. Martin, and A. J. Georges.** 1989. Biotype and Lior serogroup distribution of enteric *Campylobacter* isolated from children in Bangui (Central African Republic), and comparison with Penner serotypes. *Res. Microbiol.* **140:**489–497.
49. **Goossens, H., G. Henocque, L. Kremp, J. Rocque, R. Boury, G. Alanio, L. Vlaes, W. Hemelhof, C. Van den Borre, M. Macart, and J. P. Butzler.** 1986. Nosocomial outbreak of *Campylobacter jejuni* meningitis in newborn infants. *Lancet* **ii:**146–149.
50. **Grajewski, B. A., J. W. Kusek, and H. M. Gelfand.** 1985. Development of a bacteriophage typing system for *Campylobacter jejuni* and *Campylobacter coli. J. Clin. Microbiol.* **22:**13–18.
51. **Harris, N. V., R. J. Kimball, P. Bennett, Y. Johnson, D. Wakely, and C. M. Nolan.** 1987. *Campylobacter jejuni* enteritis associated with raw goat's milk. *Am. J. Epidemiol.* **126:**179–186.
52. **Hebert, G. A., D. G. Hollis, R. E. Weaver, M. A. Lambert, M. J. Blaser, and C. W. Moss.** 1982. 30 years of campylobacters: biochemical characteristics and a biotyping proposal for *Campylobacter jejuni. J. Clin. Microbiol.* **15:**1065–1073.
53. **Hebert, G. A., D. G. Hollis, R. E. Weaver, A. G. Steigerwalt, R. M. McKinney, and D. J. Brenner.**

1983. Serogroups of *Campylobacter jejuni, Campylobacter coli,* and *Campylobacter fetus* defined by direct immunofluorescence. *J. Clin. Microbiol.* **17**:529–538.

54. **Hershkowici, S., M. Barak, A. Cohen, and J. Montag.** 1987. An outbreak of *Campylobacter jejuni* infection in a neonatal intensive care unit. *J. Hosp. Infect.* **9**:54–59.
55. **Hirschl, A. M., H. Lior, D. Wolf, G. Stanek, M. L. Rotter, L. Wende, and H. Flamm.** 1987. Occurrence, serotypes and biotypes of thermophilic campylobacters isolated in Vienna. *Zentralbl. Bakteriol. Mikrobiol. Hyg. Ser. A* **266**:94–103.
56. **Hollander, R.** 1984. Characterization of *Campylobacter jejuni/coli* isolates from human faeces. *Zentralbl. Bakteriol. Mikrobiol. Hyg. Ser. A* **258**:128–134.
57. **Hood, A. M., A. D. Pearson, and M. Shahamat.** 1988. The extent of surface contamination of retailed chickens with *Campylobacter jejuni* serotypes. *Epidemiol. Infect.* **100**:17–25.
58. **Hudson, P. J., R. L. Vogt, J. Brodum, and C. M. Patton.** 1984. Isolation of *Campylobacter jejuni* from milk during an outbreak of campylobacteriosis. *J. Infect. Dis.* **150**:789.
59. **Hutchinson, D. N., F. J. Bolton, P. M. Hinchliffe, H. C. Dawkins, S. D. Horsley, E. G. Jessop, P. A. Robertshaw, and D. E. Counter.** 1985. Evidence of udder excretion of *Campylobacter jejuni* as the cause of milk-borne campylobacter outbreak. *J. Hyg.* (Cambridge) **94**:205–215.
60. **Hutchinson, D. N., F. J. Bolton, W. C. N. Jelley, W. G. Mathews, D. R. Telford, D. E. Counter, E. G. Jessop, and S. D. Horsley.** 1985. *Campylobacter* enteritis associated with consumption of raw goat's milk. *Lancet* **i**:1037–1038.
61. **Hutchinson, D. N., F. J. Bolton, D. M. Jones, E. M. Sutcliffe, and J. D. Abbott.** 1987. Application of three typing schemes (Penner, Lior, Preston) to strains of *Campylobacter* spp. isolated from three outbreaks. *Epidemiol. Infect.* **98**:139–144.
62. **Illingworth, D. S., and C. R. Fricker.** 1987. Rapid serotyping of campylobacters based on heat-stable antigens, using a combined passive haemagglutination/co-agglutination technique. *Lett. Appl. Microbiol.* **5**:61–63.
63. **Itoh, T., K. Saito, Y. Yanagawa, S. Sakai, and M. Ohashi.** 1982. Serological typing of thermophilic campylobacters isolated in Tokyo, abstr. 39, p. 106–110. *In* D. G. Newell (ed.), *Campylobacter: Epidemiology, Pathogenesis and Biochemistry.* MTP Press, Lancaster, United Kingdom.
64. **Johnson, K. E., C. M. Nolan, and the *Campylobacter* Laboratory Surveillance Group.** 1985. Community-wide surveillance of *C. jejuni* infection. *Diagn. Microbiol. Infect. Dis.* **3**:389–396.
65. **Jones, D. M., J. D. Abbott, M. J. Painter, and E. M. Sutcliffe.** 1984. A comparison of biotypes and serotypes of *Campylobacter* sp. isolated from patients with enteritis and from animal and environmental sources. *J. Infect.* **9**:51–58.
66. **Jones, D. M., E. M. Sutcliffe, and J. D. Abbott.** 1985. Serotyping of *Campylobacter* species by combined use of two methods. *Eur. J. Clin. Microbiol.* **4**:562–565.
67. **Kahlich, R., E. Aldova, I. Kusiak, O. Hausner, P. Roch, V. Potuznik, and V. Radovnicky.** 1989. Use of live cultures for serotyping *Campylobacter jejuni.* II. Further experience and use in an epidemiological study. *Syst. Appl. Microbiol.* **12**:306–309.
68. **Kahlich, R., E. Aldova, A. Palecek, and J. Sourek.** 1985. Use of live cultures for serotyping *Campylobacter jejuni. Syst. Appl. Microbiol.* **6**:82–85.
69. **Kaijser, B., and E. Sjogren.** 1985. *Campylobacter* strains in Sweden. *Acta Pathol. Microbiol. Immunol. Scand.* **93**:315–322.
70. **Kakoyiannis, C. K., P. J. Winter, and R. B. Marshall.** 1984. Identification of *C. coli* isolates from animals and humans by bacterial restriction endonuclease DNA analysis. *Appl. Environ. Microbiol.* **48**:545–549.
71. **Kakoyiannis, C. K., P. J. Winter, and R. B. Marshall.** 1988. The relationship between intestinal *Campylobacter* species isolated from animals and humans as determined by BRENDA. *Epidemiol. Infect.* **100**:379–387.
72. **Kaneuchi, C., M. Ashihara, K. Saito, and T. Itoh.** 1989. Serogrouping of thermophilic *Campylobacter* from gulls by slide agglutination based on heat-labile antigenic factors. *Jpn. J. Vet. Sci.* **51**:431–433.
73. **Kapperud, G., J. Lassen, S. Lauwers, and O. Rosef.** 1984. Serotyping and biotyping of *Campylobacter jejuni* and *Campylobacter coli* from sporadic cases and outbreaks in Norway. *J. Clin. Microbiol.* **19**:157–160.
74. **Karmali, M. A., B. Norrish, H. Lior, B. Heyes, A. Monteath, and H. Montgomery.** 1984. *Campylobacter* enterocolitis in a neonatal nursery. *J. Infect. Dis.* **149**:874–877.
75. **Karmali, M. A., J. L. Penner, P. C. Fleming, A. Williams, and J. N. Hennessy.** 1983. The serotype and biotype distribution of clinical isolates of *Campylobacter jejuni* and *Campylobacter coli* over a three-year period. *J. Infect. Dis.* **147**:243–246.
76. **Khakhria, R., and H. Lior.** 1987. Phagetyping of *Campylobacter jejuni,* abstr. 189, p. 134. *In* B. Kaijser and E. Falsen (ed.), *Campylobacter IV.* University of Göteborg, Göteborg, Sweden.
77. **Kiehlbauch, J. A., B. D. Plikaytis, B. Swaminathan, D. N. Cameron, and I. K. Wachsmuth.** 1991. Restriction fragment length polymorphisms in the ribosomal genes for the species identification and subtyping of aerotolerant *Campylobacter* species. *J. Clin. Microbiol.* **29**:1670–1676.
78. **Kornblatt, A. N., T. Barrett, G. K. Morris, and F. E. Tosh.** 1985. Epidemiologic and laboratory investigation of an outbreak of campylobacter enteritis associated with raw milk. *Am. J. Epidemiol.* **122**:884–889.
79. **Kosunen, T. U., B. E. Bang, and M. Hurme.** 1984. Analysis of *Campylobacter jejuni* antigens with monoclonal antibodies. *J. Clin. Microbiol.* **19**:129–133.

80. **Kosunen, T., D. Danielsson, and J. Kjellander.** 1980. Serology of *Campylobacter fetus* ss. *jejuni* ("related" campylobacters). Demonstration of strain-specific and interstrain-related antigens by immunoelectrophoresis and co-agglutination. *Acta. Pathol. Microbiol. Scand.* **88:**207–218.
81. **Kosunen, T. U., D. Danielsson, and J. Kjellander.** 1982. Serology of *Campylobacter fetus* ss. *jejuni*. 2. Serotyping of live bacteria by slide, latex and co-agglutination tests. *Acta. Pathol. Microbiol. Immunol. Scand.* **90:**191–196.
82. **Lastovica, A. J., E. Le Roux, R. V. Congi, and J. L. Penner.** 1986. Distribution of sero-biotypes of *Campylobacter jejuni* and *Campylobacter coli* isolated from paediatric patients. *J. Med. Microbiol.* **21:**1–5.
83. **Lastovica, A. J., R. B. Marshall, and J. L. Penner.** 1986. *Campylobacter* serotyping on shipped antigen extracts. *Lancet* **i:**320.
84. **Lauwers, S., and J. L. Penner.** 1984. Serotyping *Campylobacter jejuni* and *Campylobacter coli* on the basis of thermostable antigens, p. 51–59. *In* J. P. Butzler (ed.), *Campylobacter Infection in Man and Animals.* CRC Press, Inc., Boca Raton, Fla.
85. **Lauwers, S., L. Vlaes, and J. P. Butzler.** 1981. Campylobacter serotyping and epidemiology. *Lancet* **i:**158–159.
86. **Lind, L., E. Sjogren, C. Welinder-Olsson, and B. Kaijser.** 1989. Plasmids and serogroups in *Campylobacter jejuni. Acta Pathol. Microbiol. Immunol. Scand.* **97:**1097–1102.
87. **Lior, H.** 1984. New, extended biotyping scheme for *Campylobacter jejuni, Campylobacter coli,* and "*Campylobacter laridis.*" *J. Clin. Microbiol.* **20:**636–640.
88. **Lior, H.** 1984. Serotyping of *Campylobacter jejuni* and *C. coli* by slide agglutination based on heat-labile antigenic factors, p. 61–76. *In* J. P. Butzler (ed.), *Campylobacter Infection in Man and Animals.* CRC Press, Inc., Boca Raton, Fla.
88a. **Lior, H.** Personal communication.
89. **Lior, H., and A. Patel.** 1987. Improved toluidine blue-DNA agar for detection of DNA hydrolysis by campylobacters. *J. Clin. Microbiol.* **25:**2030–2031.
90. **Lior, H., D. L. Woodward, J. A. Edgar, L. J. Laroche, and P. Gill.** 1982. Serotyping of *Campylobacter jejuni* by slide agglutination based on heat-labile antigenic factors. *J. Clin. Microbiol.* **15:**761–768.
91. **Lior, H., D. L. Woodward, and R. Khakhria.** 1988. Characterization of *Campylobacter jejuni* outbreaks by 3 epidemiological typing markers, abstr. 192, p. 103–104. *In* B. Kaijser and E. Falsen (ed.), *Campylobacter IV.* University of Göteborg, Göteborg, Sweden.
92. **Logan, S. M., and T. J. Trust.** 1982. Outer membrane characteristics of *Campylobacter jejuni. Infect. Immun.* **38:**898–906.
93. **Mandatori, R., and J. L. Penner.** 1989. Structural and antigenic properties of *Campylobacter coli* lipopolysaccharides. *Infect. Immun.* **57:**3506–3511.
94. **McMyne, P. M. S., J. L. Penner, R. G. Mathias, W. A. Black, and J. N. Hennessy.** 1982. Serotyping of *Campylobacter jejuni* isolated from sporadic cases and outbreaks in British Columbia. *J. Clin. Microbiol.* **16:**281–285.
95. **McOrist, S., R. Boid, and G. H. K. Lawson.** 1989. Antigenic analysis of *Campylobacter* species and an intracellular *Campylobacter*-like organism associated with porcine proliferative enteropathies. *Infect. Immun.* **57:**957–962.
96. **Megraud, F., A. M. Gavinet, and C. Camou-Junca.** 1987. Serogroups and biotypes of human strains of *Campylobacter jejuni* and *Campylobacter coli* isolated in France. *Eur. J. Clin. Microbiol.* **6:**641–645.
97. **Melby, K., G. Storvold, R. V. Congi, and J. L. Penner.** 1985. Serotyping of *Campylobacter jejuni* isolated from sporadic cases and outbreaks in northern Norway. *Acta Pathol. Microbiol. Immunol. Scand.* **93:**83–86.
98. **Miller, I. S., F. J. Bolton, and H. C. Dawkins.** 1987. An outbreak of *Campylobacter* enteritis transmitted by puppies. *Environ. Health* **95:**11–14.
99. **Morgan, G., P. Chadwick, K. P. Lander, and K. P. W. Gill.** 1985. *Campylobacter jejuni* mastitis in a cow: a zoonosis-related incident. *Vet. Rec.* **116:**111.
100. **Moureau, P., I. Derclaye, D. Gregoire, M. Janssen, and G. R. Cornelis.** 1989. *Campylobacter* species identification based on polymorphism of DNA encoding rRNA. *J. Clin. Microbiol.* **27:**1514–1517.
101. **Munroe, D. L., J. F. Prescott, and J. L. Penner.** 1983. *Campylobacter jejuni* and *Campylobacter coli* serotypes isolated from chickens, cattle, and pigs. *J. Clin. Microbiol.* **18:**877–881.
102. **Neogi, P. K. B., and N. S. Shahid.** 1987. Serotypes of *Campylobacter jejuni* isolated from patients attending a diarrhoeal disease hospital in urban Bangladesh. *J. Med. Microbiol.* **24:**303–307.
103. **Newell, D. G.** 1986. Monoclonal antibodies directed against the flagella of *Campylobacter jejuni:* cross-reacting and serotypic specificity and potential use in diagnosis. *J. Hyg.* (Cambridge) **96:**377–384.
104. **Oosterom, J., J. R. Banffer, S. Lauwers, and A. E. Busschbach.** 1985. Serotyping of and hippurate hydrolysis by *Campylobacter jejuni* isolates from human patients, poultry and pigs in the Netherlands. *Antonie Van Leeuwenhoek* **51:**65–70.
105. **O'Sullivan, N., J. Benjamin, and M. B. Skirrow.** 1990. Lectin typing of *Campylobacter* isolates. *J. Clin. Pathol.* **43:**957–960.
106. **Owen, R. J., A. Beck, and P. Borman.** 1985. Restriction endonuclease digest patterns of chromosomal DNA from nitrate-negative *Campylobacter jejuni*-like organisms. *Eur. J. Epidemiol.* **1:**281–287.
107. **Owen, R. J., M. Costas, and C. Dawson.** 1989. Application of different chromosomal DNA restriction digest fingerprints to specific and subspecific identification of *Campylobacter* isolates. *J. Clin. Microbiol.* **27:**2338–2343.

108. **Owen, R. J., M. Costas, L. Sloss, and F. G. Bolton.** 1988. Numerical analysis of electrophoretic protein patterns of *Campylobacter laridis* and allied thermophilic campylobacters from the natural environment. *J. Appl. Bacteriol.* **65:**69–78.
109. **Owen, R. J., J. Hernandez, and F. Bolton.** 1990. DNA restriction digest and ribosomal RNA gene patterns of *Campylobacter jejuni:* a comparison with bio-, sero-, and bacteriophage-types of United Kingdom outbreak strains. *Epidemiol. Infect.* **105:**265–275.
110. **Palmer, S. R., P. R. Gully, J. M. White, A. D. Pearson, W. G. Suckling, D. M. Jones, J. C. Rawes, and J. L. Penner.** 1983. Water-borne outbreak of campylobacter gastroenteritis. *Lancet* **i:**287–290.
110a. **Patton, C.** Unpublished data.
111. **Patton, C. M., T. J. Barrett, and G. K. Morris.** 1985. Comparison of the Penner and Lior methods for serotyping *Campylobacter* spp. *J. Clin. Microbiol.* **22:**558–565.
112. **Patton, C. M., G. K. Morris, S. Erdarcan, P. Collins, and K. G. Wong.** 1986. Serotyping *Campylobacter* by coagglutination, abstr. C-83, p. 341. *Abstr. 86th Annu. Meet. Am. Soc. Microbiol.* 1986. American Society for Microbiology, Washington, D.C.
113. **Patton, C. M., I. K. Wachsmuth, G. M. Evins, J. A. Kiehlbauch, B. D. Plikaytis, N. Troup, L. Tompkins, and H. Lior.** 1991. Evaluation of 10 methods to distinguish epidemic-associated *Campylobacter* strains. *J. Clin. Microbiol.* **29:**680–688.
114. **Penner, J. L., and J. N. Hennessy.** 1980. Passive hemagglutination technique for serotyping *Campylobacter fetus* subsp. *jejuni* on the basis of soluble heat-stable antigens. *J. Clin. Microbiol.* **12:**732–737.
115. **Penner, J. L., J. N. Hennessy, and R. V. Congi.** 1983. Serotyping of *Campylobacter jejuni* and *Campylobacter coli* on the basis of thermostable antigens. *Eur. J. Clin. Microbiol.* **2:**378–383.
116. **Penner, J. L., J. N. Hennessy, and R. V. Congi.** 1984. A simplified procedure for serotyping *Campylobacter jejuni* and *Campylobacter coli,* abstr. C-52, p. 245. *Abstr. 84th Annu. Meet. Am. Soc. Microbiol.* 1984. American Society for Microbiology, Washington, D.C.
117. **Penner, J. L., J. N. Hennessy, S. D. Mills, and W. C. Bradbury.** 1983. Application of serotyping and chromosomal restriction endonuclease digest analysis in investigating a laboratory-acquired case of *Campylobacter jejuni* enteritis. *J. Clin. Microbiol.* **18:**1427–1428.
118. **Penner, J. L., A. D. Pearson, and J. N. Hennessy.** 1983. Investigation of a waterborne outbreak of *Campylobacter jejuni* enteritis with a serotyping scheme based on thermostable antigens. *J. Clin. Microbiol.* **18:**1362–1365.
119. **Prescott, J. F., and O. S. Gellner.** 1984. Intestinal carriage of *Campylobacter jejuni* and *Salmonella* by chicken flocks at slaughter. *Can. J. Comp. Med.* **48:**329–331.
120. **Preston, M. A., and J. L. Penner.** 1987. Structural and antigenic properties of lipopolysaccharides from serotype reference strains of *Campylobacter jejuni. Infect. Immun.* **55:**1806–1812.
121. **Rautelin, H., K. Koota, R. von Essen, M. Jahkola, A. Siitonen, and T. U. Kosunen.** 1990. Waterborne *Campylobacter jejuni* epidemic in a Finnish hospital for rheumatic diseases. *Scand. J. Infect. Dis.* **22:**321–326.
122. **Ritchie, A. E., J. H. Bryner, and J. W. Foley.** 1983. Phages of thermophilic *Campylobacter* spp.: isolation, morphology and utility for typing, p. 101–102. *In* A. D. Pearson, M. B. Skirrow, B. Rowe, J. R. Davies, and D. M. Jones (ed.), *Campylobacter II.* Public Health Laboratory Service, London.
123. **Rogol, M., I. Sechter, I. Braunstein, and C. B. Gerichter.** 1983. Extended scheme for serotyping *Campylobacter jejuni:* results obtained in Israel from 1980 to 1981. *J. Clin. Microbiol.* **18:**283–286.
124. **Romananiuk, P. J., and T. J. Trust.** 1987. Identification of *Campylobacter* species by Southern hybridization of genomic DNA using an oligonucleotide probe for 16S rRNA genes. *FEMS Microbiol. Lett.* **43:**331–335.
125. **Roop, R. M., II, R. M. Smibert, and N. R. Krieg.** 1984. Improved biotyping schemes for *Campylobacter jejuni* and *Campylobacter coli. J. Clin. Microbiol.* **20:**990–992.
126. **Rosef, O., G. Kapperud, S. Lauwers, and B. Gondrosen.** 1985. Serotyping of *Campylobacter jejuni, Campylobacter coli,* and *Campylobacter laridis* from domestic and wild animals. *Appl. Environ. Microbiol.* **49:**1507–1510.
127. **Rosenfield, J. A., G. J. Arnold, G. R. Davey, R. S. Archer, and W. H. Woods.** 1985. Serotyping of *Campylobacter jejuni* from an outbreak of enteritis implicating chicken. *J. Infect. Dis.* **11:**159–165.
128. **Russell, R. G., J. I. Sarmiento, J. Fox, and P. Panigrahi.** 1990. Evidence of reinfection with multiple strains of *Campylobacter jejuni* and *Campylobacter coli* in *Macaca nemestrina* housed under hyperendemic conditions. *Infect. Immun.* **58:**2149–2155.
129. **Sacks, J. J., S. Lieb, L. M. Baldy, S. Berta, C. M. Patton, M. C. White, W. J. Bigler, and J. J. Witte.** 1986. Epidemic campylobacteriosis associated with a community water supply. *Am. J. Public Health* **76:**424–428.
130. **Sagara, H., A. Mochizuke, N. Okamura, and R. Nakaya.** 1987. Antimicrobial resistance of *Campylobacter jejuni* and *Campylobacter coli* with special reference to plasmid profiles of Japanese clinical isolates. *Antimicrob. Agents Chemother.* **31:**713–719.
131. **Salama, S. M., F. J. Bolton, and D. N. Hutchinson.** 1990. Application of a new phagetyping scheme to campylobacters isolated during outbreaks. *Epidemiol. Infect.* **104:**405–411.

132. **Sandstrom, E. G., and A. K. Ruden.** 1990. Markers of *Neisseria gonorrhoeae* for epidemiological studies. *Scand. J. Infect. Dis. Suppl.* **69:**149–156.
133. **Schmid, G. P., R. E. Schaefer, B. D. Plikaytis, J. R. Schaefer, J. H. Bryner, L. A. Wintermeyer, and A. F. Kaufmann.** 1987. A one-year study of endemic campylobacteriosis in a midwestern city: association with consumption of raw milk. *J. Infect. Dis.* **156:**218–222.
134. **Selander, R. K., D. A. Caugant, H. Ochman, J. M. Musser, M. N. Gilmour, and T. S. Whittam.** 1986. Methods of multilocus enzyme electrophoresis for bacterial population genetics and systematics. *Appl. Environ. Microbiol.* **51:**873–884.
135. **Sjogren, E., K. Alestig, and B. Kaijser.** 1989. *Campylobacter* strains from Swedish patients with diarrhoea, distribution of serotypes over a five year period. *Acta Pathol. Microbiol. Immunol. Scand.* **97:**221–226.
136. **Sjogren, E., M. Johny, and B. Kaijser.** 1989. The serotype distribution of *Campylobacter* in patients with diarrhoea in Kuwait. *FEMS Microbiol. Lett.* **48:**237–239.
137. **Sjogren, E., and B. Kaijser.** 1989. Serotyping studies of *Campylobacter* from naturally colonized chickens. *Epidemiol. Infect.* **102:**215–219.
138. **Sjogren, E., G. Ruiz-Palacios, and B. Kaijser.** 1989. *Campylobacter jejuni* isolations from Mexican and Swedish patients with repeated symptomatic and/or asymptomatic diarrhoea episodes. *Epidemiol. Infect.* **102:**47–57.
139. **Skirrow, M. B.** 1987. A demographic survey of *Campylobacter, Salmonella* and *Shigella* infections in England. *Epidemiol. Infect.* **99:**647–657.
140. **Skirrow, M. B., and J. Benjamin.** 1980. Differentiation of enteropathogenic campylobacter. *J. Clin. Pathol.* **33:**1122.
141. **Slifkin, M., and R. J. Doyle.** 1990. Lectins and their application to clinical microbiology. *Clin. Microbiol. Rev.* **3:**197–218.
142. **Stelzer, W., H. Mochmann, U. Richter, and H. Dobberkau.** 1988. Characterization of *Campylobacter jejuni* and *Campylobacter coli* isolated from waste water. *Zentralbl. Bakteriol. Mikrobiol. Hyg. Ser. A* **269:**188–196.
143. **Stelzer, W., H. Mochmann, U. Richter, and H. Dobberkau.** 1989. A study of *Campylobacter jejuni* and *Campylobacter coli* in a river system. *Zentralbl. Hyg.* **189:**20–28.
144. **Taylor, D. N., M. Brown, and K. T. McDermott.** 1982. Waterborne transmission of *Campylobacter* enteritis. *Microb. Ecol.* **8:**347–354.
145. **Taylor, D. N., K. T. McDermott, J. R. Little, J. G. Wells, and M. J. Blaser.** 1983. *Campylobacter* enteritis from untreated water in the Rocky Mountains. *Ann. Intern. Med.* **99:**38–40.
146. **Taylor, N. S., M. A. Ellenberger, P. Y. Wu, and J. G. Fox.** 1989. Diversity of serotypes of *Campylobacter jejuni* and *Campylobacter coli* isolated in laboratory animals. *Lab. Anim. Sci.* **39:**219–221.
147. **Tebbutt, G. M.** 1984. A chemotyping scheme for clinical isolates of *Haemophilus influenzae. J. Med. Microbiol.* **17:**335–345.
148. **Tenover, F. C., J. S. Knapp, C. Patton, and J. J. Plorde.** 1985. Use of auxotyping for epidemiological studies of *Campylobacter jejuni* and *Campylobacter coli* infections. *Infect. Immun.* **48:**384–388.
149. **Tenover, F. C., and C. M. Patton.** 1987. Naturally occurring auxotrophs of *Campylobacter jejuni* and *Campylobacter coli. J. Clin. Microbiol.* **25:**1659–1661.
150. **Tenover, F. C., S. Williams, K. P. Gordon, N. Harris, C. Nolan, and J. J. Plorde.** 1984. Utility of plasmid fingerprinting for epidemiological studies of *Campylobacter jejuni* infections. *J. Infect. Dis.* **149:**279.
151. **Tenover, F. C., S. Williams, K. P. Gordon, C. Nolan, and J. J. Plorde.** 1985. Survey of plasmids and resistance factors in *Campylobacter jejuni* and *Campylobacter coli. Antimicrob. Agents Chemother.* **27:**37–41.
152. **Thompson, C. J., and K. A. Bettelheim.** 1989. Applications of a new method for devising bacteriological serotyping schemes. *J. Clin. Microbiol.* **27:**2391–2392.
153. **Vogt, R. L., A. A. Little, C. M. Patton, T. J. Barrett, and L. A. Orciari.** 1984. Serotyping and serology studies of campylobacteriosis associated with consumption of raw milk. *J. Clin. Microbiol.* **20:**998–1000.
154. **Wachsmuth, I. K., J. A. Kiehlbauch, C. A. Bopp, D. N. Cameron, N. A. Strockbine, J. G. Wells, and P. A. Blake.** 1991. The use of plasmid profiles and nucleic acid probes in epidemiologic investigations of foodborne, diarrheal diseases. *Int. J. Food Microbiol.* **12:**77–90.
155. **Warner, D. P., J. H. Bryner, and G. W. Beran.** 1986. Epidemiologic study of campylobacteriosis in Iowa cattle and the possible role of unpasteurized milk as a vehicle of infection. *Am. J. Vet. Res.* **47:**254–258.
156. **Whelan, C. D., P. Monaghan, R. W. A. Girdwood, and C. R. Fricker.** 1988. The significance of wild birds (*Larus* sp.) in the epidemiology of *Campylobacter* infections in humans. *Epidemiol. Infect.* **101:**259–267.
157. **Wokatsch, R., and J. Bockemuhl.** 1988. Serovars and biovars of *Campylobacter* strains isolated from humans and slaughterhouse animals in northern Germany. *J. Appl. Bacteriol.* **64:**135–140.
158. **Woldehiwet, Z., J. J. Jones, B. J. Tennant, and D. M. Jones.** 1990. Serotypes of *Campylobacter jejuni* and *Campylobacter coli* isolated from dogs. *J. Small Anim. Pract.* **31:**382–384.
159. **Wong, K. H., S. K. Skelton, and J. C. Feeley.** 1986. Strain characterization and grouping of *Campylobacter jejuni* and *Campylobacter coli* by interaction with lectins. *J. Clin. Microbiol.* **23:**407–410.
160. **Wong, K. H., S. K. Skelton, C. M. Patton, J. C. Feeley, and G. Morris.** 1985. Typing of heat-sta-

ble and heat-labile antigens of *Campylobacter jejuni* and *Campylobacter coli* by coagglutination. *J. Clin. Microbiol.* **21**:702–707.
161. **Yan, W., N. Chang, and D. E. Taylor.** 1991. Pulsed-field gel electrophoresis of *Campylobacter jejuni* and *Campylobacter coli* genomic DNA and its epidemiologic application. *J. Infect. Dis.* **163**:1068–1072.
162. **Yogasundram, K., S. M. Shane, and K. S. Harrington.** 1989. Prevalence of *Campylobacter jejuni* in selected domestic and wild birds in Louisiana. *Avian Dis.* **33**:664–667.

IV. PATHOGENESIS OF CAMPYLOBACTER INFECTIONS

CHAPTER 13

In Vivo Models of Enteric Campylobacteriosis: Natural and Experimental Infections

JAMES G. FOX

A brief overview of naturally occurring enteric campylobacteriosis and the use of selected mammalian animal models for the study of campylobacteriosis will be provided to alert the investigator to their potential value in his or her research.

DEFINITION AND SELECTION OF APPROPRIATE IN VIVO MODELS

Several papers have been published on the importance of selecting the proper animal model to study a particular human disease (16, 38, 44). Criteria for selection of the animal model suggested by these authors include the following: (i) it reproduces the pathology of the disease being studied; (ii) it is readily available commercially in sufficient numbers; (iii) it can be easily transported or exported; (iv) it is easy to maintain and handle in laboratories; (v) it is well characterized biologically; (vi) its disease status is established; and (vii) it has a sufficient life span for the study in question (51, 82).

It is also important to exploit diseases that occur naturally in a variety of animal species and that closely mimic similar diseases in humans. In addition, issues such as cost, animal welfare, public concern, and animal legislation regarding the use of certain species may in part dictate the selection of a given species for a particular study (51, 82).

During the past two decades, there have been numerous publications by investigators attempting to establish appropriate models for the study of enteric campylobacteriosis. Although investigators have successfully established intestinal colonization of several species of animals with *Campylobacter jejuni* and *Campylobacter coli,* few studies have reproduced the clinical diarrheal disease associated with acute *C. jejuni* infection in humans. Clinical diarrheal disease, however, has been reproduced in macaques and is described elsewhere in this volume. Another important, useful model for studying colonization by *C. jejuni* and protective immunity is the rabbit surgical model, which is also discussed in this volume.

In selecting animal models for *Campylobacter* research, it is imperative that the species chosen has no preexisting colonization by *Campylobacter* species in the gastrointestinal tract; equally importantly, the immune status of the animal to previous or current *Campylobacter* infection must be quantified. In selecting the appropriate model, the availability of immune reagents (e.g., conjugated immunologlobins [Igs], assays for secretory immunoglobulin A [IgA], monoclonal antibodies to lymphocyte subclasses) is an important consideration when studies require monitoring some aspect of the immune response of the species.

When screening animals for enteric campylobacteriosis, it is important not only to identify various campylobacters to the species level, but also to identify newly recognized enteric *Helicobacter* species that may share antigenic features with campylobacters; their presence in the intestines of animals may interfere with immunological profiles being proposed for the species in question (46).

Other microbial agents in the test animal, as well as environmental variables, may also interfere with the model system. Prior knowledge of the health status of the animals being selected, routine health surveillance, and the use of com-

James G. Fox, Division of Comparative Medicine, Massachusetts Institute of Technology, Cambridge, Massachusetts 02139.

mercially reared and barrier-maintained animals will help determine the ultimate success of the model being used. Not only can intercurrent pathogens cause clinical disease, but also host defenses may be altered or compromised. Insidious or latent infections may affect immunological parameters or other biological systems (59). For example, a synergistic effect has been postulated between *C. jejuni* and other enteropathogens such as enteroinvasive *Salmonella* sp., *Shigella* sp., and *Escherichia coli* (12). Recently, a study showed a significant increase in *C. jejuni* invasion of HEp-2 cells preinfected with enteroviruses such as echovirus 7 and coxsackievirus B3, whereas poliovirus and swine enterovirus had no effect on *C. jejuni* invasive properties in the same in vitro system (43).

NATURAL COLONIZATION AND PREVALENCE OF ENTERIC CAMPYLOBACTERS IN ANIMALS

Successful *C. jejuni* or *C. coli* colonization of several species of laboratory animals is not surprising, given the number of domestic and wild animals and birds that are naturally colonized by a variety of enteric *Campylobacter* species (8, 47, 54, 63, 66, 67). For example, *C. jejuni* intestinal colonization of chickens and, to a lesser extent, turkeys, with subsequent contamination of the carcasses of the birds, accounts for the greatest single risk of infection in humans in the United States. Indeed, recent *C. jejuni* milkborne infection in humans, associated with foil-capped milk bottles that had been delivered to residences and had been pecked open by birds with beaks contaminated with *C. jejuni*, provides an example of the variety and importance of animals and birds as *Campylobacter* reservoirs (36). Dogs and cats also present zoonotic risk to pet owners and animal technicians; this happens particularly with younger animals, with and without diarrhea, when they shed *C. jejuni*, *C. coli*, or *C. upsaliensis* in their feces (8, 10, 17, 18, 24, 26, 29, 31, 50, 74, 75).

Lagomorphs and rodents, particularly hamsters (from certain vendors but not others), commonly shed *C. jejuni* and *C. coli*, as well as *C. hyointestinalis* and *Helicobacter* (*Campylobacter*) *cinaedi* and other *Campylobacter*-like organisms in their feces, sometimes for protracted periods and without clinical signs of disease (32–34, 63, 78).

Various nonhuman primates, including old-world species, such as macaques, patas, and baboons, as well as new-world monkeys, marmosets, and squirrel and owl monkeys, commonly shed campylobacters, particularly during quarantine; newly captured primates routinely become infected while being housed at trapping stations in their country of origin (11, 53, 70, 79–81). Endemic enteric campylobacteriosis is also commonly observed, as pointed out by Russell et al., in captive primate colonies, where constant reinfection and colonization by *Campylobacter* species occurs (71–73). Endemic campylobacteriosis also occurs when other laboratory animal species, such as dogs, ferrets, and cats, are housed in groups in environments where fecal contamination occurs frequently (23, 24, 26, 27, 30). Colonization with multiple Penner serotypes of *C. jejuni* and *C. coli* is also common (26, 54, 73).

IN VIVO CAMPYLOBACTERIOSIS MODELS

The rapid progress of in vivo models of enteric campylobacteriosis in defining the pathophysiology of *C. jejuni* and *C. coli* has been severely curtailed by the lack of an animal model which fulfills the criteria mentioned above. As reviewed initially by Fox in 1982 (22) and then by Newell in 1984 (55) and Walker et al. in 1986 (83), many different species have been used in an attempt to establish a model system which would mimic the enteric disease in humans.

Examination of animal species in which natural *C. jejuni*/*C. coli*-associated diarrhea has been documented provides an insight into species in which experimental infections with *C. jejuni* and *C. coli* have succeeded in producing diarrheal illness (23, 27, 28, 50, 72, 79). Although in many cases cats and dogs are asymptomatic carriers of *Campylobacter* spp., the clinical syndrome, when present, occurs most frequently in dogs less than 6 months of age. *Campylobacter*-associated diarrhea has a wide clinical spectrum in dogs as well as humans, ranging from loose feces to watery diarrhea to bloody mucoid diarrhea (28, 30). Acute campylobacteriosis that develops in puppies and some adult dogs is manifest by mucus-laden, watery, or bile-streaked diarrhea (with or without blood and leukocytes) lasting 5 to 15 days, partial anorexia, and occasional vomiting. Elevated temperature and leukocytosis may also be present (27, 28, 30, 50). In certain cases, diarrhea can be chronic for 2 weeks or more, be intermittent, or in some cases be present for several months (17).

Experimental dosing with *C. jejuni* in random-source kittens and puppies resulted in minimal clinical signs of diarrhea, even though the strain caused diarrhea in the researcher, who unintentionally infected himself (64). Similar results have been noted in studies involving adult dogs (48). Prescott and Brun-Mosch, however, successfully produced mild diarrhea in gnotobiotic puppies by oral inoculation of *C. jejuni* (62). At necropsy 43 h postinoculation, the colons of two animals were congested and edematous and contained fluid (62). Microscopically, the colons and ceca showed decreases in epithelial cell height, brush borders, and numbers of goblet cells; hyperplasia of epithelial glands resulted in a thickened mucosa. Subepithelial congestion, hemorrhage, and inflammatory infiltrate were also seen (62). Use of germfree dogs is limited by cost and lack of gnotobiotic facilities.

Mink raised commercially are known to develop severe *C. jejuni/C. coli*-associated colitis (37). The ferret, another carnivore belonging to the family Mustelidae, is being used increasingly in biomedical research. Ferrets reared commercially and sold for research purposes commonly shed *C. jejuni* in their feces (23). Young weanling ferrets have *C. jejuni*-associated mucoid, sometimes bloody or watery diarrhea lasting from 5 to 10 days. Recently, this model has been used to study *C. jejuni*-induced diarrhea and its relationship to acquired and maternal immunity (4, 5, 25). In this model, self-limiting diarrhea can be produced consistently. As shown in the primate model of Russell et al. (69) and the removable intestinal tie adult rabbit diarrhea (RITARD) model (61), acquired immunity provides at least partial resistance to infection, manifested mainly by shortened periods of *C. jejuni* colonization and development of serum antibodies; these antibodies do not prevent colonization by *C. jejuni,* but do provide immunity against diarrheal illness (4, 5). A mild colitis is seen histologically in infected ferrets (5, 25). However, concurrent cryptosporidiosis, although reported to be nonpathogenic in ferrets, makes interpretation of the lesions more difficult in some *C. jejuni*-infected ferrets (65). Although raising germfree ferrets is possible, it is costly and time-consuming. The commercial availability of specific-pathogen-free ferrets, therefore, without prior exposure to *C. jejuni* and free of intercurrent infection, is needed before this model can be fully utilized (49).

Laboratory mice and rats do not normally have *C. jejuni* as a member of the enteric flora. However, mice (and to a lesser extent, rats) have been used in numerous experiments involving *C. jejuni,* because of their availability commercially, ease of housing and handling, defined microbial flora, and in many cases prescribed genetic traits (51). With few exceptions, oral dosing of *C. jejuni* in mice of different strains (both inbred and outbred) results in intestinal colonization and in some cases bacteremia, but the organism usually does not cause clinical diarrhea (1, 2, 7, 19). Pretreatment with oral antibiotics can prolong the colonization. Continued debate focuses on whether *C. jejuni* in the mouse intestine colonizes the mucus in intestinal crypts or whether adherence to mucus epithelial cells also occurs (45, 57, 58). The mouse model also has highlighted the essential nature of the flagella in colonization of the intestinal mucosa (1, 2, 52, 57). This was also verified recently in *C. jejuni* colonization studies in the hamster (3). Also noteworthy are studies demonstrating protection against colonization in offspring of female mice immunized with the homologous strain of *C. jejuni;* immunity was conferred through IgG antibodies in the milk of the dam (1, 2). Similarly, 39 of 68 (57%) offspring of female mice vaccinated with a particular Lior serotype were protected from intestinal colonization when challenged orally with a heterologous strain. In contrast, none of the infant mice challenged with a strain carrying the same heat-stable antigen (i.e., of the same Penner serotype as the vaccine strain) were afforded protection against colonization (1, 2). However, the use of passive immunization with monoclonal antibodies was not protective when directed against flagellar antigens (56).

Some authors have been successful in developing diarrhea in infant mice dosed intragastrically (39). One of three strains of *C. jejuni* caused severe diarrhea in 36 of 42 mice after virulence enhancement of the organisms (in iron dextran) by serial intraperitoneal passage in mice (39). Intraperitoneal injection of mice with 10^6 CFU of *C. jejuni* produced a self-limiting diarrhea characterized by soft mucoid stools, blood, and fecal leukocytes in outbred Swiss mice or inbred BALB/c mice (77). Higher doses ($>10^9$ CFU) killed the mice in 48 h. The model was proposed for virulence studies of *C. jejuni.*

Immunocompromised mice, such as athymic nude mice and gamma-irradiated mice, are also colonized by *C. jejuni* when challenged orally (76, 85–87). Athymic nude mice were colonized in the epithelial surface of the intestine, whereas irradiation allowed intracellular infection of BALB/c mice. The utility of these particular models requires further investigation.

Of recent interest is the finding of hepatitis in mice 1 to 2 months after oral dosing with *C.*

jejuni (41, 42). Tissue culture studies with mouse hepatocytes demonstrated that low concentrations of factors isolated from whole-cell lysates of *C. jejuni* and purified by column chromatography caused the release of hepatic enzymes and that higher concentrations induced cytolysis (42). These effects were neutralized by antisera to the factor, but not by antisera to lipopolysaccharide of *C. jejuni* or heat-labile enterotoxin of *E. coli* (42). Unfortunately, information on whether *C. jejuni*-infected mice (or mice used for antisera) were also infected with other pathogens infecting their livers, particularly mouse hepatitis virus, was not provided (59).

The RITARD model, which is fully described by Walker et al. (this volume), has proved very useful in studies of intestinal colonization and development of immunization strategies (83, 84). Like the mouse, the rabbit model, through oral challenge studies, has shown the importance of cross-strain protection (using the Lior serotype), thus implicating the flagellum as a protective antigen. In contrast, *C. jejuni*-immunized rabbits challenged with matched Penner-unmatched Lior strains showed little protection (61). Furthermore, an aflagellated mutant of *C. jejuni* failed to colonize rabbits, regardless of the route of administration (61). A single feeding of this aflagellated strain did not protect rabbits against challenge with the parent strain, but three feedings of the mutant strain did, indicating that antigens not located on the flagella can also produce protection against homologous flagellated strains (61). The model is also very useful in measuring the secretory IgA response to *C. jejuni* oral inoculation (13, 14). Recent studies with the RITARD model have also demonstrated that the M cell, an important antigen-processing cell found in the epithelial layer over intestinal Peyer's patches, is a probable route for systemic spread of *C. jejuni* (84).

In experimental studies conducted with human volunteers, *C. jejuni* 81–176 caused higher attack rates and a greater number and volume of stools than did *C. jejuni* A 3249 (6). However, similar clinical outcomes were noted when the two strains were inoculated into RITARD rabbits (i.e., illness in all animals, with three deaths in each test group) (6). This suggests that the two strains were of equal virulence or, alternatively, that the RITARD rabbit model was relatively insensitive to strain differences (6). Perhaps the age and source of the rabbit, as well as in vitro growth conditions of the *C. jejuni* strain, also may affect the clinical course of the disease in individual experiments. This model, as Walker notes, requires surgical intervention and is time-consuming (see Walker et al., this volume). Also, because rabbits are susceptible to a variety of infectious enteropathies, the source, health status, and housing conditions of the rabbits will also influence the success of this model when used by other investigators.

The nonhuman primate, albeit the most expensive of the models and limited in supply, has many of the clinical and epidemiological features noted in naturally occurring human campylobacteriosis, particularly for patients suffering from the disease in third-world countries. As with other species maintained in communal environments, where fecal-oral contamination is frequent, *Campylobacter* infection is widespread in many colonies of nonhuman primates (11, 22, 35, 53, 70, 71, 72, 79–81). Although detailed epidemiologic data in these species are lacking, episodes of *Campylobacter*-associated diarrhea or asymptomatic infection have been documented in *Macaca mulatta, Macaca fascicularis,* Patas monkeys, and marmosets. In a study of the epidemiology of diarrhea in colony-born *Macaca nemestrina,* 205 neonates and infants in an infant research laboratory, plus 248 neonates, juveniles, and adolescents up to 4 years of age, housed in a different facility, were commonly diagnosed with *Campylobacter, Shigella,* and *Crytosporidium* infections (71). Chronic diarrhea was noted in 10% of the animals. More recently, Russell et al. explored the prevalence of *Campylobacter* spp. in infant *M. nemestrina* animals, with and without diarrhea, housed in a nursery under hyperendemic conditions. They determined by using serotyping, DNA hybridization, and polyacrylamide gel electrophoresis that during a 12-month period, multiple reinfections with different strains of *C. jejuni* and *C. coli* occurred (73). The duration of infection with a particular strain averaged 3 to 4 weeks; *C. jejuni* and *C. coli* infection correlated with diarrhea in infants from 1 to 4 months of age (73). The 3- to 4-week course of infection with a particular strain is similar to the course of infection with a particular strain in susceptible humans and in experimentally infected infant *M. nemestrina* (9, 68). Also, isolation of multiple serotypes over time is similar to that found in children during a 12-week study in Thailand. Infant primates were infected at an early age, particularly if they had been nursed by their mothers. Infants raised in the nursery in isolettes did not become infected until moved into single cages in a holding room. Finger contact and aerosolization of feces during cleaning probably accounted for fecal-oral transmission in this setting. Interestingly, in this study, infants were also infected with nalidixic acid-resistant (Nal^r) campylobacters; the duration of infection with those strains was only 1 ± 1.4 weeks. These isolates have been subsequently identified as *C. fetus* subsp. *fetus, C. hyointestinalis,* and *C. butzleri* (40, 68). Their significance as a cause of primary diarrhea in *Macaca* species requires further analysis.

Earlier experimental studies in *Macaca* species suggested that these animals were susceptible to both colonization with campylobacters and also, in some cases, diarrhea following inoculation of the organism (60; J. Melling, cited in reference 15). Three *M. fascicularis* animals inoculated orally with thermophilic campylobacters isolated from diarrheic nonhuman primates did not develop diarrhea but had either partial or complete anorexia 1 week postinoculation. Two of the animals shed the organism for 5 and 6 weeks (80). These studies were followed by a more controlled and detailed study, in which eight young rhesus monkeys (*Macaca mulatta*) were infected orally with a human strain of *C. jejuni* (20). The disease induced was mild, with inappetence and diarrhea of short duration, but prolonged intermittent excretion of the bacteria in the feces occurred. Bacteremia generally was present for 2 to 3 days, and later the organisms were localized in the liver and gallbladder. When challenged with the same strain, animals that had recovered showed no clinical symptoms and no bacteremia and excreted the organisms in the feces for only 3 days. At necropsy, lesions attributable to *C. jejuni* were not observed in any portion of the gastrointestinal tract (20).

More recently, as discussed by Russell (this volume), a well-controlled and designed study in infant *M. nemestrina* animals demonstrated the usefulness of this model in studying enteric campylobacteriosis (68). The experiment is particularly relevant, given that the strain used, 81-176 (Penner serotype 23/36), was isolated initially during an outbreak of milk-borne campylobacteriosis in Minnesota and later used in experimental infections of humans (6). Four infant pig-tail macaques, 3.5 to 4 months old and specific pathogen (i.e., *Campylobacter* and *Shigella*) free, when inoculated with strain 81-176 (3×10^{11} CFU), developed acute diarrheal illness, lasting approximately 7 to 11 days. The illness was characterized by fluid diarrhea, bloody feces, and fecal leukocytes (68). Histologically, the animals had an acute colitis, but no small-intestine abnormalities. The *C. jejuni* strain was present 2 to 4 weeks postchallenge. Infants also developed IgG, IgA, and IgM titers to *C. jejuni* after experimental challenge. Partial immunity protection was noted by the appearance of mild diarrhea after rechallenge of the infants with the homologous strain or with a heterologous *C. jejuni* strain, 79-168. Four 1-year-old *M. nemestrina* animals, which had previously experienced several infections with *Campylobacter* species and preexisting *C. jejuni* antibody titers, did not develop diarrhea when dosed with *C. jejuni* 81-176 (68).

Interestingly, infant *M. nemestrina* animals have been recently used as a model to study diarrheal disease caused by *H. cinaedi* and *H. fennelliae* (21). Both organisms caused acute watery diarrhea and bacteremia 3 to 7 days postinoculation in 12- to 25-day-old macaques. After resolution of clinical signs, the stools were positive for the organism for >3 weeks postinoculation (21).

In summary, results of in vivo studies in rodents, lagomorphs, carnivores, and nonhuman primates have established several important criteria necessary for enteric colonization of *C. jejuni* in mammalian hosts. The requirement of flagella on *C. jejuni* for colonization has been clearly documented. Also, flagellin plays a major antigenic role during colonization and development of colonization resistance to subsequent rechallenge with *C. jejuni* in both the rabbit and mouse models. Therefore, it is important for investigators to know the Lior serotype in designing in vivo challenge studies. Also, other surface antigens probably play a role in developing immunity. Thus far, *M. nemestrina* and perhaps the ferret offer useful models to study host-organism interaction, development of intestinal lesions, and conferred immunity. Both of these models, however, need development of species-specific immunological reagents, as well as the commercial availability of specific-pathogen-free animals. As noted by Russell et al., additional studies are required to characterize the mechanisms of *C. jejuni*-induced colitis and to define the mucosal immunity to *C. jejuni* infection (69). Also, the importance of flagellin antigen in effecting protective immunity in the primate and ferret must be documented. Future in vivo experiments will require careful characterization of the infecting strain and, if possible, more general use of well-characterized strains, such as strain 81-176, previously validated in human experimental trials and other in vivo models (6, 69). The role and importance of the antigen-processing M cell in bacteremia noted in several animal models also needs further study (84). The need for validated in vitro characterization of virulence markers, prior to initiation of in vivo studies, continues to be of paramount importance. Hopefully, by the judicious use of animal models in the next decade, further progress can be made in our understanding of the pathogenesis of and the prospects of a protective vaccine for this important enteric pathogen.

REFERENCES

1. **Abimiku, A. C., and J. M. Dolby.** 1988. Cross-protection of infant mice against intestinal colonization by *Campylobacter jejuni:* importance of heat-labile serotyping (Lior) antigens. *J. Med. Microbiol.* **26:**265–268.
2. **Abimiku, A. C., J. M. Dolby, and S. P. Borriello.** 1989. Comparison of different vaccines and induced immune response against *Campylobacter jejuni* colonization in the infant mouse. *Epidemiol. Infect.* **102:**271–280.
3. **Aguero-Rosenfeld, M. E., X.-H. Yang, and I. Nachamkin.** 1990. Infection of adult Syrian hamsters with flagellar variants of *Campylobacter jejuni. Infect. Immun.* **58:**2214–2219.
4. **Bell, J. A., and D. D. Manning.** 1990. A domestic ferret model of immunity to *Campylobacter jejuni*-induced enteric disease. *Infect. Immun.* **58:**1848–1852.
5. **Bell, J. A., and D. D. Manning.** 1991. Evaluation of *Campylobacter jejuni* colonization of the domestic ferret intestine as a model of proliferative colitis. *Am. J. Vet. Res.* **52:**826–832.
6. **Black, R. E., M. M. Levine, M. L. Clements, T. P. Hughes, and M. J. Blaser.** 1988. Experimental *Campylobacter jejuni* infection in humans. *J. Infect. Dis.* **157:**472–479.
7. **Blaser, M. J., D. J. Duncan, and P. F. Smith.** 1984. Pathogenesis of *Campylobacter* infection: clearance of bacteremia in mice. *Microecol. Ther.* **14:**103–108.
8. **Blaser, M. J., F. M. LaForce, N. A. Wilson, and W. L. L. Wang.** 1980. Reservoirs for human campylobacteriosis. *J. Infect. Dis.* **141:**665–669.
9. **Blaser, M. J., R. B. Parsons, and W.-L. L. Wang.** 1980. Acute colitis caused by *Campylobacter fetus* ss *jejuni. Gastroenterology* **78:**448–453.
10. **Blaser, M. J., S. H. Weiss, and T. J. Barrett.** 1982. *Campylobacter* enteritis associated with a healthy cat. *JAMA* **816:**247.
11. **Bryant, J. L., H. F. Stills, R. H. Lentsch, and C. C. Middleton.** 1983. *Campylobacter jejuni* isolated from Patas monkeys with diarrhea. *Lab. Anim. Sci.* **33:**303–305.
12. **Bulkholm, G., and G. Kapperud.** 1987. Expression of *Campylobacter* invasiveness in cell cultures coinfected with other bacteria. *Infect. Immun.* **55:**2816–2821.
13. **Burr, D. H., M. B. Caldwell, A. L. Bourgeois, H. P. Morgan, R. Wistar, Jr., and R. I. Walker.** 1988. Mucosal and systemic immunity to *Campylobacter jejuni* in rabbits after gastric inoculation. *Infect. Immun.* **56:**99–105.
14. **Burr, D. H., D. T. Kerner, G. S. Blanco, A. L. Bourgeois, and R. Wistar, Jr.** 1987. Gastric lavage: a simple method to obtain IgA-rich intestinal secretions from the rabbit. *J. Immunol. Methods* **99:**277–281.
15. **Butzler, J. P., and M. B. Skirrow.** 1979. *Campylobacter* enteritis. *Clin. Gastroenterol.* **8:**737–765.
16. **Cheville, N. F.** 1980. Criteria for development of animal models of diseases of the gastrointestinal system. *Am. J. Pathol.* **101:**S67–S76.
17. **Davies, A. P., C. J. Gebhart, and S. A. Meric.** 1984. *Campylobacter*-associated chronic diarrhea in a dog. *J. Am. Vet. Med. Assoc.* **184:**469.
18. **Fernie, D. S., and R. W. A. Park.** 1977. Isolation and nature of campylobacters (microaerophic vibrios) from laboratory and wild rodents. *J. Med. Microbiol.* **10:**325–329.
19. **Field, L. H., J. L. Underwood, L. M. Pope, and L. J. Berry.** 1981. Intestinal colonization of neonatal animals by *Campylobacter fetus* subsp. *jejuni. Infect. Immun.* **33:**884–892.
20. **Fitzgeorge, R. B., A. Baskerville, and K. P. Lander.** 1981. Experimental infection of rhesus monkeys with a human strain of *Campylobacter jejuni. J. Hyg.* **86:**343–351.
21. **Flores, B. M., C. L. Fennell, L. Kuller, M. A. Bronsdon, W. R. Morton, and W. E. Stamm.** 1990. Experimental infection of pig-tailed macaques (*Macaca nemestrina*) with *Campylobacter cinaedi* and *Campylobacter fennelliae. Infect. Immun.* **58:**3947–3953.
22. **Fox, J. G.** 1982. *Campylobacter*iosis—a 'new' disease in laboratory animals. *Lab. Anim. Sci.* **32:**625–637.
23. **Fox, J. G., J. I. Ackerman, and C. E. Newcomer.** 1983. Ferret as a potential reservoir for human campylobacteriosis. *Am. J. Vet. Res.* **44:**1049–1052.
24. **Fox, J. G., J. I. Ackerman, and C. E. Newcomer.** 1985. The prevalence of *Campylobacter jejuni* in random source cats used in biomedical research. *J. Infect. Dis.* **151:**743–744.
25. **Fox, J. G., J. I. Ackerman, N. S. Taylor, M. Claps, and J. C. Murphy.** 1987. *Campylobacter jejuni* infection in the ferret: an animal model of human campylobacteriosis. *Am. J. Vet. Res.* **48:**85–90.
26. **Fox, J. G., M. C. Claps, N. S. Taylor, and J. I. Ackerman.** 1988. *Campylobacter jejuni/coli* in commercially reared beagles: prevalence and serotypes. *Lab. Anim. Sci.* **38:**262.
27. **Fox, J. G., S. Krakowka, and N. S. Taylor.** 1985. Acute-onset *Campylobacter*-associated gastroenteritis in adult beagles. *J. Am. Vet. Med. Assoc.* **187:**1268–1271.
28. **Fox, J. G., K. O. Maxwell, and J. I. Ackerman.** 1984. *Campylobacter jejuni*-associated diarrhea in commercially reared beagles. *Lab. Anim. Sci.* **34:**151.
29. **Fox, J. G., K. O. Maxwell, N. S. Taylor, C. D. Runsick, and P. Edmonds.** 1989. *Campylobacter upsaliensis* isolated from cats as identified by DNA relatedness and biochemical features. *J. Clin. Microbiol.* **27:**2376–2378.

30. **Fox, J. G., R. Moore, and J. I. Ackerman.** 1983. *Campylobacter jejuni*-associated diarrhea in dogs. *J. Am. Vet. Med. Assoc.* **183:**1430–1433.
31. **Fox, J. G., N. S. Taylor, J. L. Penner, B. Shames, R. V. Gurgis, and F. Thomson.** 1989. Investigation of zoonotic acquired *Campylobacter jejuni* enteritis with serotyping and restriction endonuclease DNA analysis. *J. Clin. Microbiol.* **27:**2423–2425.
32. **Fox, J. G., S. Zanotti, and H. V. Jordan.** 1981. The hamster as a reservoir of *Campylobacter jejuni. J. Infect. Dis.* **143:**856.
33. **Gebhart, C. J., C. L. Fennell, M. P. Murtaugh, and W. E. Stamm.** 1989. *Campylobacter cinaedi* is normal intestinal flora in hamsters. *J. Clin. Microbiol.* **27:**1692–1694.
34. **Gebhart, C. M., P. Edmonds, G. E. Ward, H. J. Kurtz, and D. J. Brenner.** 1985. *Campylobacter hyointestinalis* sp. nov.: a new species of *Campylobacter* found in the intestines of pigs and other animals. *J. Clin. Microbiol.* **21:**715–720.
35. **Goodwin, T., M. R. Adams, N. D. M. Lehner, and C. P. Jerome.** 1983. *Campylobacter* enteritis in Patas monkeys. *Lab. Anim. Sci.* **33:**481.
36. **Hudson, S. J., N. F. Lightfoot, J. C. Coulson, K. Russell, P. R. Sisson, and A. O. Sobo.** Jackdaws and magpies as vectors of human *Campylobacter* infection. *Epidemiol. Infect.*, in press.
37. **Hunter, D. B., J. F. Prescott, D. M. Hoover, G. Hlywka, and J. A. Kerr.** 1986. *Campylobacter* colitis in ranch mink in Ontario. *Can. J. Vet. Res.* **50:**47–53.
38. **Jones, T. C.** 1980. The value of animal models. *Am. J. Pathol.* **101:**S3–S9.
39. **Kazmi, S. U., B. S. Roberson, and N. J. Stern.** 1984. Animal-passed, virulence-enhanced *Campylobacter jejuni* causes enteritis in neonatal mice. *Curr. Microbiol.* **11:**159–164.
40. **Kiehlbauch, J. A., D. J. Brenner, M. A. Nicholson, C. N. Baker, C. M. Patton, A. G. Steigerwalt, and I. K. Wachsmuth.** 1991. *Campylobacter butzleri* sp. nov. isolated from humans and animals with diarrheal illness. *J. Clin. Microbiol.* **29:**376–385.
41. **Kita, E., N. Katsui, K. Nishi, M. Emoto, Y. Yanagase, and S. Kashiba.** 1986. Hepatic lesions in experimental *Campylobacter jejuni* infection of mice. *J. Gen. Microbiol.* **132:**3095–3103.
42. **Kita, E., D. Oku, A. Hamuro, F. Nishikawa, M. Emoto, Y. Yagyu, N. Katsui, and S. Kashiba.** 1990. Hepatotoxic activity of *Campylobacter jejuni. J. Med. Microbiol.* **33:**171–182.
43. **Konkel, M. E., and L. A. Joens.** 1990. Effect of enteroviruses on adherence to and invasion of HEp-2 cells by *Campylobacter* isolates. *Infect. Immun.* **58:**1101–1105.
44. **Leader, R. W., and G. A. Padgett.** 1980. The genesis and validation of animal models. *Am. J. Pathol.* **101:**S11–S16.
45. **Lee, A., J. L. O'Rourke, P. J. Barrington, and T. J. Trust.** 1986. Mucus colonization as a determinant of pathogenicity in intestinal infection by *Campylobacter jejuni:* a mouse cecal model. *Infect. Immun.* **51:**536–546.
46. **Lee, A., M. W. Phillips, J. O'Rourke, B. Pasteur, F. E. Dewhirst, G. L. Fraser, J. G. Fox, L. I. Sly, P. J. Romaniuk, T. J. Trust, and S. Kouprach.** 1992. *Helicobacter muridarum* sp. nov., a microaerophilic helical bacterium with a novel ultrastructure isolated from the intestinal mucosa of rodents. *Int. J. Syst. Bacteriol.* **42:**27–36.
47. **Luechtefeld, N. W., R. C. Cambre, and W.-L. L. Wang.** 1981. Isolation of *Campylobacter fetus* subsp. *jejuni* from zoo animals. *J. Am. Vet. Med. Assoc.* **179:**1119–1122.
48. **Macartney, L., I. A. P. McCandlish, R. R. Almasat, and D. J. Taylor.** 1972. Natural and experimental infections with *Campylobacter jejuni* in dogs, p. 172. *In* D. G. Newell (ed.), *Campylobacter: Epidemiology, Pathogenesis and Biochemistry.* MTP Press, Lancaster, England.
49. **Manning, D. D., and J. A. Bell.** 1990. Derivation of gnotobiotic ferrets: perinatal diet and hand-raising requirements. *Lab. Anim. Sci.* **40:**51–55.
50. **McOrist, S., and J. W. Browning.** 1982. Carriage of *Campylobacter jejuni* in healthy and diarrhoeic dogs and cats. *Aust. Vet. J.* **58:**33–34.
51. **Migaki, G., and C. C. Capen.** 1984. Animal models in biomedical research, p. 667–695. *In* J. G. Fox, B. J. Cohen, and F. M. Loew (ed.), *Laboratory Animal Medicine.* Academic Press, Inc., Orlando, Fla.
52. **Morooka, T., A. Umeda, and K. Amako.** 1985. Motility as an intestinal colonization factor for *Campylobacter jejuni. J. Gen. Microbiol.* **131:**1973–1980.
53. **Morton, W. R., M. Bronsdon, G. Mickelsen, G. Knitter, S. Rosenkranz, L. Kueller, and D. Sajuthi.** 1983. Identification of *Campylobacter jejuni* in *Macaca fascicularis* imported from Indonesia. *Lab. Anim. Sci.* **33:**187–188.
54. **Munroe, D. L., J. F. Prescott, and J. L. Penner.** 1983. *Campylobacter jejuni* and *Campylobacter coli* serotypes isolated from chickens, cattle, and pigs. *J. Clin. Microbiol.* **18:**877–881.
55. **Newell, D. G.** 1984. Experimental studies of *Campylobacter* enteritis, p. 113–132. *In* J. P. Butzler (ed.), *Campylobacter Infection in Man and Animals.* CRC Press, Inc., Boca Raton, Fla.
56. **Newell, D. G.** 1986. Monoclonal antibodies directed against the flagella of *Campylobacter jejuni:* production, characterization and lack of effect on the colonization of infant mice. *J. Hyg.* **96:**131–141.
57. **Newell, D. G., H. McBride, and J. M. Dolby.** 1985. Investigations on the role of flagella in the colonization of infant mice with *Campylobacter jejuni* and attachment of *Campylobacter jejuni* to human epithelial cell lines. *J. Hyg.* **95:**217–227.
58. **Newell, D. G., and A. Pearson.** 1984. The invasion of epithelial cell lines and the intestinal epithelium of infant mice by *Campylobacter jejuni/coli. J. Diarrhoeal Dis. Res.* **2:**19–26.
59. **Pakes, S. P., L. Yue-Shoung, and P. C. Meunier.** 1984. Factors that complicate animal research, p. 649–665. *In* J. G. Fox, B. J. Cohen, and F. M. Loew (ed.), *Laboratory Animal Medicine.* Academic Press, Inc., Orlando, Fla.
60. **Park, C.** 1979. Personal communication.

61. **Pavlovskis, O. R., D. M. Rollins, R. L. Haberberger, A. E. Green, L. Habash, S. Strocko, and R. I. Walker.** 1991. Significance of flagella in colonization resistance of rabbits immunized with *Campylobacter* spp. *Infect. Immun.* **59**:2259–2264.
62. **Prescott, J. F., and I. K. Barker.** 1980. *Campylobacter* colitis in gnotobiotic dogs. *Vet. Rec.* **107**:314.
63. **Prescott, J. F., and C. W. Brun-Mosch.** 1981. Carriage of *Campylobacter jejuni* in healthy and diarrheic animals. *Am. J. Vet. Res.* **42**:164–165.
64. **Prescott, J. F., and M. A. Karmali.** 1978. Attempts to transmit *Campylobacter* enteritis to dogs and cats. *Can. Med. Assoc. J.* **119**:1001.
65. **Rehg, J. E., F. Gigliotti, and D. C. Stokes.** 1988. Cryptosporidiosis in ferrets. *Lab. Anim. Sci.* **38**:155–158.
66. **Rosef, O., B. Gondrosen, G. Kapperud, and B. Underal.** 1983. Isolation and characterization of *Campylobacter jejuni* and *Campylobacter coli* from domestic and wild mammals in Norway. *Appl. Environ. Microbiol.* **46**:855–859.
67. **Rosef, O., G. Kapperud, S. Lauwers, and B. Gondrosen.** 1985. Serotyping of *Campylobacter jejuni, Campylobacter coli,* and *Campylobacter laridis* from domestic and wild animals. *Appl. Environ. Microbiol.* **49**:1507–1510.
68. **Russell, R. G.** Personal communication.
69. **Russell, R. G., M. J. Blaser, J. I. Sarimento, and J. Fox.** 1989. Experimental *Campylobacter jejuni* infection in *Macaca nemestrina. Infect. Immun.* **57**:1438–1444.
70. **Russell, R. G., D. A. Brian, A. Lenhard, L. N. D. Potgieter, D. Gillespie, and N. K. Clapp.** 1985. Coronavirus-like particles and *Campylobacter* in marmosets with diarrhea and colitis. *Dig. Dis. Sci.* **30**:72S–77S.
71. **Russell, R. G., L. Krugner, C.-C. Tsai, and R. Ekstrom.** 1988. Prevalence of *Campylobacter* in infant, juvenile, and adult laboratory primates. *Lab. Anim. Sci.* **38**:711–714.
72. **Russell, R. G., S. L. Rosenkranz, L. A. Lee, H. Howard, R. F. DiGiacomo, M. A. Bronsdon, G. A. Blakely, C.-C. Tsai, and W. R. Morton.** 1987. Epidemiology and etiology of diarrhea in colony-born Macaca nemestrina. *Lab. Anim. Sci.* **37**:309–316.
73. **Russell, R. G., J. I. Sarmiento, J. Fox, and P. Panigrahi.** 1990. Evidence of reinfection with multiple strains of *Campylobacter jejuni* and *Campylobacter coli* in *Macaca nemestrina* housed under hyperendemic conditions. *Infect. Immun.* **58**:2149–2155.
74. **Sandstedt, K., J. Ursing, and M. Walder.** 1983. Thermotolerant *Campylobacter* with no or weak catalase activity isolated from dogs. *Curr. Microbiol.* **8**:209–213.
75. **Skirrow, M. B., G. L. Turnbull, R. E. Walker, and S. E. J. Young.** 1980. *Campylobacter jejuni* enteritis transmitted from cat to man. *Lancet* **i**:1188. (Letter.)
76. **Sosula, L., E. M. Nicholls, and M. Skeen.** 1988. Ultrastructure of *Campylobacter jejuni* in gamma-irradiated mouse jejunum. *Am. J. Pathol.* **131**:125–131.
77. **Stanfield, J. T., B. A. McCardell, and J. M. Madden.** 1987. *Campylobacter* diarrhea in an adult mouse model. *Microb. Pathog.* **3**:155–165.
78. **Stills, H. F., Jr., R. R. Hook, Jr., and D. A. Kinden.** 1989. Isolation of a *Campylobacter*-like organism from healthy Syrian hamsters (*Mesocricetus auratus*). *J. Clin. Microbiol.* **27**:2497–2501.
79. **Tribe, G. W., and M. P. Fleming.** 1983. Biphasic enteritis in imported cynomolgus (Macaca fascicularis) monkeys infected with *Shigella, Salmonella* and *Campylobacter* species. *Lab. Anim. Sci.* **17**:65–69.
80. **Tribe, G. W., and A. Frank.** 1980. *Campylobacter* in monkeys. *Vet. Rec.* **106**:365–366.
81. **Tribe, G. W., P. S. Mackenzie, and M. P. Fleming.** 1979. Incidence of thermophilic *Campylobacter* species in newly imported simian primates with enteritis. *Vet. Rec.* **105**:333.
82. **Van Citters, R.** 1973. The role of animal research in clinical medicine, p. 3–8. *In* U.S. Department of Health, Education, and Welfare publication no. NIH 72-333. National Institutes of Health, Bethesda, Md.
83. **Walker, R. I., M. Caldwell-Blake, E. C. Lee, P. Guerry, T. Trust, and G. M. Ruiz-Palacios.** 1986. Pathophysiology of *Campylobacter* enteritis. *Microbiol. Rev.* **50**:81–94.
84. **Walker, R. I., E. A. Schmauder-Chock, and J. L. Parker.** 1988. Selective association and transport of *Campylobacter jejuni* through M cells of rabbit Peyer's patches. *Can. J. Microbiol.* **34**:1142–1147.
85. **Yrios, J. W., and E. Balish.** 1986. Colonization and infection of athymic and euthymic germfree mice by *Campylobacter jejuni* and *Campylobacter fetus* subsp. *fetus. Infect. Immun.* **53**:378–383.
86. **Yrios, J. W., and E. Balish.** 1986. Immune response of athymic and euthymic germfree mice to *Campylobacter* spp. *Infect. Immun.* **54**:339–346.
87. **Yrios, J. W., and E. Balish.** 1986. Pathogenesis of *Campylobacter* spp. in athymic and euthymic germfree mice. *Infect. Immun.* **53**:384–392.

CHAPTER 14

Studies of *Campylobacter* Infection in the Adult Rabbit

RICHARD I. WALKER, DAVID M. ROLLINS, AND DONALD H. BURR

INTRODUCTION

In the early 1980s *Campylobacter* species were clearly emerging as a major cause of diarrheal disease. However, nothing was known about the colonization and pathogenesis factors of these organisms, nor were sufficient data available to permit development of immunoprophylactic measures against them. For these reasons we began a search for small laboratory animal models which would be amenable for these evaluations. We found that adult rabbits were suitable for investigation of some pathophysiologic and immunologic processes associated with *Campylobacter jejuni* infection.

COLONIZATION AND PATHOGENESIS IN THE RABBIT MODEL

RITARD Model

Spira et al. (27, 28) developed the removable intestinal tie adult rabbit diarrhea (RITARD) model to study the pathogenesis of *Vibrio cholerae* and enterotoxigenic *Escherichia coli*. A key factor in the RITARD model is that colonization of the mucosa is enhanced through the temporary inhibition of normal peristaltic clearance mechanisms. Caldwell et al. (7, 8) applied the RITARD procedure to studies with *Campylobacter* spp. In this procedure, the abdomen of a young rabbit is opened surgically under general anesthesia and aseptic conditions. The cecum is ligated with umbilical tape near the ileocecal junction, and a slip knot used to gently ligate the terminal ileum immediately anterior to the mesoappendix. A 10-ml sample of *C. jejuni* culture of approximately 10^9 CFU is injected into the mid-small bowel. The incision is closed in two layers, and the loose ends of the slip knot are brought out through the incision. Four hours after surgery, the slip knot is released and additional sutures are placed as needed.

The RITARD model is the key to the design of subsequent experiments described in this report. In early studies this procedure was performed on young (1-kg) rabbits so that pathogenic phenomena might be best observed. For studies of immune responses, young rabbits were first orally immunized with organisms and then, approximately 30 days later, challenged with bacteria administered via the RITARD procedure (Table 1). For oral immunization, rabbits are treated with cimetidine and oral bicarbonate to reduce gastric acidity and then intragastrically inoculated with 10^9 CFU. These animals become colonized for 1 to 2 weeks depending on the bacterial strain. No sign of disease is observed following these infections, but bacteremia occurs in many cases.

Colonization

In addition to the pathophysiologic and immunologic consequences in the rabbit of challenge with *Campylobacter* spp., the mucosal environment has significant effects on the physiology of the organism. *Campylobacter* motility and the flagellar protein are thought to facilitate colonization of the mucous lining of the intestinal tract (22). The colonization potential of wild-type motile *C. jejuni* was compared with that of motile and nonmotile variants. A spontaneously isolated, nonmotile, nonflagellated variant colonizes the intestinal tract of infant mice for a shorter duration than a flagellated, nonmotile variant or the wild-type strain does. When nonflagellated variants of such strains are used to infect either rabbits or humans, only flagellated cells can be recovered from fecal samples,

Richard I. Walker, David M. Rollins, and Donald H. Burr, Enteric Diseases Program, Naval Medical Research Institute, Bethesda, Maryland 20889–5055.

TABLE 1. Postchallenge events in rabbits administered *Campylobacter* spp.

Fed only
Shed *Campylobacter* cells for 1 to 2 wk depending on bacterial strain
No evidence of disease
Immune response
Bacteremia
Colonization obtained with as few as 10^2 organisms
Fed and then fed again
Rapid clearance not seen
RITARD only in young rabbits
Shed organisms for 1 to 2 wk depending on bacterial strain
Bacteremia
Mucous diarrhea after 3 to 5 days
Death in 56% of animals (associated with dehydration)
RITARD in orally immunized older rabbits
Shed organism for <3 days following homologous challenge
No disease or death following challenge, even in nonimmune group
No heterologous protection outside Lior serogroup
No bacteremia following homologous challenge
Immunity to colonization present at 9 months

suggesting that nonflagellated forms are less able to colonize the host (2, 9).

Recent work has further established that flagella are necessary for prolonged colonization of rabbits. An isogenic nonflagellated deletion mutant failed to colonize after challenge via the feeding or RITARD procedure (25). As discussed below, a single feeding with flagellated organisms induces protective immunity. In contrast, a single feeding with nonflagellated organisms is not sufficient to render rabbits immune to colonization when challenged again with the flagellated parent strain. However, if the nonflagellated mutant was fed to the rabbits three times at 48-h intervals, protection was observed against the parent strain but not against other strains of the same Lior serotype. Flagellated organisms also induce protection against other strains of the same Lior serotype (see below).

Some *Campylobacter* strains undergo a bidirectional transition, between flagellated and nonflagellated phenotypes (9). By using motility media it was shown in vitro that the frequency of the switch was 5.9×10^{-3} in the Fla^+-to-Fla^- direction and 8.0×10^{-7} in the Fla^--to-Fla^+ direction. The frequency of the shift from Fla^+ to Fla^- is very high during growth in laboratory media; however, the Fla^--to-Fla^+ shift clearly predominated in the rabbit intestine. When rabbits are infected with Fla^- phenotypes by the RITARD procedure, only motile *C. jejuni* organisms can be isolated 96 h after infection. Although the Fla^+ form predominates in vivo, it could not be determined whether this was due to an increase in the switching frequency or a result of selection for the flagellated form. Selection of the Fla^+ phenotype may be associated with enhanced ability to colonize. This bidirectional switch suggests that the ability to reversibly express flagella is inherent in the wild-type strain and is not just a peculiarity of the Fla^- variants.

Antigenic variation of flagella also occurs in the mucosal environment. *Campylobacter* strains reversibly express two distinct flagellin types, designated as phase 1 and phase 2, that are distinguishable antigenically and by differences in the apparent molecular weight of the flagellin subunit (19). Since the flagellum has been implicated as a virulence determinant of *Campylobacter* spp. (22, 29), the ability to undergo antigenic variation in experimentally infected rabbits was investigated.

Cultures of *Campylobacter* cells producing antigenic phase 1 or phase 2 flagella were used to infect rabbits by the RITARD procedure. After challenge, campylobacters isolated from the stools of infected rabbits were analyzed for both the molecular weight of the flagellin produced and the DNA pattern obtained in Southern blot hybridization analysis. When animals were challenged with organisms of either phase, isolates of the other configuration were detected within several days, although a definite preference for the phase 2 configuration was noted. The data demonstrate that antigenic variation of flagella occurs in vivo and that it correlates with the same DNA rearrangement previously described to be associated with in vitro flagellar variation (13). The observed flagellar changes suggest a role for phase 2 flagella in pathogenesis, although no major differences in symptoms were observed between animals infected with either the phase 1 or phase 2 cells. All rabbits infected with phase 2 cells excreted *Campylobacter* organisms sooner after infection than did the animals infected with phase 1 cells, suggesting that phase 2 cells may have an advantage in establishing an infection or in their ability to survive in the host.

Pathogenesis

Infection after RITARD challenge

When 55 young rabbits received *C. jejuni*, 34 animals developed diarrhea and 29 died, resulting in an overall attack rate of 62% and a mortality rate of 53% (7, 8). The onset of diarrhea occurred after the first 24 to 48 h and was remarkable in its consistent mucous content. All control rabbits had normal pellet stools from day 1 to the end of the 2-week observation period.

Rectal swabs were negative for *C. jejuni* before challenge. All swabs from infected animals were positive at 24 h and remained positive throughout the 2 weeks that samples were taken. All rectal swabs from control animals were negative for *C. jejuni.*

Bacteremia with *C. jejuni* was seen in 26 of 27 (96.3%) rabbits from which samples were taken 24 h after challenge, but it diminished in incidence during the following 3 days. Of 24 rabbits, 13 (54.2%) were positive at 48 h, but only 5 of 19 (26.3%) were positive at 96 h. All blood cultures from control rabbits were negative.

Clinical signs

Blood samples were obtained from 30 rabbits. Complete blood counts, including platelet counts, were unremarkable. Liver function tests were likewise unaffected, except for nonspecific changes in four animals near death. The creatinine levels in serum were minimally elevated only in rabbits with extreme azotemia.

The major blood abnormalities occurred in blood urea nitrogen and pH. If azotemia is conservatively defined as a blood urea nitrogen level greater than 50 (normal, 17.6 ± 4.4), 6 of 9 (66.7%) rabbits were azotemic on the day of death, compared with 3 of 33 (9.1%) at 1 to 3 days before death ($P = 0.001$). Similarly, if acidosis is defined as a pH less than 7.26 or a CO_2 level in serum less than 10 (normal, 22.8 ± 3.2), 6 of 9 (66.7%) were acidotic on the day of death compared with 2 of 33 (6.1%) on a previous day ($P = 0.0003$).

Pathology

Abnormal histology was present in seven of eight infected rabbits examined (7, 8). Lesions ranged from mild inflammatory infiltrates to frank epithelial necrosis. Such lesions were not seen in control animals studied. Lesions in infected animals were restricted to the terminal ileum, the unligated portion of the cecum, and the colon. Lesions seen in the cecum were often diffuse and more severe than those in other affected areas. Ileal and colonic lesions were usually multifocal and microscopic. Goblet cell hyperplasia was noted in six rabbits. This consisted of loss of mucus compared with normal goblet cells and signs of intense proliferative activity such as increased mitotic figures, architectural disarray, and increased nuclear material. Organisms were not demonstrated within the lesions by the Warthin-Starry stain. Sections of the liver, lungs, kidneys, and adrenal glands from infected animals werc unchanged from those of control rabbits.

Examination by scanning electron microscopy (SEM) and transmission electron microscopy (TEM) showed *Campylobacter* cells in the mucus and in close association with the brush border (unpublished data). Numerous organisms were found in the crypts. However, no organisms were seen clearly attached to the epithelium or making any kind of penetration of the epithelial cells. These electron microscopy findings are consistent with observations for *Campylobacter* cells in mice (16).

M-cell interactions

Since no remarkable bacterial interactions were seen with absorptive epithelial cells in the intestine, Peyer's patches in ligated rabbit ileal loops were examined (30). These studies were done because knowledge of possible M-cell–*Campylobacter* cell interactions could contribute to our understanding of the pathogenesis of the disease as well as to the development of oral vaccines against this organism. M cells are important antigen-sampling structures found in the epithelial layer over lymphoid follicles of the gastrointestinal mucosa (26). Sincc their initial description (23), these cells have been shown to interact with a number of pathogens (14, 15, 24).

When Peyer's patches were examined, associations between *Campylobacter* cells and the host were found. In a specimen fixed 15 min after inoculation of *Campylobacter* organisms into the intestinal loop, the bacteria were seen selectively associated with M cells.

The specificity of the attachment of *Campylobacter* cells to M cells after a 15-min incubation was also observed by SEM. Numerous *Campylobacter* cells were seen adhering to certain areas while leaving the absorptive epithelial cells uncovered. These covered areas were identified as M cells by using TEM. With TEM the bacteria were clearly observed in association with the luminal surface of the M cells, but not the absorptive cells.

Vacuoles containing *Campylobacter* cells could be seen in the M cells. Bacteria were rapidly transported to lymphoid cells, presumably macrophages. Bacteria were often free in large groups between cells in the lymphoid follicle (Fig. 1).

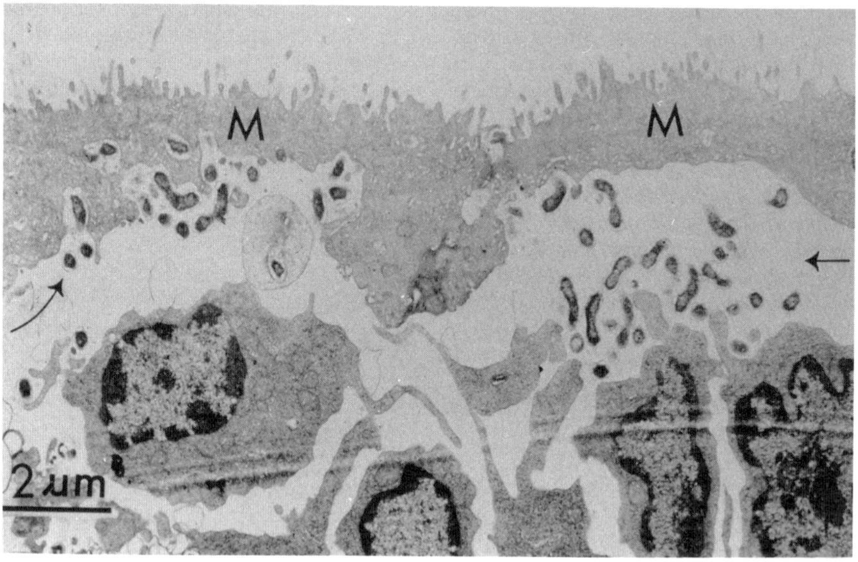

FIGURE 1. Transmission electron micrograph showing campylobacters (arrows) which have passed from the lumen, through the M cell (M), and into the underlying follicle. Bar, 2 μm.

Potential virulence mechanisms

The virulence mechanisms of *C. jejuni* responsible for the infectious processes initiated by the RITARD procedure cannot be determined from the present studies. However, it appears that microbial activities occurring at the intestinal level are more significant than extraintestinal invasion. Diarrhea was highly associated with mortality. Eighty-five percent of the animals which developed diarrhea died within 1 to 5 days of onset. Although the definitive cause of death in the rabbits was not determined, azotemia and acidosis were statistically correlated with the day of death. Severe dehydration is the most likely explanation of these findings, since other etiologies of azotemia and acidosis, such as renal failure and significant loss of blood into the gastrointestinal tract, were eliminated.

Levine et al. have categorized enteric pathogens into five groups on the basis of the mechanisms by which they produce disease (17). *Campylobacter* spp. can exhibit clinical characteristics resembling three of these mechanisms (29). The first type of mechanism involves toxin-induced disease, classically represented by *Vibrio cholerae.* The second type of mechanism, typified by *Shigella* spp., involves penetration of the intestinal epithelium and bacterial proliferation therein. Cells are damaged and die, but the lesion remains superficial and mesenteric adenitis and bacteremia seldom occur. The third pathogenic mechanism, termed translocation, is characterized by *Salmonella* and *Yersinia* spp. In translocation, the organisms penetrate the intestinal mucosa, resulting in minimal damage, and proliferate in the lamina propria and mesenteric lymph nodes. Frank dysentery and profuse watery diarrhea may represent two ends of the clinical spectrum, or the variation in symptoms may be the result of different mechanisms predominating for different strains, such as those seen for various types (e.g., enteropathogenic, enterotoxigenic, and enteroinvasive) of *E. coli* enteritis.

DEVELOPMENT OF IMMUNE RESPONSES

Evidence for Immunity

Prospective epidemiologic and human challenge studies suggest that protective immunity develops after *C. jejuni* infection and that vaccination for *Campylobacter* enteritis is possible (2, 12). Human volunteers fed *C. jejuni* cells become infected and respond with the development of specific serum immunoglobulin G (IgG), IgM, and IgA to *Campylobacter* spp. (2). When 20 adult volunteers were fed 10^8 or 10^9 organisms, diarrhea developed in 9 of these 20. When 7 of these volunteers who had been ill were rechallenged later with the same organism, none developed disease, whereas 6 of 12 nonimmunized volunteers developed diarrhea.

The development of anti-*Campylobacter* antibodies with age in endemic areas suggests that protective immunity in humans reflects the appearance of a specific anti-*Campylobacter* serum or intestinal antibody response (3, 4). The development of *Campylobacter* immunity in young children living in these endemic areas may explain the frequent isolation of *C. jejuni* from apparently healthy older children and also the age-associated decrease in the *C. jejuni* illness/infection ratio found in Bangladesh and in other developing countries (12).

Initial studies in the rabbit also demonstrated that immunity develops after *C. jejuni* infection (8). After oral inoculation, these rabbits became resistant to intestinal colonization and bacteremia when challenged with the same strain by the RITARD procedure.

Intestinal Lavage Technique

Repeated monitoring of antigen-specific mucosal immune responses in rabbits has been hindered by the lack of simple monitoring methods. To overcome previous difficulties, a lavage procedure was adapted for use with the rabbit as a method for the repeated sampling of intestinal secretions (6). In this procedure, rabbits are anesthetized, fed four doses of an isotonic salt solution, and injected intraperitoneally with pilocarpine to stimulate intestinal motility. Diarrheal secretions from individual rabbits are collected, expressed through gauze, heat treated, processed with bacterial and protease inhibitors, and stored at −20°C until assayed. The volume of material recovered per animal ranged from several milliliters to up to 50 ml. Following the procedure, the animals recover completely, with no observable side effects. During the course of some experiments, rabbits underwent repeated lavages at weekly intervals for up to 3 months.

The lavage procedure was used to study the mucosal response of rabbits to *Campylobacter* infection. Groups of rabbits were inoculated intragastrically and then challenged approximately 1 month later with either homologous or heterologous strains via the RITARD procedure (5). One week before gastric feeding and subsequently at weekly intervals after primary and secondary infection, intestinal lavage secretions and serum samples were collected and assayed for *Campylobacter*-specific IgA, IgM, and IgG antibodies. Primary and secondary intestinal (IgA) and serum (IgA, IgM, and IgG) antibody response kinetics were determined. After oral and RITARD challenge, rectal swabs and blood specimens were cultured for *C. jejuni* to monitor infection.

Specific anti-*Campylobacter* antibody in lavage or serum samples was measured by enzyme-linked immunosorbent assay (ELISA) with microwell plates that were coated with either glycine extracts or crude flagellar antigens of various *Campylobacter* strains (18). In early experiments goat anti-rabbit immunoglobulin was used. In later experiments, mouse monoclonal anti-rabbit antibody was used. The isotype specificity of each antiserum was indicated by ELISA and Western immunoblot analysis.

Antibody Response

The time course of anti-*Campylobacter* intestinal and serum antibody responses after primary oral immunization showed that *C. jejuni* strains differed in their ability to stimulate primary mucosal and serum antibody responses (5). Anti-*Campylobacter* intestinal IgA titers rose within the first week and then declined with some strains. IgA titers in serum rose more slowly but persisted longer. No anti-*Campylobacter*-specific IgG or IgM was detected in intestinal secretions following infection, although titers in serum increased significantly for both. The IgM response peaked at 1 to 2 weeks and then declined (unpublished data), whereas the IgG response in serum declined more slowly.

Both homologous and heterologous challenge groups developed a detectable secondary intestinal IgA response after RITARD challenge. Following the RITARD challenge, no secondary IgM response was observed. The kinetics of the IgG response in serum to *Campylobacter* spp. were similar to those of the IgM response, although the IgG titer rose more slowly. In both the homologous and heterologous challenge groups, no anti-*Campylobacter* IgG or IgM was detected in intestinal secretions after secondary infection.

For some strains of *C. jejuni,* primary oral challenge with whole-cell *Campylobacter* preparations did not induce any detectable mucosal IgA immune response. However, the immune system was apparently primed by this oral immunization, since, upon secondary challenge, significantly higher titers were observed in these animals than in those that had not received an immunizing dose (5, 25). Immunized rabbits attained a 2-log-higher IgA titer than did nonimmunized control animals.

Intestinal IgA titer consistently peaked approximately 7 days after RITARD challenge, independent of the immunization regimen (5, 25). By day 14 the immune response was greatly reduced, and by day 21 no mucosal IgA could be detected. The kinetics of this post-RITARD response were compared for immune and nonimmune animals. It was expected that immune rabbits would demonstrate a more rapid increase in IgA titer, i.e., a memory response, since their immune system had been previously primed by oral challenge. As predicted, the early mucosal immune response was more pronounced in immunized animals than in nonimmune rabbits (25).

Colonization Resistance

To determine whether the self-limiting colonization produced by oral feeding with *C. jejuni* protected animals against recolonization, separate groups of rabbits were first inoculated with *C. jejuni* via gastric intubation and monitored for intestinal colonization. One month after feeding, when no animals remained colonized with *C. jejuni,* rabbits were challenged via the RITARD procedure with either the same or a heterologous organism (5). In all homologous challenge groups the duration of colonization after challenge by the RITARD procedure was significantly shorter in previously immunized animals than in nonimmune control animals that were given only sterile broth before RITARD challenge. In all groups, the majority of rabbits had negative fecal swabs by 2 days after the RITARD challenge as compared with 7 to 14 days of colonization for nonimmunized animals.

Colonization resistance against challenge with the homologous strain persisted for an extended period. A single oral feeding protected animals against recolonization when challenged up to 9 months after immunization (unpublished data). To determine the dose of *C. jejuni* required to induce protective immunity, separate groups of rabbits were orally inoculated with graded doses of *C. jejuni* and, 1 month later, challenged with the homologous organism via the RITARD procedure. Rabbits that were fed as few as 100 organisms became intestinally colonized and resistant to recolonization (unpublished data). Although colonization resistance occurred when rabbits were challenged with the homologous strain, animals were not resistant to recolonization when challenged with heterologous organisms (5). As expected from the colonization results, rabbits immunized with *C. jejuni* varied in their resistance to bacteremia when challenged with homologous or heterologous bacteria. Rabbits given gastric inoculations and challenged with the same organism had no bacteremia, whereas the frequencies of bacteremia in animals challenged with heterologous cells were not significantly different from those observed in nonimmune animals.

Recent data indicate that the Lior serotype can be used to predict cross-protection among *Campylobacter* strains following oral immunization (1, 25). Immunized rabbits become resistant to colonization by *Campylobacter* strains of the same Lior serotype after challenge with 10^{10} CFU by the RITARD procedure. Immunized rabbits are not protected against strains of Lior serotype that differ from the immunizing serotype. Similar observations have been made in infant mice (1).

Secondary challenge of orally immunized rabbits with strains of the matched Penner and unmatched Lior serotype resulted in limited protection (25). Protection could be obtained, but only if the secondary challenge dose was reduced to 10^4 CFU. The Penner antigen is generally considerable to be lipopolysaccharide (LPS). Intestinal lavage from immune rabbits, known to be high in anti-*Campylobacter* mucosal IgA, recognizes a heavy LPS band in Western blot procedures (unpublished data).

Role of IgA in Colonization Resistance

The role of secretory IgA in gastrointestinal immune responses remains unclear. This molecule prevents adherence of *V. cholerae* (11) and enterotoxigenic *E. coli* (20) to intestinal epithelium. Anti-*Campylobacter* IgA in the gut may also afford protection by preventing the interaction of these organisms with intestinal epithelial cells.

In vitro assay

An in vitro assay was used to assess the interactions of *C. jejuni* with tissue culture cells overlaid with mucus from nonimmune rabbits and from rabbits previously challenged with the organism (21). An overlay of intestinal mucus from nonimmune rabbits was a greater impediment to adherence of *Campylobacter* cells to INT 407 cells than was an overlay of bovine serum albumin (BSA). Mucus obtained from rabbits previously colonized with *C. jejuni* was more effective in preventing bacterial adherence to the underlying INT 407 cells than was mucus from noncolonized, nonimmune rabbits.

The ability of mucus from rabbits previously colonized with *Campylobacter* spp. to effectively block cell adherence suggested that antibodies in the mucus could be associated with this phenomenon. To determine whether this was the case, mucus from immune rabbits was adsorbed with whole-cell preparations of *C. jejuni* before being used in the mucus inhibition assay. Cell-adsorbed mucus from immune rabbits was no longer able to prevent the adherence of *C. jejuni*. However, adsorption of immune mucus on *E. coli* K-12 had no effect on the ability of immune mucus to impede *C. jejuni*. Adsorption of immune mucus on whole-cell preparations of *C. jejuni* significantly reduced the levels of secretory IgA, whereas adsorption with *E. coli* K-12 cells had no effect.

Antibodies directed against antigens other than the flagella must contribute to retention of the bacteria within the mucus layer. Lavage fluid collected from immune rabbits was adsorbed on flagella and used in subsequent inhibition assays. Secretory IgA ELISAs showed a fourfold reduction in secretory IgA against the flagella, but this reduced antibody level failed to significantly increase the number of *C. jejuni* cells able to reach the INT 407 cells in the mucus inhibition assay.

Campylobacter cells in tissue culture wells containing immune mucus tended to aggregate into large clumps, whereas *Campylobacter* cells in normal mucus or BSA did not (unpublished data). *Campylobacter* cells trapped within the immune mucus layers remained viable. Aggregates of *Campylobacter* cells collected from some of the wells and streaked onto blood agar plates produced heavy lawns of bacterial growth. This trapping phenomenon may facilitate rapid clearance of *Campylobacter* cells from the gut.

In vivo assay

Immune rabbits clear the organism from the gut much more rapidly, generally within 1 day, than do nonimmune animals. This clearance may be associated with an enhanced mucosal IgA response. This hypothesis is supported by our finding that by day 7 post-RITARD, a 2-log-greater IgA titer is attained in animals given prior oral immunization than in nonimmunized animals (25).

Immune Response following Inoculation with Nonliving Preparations

Traditional approaches to oral vaccines against intestinal pathogens have favored living preparations owing to the relatively poor immunogenicity of nonliving materials. However, new advances in immunotechnology have made possible a major breakthrough in control of diarrheal diseases. These advances include mucosal adjuvants to enhance immunogenicity of nonliving microbial antigens and various microvesicle preparations which will deliver these antigens to appropriate lymphoid tissues in the gut. With these adjuvant and delivery systems, it is now possible to exploit the simplicity and safety of nonliving antigen preparations.

Recombinantly produced heat-labile toxin of enterotoxigenic *E. coli* (10) has recently been shown to greatly enhance the immune response to orally administered antigen. When this adjuvant was administered orally in subtoxic amounts with *Campylobacter* antigen, subsequent protection was obtained against colonization by live organisms (unpublished data). When rabbits were fed three times with 100 μg of sonicated whole-cell *Campylobacter* antigen and 25 μg of heat-labile toxin, colonization following RITARD challenge with 10^9 CFU was reduced to less than 3 days, compared with more than 7 days in control groups.

CONSIDERATIONS FOR FUTURE RESEARCH

Studies of *Campylobacter* infections in rabbits are enabling development of vaccines against this pathogen. The value of such a vaccine is indicated by the importance of this pathogen as a cause of diarrhea in humans. The goal of a *Campylobacter* vaccine is now more practical owing to new advances in immunotechnology which make it possible to exploit the safety and simplicity of nonliving antigen preparations for inducing mucosal immunity. Since relatively little is known about which *Campylobacter* antigens are protective, the first vaccine candidate for this organism to go into initial evaluations in human volunteers will be killed whole-cell preparations mixed with an adjuvant, such as described in this report. After protective antigens are identified, a second generation of subunit vaccines for *Campylobacter* spp. can be considered.

The rabbit has been useful in immunization studies because it naturally clears the organism and develops an immune response to this exposure. Unfortunately, challenge studies of immune animals require the use of the RITARD procedure to demonstrate acceleration of the clearance process. The tying off of the cecum from the intestinal tract, as occurs during the RITARD procedure, apparently is necessary for colonization resistance to be observed.

Although colonization resistance in immunized rabbits is a valid demonstration of protection, it is possible that protection against disease occurs without reflecting any change in the length of time that organisms are shed. For this reason, a natural and, hopefully, less laborious animal model which can also demonstrate protection against disease in immunized animals would be useful.

In contrast to other major enteric pathogens, relatively little is known about the virulence properties of *Campylobacter* spp. A model for studying *Campylobacter* infections which readily develops disease will enable pathogenic processes to be better understood. The rabbit model has, however, made possible a better understanding of the colonization process. Use of various flagellar mutant and hybrid *Campylobacter* strains has shown the importance of the flagellum in the colonization process and may soon show whether flagellar antigen can contribute significantly to immunoprotection in the RITARD model.

Colonization resistance in the rabbit has been used to establish that immunoprotection among *Campylobacter* strains can be predicted on the basis of Lior serotype. This finding is important to vaccine construction, because it indicates that a cocktail of serotypes will be needed. The number of Lior serotypes that have been identified continues to rise and now is over 120. However, it may be possible to identify a limited number of clinically significant serogroups found in various geographical areas.

A final consideration for future research which will contribute to vaccine development stems from the observations that as few as 100 CFU of *Campylobacter* organisms can colonize a rabbit and that changes in flagellar physiology and antigenicity occur during colonization. These data show that *Campylobacter* spp. can readily colonize and multiply in the gut and are influenced by the mucosal environment. If the organism is to be grown in fermentors for production of killed vaccines which optimally express relevant antigens, it will be necessary to know more about the physiology of *Campylobacter* spp. and how they respond to factors which may be found in the gut environment.

REFERENCES

1. **Abimiku, A. C., and J. M. Dolby.** 1988. Cross-protection by *Campylobacter jejuni:* importance of heat-labile serotyping (Lior) antigens. *J. Med. Microbiol.* **26:**265–268.
2. **Black, R. E., M. M. Levine, M. L. Clements, J. B. Hughes, and M. J. Blaser.** 1988. Experimental *Campylobacter jejuni* infections in humans. *J. Infect. Dis.* **157:**472–479.
3. **Blaser, M. J., R. E. Black, D. J. Duncan, and J. Amer.** 1985. *Campylobacter jejuni*-specific serum antibodies are elevated in healthy Bangladeshi children. *J. Clin. Microbiol.* **21:**164–167.
4. **Blaser, M. J., D. N. Taylor, and P. Echeverria.** 1986. Immune response to *Campylobacter jejuni* in a rural community in Thailand. *J. Infect. Dis.* **153:**249–254.
5. **Burr, D. H., M. B. Caldwell, A. L. Bourgeois, H. P. Morgan, R. Wistar, Jr., and R. I. Walker.** 1988. Mucosal and systemic immunity to *Campylobacter jejuni* in rabbits after gastric inoculation. *Infect. Immun.* **55:**99–105.
6. **Burr, D. H., D. T. Kerner, G. S. Blanco, A. L. Bourgeois, and R. Wistar, Jr.** 1987. Gastric lavage: a simple method to obtain IgA-rich intestinal secretions from the rabbit. *J. Immunol. Methods* **99:**277–281.
7. **Caldwell, M. B., P. Guerry, E. C. Lee, J. P. Burans, and R. I. Walker.** 1985. Reversible expressions of flagella in *Campylobacter jejuni. Infect. Immun.* **50:**941–943.
8. **Caldwell, M. B., R. I. Walker, and S. D. Stewart.** 1983. Development of an adult rabbit model of campylobacter infection suitable for testing immune responses to disease, p. 114. *In* A. D. Pearson, M. B. Skirrow, B. Rowe, J. R. Davies, and D. M. Jones (ed.), *Campylobacter II.* Public Health Laboratory Service, London.
9. **Caldwell, M. B., R. I. Walker, S. D. Stewart, and J. E. Rogers.** 1983. Simple adult rabbit model for *C. jejuni* enteritis. *Infect. Immun.* **42:**1176–1182.
10. **Clements, J. D., N. M. Hartzog, and F. L. Lyon.** 1988. Adjuvant activity of *Escherichia coli* heat-labile enterotoxin and effect on the induction of oral tolerance in mice to unrelated protein antigens. *Vaccine* **6:**269–277.
11. **Fubura, E. S., and R. Freter.** 1973. Protection against enteric bacterial infection by secretory IgA antibodies. *J. Immunol.* **111:**395–403.
12. **Glass, R. I., B. J. Stoll, M. I. Huq, M. J. Struelens, M. J. Blaser, and A. K. G. Kibriya.** 1983. Epidemiologic and clinical features of endemic *Campylobacter jejuni* infection in Bangladesh. *J. Infect. Dis.* **148:**292–296.
13. **Harris, L. A., S. M. Logan, P. Guerry, and T. J. Trust.** 1987. Antigenic variation of *Campylobacter* flagella. *J. Bacteriol.* **169:**5066–5071.
14. **Inman, L. R., and J. R. Cantey.** 1983. Specific adherence of *Escherichia coli* (strain RDEC-1) to membranous (M) cells of the Peyer's patch in *Escherichia coli* diarrhea in the rabbit. *J. Clin. Invest.* **71:**1–8.
15. **Kohbata, S., H. Yokoyama, and E. Yabuuchi.** 1986. Cytopathogenic effect of *Salmonella typhi* GI FU 10007 on M cells of murine ileal Peyer's patches in ligated ileal loops: an ultrastructural study. *Microbiol. Immunol.* **30:**1225–1237.
16. **Lee, A., J. L. O'Rourke, P. J. Barrington, and T. J. Trust.** 1986. Mucus colonization by *Campylobacter jejuni:* a mouse cecal model. *Infect. Immun.* **51:**536–546.

17. **Levine, M. M., J. B. Kaper, R. E. Black, and M. L. Clements.** 1983. New knowledge on pathogenesis of bacterial enteric infection as applied to vaccine development. *Microbiol. Rev.* **47:**510–550.
18. **Logan, S. M., P. Guerry, D. M. Rollins, D. H. Burr, and T. J. Trust.** 1989. In vivo antigenic variation of *Campylobacter* flagellin. *Infect. Immun.* **57:**2583–2585.
19. **Logan, S. M., and T. J. Trust.** 1983. Molecular identification of surface protein antigens of *Campylobacter jejuni. Infect. Immun.* **42:**675–682.
20. **McNabb, P. C., and T. B. Tomasi.** 1981. Host defense mechanisms at mucosal surfaces. *Annu. Rev. Microbiol.* **35:**477–496.
21. **McSweegan, E., D. H. Burr, and R. I. Walker.** 1987. Intestinal mucus gel and secretory antibody are barriers to *Campylobacter jejuni* adherence to INT 407 cells. *Infect. Immun.* **55:**1431–1435.
22. **Newell, D. G., H. McBride, and J. M. Dolby.** 1983. The significance of flagella in the pathogenesis of *Campylobacter jejuni,* p. 109. *In* A. D. Pearson, M. B. Skirrow, B. Rowe, J. R. Davies, and D. M. Jones (ed.), *Campylobacter II.* Public Health Laboratory Service, London.
23. **Owen, R. L., and A. L. Jones.** 1974. Epithelial cell specialization within human Peyer's patches: an ultrastructural study of intestinal lymphoid follicles. *Gastroenterology* **66:**189–203.
24. **Owen, R. L., N. F. Pierce, R. T. Apple, and W. C. Cray, Jr.** 1986. M cell transport of *Vibrio cholerae* from the intestinal lumen into Peyer's patches: a mechanism for antigen sampling and for microbial transepithelial migration. *J. Infect. Dis.* **153:**1108–1118.
25. **Pavlovskis, O. R., D. M. Rollins, R. L. Haberberger, Jr., A. E. Green, L. Habash, S. Strocko, and R. I. Walker.** 1991. Significance of flagella in colonization resistance of rabbits immunized with *Campylobacter* spp. *Infect. Immun.* **59:**2259–2264.
26. **Sneller, M. C., and W. Strober.** 1986. M cells and host defense. *J. Infect. Dis.* **154:**737–741.
27. **Spira, W. M., and R. B. Sack.** 1982. Kinetics of early cholera infection in the removable intestinal tie-adult rabbit diarrhea model. *Infect. Immun.* **35:**952–957.
28. **Spira, W. M., R. B. Sack, and J. L. Froehlich.** 1981. Simple adult rabbit model for *Vibrio cholerae* and enterotoxigenic *Escherichia coli* diarrhea. *Infect. Immun.* **32:**739–747.
29. **Walker, R. I., M. B. Caldwell, E. C. Lee, P. Guerry, T. J. Trust, and G. M. Ruiz-Palacios.** 1986. Pathophysiology of *Campylobacter* enteritis. *Microbiol. Rev.* **50:**81–94.
30. **Walker, R. I., E. A. Schmauder-Chock, J. L. Parker, and D. Burr.** 1988. Selective association and transport of *Campylobacter jejuni* through M cells of rabbit Peyer's patches. *Can. J. Microbiol.* **34:**1142–1147.

CHAPTER 15

Campylobacter jejuni Colitis and Immunity in Primates: Epidemiology of Natural Infection

ROBERT G. RUSSELL

INTRODUCTION

Experimental challenge of pig-tailed macaques (*Macaca nemestrina*) with a known virulent strain of *Campylobacter jejuni* produced acute diarrheal disease that was self-limiting. Intestinal biopsies from affected animals showed an acute colitis, similar to the colon lesions reported in biopsies of humans with acute *C. jejuni* infection (10).

In addition to the relevance of the experimental challenge studies for an animal model of the human disease, studies with pig-tailed macaques and cotton-top tamarins *(Saquinus oedipus)* have attempted to address the practical issue of the etiologic significance of *Campylobacter* spp. in diarrheal disease affecting primates housed in animal facilities. An understanding of the epidemiology of *Campylobacter* infections in primate colonies is important for a number of reasons: (i) because of the possible clinical importance for health care of the animals housed in facilities, (ii) because of possible zoonotic spread to animal handlers, and (iii) the use of macaques for *Campylobacter* research requires an adequate understanding of the natural infection in order to use the model effectively.

We have investigated the epidemiology of the course of natural infection within individual animals exposed to natural infection. The correlation between infection and diarrheal disease was investigated. Because infection appears to be widespread in many animal colonies (3, 5, 6, 9, 12, 14), studies of experimental natural infection in laboratory-housed primates included the following.

(i) A longitudinal study of infant macaques was conducted in a nursery housing approximately 100 infants. Sixteen animals were studied from birth to 1 year of age. Infants were separated from the mother at birth and artificially reared. They were housed in individual cages and had brief daily periods of socialization with three other infants for 1 h per day. Rectal swabs from each infant were cultured weekly for 12 months. The duration of study to complete investigations on all 16 infants was 23 months. This study was conducted in the Infant Primate Research Laboratory at the Washington Regional Primate Research Center.

(ii) A prospective study was conducted with groups of 8 to 10 mother-infant pairs. Samples from the infants and mothers were cultured weekly from the birth of the infant until weaning at 4 months old. This study was conducted at the Primate Field Station affiliated with the Washington Regional Primate Center.

(iii) A prospective study of cotton-top tamarins was conducted to investigate the occurrence of *Campylobacter* infection in twins reared in two separate locations at the same Primate Center. The infection data were correlated with the episodes of diarrhea. This study was conducted at the New England Regional Primate Research Center.

CAMPYLOBACTER SPP. CULTURED FROM MACAQUES

The *Campylobacter* spp. cultured from naturally infected infant macaques in the nursery included *C. jejuni, C. coli, C. fetus* subsp. *fetus, C. butzleri*, and *C. hyointestinalis.*

In our studies the bacteriologic culture methods have been directed mainly toward iso-

Robert G. Russell, Department of Pathology and Program of Comparative Medicine, School of Medicine, University of Maryland, Baltimore, Maryland 21201.

TABLE 1. Summary of clinical diarrhea in four infant *M. nemestrina* monkeys challenged with 10^{11} CFU of *C. jejuni* 81-176

Clinical signs	Experimental results[a]
Onset of diarrhea (h after inoculation)	34 ± 5.0
Peak of diarrhea (days after inoculation)	4 ± 0.1
Duration of diarrhea (days after inoculation)	9 ± 0.9
Presence of (no. positive/total)	
Occult blood	4/4
Bacteremia	3/4
Fecal leukocytes	1/4
Vomition	3/4

[a] Expressed as mean ± standard error of the mean.

lation of *C. jejuni* and *C. coli*. Therefore, the relative frequencies of isolation of the various *Campylobacter* species cannot be estimated at this time. However, it appears that all species identified so far commonly cause infection in both facilities (i.e., the nursery and field station) of the Washington Regional Primate Research Center.

CLINICAL SIGNS OF DIARRHEAL DISEASE IN *M. NEMESTRINA*

Experimental Challenge in Infant *M. nemestrina*

Four macaques were delivered by cesarean section and reared in isolation from other monkeys. The room housing the neonates had restricted entry to personnel. Animal attendants wore protective clothing including coveralls, masks, gloves, and boots when entering the room. The neonates were housed individually in Perspex-partitioned cages.

The four infants were challenged with a virulent strain of *C. jejuni*. Two of the infants were 3.5 months old and the other two were 4.5 months old. *C. jejuni* 81-176, used in these experimental challenge studies, was isolated from humans during an outbreak of campylobacteriosis in Minnesota, traced to consumption of contaminated raw milk (7). The organism caused diarrhea in human volunteers who were administered doses of 10^6 to 10^9 CFU (1).

All four infants developed acute diarrhea 24 to 36 h after administration of 10^{11} CFU of *C. jejuni* 81-176 via the intragastric route. The clinical signs are summarized in Table 1. All infants had grade 3 diarrhea (i.e., semiformed feces that took the form of the container), which developed into grade 4 diarrhea (fluid, watery feces). The fecal dry weight decreased from preinfection levels of 14% (± 1.5%, standard deviation) to 2.0% (± 0.6%) during diarrhea. One infant had bloody diarrhea with fecal leukocytes. Determination of the number of *C. jejuni* organisms in diarrheal specimens demonstrated large numbers of organisms (approximately 4×10^{10} CFU/g) at 48 h postinfection. High titers of *C. jejuni* (approximately 3×10^7 to 8×10^8 CFU/g) were recovered between days 3 and 11 postinfection. The titers declined to 5×10^2 to 8×10^3 CFU/g in infants that remained positive on days 15 to 21 as they cleared the infection. The results are summarized in Fig. 1. Rectal swabs from all four infants were negative by day 30 postinfection. The experimental challenge studies demonstrate that *C. jejuni* causes a self-limiting diarrheal illness in *M. nemestrina* (10). The severity of the diarrhea and the clinical course were analogous to those of the acute diarrheal disease in humans after food-borne infection.

Experimental Challenge of *M. fascicularis*

Four infant (6-month-old) cynomolgus monkeys were challenged with 10^{10} CFU of *C. jejuni* 81-176. Titers of 3×10^5 to 3×10^7 CFU/g were recovered from stool samples at 24 to 72 h postchallenge. Infants cleared the infection by days 20 to 35 postchallenge. None of the infants developed diarrhea. The acute diarrhea we observed in 3.5- to 4.5-month-old macaques was not seen in experimentally challenged nonimmune 6-month-old cynomolgus monkeys. It is not known whether the differences observed are indicative of species differences in susceptibility or whether other factors influenced the outcome. For example, the cynomolgus monkeys were slightly older and no macaque controls were used to monitor the challenge dose.

Role of *C. jejuni* and *C. coli* in Diarrhea Affecting Laboratory-Housed *M. nemestrina*

The prevalence of diarrhea in laboratory-housed macaques is variable within different age groups and under different management conditions. Our epidemiologic studies demonstrated a much higher prevalence of episodes of diarrhea among neonates (i.e., <1 month old) that had been separated from their mothers and reared artificially in an infant primate nursery than in neonates at another facility where neonates were nursed by their mothers (12). The prevalence of diarrheal episodes was also higher in infants of 1 to 6 months old in the nursery facility than in infants nursed by their mothers until weaning at 4 months old (Table 2).

The results of a prospective study in the nursery facility in which 16 infants were studied from birth to 1 year old showed that the onset of *C. jejuni* or *C. coli* infection correlated with the onset of diarrhea in approximately 13% of the episodes in neonates less than 1 month old. The mean age at initial *Campylobacter* infection in the nursery was 7.3 ± 3.5 weeks. In infants between 1 and 6 months old, *C. jejuni* and *C. coli* infections correlated with diarrheal episodes in approximately 25% of the diarrheal episodes (Table 3). All of the episodes of diarrhea which correlated with *C. jejuni*/*C. coli* infection occurred in infants less than 4 months old (13). Diarrhea was usually either soft and semiformed or fluid and watery. The results of the prospective study at the Primate Field Station facility

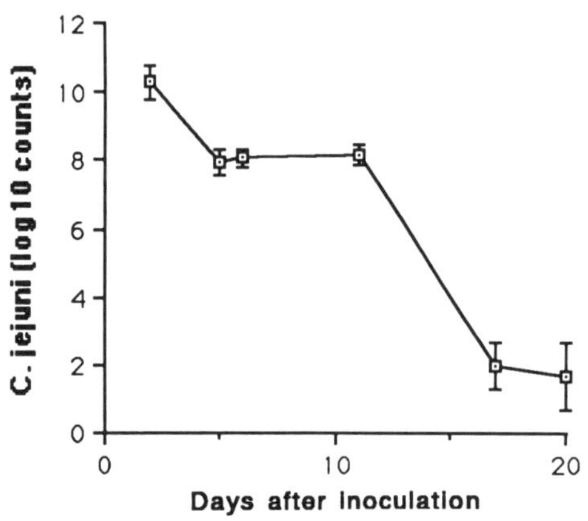

FIGURE 1. Intestinal titers of *C. jejuni* after challenge with strain 81-176. The titers immediately after challenge were $>10^{10}$ CFU/g (wet fecal weight). The titers declined progressively with clearance by 3 to 4 weeks postchallenge.

TABLE 2. Age-specific incidence of cases of diarrhea in colony-born macaques in a nursery facility where infants were artificially reared compared with the incidence in infants nursed by their mothers

Age (mo)	Incidence of diarrhea (cases/1,000 animal-days)[a] in animals: Artificially reared	Nursed by mother
<1	18.6	0.8
>1–6	2.0	0.8
>6–12	0.1	1.4

[a] A case is defined as the first episode of diarrhea. Incidence is expressed as the number of cases divided by the population at risk (i.e., cumulative animal-days of colony-born macaques until they developed diarrhea).

where infants were nursed and raised by their mothers contrasted markedly with observations of the diarrheal disease problems in the nursery facility. During the longitudinal study of 23 mother-infant pairs (from birth to weaning of the infants at 4 months old), none of the infants had episodes of diarrhea (Table 3). All of the infants were infected with *C. jejuni* or *C. coli* within the first 1 to 2 weeks of life and remained infected throughout the 4 months of observation. These results suggest a protective effect against diarrhea associated with maternal nursing of neonatal and infant macaques in captivity.

Campylobacter Infection in Cotton-Top Tamarins

A prospective epidemiologic study was conducted to investigate *Campylobacter* sp. infection in cotton-top tamarins housed in two buildings at the same primate facility. The two populations of *S. oedipus* studied were age-matched twin siblings. The overall objectives were an evaluation of (i) the effect of location and associated husbandry on the incidence of *Campylobacter* infections in the main facility compared with an annex facility located at some distance (1,000 m) from the main facility, (ii) the effect of different diets, (iii) correlation with clinical history, and (iv) correlation with colon biopsy results. Traffic patterns of personnel were controlled and protective clothing was worn by personnel in the annex.

No *C. jejuni* or *C. coli* organisms were cultured from 11 tamarins in the annex. None of them exhibited diarrhea. In the main facility seven tamarins were housed initially in the nursery. Only one infant was infected with *C. jejuni* in the nursery. After the infants were weaned and

TABLE 3. Association of *C. jejuni* and *C. coli* with episodes of diarrhea in neonatal and infant macaques during prospective studies in a nursery facility where infants were housed singly and artificially reared and in a study of mother-infant pairs

Location	Age group (mo)	Total no. of episodes of diarrhea[a]	Diarrheal episodes correlating with initial diarrhea[a]
Nursery (singly housed infants[b])	<1	27.7	3.7
	<1–6	5.4	1.5
Mother-infant pairs[c]	0–6	0	0

[a] Episodes per 1,000 animal-days.
[b] Mean age of initial infection in nursery-reared infants was 7.3 ± 3.5 weeks.
[c] Mean age of initial infection in infants nursed by their mothers was 1 week.

moved to animal rooms, they were infected with different strains of *C. jejuni* and *C. coli*. Over a 5-month period the seven infants experienced four reinfections with different strains of *C. jejuni* and *C. coli*.

In contrast to the observations in the nursery at the Washington Regional Primate Research Center, where infant macaques had negative cultures for very brief periods (mean, 2.0 ± 1.5 weeks) before becoming reinfected, the duration of negative cultures between reinfections of the tamarins at the New England Regional Primate Research Center was usually 8 to 11 weeks, and in some instances reinfections occurred at approximately monthly intervals.

Whereas no diarrhea was seen in the infants in the annex, four of the infants in the main facility had diarrhea. Diarrhea correlated with initial *C. jejuni* infection in three infants, and an episode of diarrhea coincided with the first reinfection of another infant at approximately 4 weeks of age.

The etiologic significance of *C. jejuni* in diarrheal disease of *S. oedipus* has not been determined. Colitis and diarrhea are important clinical problems in these animals. The preliminary results of the epidemiologic studies indicate that further studies of the clinical and pathologic findings of *C. jejuni* infection of *S. oedipus* under controlled experimental conditions are warranted.

In summary, the experimental challenge studies demonstrated that *C. jejuni* 81-176 caused acute diarrhea in infant macaques from 3.5 to 4.5 months old. The experimentally induced diarrheal disease in these animals was self-limiting. The observations in two primate facilities show that both old-world primates *(M. nemestrina)* and new-world primates *(S. oedipus)* are commonly infected with *Campylobacter* spp., particularly *C. jejuni* and *C. coli*. The incidence of infection and reinfection was different at each facility. Reinfection was less common in *S. oedipus* at the New England Regional Primate Research Center. This suggests that the incidence and pattern of infection may vary with the location and with different husbandry practices.

The correlations of clinical diarrheal disease with the onset of *Campylobacter* infection in individual animals must be interpreted with caution. The observations indicate that an etiologic role in some cases of diarrhea cannot be excluded. However, infections which correlated with clinical diarrhea could be coincidental. Also, the virulence properties of the isolates have not been determined. The lack of understanding of virulence mechanisms and the absence of laboratory tests to screen for virulence traits in *C. jejuni* are serious drawbacks in the current status of *Campylobacter* research.

INTESTINAL PATHOLOGY IN INFECTED INFANT *M. NEMESTRINA*

Histologic examination of biopsies from the jejunum, ileum, and colon at 48 to 72 h postchallenge demonstrated acute inflammation in the large intestine, with no lesions in the small intestine. This indicates that *C. jejuni*-mediated inflammation of the intestinal tract is a disease of the large intestine. The colitis was characterized by intense diffuse infiltration of neutrophils in the mucosa. There was damage to the epithelium in some crypts. Neutrophils were present in the lumen of the crypts. The luminal epithelium exhibited degeneration and necrosis with replacement of the columnar epithelium by a flattened epithelium, accompanied by loss of goblet cells (Fig. 2). The histologic lesions in the colon of *M. nemestrina* (10) are similar to the pathologic changes reported in humans with *C. jejuni* colitis (2, 4, 8).

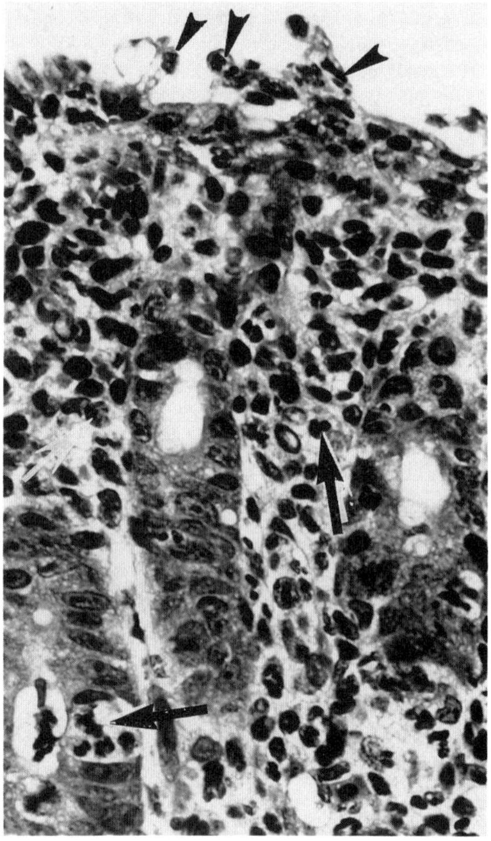

FIGURE 2. Histology of colitis in infant macaques at 48 h postinfection. There is necrosis of the luminal epithelium (arrowheads). Moderate numbers of neutrophils are present in the lamina propria and infiltrating into the glandular epithelium (arrows).

Electron microscopy of the colon shows superficial damage to the luminal colonic epithelium (Fig. 3). Invasive extracellular organisms were observed in the submucosa.

COURSE OF *CAMPYLOBACTER* INFECTION IN *M. NEMESTRINA*

Duration of Infection after Experimental Challenge and Rechallenge

The organism was recovered for 17 to 21 days postinfection from two infant macaques. All four infants studied were negative for *C. jejuni* 81-176 by day 30 postchallenge. The mean duration of excretion was estimated to be 23 days. After rechallenge of two infants 30 days after the initial challenge, the organism was recovered for 7 to <9 days from the respective infants. These results indicate a shorter duration of excretion after rechallenge with the homologous strain of *C. jejuni*.

Longitudinal Study of the Epidemiology of Infection in Housed *M. nemestrina*

A longitudinal epidemiologic study was performed to investigate the reasons for the persistent isolation of *C. jejuni* and *C. coli* from individual animals in all age groups at the Primate Center, including infants and older adults. The prospective study in which samples from infants from birth to 1 year old were cultured weekly showed that animals at the Washington Regional Primate Research Center were constantly reinfected under the hyperendemic conditions of *Campylobacter* infection in the nursery facility (13). The infants experienced infection with a mean of 7.9 ± 1.7 strains of *C. jejuni* or *C. coli* from birth to 1 year old. The individual strains were characterized by differences in Penner serotyping, Lior serotyping, whole-cell polyacrylamide gel electrophoresis protein profile, DNA hybridization (*C. jejuni* or *C. coli*), and hippurate hydrolysis (positive or negative). The repeated isolation of strains with different features is illustrated in Fig. 4 for one of the infants.

The duration of infection with a particular strain of *C. jejuni* or *C. coli* in individual animals varied from 1 to 11 weeks. The mean duration of infection per strain was 3 to 4 weeks. The duration of natural infection in infants in the nursery was therefore similar to the course of experimental infection in acute infections of nonimmune infant macaques.

The high prevalence of infection we observed in animals of various age groups (11) and the continual reinfection observed in the longitudinal studies (13) are explained by diversity among the *C. jejuni* and *C. coli* strains, high levels of environmental contamination, and excretion of large numbers of organisms by infected animals. Our data show that infected animals may excrete 10^2 to 10^9 CFU/g in the feces. The results indicate that intestinal colonization is not inhibited by previous *Campylobacter* infection. Although there was evidence from experimental studies that the duration of excretion of the homologous strain may be shorter after rechallenge, a shortened period of excretion was not observed in naturally infected animals, which were generally reinfected with different strains.

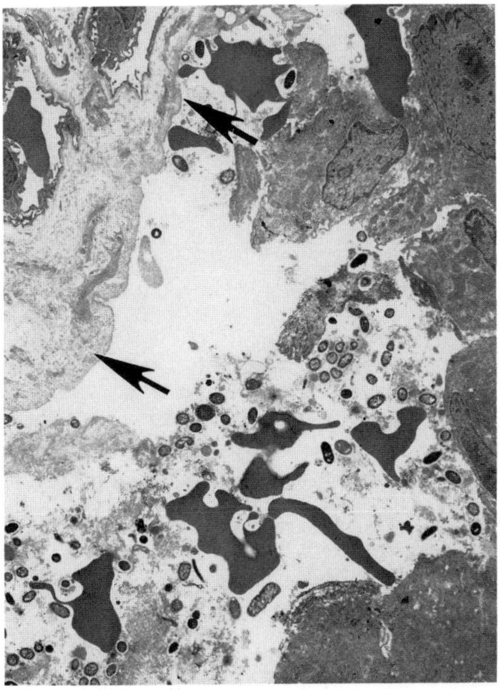

FIGURE 3. Electron micrograph showing local erosion of the luminal epithelium (arrows). Epithelial cells have lost the brush border. Erythrocytes and bacteria are present in the lumen.

IMMUNITY FOLLOWING *CAMPYLOBACTER* INFECTION IN *M. NEMESTRINA*

Experimental Challenge Experiments

The nonimmune infant macaques which developed diarrhea after challenge at 3.5 and 4.5 months old (i.e., 14 and 18 weeks old) did not exhibit clinical signs of diarrheal disease when rechallenged 30 days after the initial infection. This suggests that protective immunity developed with the initial episode of diarrhea. High titers of the organism were recovered in the stool following rechallenge. The duration of excretion was 1 week. This was shorter than the 3- to 4-week duration of excretion after the initial challenge.

The humoral immunoglobulin G (IgG), IgM, and IgA responses to the initial experimental challenge with *C. jejuni* 81-176 are shown in Fig. 5. The IgG levels were significantly elevated ($P < 0.01$) at day 21 postchallenge in all infants. The IgM titers also increased from day 0 to day 27 postinfection. There was no significant increase in IgA titers in serum.

After rechallenge (of previously infected infant macaques) on day 30 after the initial challenge, infants showed elevated titers of IgG and IgM on days 14 and 23 postrechallenge (i.e., days 44 and 53 after the initial challenge), indicating an anamnestic response. The IgA titers were elevated on day 7 postrechallenge and continued to rise through day 21 (Fig. 6).

Immunity in Spontaneously Infected *M. nemestrina*

During the prospective epidemiologic study of *Campylobacter* infection and reinfection, serum specimens were collected at monthly intervals for serologic studies. Each infant was its own control for the course of antibody titers over the 12 months each infant was studied.

The IgG titers measured by enzyme-linked immunosorbent assay decreased from birth to the lowest titer at approximately 8 weeks old. This is explained by the decreasing titer of passively acquired anti-*C. jejuni* IgG. Subsequent elevation in titers of IgG, IgM, and IgA in serum corresponded to active infection with *C. jejuni* and *C. coli* in immunocompetent animals (Fig. 7).

The bacterial titers in serum in macaques in the nursery which experienced continuous natural reinfections remained elevated, but with fluctuations. In general, the stimulation of further elevations in titers corresponded to anamnestic responses associated with the recurrent reinfections (Fig. 7). This is analogous to the anamnestic response in infant macaques after a single rechallenge infection (Fig. 6).

The data from the longitudinal study show that elevation of titers in serum occurs with experimental and natural reinfections and that there is persistent elevation of titers with repeated reinfections. Further studies are needed to obtain a better understanding of the immunologically important antigens for eliciting a protective immune response.

A challenge study was conducted with four 1-year-old macaques from the longitudinal study, similar to the infant illustrated in Fig. 4. During the longitudinal study the four infants were reinfected with multiple strains of *C. jejuni* and *C. coli* from birth to 1 year old. After challenge with *C. jejuni* 81-176, none of the 1-year-old immune infants developed diarrhea.

Further evidence for acquired immunity in naturally infected monkeys was obtained by correlating known reinfections with clinical records of diarrheal episodes in each of the 16 infants participating in the longitudinal study. None of

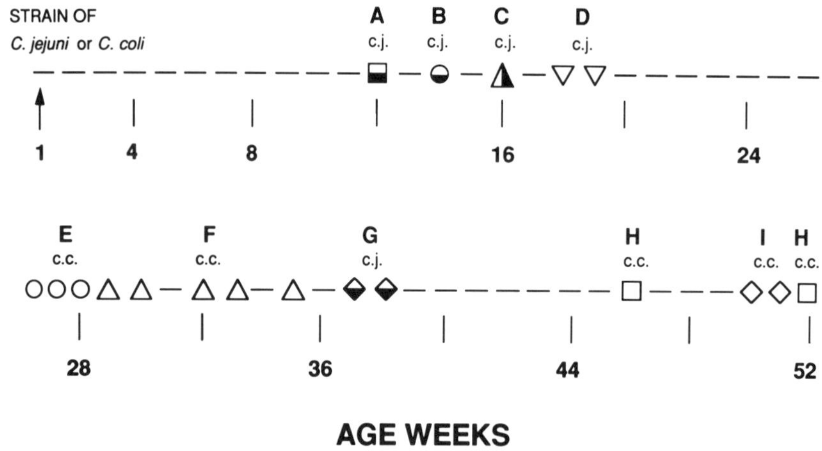

FIGURE 4. Reinfections of an infant in the nursery facility with nine different strains of *C. jejuni* and *C. coli* (designated A to H and indicated by different symbols in the diagram). *C. jejuni* (c.j.) and *C. coli* (c.c.) strains were differentiated by DNA probes, hippurate hydrolysis, Penner and Lior serotyping, and whole-cell protein profiles on polyacrylamide gel electrophoresis (13).

the infants over 4 months old showed diarrhea associated with *C. jejuni* or *C. coli* reinfection. These data are consistent with the hypothesis that infants over 4 months of age, with elevated titers of humoral Ig, have protective immunity against diarrhea. Further studies are needed to define the immunologic basis of protective immunity.

Evidence for passive protective immunity was implied by the observation that none of the 23 neonates nursed by their mothers developed diarrhea. Serology tests of colostrum from nursing mothers showed that five of eight colostrum samples had anti-*C. jejuni* antibodies. Although other factors such as the virulence of the isolates were not investigated, these observations may indicate that nursing provides passive protection against diarrheal disease in colonized infants. Six of eight mothers had elevated levels of anti-*C. jejuni* IgA antibodies in their colostrum.

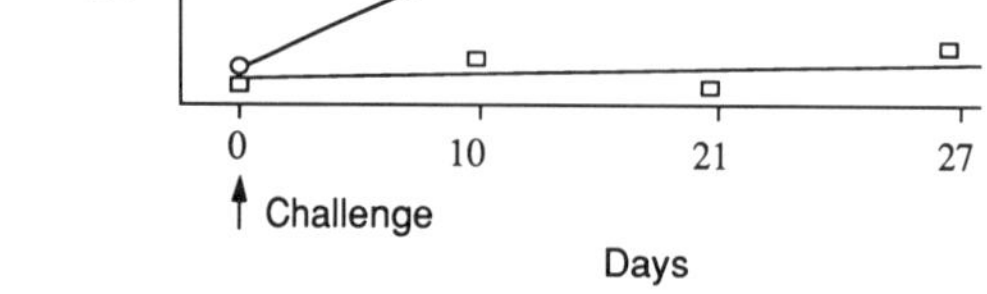

FIGURE 5. Humoral immune response following infection of 3.5- and 4.5-month-old macaques with *C. jejuni* 81-176. There was elevation in IgG (■) and IgM (○) titers. There was no detected elevation in IgA (□) titers. OD_{492}, optical density at 492 nm.

CHARACTERIZATION OF *C. JEJUNI* AND *C. COLI* IN LABORATORY PRIMATES

A total of 112 isolates of *C. jejuni* and *C. coli* from eight of the infants in the longitudinal study in the nursery facility were analyzed by DNA hybridization with *C. jejuni* and *C. coli* probes, by Penner and Lior serotyping, and by whole-cell protein profiles in sodium dodecyl sulfate-polyacrylamide gel electrophoresis. These analyses showed considerable diversity among the strains infecting infants in the nursery. Each of the eight infants experienced infection with a mean of 7.9 ± 1.7 strains of *C. jejuni* and *C. coli*. Of the 112 isolates studied, 63 were identified, which represented all of the *C. jejuni* and *C. coli* strains with different characteristics that were isolated from each of the eight infants. The Penner serotyping and DNA hybridization results for these 63 isolates are summarized in Table 4. Of the 63 isolates serotyped by the Penner method, 44 fell into 10 different serotypes and 19 were serotype negative. The serotypes were 46, 38, 34, 30, 24, 19, 8, 5, 4, and 30/34.

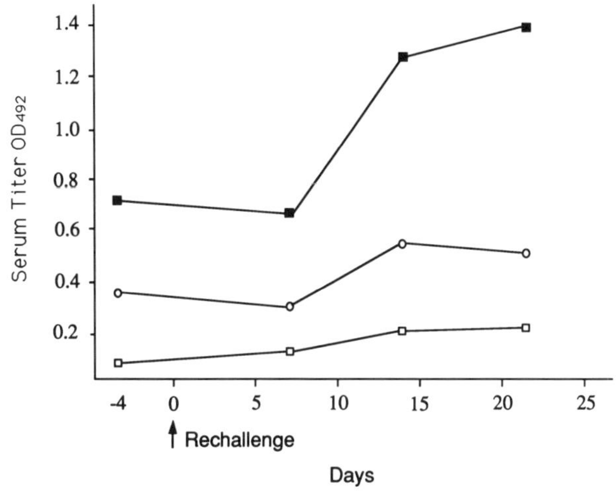

FIGURE 6. Anamnestic response in IgG (■) and IgM (○) levels in serum after rechallenge of infant macaques with *C. jejuni* 81-176. The IgA levels (□) were also elevated following rechallenge. OD_{492}, optical density at 492 nm.

Of the 63 isolates, 28 were distributed among nine serotypes by the Lior method (serotypes 2, 7, 11, 15, 29, 36, 44, 79, and 115).

Within some serotype categories, isolates examined by DNA hybridization included *C. jejuni* and *C. coli*. Both *C. jejuni* and *C. coli* occurred in Penner serotypes 34, 30, 24, and 5 and Lior serotype 2. These observations indicate that at least some Penner and Lior serotypes are not species-specific antigens.

SUMMARY AND CONCLUSIONS

The clinical signs of colitis caused by virulent *C. jejuni* infection in infant nonimmune macaques are manifested as soft catarrhal, fluid watery, and sometimes bloody diarrhea. The clinical diarrhea lasts approximately 7 to 10 days, and the infection is usually cleared by 3 to 4 weeks postinfection. Anti-*C. jejuni*-specific humoral IgG and IgM antibody titers became elevated by day 10 postinfection. The IgG levels were decreasing at 4 weeks postinfection.

The infants did not exhibit diarrhea after rechallenge, and they developed an anamnestic antibody response. *C. jejuni* was recovered for 1 to 1.5 weeks after rechallenge.

Epidemiologic studies demonstrated considerable diversity in the isolates infecting macaques and tamarins in primate colonies. Reinfection with different strains is common. Intestinal colonization after reinfection lasted approximately 3 to 4 weeks. The infants which developed active immunity appeared to be protected against diarrheal disease with recurrent infections. The humoral antibody levels remained elevated in infants experiencing continual reinfection. These infants did not develop diarrhea after challenge with virulent *C. jejuni* 81-176.

The infant *M. nemestrina* offers a suitable animal model for pathogenesis and immunity studies of *C. jejuni*. Challenge studies have been conducted only with small numbers of *M. nemestrina* infants so far. Further experimental challenge studies are warranted to define the dose range causing clinical diarrhea, the age range of susceptibility, and the development and duration of mucosal immunity. Because infection is hyperendemic in some colonies, infants for experimental challenge studies should be raised in isolation to ensure they are not infected.

The epidemiologic studies must be interpreted with caution. Although there appears to be a correlation between clinical diarrhea with onset of infection, especially in infants less than 4 months old, the virulence and dose of the strains infecting the infants is not known. Approximately half of the infections in the infant macaques were caused by *C. coli*. The etiologic significance of this species has not been defined in this *M. nemestrina* model.

FUTURE STUDIES

At present the virulence mechanisms of *C. jejuni* are still not well defined. The acute colitis

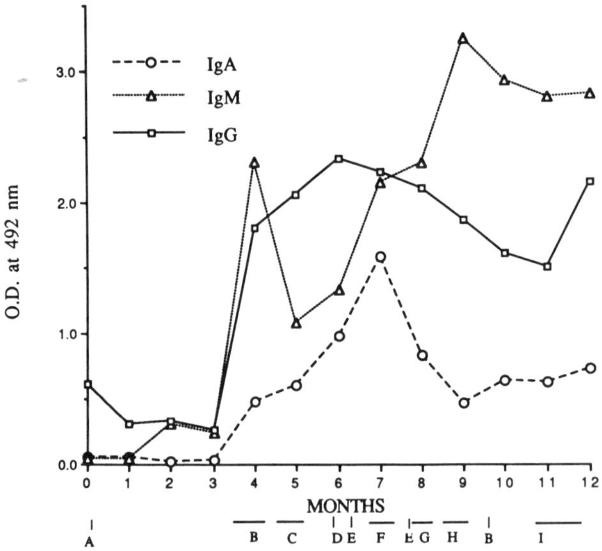

FIGURE 7. IgG, IgM, and IgA antibody levels remain elevated in an infant macaque experiencing multiple naturally occurring reinfections with *C. jejuni* and *C. coli.* This infant was infected with strains A to I, detected by weekly cultures from birth to 12 months old, during a prospective study conducted in a nursery facility. O.D., optical density.

is indicative of invasion. However, further studies are needed to define the invasion process. To better understand the pathogenesis of the diarrheal disease, virulence factors must be determined and suitable laboratory methods (e.g., DNA probes) are needed for detecting virulence factors in isolates of *C. jejuni* and *C. coli.*

Studies in the infant *M. nemestrina* model indicate that immunity protects against rechallenge. Because infant macaques less than 4 months old appear to be the most susceptible, it is important to develop practical methods for providing protection against disease, by either passive or active immunity. *M. nemestrina* provides a suitable model for studies to define the protective immune response. The protective and immunologic antigens must be defined. The extent of cross-protection between strains must be determined.

REFERENCES

1. **Black, R. E., M. M. Levine, M. L. Clements, T. P. Hughes, and M. J. Blaser.** 1988. Experimental Campylobacter jejuni infection in humans. *J. Infect. Dis.* **157:**472–479.
2. **Blaser, M. J., R. B. Parsons, and W.-L. L. Wang.** 1980. Acute colitis caused by *Campylobacter fetus ss jejuni. Gastroenterology* **78:**448–453.
3. **Bryant, J. L., H. F. Stills, R. H. Lentsch, and C. C. Middleton.** 1983. *Campylobacter jejuni* isolated

TABLE 4. Characterization of 63 isolates of *C. jejuni* and *C. coli* from eight infants by DNA hybridization and serotyping by the Penner and Lior methods

Method and result	No. (%) of isolates
Positive *C. jejuni* probe	32 (51)
Positive *C. coli* probe	31 (49)
Penner serotyped	44 (70)
Negative serotyping by Penner method	19 (30)
Lior serotyped	28 (44)
Negative serotyping by Lior method	35 (56)
Negative by Penner and Lior methods	15 (24)

from Patas monkeys with diarrhea. *Lab. Anim. Sci.* **33**:303–305.
4. **Colgan, T., J. R. Landert, A. Newman, and S. C. Luk.** 1980. *Campylobacter jejuni* enterocolitis: a clinicopathologic study. *Arch. Pathol. Lab. Med.* **104**:571–574.
5. **Fitzgeorge, R. B., A. Baskerville, and K. P. Lander.** 1981. Experimental infection of Rhesus monkeys with a human strain of *Campylobacter jejuni. J. Hyg.* **86**:343–351.
6. **Goodwin, T., M. R. Adams, N. D. M. Lehner, and C. P. Jerome.** 1983. *Campylobacter* enteritis in Patas monkeys. *Lab. Anim. Sci.* **33**:481.
7. **Korlath, J. A., M. T. Osterholm, L. A. Judy, J. C. Forfang, and R. A. Robinson.** 1985. A point-source outbreak of campylobacteriosis associated with consumption of raw milk. *J. Infect. Dis.* **152**:592–596.
8. **Lambert, N. E., P. F. Schofield, A. G. Ironside, and B. K. Mandal.** 1979. *Campylobacter* colitis. *Br. Med. J.* **1**:857–859.
9. **Morton, W. R., M. Bronsdon, G. Mickelsen, G. Knitter, S. Rosenkranz, L. Kueller, and D. Sajuthi.** 1983. Identification of *Campylobacter jejuni* in *Macaca fascicularis* imported from Indonesia. *Lab. Anim. Sci.* **33**:187–188.
10. **Russell, R. G., M. J. Blaser, J. I. Sarmiento, and J. Fox.** 1989. Experimental *Campylobacter jejuni* infection in *Macaca nemestrina. Infect. Immun.* **57**:1438–1444.
11. **Russell, R. G., L. Krugner, C.-C. Tsai, and R. Ekstrom.** 1988. Prevalence of Campylobacter in infant, juvenile, and adult laboratory primates. *Lab. Anim. Sci.* **38**:711–714.
12. **Russell, R. G., S. L. Rosenkranz, L. A. Lee, H. Howard, R. F. DiGiacomo, M. A. Brondson, G. A. Blakely, C.-C. Tsai, and W. R. Morton.** 1987. Epidemiology and etiology of diarrhea in colony-born *Macaca nemestrina. Lab. Anim. Sci.* **37**:309–316.
13. **Russell, R. G., J. I. Sarmiento, J. Fox, and P. Panigrahi.** 1990. Evidence of reinfection with multiple strains of *Campylobacter jejuni* and *Campylobacter coli* in *Macaca nemestrina* housed under hyperendemic conditions. *Infect. Immun.* **58**:2149–2155.
14. **Tribe, G. W., and M. P. Fleming.** 1983. Biphasic enteritis in imported cynomolgus *(Macaca fascicularis)* monkeys infected with *Shigella, Salmonella* and *Campylobacter* species. *Lab. Anim.* **17**:65–69.

CHAPTER 16

Pathogenesis of *Campylobacter* Infection: In Vitro Models

GUILLERMO M. RUIZ-PALACIOS

The mechanisms by which *Campylobacter* spp. induce disease are not well understood. Three mechanisms by which *Campylobacter jejuni* induces illness have been postulated on the basis of the clinical syndromes: (i) adherence and production of enterotoxins, inducing secretory diarrhea; (ii) invasion and proliferation within the intestinal epithelium, inducing cell damage and an inflammatory response clinically manifested as dysentery and inflammatory diarrhea with fecal leukocytes; and (iii) translocation, in which the organism penetrates the intestinal mucosa, causing minimal damage, and proliferates in the lamina propria and mesenteric lymph nodes, with further extraintestinal infections such as meningitis, cholecystitis, urinary tract infection, and mesenteric adenitis. There is clinical and laboratory evidence that supports the existence of these three mechanisms, although it is not conclusive. In addition, recent cohort studies have shown that susceptible children may be infected with *Campylobacter* spp. without becoming ill, further suggesting that there may be nonpathogenic strains.

In vitro studies have demonstrated that *C. jejuni* is capable of adhering to several cell lines, and a correlation between in vitro cell adherence and illness has been found. Furthermore, the ability of some clinical isolates to penetrate cells has been demonstrated in in vitro assays. The in vitro studies discussed in this section of this volume shed some light on the understanding of the host-bacterium interaction and the induction of illness in *Campylobacter* infections. Assays of *Campylobacter* association with eucaryotic cells seem useful in differentiating virulent from nonvirulent strains; a significant association was found between illness and the isolation of a cell-associated strain. Furthermore, from virulent strains that associated to eucaryotic cells, a subgroup that only adhered to but did not penetrate the cell was identified in association with noninflammatory diarrhea, whereas a second subgroup, which penetrated the cells, was found in association with inflammatory diarrhea. Supporting the importance in pathogenesis of adherence and invasion is the finding of a putative invasion-related antigen, defined as a surface-exposed protein of 26 kDa, which may play a key role in *C. jejuni*-host cell interaction and ultimate cell penetration. Moreover, specific receptor analogs for *C. jejuni* invasive strains have been found in abundance in human milk and have been characterized as fucosylated oligosaccharides. It would be very interesting to see whether the 27-kDa surface protein interacts with the milk receptor analogs. Another finding that must be elucidated is whether cell attachment of strains identified as adherent/noninvasive in one of the studies involves antigens different from the 27-kDa surface protein. It seems necessary to extend these studies to confirm findings by Fauchère and Ruiz-Palacios.

Although several groups have demonstrated the presence of enterotoxin that induces intraluminal fluid accumulation and reacts with anticholera toxin antibodies, its clinical relevance remains controversial. Two studies presented in this section found that approximately half of the strains tested produce the toxin, detected by in vitro assays with CHO cells or by an immunoassay with monoclonal antibodies raised against the toxin.

The ability to induce illness seemed to be related to enterotoxin production; strains found to be strong toxin producers were more likely

Guillermo M. Ruiz-Palacios, Department of Infectious Diseases, National Institute of Nutrition, Mexico City 14000 D.F., Mexico.

to be isolated from individuals with diarrhea. On the other hand, two independent studies were unable to demonstrate enterotoxin production in isolates from developed and developing nations or an antibody response to adenylate cyclase-related toxins. This may show that the lack of isolation of enterotoxigenic strains is not related to a specific geographic region. It is essential that discrepancies in identifying enterotoxigenic strains be clarified and the role of enterotoxin in human disease be defined. Differences in the results presented in different chapters in this section may be due to problems with the methods used to induce toxin production in strains tested or may perhaps be laboratory artifacts. The best way to solve this controversy is to exchange strains and details of methods between the groups.

Finally, although a cytotoxin is consistently found in *Campylobacter* isolates and some of its biological characteristics have been defined (Guerrant et al., this volume), the role of the cytotoxin in producing illness is not known. Since the cytotoxin has already been purified, it is important to set up sensitive and specific experiments to quantify its production among isolates and to correlate it with disease in well-defined clinical syndromes.

Are we talking about a single pathogen or about subgroups of the same species that, as in *Escherichia coli,* have different pathogenic mechanisms and also include some strains that are nonpathogenic? I believe that this is the most exciting question that arises from the data presented in this section. Research in the area of *Campylobacter* pathogenesis is in its infancy, and there seems to be a promising future for the understanding of the mechanisms by which this organism interacts with the host and induces disease. It is sad to see that, at this point, attention is being diverted from these promising concepts to other, more fashionable areas of research, since *Campylobacter* species are unquestionably among the most common agents of diarrhea in both developing and developed regions of the world.

CHAPTER 17

In Vitro Models for Studying *Campylobacter jejuni* Infections

RICHARD L. GUERRANT, GUODONG FANG, ROSS A. PENNIE, AND RICHARD D. PEARSON

EARLY STUDIES OF *C. FETUS* AND *C. JEJUNI* FOR ENTEROTOXINS, CYTOTOXINS, AND INVASIVENESS

Although *Campylobacter* spp. were recognized as a likely cause of diarrhea by Dekeyser et al. in 1972 (7) and even earlier (1957) by King (20), our interests began in 1976 and 1977 with bloodstream *Campylobacter* isolates at the University of Virginia Hospital and at the New York Hospital and Cornell Medical Center (13). Before they were cultured widely from fecal specimens, the few *Campylobacter jejuni* isolates from the bloodstream were overshadowed by *C. fetus,* the predominant cause of *Campylobacter* bacteremia among pregnant patients or patients with underlying conditions such as cirrhosis, alcoholism, diabetes mellitus, or gastrectomy (Table 1) (13). The association of both *C. jejuni* and *C. fetus* bacteremic infections with gastrointestinal symptoms in 80 and 38% of patients, respectively, prompted us to examine our isolates and several from Robert Smibert, Virginia Polytechnic Institute and State University, Blacksburg, Va., for recognized enterotoxins, cytotoxins, and invasiveness traits by using CHO cells, suckling mice, ligated rabbit ileal segments, and guinea pig conjunctivitis (Sereny) tests, respectively (6, 9, 12, 36).

As shown in Table 2, 48-hour tryptic soy blood broth culture filtrates of eight strains of *C. fetus* and three strains of *C. jejuni* failed to show any choleralike elongation of CHO cells. Interestingly, however, the three *C. jejuni* isolates and four of seven *C. fetus* isolates showed significant cytotoxicity (as determined by trypan blue uptake) in comparison with controls. Furthermore, whole tryptic soy broth cultures of three of the *C. fetus* isolates caused no fluid secretion or histologic alterations in 18-h ligated rabbit ileal loops, and blood agar plate-grown cultures were negative in the guinea pig conjunctivitis (Sereny) test for invasiveness.

IN VITRO STUDIES OF *C. JEJUNI* SUSCEPTIBILITY TO SERUM

Thereafter, because *C. jejuni* was much more commonly observed as an enteric rather than a bloodstream pathogen, its susceptibility to serum was examined (30). Although fresh normal serum produced only a slight (0.2-log) mean reduction (range, 0.1 to 0.3) in viable *C. jejuni* numbers, convalescent-phase serum produced a 2.7- to 4.4-$\log_{10}$ kill (mean, 3.7) of the homologous strains (Fig. 1). In contrast, heterologous immune convalescent-phase serum exhibited a slight (0.3-log) mean reduction in *C. jejuni* viability (range, 0.1 to 1.1; $n = 6$). Homologous acute-phase serum (taken 1.5 to 2 days after the onset of diarrheal illness) produced a variable, 0- to 3.8-log reduction (mean, 1.8) in viable organisms. The effects of heterologous acute-phase serum were similar to those of nonimmune serum, exhibiting a 0- to 0.4-log reduction ($n = 5$) (mean, 0.3). Complement was responsible for the bactericidal effects of acute-phase homologous and convalescent-phase sera; bacterial killing was abrogated by heat inactivation of serum at 56°C for 30 min or by EDTA chelation. The role of the classical pathway in complement activation was demonstrated by abrogation of kill-

Richard L. Guerrant, Guodong Fang, Ross A. Pennie, and Richard D. Pearson, Division of Geographic Medicine, University of Virginia School of Medicine, Charlottesville, Virginia 22908.

TABLE 1. *Campylobacter* bacteremia: summary of 91 cases[a]

Parameter	Result for: *C. fetus*	*C. jejuni*	*Campylobacter* spp.[b]
n (60 to 87% male)	50	10	31
Age (yr) and % of patients	96% > 14 yr	60% < 1 yr	89% > 14 yr
Underlying disease	72%	40%	29%
Farm or animal exposure	26%	0	19%
Signs and symptoms			
Fever	96%	60%	97%
Gastrointestinal[c]	38%	80%	35%
Hepatosplenomegaly or jaundice	44%	10%	19%
Neurologic	28%	10%	16%
Rash	2%	20%	13%
Arthritis	12%	30%	7%
Mortality	26%	20%	10%

[a] From reference 13.
[b] Species uncertain.
[c] Diarrhea, nausea, vomiting, abdominal pain.

ing following magnesium ethylene glycol-bis (β-aminoethyl ether)-*N,N,N′,N′*-tetraacetate (Mg-EGTA) chelation and by reconstitution experiments with heat-inactivated serum, C2-deficient serum, and purified C2.

Furthermore, the requirement for specific antibody for the serum bactericidal effect was indicated by the loss of bactericidal activity when immune sera were adsorbed with homologous, but not with heterologous, whole *C. jejuni*

TABLE 2. Studies of enterotoxinlike and cytotoxin effects on CHO cells in vitro

Toxin[a]	CT/LT-like effect (% of cells elongated)	Cytotoxic effect (% of cells trypan blue positive)
Cholera toxin (CT)	33.0	7.0
E. coli 334 (LT)	25.0	14
E. coli 10405 (control)	1.3	7
C. fetus		
CF	2.5	12
NB	3.0	6
GM	1.5	15
NJ	5.0	NT[b]
RS/P	6.0	18.5
RS/B	8.0	21.5
11669	2.0	29.0
319-A-77	4.0	27.5
C. jejuni		
H641	6.0	17.0
B7619	6.5	17.5
H840	5.5	17.5

[a] *C. fetus* CF, NB, and GM were also tested and found to be negative for LT in 18-h rabbit ileal segments (<0.2 ml/cm versus 1.06 ml/cm for *E. coli* 334), for ST in suckling mice (gut/remaining body weight = 0.0620, 0.0607, and 0.0618, respectively, versus 0.1279 for ST *E. coli* B44), and for invasiveness in the guinea pig conjunctivitis (Sereny) test.
[b] NT, not tested.

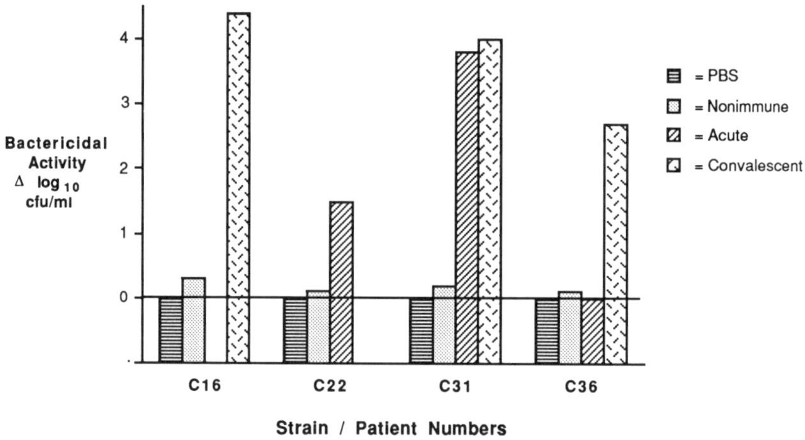

FIGURE 1. Killing of *C. jejuni* by immune sera.

cells. The presence of specific antibody in convalescent-phase serum was further documented by agglutination of only homologous *C. jejuni* suspensions by heat-inactivated serum. Finally, because *C. jejuni* often produces an inflammatory diarrhea with polymorphonuclear neutrophils (PMN) present in fecal smears, we examined the interaction of *C. jejuni* with PMN. Studies with human PMN suggested that the ingestion and killing of two *C. jejuni* strains were modest and variable in the presence of heat-inactivated homologous serum (0 to 24% mean PMN association and 0 to 22% mean percent killing), in contrast to the 92% association and 82% killing of *Staphylococcus aureus* 502A by PMN in these experiments.

The potent, antibody-dependent, rapidly developing bactericidal effects of serum may help limit most *C. jejuni* infections to the intestinal tract, as suggested by Johnson et al. (17), who reported a patient with systemic lupus erythematosus and immunoglobulin deficiency who had repeated positive stool and blood cultures for *C. jejuni* for months until *C. jejuni*-specific immunoglobulin G was detectable in the serum. Similar persistent *C. jejuni* infections have been reported in several patients with human immunodeficiency virus infection (2, 8, 33).

TYPE OF DIARRHEA CAUSED BY *C. JEJUNI* INFECTIONS

With the continued development of clinical experience with *C. jejuni,* it became increasingly evident that the majority of patients with *C. jejuni* diarrhea in industrialized countries had an inflammatory colitis characterized by numerous fecal PMN in 78 to 93% of cases (3, 39) and bloody diarrhea in 60 to 65% of cases (3, 5) (Table 3). This is in striking contrast to the watery, noninflammatory diarrhea often seen in tropical areas (10, 37), where choleralike enterotoxin has been associated with *C. jejuni* (35) and where asymptomatic infection rates may be very high (up to 39%) (4, 10). These findings suggest that striking differences in virulence traits may exist in *C. jejuni* from different geographic areas. In

TABLE 3. Clinical presentations of *C. jejuni* infections[a]

Geographical location	% of patients whose diarrhea is caused by *C. jejuni*	% of *C. jejuni* diarrhea patients with: Fecal PMN	Blood in stools	% of *C. jejuni* patients with asymptomatic infection
Industrialized countries	4.6–13.9	78–93	60–65	<1.3
Developing countries	2–35	22–46	5–17	0–39[b]

[a] Data from references 3, 4, 10, 38, and 39.
[b] Percentage depends on age (39% for those <2 years old).

addition, the data suggest that important differences in host susceptibility and immunity may exist.

Because most episodes of recognized *C. jejuni* diarrhea in Virginia are inflammatory, we further explored the possibility that a Shiga-like or *Clostridium difficile*-like cytotoxin might be produced by local *C. jejuni* isolates. Investigators in our laboratory have been interested in the effects of enteric bacterial toxins on cells in tissue culture, ranging from CHO cell elongation in response to the adenylate cyclase-activating choleralike *E. coli* heat-labile toxin (12) to the cytopathic effects of *Clostridium difficile* toxin B, pertussis toxin, and other cytotoxins (Table 4) (11, 15, 16, 18, 19, 21–23, 24, 27, 29, 34, 40, 41). Consequently, we examined *C. jejuni* culture filtrates for cytotoxic effects.

STUDIES OF *C. JEJUNI* CYTOTOXIN

Twelve *C. jejuni* isolates from individuals with inflammatory diarrhea seen at the University of Virginia Medical Center were grown in pure culture on sheep blood agar plates for 48 h at 42°C in an atmosphere of reduced oxygen and increased carbon dioxide (14, 14a, 31). Colonies were harvested and suspended in phosphate-buffered saline to a McFarland no. 10 standard that represented approximately 3 × 10^9 organisms per ml. Bacteria were then centrifuged at 2,500 rpm (1,200 × *g*) for 20 min, and the supernatants were passed through a 0.22-μm filter. *C. jejuni* filtrates were then placed on HeLa or CHO cells in F-12 tissue culture medium in 96-well, flat-bottom tissue culture plates. Filtrates were added within 2 to 3 h of the cells being plated. The plates were read for cytotoxicity by phase-contrast microscopy after 24 h with and without trypan blue staining and confirmed after methanol fixation and Giemsa staining.

Neutralization studies were done with 1:10 dilutions of antiserum against Shiga toxin (provided by Alison O'Brien, Uniformed Services University for Health Sciences, Bethesda, Md.) or 1:25 dilutions of anti-*Clostridium difficile* antiserum (provided by Tracey Wilkins, Virginia Polytechnic Institute and State University). The antisera were incubated for 30 min at 37°C with various dilutions of the *C. jejuni* filtrates prior to placing the toxin-antitoxin mixture on the tissue culture cell monolayers.

In addition, 1 ml each of undiluted, polymyxin-treated culture filtrates of *C. jejuni* cytotoxin were studied in 4- to 6-cm ligated rabbit ileal loop segments, which were examined for volume:length ratios at 6 and 18 h (9). Five-day-old suckling mice were also inoculated intragastrically with 0.1 ml of polymyxin-treated culture filtrates, and the gut:body weight ratios were determined after 3 h as described by Dean et al. (6).

Whereas polymyxin without bacteria appeared cytotoxic to HeLa cells only when undiluted (1 mg/ml) or at a dilution of 1:2, 5 of the 12 *C. jejuni* isolates (representing at least two different serotypes) had a cytolethal effect on HeLa cells at 1:4 or greater dilutions. Although slight amounts of cytotoxicity from 4 of these 12 strains were noted in CHO cells, only strain C-31 (serotype 6, biotype IV) (25, 26) consistently exhibited cytotoxic activity (a killing of 50% of cells) at dilutions of 1:32 to 1:128 (Fig. 2). Although no significant cytotoxicity was noted in untreated culture filtrates of strain C-31, sonication of strain C-31 produced cytotoxic effects that approached those seen with polymyxin treatment of this strain. Additional studies were done with the more potent cytotoxic culture filtrates of strain C-31.

To test the heat lability of this material, fresh preparations of *C. jejuni* C-31 filtrates were kept frozen or refrigerated or heated to 50 to 100°C for 30 to 120 min. Whereas treatment at 50°C for 30 min destroyed little of the cytotoxic activity, treatment at 60°C for 30 min or longer abrogated well over half the cytotoxic activity. Treatment at 50°C for 2 h almost completely

TABLE 4. Microbial toxins from enteric pathogens

Type	Examples	Tissue culture, effects
Secretory enteroroxins, acting via		
Cyclic AMP	CT, LT	"Cytotonic"
Cyclic GMP	STa	–
Unclear (? Ca^{2+})	STb, *C. difficile* toxin A	–, ±
Cell-releasing toxins	*E. histolytica*	Release, rinsible
Cytotoxic toxins	*C. difficile* toxin B, Shiga toxin	Irreversible cell damage

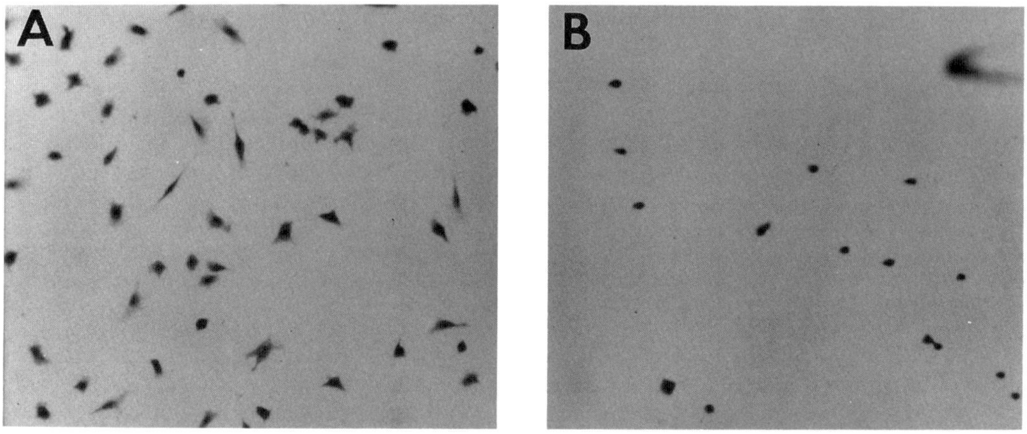

FIGURE 2. Effect of C31 cytotoxin (1:32 dilution) on CHO cells (B) compared with normal CHO cells (A) stained with Giemsa stain.

abolished cytotoxic activity, as did treatment at 70, 80, or 100°C for 30 min.

Treatment of *C. jejuni* filtrates with 0.25% trypsin also destroyed 60 to 70% of the cytotoxic activity, an effect that was completely abolished if the trypsin was previously incubated with trypsin inhibitor. In contrast, treatment of *C. jejuni* C-31 cytotoxin with the protease inhibitor phenylmethylsulfonyl fluoride failed to significantly reduce the cytotoxic activity.

To estimate the size of *C. jejuni* cytotoxin, the crude culture filtrate was placed in SP dialysis tubing (D-16151-1; Scientific Products, McGaw Park, Ill.) with a molecular weight cutoff of 12,000 to 14,000. After dialysis against phosphate-buffered saline for 72 h, the cytotoxic activity was found to be fully retained in the dialysis tubing.

To determine whether *C. jejuni* cytotoxin was immunologically similar to Shiga or *Clostridium difficile* cytotoxins, we incubated 1:4 and 1:8 dilutions of *C. jejuni* C-31 filtrate with Shiga antitoxin at 1:10 or anti-*Clostridium difficile* toxins (A plus B) at 1:25. In contrast to the ability of these antisera to completely neutralize the effects of the respective Shiga or *Clostridium difficile* toxins on HeLa and CHO cells, neither antiserum had any neutralizing effect on the cytotoxicity of *C. jejuni* C-31 on HeLa or CHO cells. Likewise, antiserum prepared by Strockbine et al. (38) against an immunologically distinct Shiga-like toxin II also failed to neutralize *C. jejuni* C-31 cytotoxin, indicating that *C. jejuni* cytotoxin is immunologically distinct from these other recognized cytotoxins.

Finally, to further examine the nature of *C. jejuni* cytotoxin binding to target CHO cells, we studied the effects of the *C. jejuni* culture filtrate in the presence or absence of 12 monosaccharides or disaccharides at 4 g/dl. Only D-galactose, *N*-acetylglucosamine, and *N*-acetylneuraminic acid showed a fourfold or greater inhibition of *C. jejuni* cytotoxicity (Table 5). Minimal or no effects were seen with dextrose, L-fucose, D-mannose, *N*-actylgalactosamine, xylose, sucrose, lactose, and maltose.

To further examine the effects of *C. jejuni* cytotoxin, we removed a 1:16 dilution of toxin after 30 s, 1 min, 10 min, 30 min, or 1 to 10 h. These experiments consistently revealed that the

TABLE 5. Effect of 4 g of carbohydrates per dl on *C. jejuni* C-31 toxicity

Carbohydrate	Mean reciprocal titer[a]
None (control)	64
D-Galactose	113
N-Acetylglucosamine	113
N-Acetylneuraminic acid	16
Dextrose	32
L-Fucose	32
D-Mannose	32
N-Acetylgalactosamine	32
Xylose	64
Sucrose	64
Lactose	64
Maltose	64

[a] The greatest dilution at which ≥50% of CHO cells are killed.

toxin at this marginally effective dose had to remain on these cells for a minimum of 5 to 10 h for the full cytotoxic effect to be seen. Furthermore, the cytotoxic effects were considerably more impressive when the tissue culture cells were plated for 3 h than when the cells were left for longer periods before exposure to the toxin.

CONCLUSIONS

We found that 5 of 12 isolates of *C. jejuni* from patients with invasive, inflammatory enteritis in Charlottesville, Va., produced a cytotoxin that was released by polymyxin or by sonication. This cytotoxin had a cytolethal effect on HeLa, CHO, and colonic carcinoma cells (T84) (data not shown). The *C. jejuni* cytotoxin was heat labile at 70°C or greater, partially trypsin sensitive, and nondialyzable through a membrane with a 12,000 to 14,000 molecular weight cutoff. This finding was supported by results of preliminary ACA 34 column chromatography, which suggested that the cytotoxic fraction was in the 50,000 to 70,000 molecular weight range when kept from aggregation by 0.5 μg of polymyxin per ml (data not shown). Several features distinguish *C. jejuni* cytotoxin from Shiga-like toxins I and II and *Clostridium difficile* cytotoxins. Potent antisera raised against these respective purified cytotoxins, which fully neutralized their respective cytotoxins, had no effect on the *C. jejuni* cytotoxin at dilutions of 1:4 on HeLa cells or at 1:8 to 1:16 on CHO cells. Furthermore, the wider range of cells affected by *C. jejuni* cytotoxin is different from the HeLa cell specificity of Shiga toxin. The striking cytolethal effect of *C. jejuni* cytotoxin seen by trypan blue uptake by affected cells is also different from the cytopathic effect of *Clostridium difficile* cytotoxin (24). A similar, heat-labile, 68-kDa CHO cell cytotoxin from *C. jejuni* has recently been reported by Mahajan and Rogers (28), who have prepared neutralizing monoclonal antibody to the cytotoxin.

Finally, in preliminary attempts to discern the ability of specific carbohydrates to inhibit *C. jejuni* cytotoxicity, only D-galactose, *N*-acetylglucosamine, and *N*-acetylneuraminic acid, at 4 g/dl, significantly inhibited the *C. jejuni* cytotoxin effects (Table 5). Further work is needed to clarify the mechanisms of cytotoxicity and the receptor for this potentially important *C. jejuni* cytotoxin. Although preliminary observations failed to confirm any hemolytic activity with this cytotoxin, in contrast to *Aeromonas* strains, in which hemolysin and cytotoxicity are closely correlated, if not identical (1, 24), several potential mechanisms such as phospholipase activities warrant further exploration.

In summary, certain *C. jejuni* isolates produce a cytolethal, nondialyzable, trypsin- and heat-labile cytotoxin that is immunologically distinct from Shiga and *Clostridium difficile* toxins. The *C. jejuni* cytotoxin may contribute to the inflammatory dysentery produced by *C. jejuni,* but its precise role in the pathogenesis of human disease remains unclear, especially in light of the lack of demonstrable neutralizing antibody associated with natural disease (32). It is clear that the pathogenesis of *C. jejuni* diarrhea, the roles of specific *C. jejuni* enterotoxins and cytotoxins, and the invasiveness traits of the bacteria require further study.

Acknowledgments. This work was supported in part by grants from the Rockefeller Foundation and from the International Development Research Council of Canada. We thank Leah Barrett and Yatta Jacob for technical assistance and for their help in preparing the manuscript.

REFERENCES

1. **Asao, T., Y. Kinoshita, S. Kozaki, T. Uemura, and G. Sakaguchi.** 1984. Purification and some properties of *Aeromonas hydrophila* hemolysin. *Infect. Immun.* **46:**122–127.
2. **Bernard, E., P. M. Roger, D. Carles, V. Bonaldi, J. P. Fournier, and P. Dellamonica.** 1989. Diarrhea and *Campylobacter* infections in patients infected with the human imunodeficiency virus. *J. Infect. Dis.* **159:**143–144.
3. **Blaser, M. J., I. D. Berkowitz, F. M. La Force, J. Cravens, L. B. Reller, and W.-L. L. Wang.** 1979. *Campylobacter* enteritis: clinical and epidemiologic features. *Ann. Intern. Med.* **91:**179–185.
4. **Blaser, M. J., R. I. Glass, M. I. Huq, B. Stoll, G. M. Kibriya, and A. R. M. A. Alim.** 1980. Isolation of *Campylobacter fetus* subsp. *jejuni* from Bangladeshi children. *J. Clin. Microbiol.* **12:**744–747.
5. **Blaser, M. J., J. G. Wells, R. A. Feldman, H. M. Pollock, and J. R. Allen.** 1983. *Campylobacter* enteritis in the United States. *Ann. Intern. Med.* **98:**360–365.
6. **Dean, A. G., Y.-C. Ching, R. G. Williams, and L. B. Harden.** 1972. Test for *Escherichia coli* enterotoxin using infant mice: application in a study of diarrhea in children in Honolulu. *J. Infect. Dis.* **125:**407–411.
7. **Dekeyser, P., M. Gossuin-Detrain, J. P. Butzler, and J. Sternon.** 1972. Acute enteritis due to related *Vibrio:* first positive stool cultures. *J. Infect. Dis.* **125:**390.
8. **Dworkin, B., G. P. Wormser, R. A. Abdoo, F. Cabello, M. E. Aguero, and S. L. Sivak.** 1986. Persistence of multiple antibiotic-resistant *Campylobacter jejuni* in a patient with acquired

immune deficiency syndrome. *Am. J. Med.* **80**:965–970.
9. **Evans, D. G., D. J. Evans, and N. F. Pierce.** 1973. Difference in the response of rabbit small intestine to heat-labile and heat-stable enterotoxins of *Escherichia coli. Infect. Immun.* **7**:873–880.
10. **Glass, R. I., B. J. Stoll, and M. I. Huq.** 1983. Epidemiologic and clinical features of endemic *Campylobacter jejuni* infection in Bangladesh. *J. Infect. Dis.* **148**:292–296.
11. **Guerrant, R. L.** 1985. Microbial toxins and diarrhoeal diseases. *CIBA Found. Symp.* **112**:1–13.
12. **Guerrant, R. L., L. L. Brunton, R. C. Schnaitman, L. I. Rebhun, and A. G. Gilman.** 1974. Cyclic adenosine monophosphate and alteration of Chinese hamster ovary cell morphology: a rapid, sensitive in vitro assay for the entertoxins of *Vibrio cholerae* and *Escherichia coli.* Infect. Immun. **10**:320–327.
13. **Guerrant, R. L., R. G. Lahita, W. C. Winn, Jr., and R. B. Roberts.** 1978. Campylobacteriosis in man: pathogenic mechanisms and review of 91 bloodstream infections. *Am. J. Med.* **65**:584–592.
14. **Guerrant, R. L., C. A. Wanke, R. A. Pennie, L. J. Barrett, A. A. M. Lima, and A. D. O'Brien.** 1987. Production of a unique cytotoxin by *Campylobacter jejuni. Infect. Immun.* **55**:2526–2530.
14a. **Guerrant, R. L., C. A. Wanke, R. A. Pennie, C. J. Barrett, A. A. M. Lima, and A. D. O'Brien.** *Twenty-Second U.S.-Japan Cholera Symposium, 1986*, in press.
15. **Hewlett, E. L., K. T. Sauer, G. A. Myers, J. L. Cowell, and R. L. Guerrant.** 1983. Induction of a novel morphologic response in Chinese hamster ovary cells by pertussis toxin. *Infect. Immun.* **40**:1198–1203.
16. **Hughes, S., G. Warhurst, L. A. Turnberg, N. B. Higgs, L. G. Giugliano, and B. S. Drasar.** 1983. *Clostridium difficile* toxin-induced intestinal secretion in rabbit ileum *in vitro. Gut* **24**:94–98.
17. **Johnson, R. J., C. Nolan, S. P. Wang, W. R. Shelton, and M. J. Blaser.** 1984. Persistent *Campylobacter jejuni* infection in an immunocompromised patient. *Ann. Intern. Med.* **100**:832–834.
18. **Kennedy, D. J., R. N. Greenberg, J. A. Dunn, R. Abernathy, J. S. Ryerse, and R. L. Guerrant.** 1984. Effects of *Escherichia coli* heat-stable enterotoxin STb on intestines of mice, rats, rabbits, and piglets. *Infect. Immun.* **46**:639–643.
19. **Keusch, G. T., and M. Jacewicz.** 1975. The pathogenesis of *Shigella* diarrhea. V. Relationships of Shiga enterotoxin, neurotoxin and cytotoxin. *J. Infect. Dis.* **131**:S33–S39.
20. **King, E. O.** 1957. Human infections with *Vibrio fetus* and a closely related *Vibrio. J. Infect. Dis.* **101**:119.
21. **Libby, J. M., B. S. Jortner, and T. D. Wilkins.** 1982. Effects of the two toxins of *Clostridium difficile* in antibiotic-associated cecitis in hamsters. *Infect. Immun.* **36**:822–829.
22. **Lima, A. A. M., L. J. Barrett, B. J. Freij, J. D. Nelson, M. Conway, and R. L. Guerrant.** 1986. Production of cytotoxin and enterotoxin by *Aeromonas* from young children with diarrhea. *Clin. Res.* **34**:524.
23. **Lima, A. A. M., D. J. Innes, K. Chadee, D. M. Lyerly, T. D. Wilkins, and R. L. Guerrant.** 1989. *Clostridium difficile* toxin A: early sequential histopathologic effects in rabbit small intestine. *Lab. Invest.* **61**:419–425.
24. **Lima, A. A. M., D. M. Lyerly, T. D. Wilkins, D. J. Innes, and R. L. Guerrant.** 1988. Effects of *Clostridium difficile* toxins A and B in rabbit small and large intestine in vivo and on cultured cells in vitro. *Infect. Immun.* **56**:582–588.
25. **Lior, H.** 1984. New, extended biotyping scheme for *Campylobacter jejuni, Campylobacter coli,* and *Campylobacter laridis. J. Clin. Microbiol.* **20**:636–640.
26. **Lior, H., D. L. Woodward, J. A. Edgar, L. J. Laroche, and P. Gill.** 1982. Serotyping of *Campylobacter jejuni* by slide agglutination based on heat-labile antigenic factors. *J. Clin. Microbiol.* **15**:761–768.
27. **Lushbaugh, W. B., A. B. Kairalla, J. R. Cantey, A. F. Hofbaur, and F. E. Pittman.** 1979. Isolation of a cytotoxin-enterotoxin from *Entamoeba histolytica. J. Infect. Dis.* **139**:9–17.
28. **Mahajan, S., and F. G. Rogers.** 1990. Isolation, characterization, and host-cell-binding properties of a cytotoxin from *Campylobacter jejuni. J. Clin. Microbiol.* **28**:1314–1320.
29. **O'Brien, A. D., T. A. Lively, T. W. Chang, and S. L. Gorbach.** 1983. Purification of shigella dysenteriae 1 (shiga)-like toxin from *Escherichia coli* O157:H7 strain associated with haemorrhagic colitis. *Lancet* **i**:573.
30. **Pennie, R. A., R. D. Pearson, L. J. Barrett, and R. L. Guerrant.** 1986. Susceptibility of *Campylobacter jejuni* to strain-specific bactericidal activity in sera of infected patients. *Infect. Immun.* **52**:702–705.
31. **Pennie, R. A., J. N. Zunino, E. Rose, and R. L. Guerrant.** 1984. An economical, simple method for the production of the gaseous environment required for the cultivation of *Campylobacter jejuni. J. Clin. Microbiol.* **20**:320–322.
32. **Perez-Perez, G. L., D. L. Cohn, R. L. Guerrant, C. M. Patton, L. B. Reller, and M. J. Blaser.** 1989. Clinical and immunologic significance of cholera-like toxin and cytotoxin production by *Campylobacter* species in patients with acute inflammatory diarrhea in the USA. *J. Infect. Dis.* **160**:460–467.
33. **Perlman, D. M., N. M. Ampel, R. B. Schifman, D. L. Cohn, C. M. Patton, M. L. Aguirre, L. W.-L. Wang, and M. F. Blaser.** 1988. Persistent *Campylobacter jejuni* infections in patients infected with human immunodeficiency virus (HIV). *Ann. Intern. Med.* **108**:540–546.
34. **Ravdin, J. I., B. Y. Croft, and R. L. Guerrant.** 1980. Cytopathogenic mechanisms of *Entamoeba histolytica. J. Exp. Med.* **152**:377–390.
35. **Ruiz-Palacios, G. M., J. Torres, N. I. Torres, E. Escamilla, B. R. Ruiz-Palacios, and J. Tomayo.** 1983. Cholera-like enterotoxin produced by *Campylobacter jejuni. Lancet* **ii**:250–253.

36. **Sereny, B.** 1955. Experimental shigella keratoconjunctivitis: a preliminary report. *Acta Microbiol. Acad. Sci. Hung.* **2**:293.
37. **Stoll, B. J., R. I. Glass, H. Banu, M. I. Huq, M. U. Khan, and M. Ahmed.** 1983. Value of stool examination in patients with diarrhoea. *Br. Med. J.* **286**:2037–2040.
38. **Strockbine, N. A., L. R. M. Marques, J. W. Newland, H. W. Smith, R. K. Holmes, and A. D. O'Brien.** 1986. Two toxin-converting phages from *Escherichia coli* O157:H7 strain 933 encode antigenically distinct toxins with similar biologic activities. *Infect. Immun.* **53**:135–140.
39. **Thorson, S. M., J. A. Lohr, S. Dudley, and R. L. Guerrant.** 1985. Value of methylene blue examination, dark-field microscopy, and carbol-fuchsin Gram stain in the detection of *Campylobacter* enteritis. *J. Pediatr.* **106**:941–943.
40. **Weikel, C. S., H. N. Nellans, and R. L. Guerrant.** 1986. The *in vivo* and *in vitro* effects of a novel enterotoxin, STb, produced by *Escherichia coli*. *J. Infect. Dis.* **153**:893–901.
41. **Weikel, C. S., J. J. Sando, and R. L. Guerrant.** 1985. Stimulation of porcine jejunal ion secretion *in vivo* by protein kinase-C activators. *J. Clin. Invest.* **76**:2430–2435.

CHAPTER 18

In Vitro Study of Virulence Factors of Enteric *Campylobacter* spp.

J.-L. FAUCHÈRE, M. KERVELLA, A. ROSENAU, J. M. PAGÈS, AND C. FENDRI

INTRODUCTION

Campylobacter jejuni and the other thermophilic *Campylobacter* species are frequent enteric pathogens, which cause diarrhea or enteritis in all parts of the world. Isolation and diagnosis of these organisms by conventional microbiological methods are now routinely performed in most laboratories. However, the pathophysiology of *Campylobacter* infections is still poorly understood, and this has confounded the prevention and treatment of campylobacteriosis. The clinical polymorphism of *Campylobacter* enteritis may be partly due to differences in virulence properties from strain to strain, and it would be of interest to be able to identify virulence markers easily. Treatment and prevention of *Campylobacter* enteritis should be monitored more efficiently and logically with a better knowledge of virulence properties. Moreover, the identification of the bacterial components associated with the virulence properties could lead to both new diagnostic and new prophylactic approaches.

Clinical signs, experimental infections, and epidemiologic studies suggest that differences in the expression of pathogenicity of *Campylobacter* species result from a combination of different bacterial properties and host responses. *Campylobacter* species are often associated with fever and bloody diarrhea, characteristic of an invasive organism; occasionally, they are associated with watery diarrhea, consistent with an enterotoxin-producing organism; and sometimes they have been found in healthy carriers (7). In animal models, *C. jejuni* selectively associates with M cells of Peyer's patches (17) and has also been observed closely associated with or internalized in enterocytes (6, 8, 14). In addition, *Campylobacter* species may be well adapted to the mucus environment of the intestinal crypts (12). Finally, one of the least understood aspects of *Campylobacter* virulence is the nature of interactions of these organisms or their products with intestinal cells.

In the past 10 years, several in vitro models have been developed to study the pathogenicity of *C. jejuni* (16). A prerequisite for the relevance of these models should be their correlation with the expression of pathogenicity in humans. In the last several years, we developed models studying the interaction between *C. jejuni* and epithelial cell lines (5). We defined different pathovars on the basis of in vitro putative virulence properties, correlated these pathovars with expression of virulence in humans (7), and then identified the bacterial components involved in those bacterial properties (4).

INTERACTION BETWEEN *CAMPYLOBACTER* CELLS OR PRODUCTS AND DIFFERENT CELL LINES

Campylobacter cells may colonize the intestinal mucus, but stable colonization of the intestinal tract implies a close association between bacteria and intestinal cells. Cell-associated bacteria may adhere to intestinal cells, and they may also invade these cells with or without conse-

J.-L. Fauchère, Microbiologie A, CHRU, 86021 Poitiers, France. **M. Kervella,** Laboratoire de Bactériologie, CHU Necker-Enfants Malades, 75730 Paris Cédex, France. **A. Rosenau,** Faculté des Sciences, Université de Tours, 37200 Tours, France. **J. M. Pagès,** Centre National de la Recherche Scientifique, Marseilles, France. **C. Fendri,** Hôpital Charles Nicolle, Tunis, Tunisia.

quences for the host cells. Models of interactions between *C. jejuni* and epithelial cell lines are often used to study these phenomena.

Definition of Different *Campylobacter* Pathovars

The strains used in this study were collected either in the Paris metropolitan area or in Tunisia from patients whose clinical status was well characterized on the basis of nonsubjective clinical signs, i.e., fever (temperature ⩾38°C), diarrhea (watery or unformed stools), and/or macroscopic or microscopic blood in feces. On the basis of these symptoms, we defined three groups of patients: (i) nonfebrile nondiarrheic, (ii) nonfebrile diarrheic, and (iii) febrile diarrheic with blood in feces. These patients were aged from 1 month to 30 years (median, 3 years).

We developed an in vitro assay for association of *Campylobacter* organisms with cultivated cells (5). In this assay, bacterial cells are suspended in minimal essential medium and are incubated with a HeLa cell monolayer (10^3 to 10^4 bacteria per cell) for 1 h at 37°C to allow bacterial adhesion. The cell monolayer is then washed and reincubated for 3 h to allow bacterial invasion. After washing, the target cells are fixed and the cell-associated bacteria are revealed either by Giemsa staining or by immunodetection with a rabbit anti-*Campylobacter* serum. A *Campylobacter* strain is considered associative or nonassociative on the basis of the presence or absence of cell-associated bacteria; this is quantified by determining the mean number of bacteria attached per HeLa cell (association index). The 49 studied strains appeared to cluster into two groups. The first group included 25 (51%) nonassociative strains (phenotype a) with a low association index (range, 0 to 2; mean ± standard deviation [SD], 0.5 ± 0.3), and the second group included 24 (49%) associative strains (phenotype A) showing a high association index (range, 3.5 to 8.3; mean ± SD, 4.9 ± 1.9). These results support the existence of two different *Campylobacter* phenotypes (a and A) in relation to in vitro association with epithelial cells.

The culture supernatants from the same strains were tested for elongation of Chinese hamster ovary cells (CHO) by previously described methods (1, 9). The ability to elongate CHO (E phenotype) has been associated with the release of a heat-labile choleralike toxin (15). Of the supernatants from the 49 strains, 25 (43%) elongated the CHO cells at a 1:128 dilution (E phenotype) whereas the supernatants from the 28 (57%) other strains did not elongate CHO at any dilution tested (e phenotype) (7).

Using the presence of these two markers (A and E), which are expressed independently in individual strains, we defined four *Campylobacter* pathovars: pathovars AE (associative elongating strains), Ae (associative nonelongating strains), aE (nonassociative elongating strains) and ae (nonassociative nonelongating strains). The relationship between the pathovar and the clinical presentation of enteritis is shown in Table 1. Of the 11 nondiarrheic, nonfebrile patients, 10 (91%) carried a strain of the ae phenotype, whereas of the 38 diarrheic patients, only 7 (18%) carried this phenotype ($P = 4 \times 10^{-5}$). In addition, of the 29 febrile patients, 21 (72%) carried a strain with the A marker, whereas among the 20 nonfebrile patients, only 3 (15%) carried a strain with this marker ($P = 0.05$). Thus, the ae phenotype was associated with asymptomatic infection. The A marker was associated with febrile diarrhea. The E marker was not related to a particular symptomatic expression (7).

We further focused our studies on the associative properties of *Campylobacter* strains.

Relationship between Associative *Campylobacter* spp. and the Host Cell

Similar to other enteropathogens, associative and nonassociative *Campylobacter* strains may have different types of relationship with host enterocytes. Associative bacteria may adhere to the host cell membrane, and they may also invade this cell with or without consequences for the host cell. It has been demonstrated that associative *Campylobacter* strains

TABLE 1. Prevalence of enteric *Campylobacter* pathovars in different categories of patients

Clinical presentation	Total no.	Prevalence of pathovar: AE	Ae	aE	ae
Diarrhea and fever	29	11 (38.0%)	10 (34.5%)	3 (10.3%)	5 (17.2%)
Diarrhea, no fever	9	2 (22.2%)	1 (11.1%)	4 (44.5%)	2 (22.2%)
No diarrhea, no fever	11	0 (0.0%)	0 (0.0%)	1 (9.0%)	10 (91.0%)

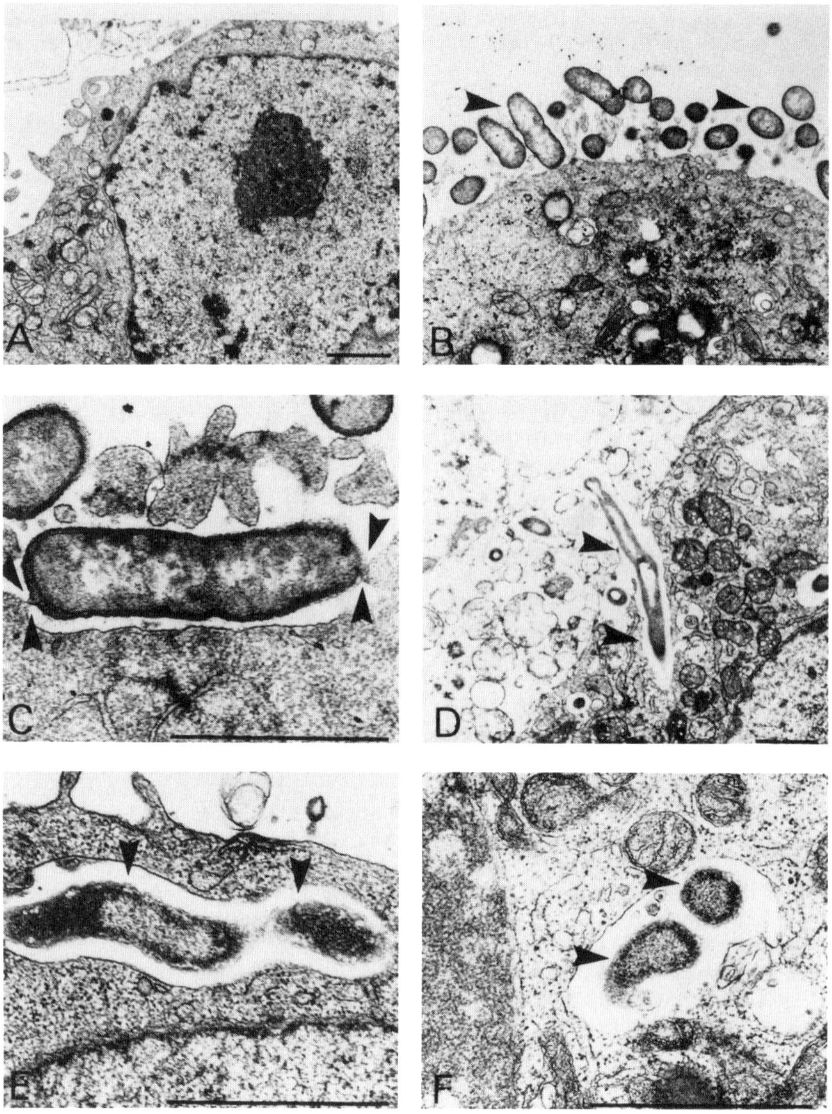

FIGURE 1. Electron micrographs of HeLa cells inoculated with *Campylobacter* cells (from reference 5). (A) Nonassociative strain. (B to F) Associative strain. Multiple bacteria (arrows) in various stages of internalization. Panels B and C show adhesion to the HeLa cell membrane; panel D shows internalization of bacteria; panels E and F show bacteria in phagosomes. Bars, 1 μm.

associate with various cell lines including HeLa, INT 407, and HEp-2 (16). Moreover, the use of an in vitro enterocyte-differentiated cell line, CaCo-2, permits expression of the same associative properties (13). To assess the invasive capacity of 20 associative strains, we enumerated total associated bacteria and intracellular bacteria after killing extracellular bacteria by suitable treatment of infected HeLa cells with gentamicin (5). The percentages of intracellular viable bacteria ranged from 18 to 80% (mean ± SD, 46% ± 26%). In contrast, the same assay performed with nonassociative strains showed percentages of internalized bacteria ranging from 0 to 5% (mean ± SD, 0.97% ± 2%). Transmission electron microscopy of HeLa cells infected with associative strains showed bacteria either in close association with the cell membrane or internalized inside cytoplasmic vacuoles (Fig. 1). Cytochalasin B, which inhibits particle engulfment by both professional and nonprofessional phagocytic cells, inhibited the association of *Campylobacter* spp. with HeLa cells. Likewise, dinitrophenol, which is well known to deprive cells of energy, inhibited the association of *Campylobacter* spp. with those cells (13). When we monitored the number of intracellular viable *Campylobacter* cells over time, we observed a regular decrease in the number of viable internalized bacteria, and after 24 h no viable bacteria were detected in the host cells. From these data, it can be concluded that associative strains of *C. jejuni* adhere mostly to epithelial cells in vitro; adhering bacteria can be internalized by a phagocytosislike mechanism, but the internalized bacteria do not grow in the host cells, which seem not to be profoundly damaged. We therefore decided to study the adherence phenomenon in more detail.

BACTERIAL COMPONENTS INVOLVED IN *CAMPYLOBACTER* ADHERENCE TO EPITHELIAL CELLS

Attachment of OMP to HeLa Cell Membranes

Bacterial adhesion to the cellular membrane may involve surface-exposed bacterial structures. Consequently, we investigated the components of the entire bacterial outer membrane (OM) for attachment to HeLa cell membranes (4). Bacterial OMs were prepared by the sodium lauryl sarcosinate method (4). By this method, OM proteins (OMPs) incorporated in microvesicles are structurally similar to OMs and retain their native configuration. After the Sarkosyl had been removed, a standard quantity of OMP preparations was incubated for 2 h at 37°C with HeLa cell monolayers. After the mixture was washed, the bulk of HeLa cells bearing OM vesicles were removed by using sodium dodecyl sulfate (SDS), separated by SDS-polyacrylamide gel electrophoresis (PAGE), and immunoblotted by using an anti-whole-bacterial-cell rabbit antiserum that had been previously absorbed on HeLa cells and shown to recognize only *Campylobacter* antigens. Under these conditions, the OM-like microvesicles bearing sufficient quantities of a hypothetical adhesin for binding to the HeLa cells can be resolved by immunoblot, along with small amounts of various OMPs which were originally aggregated with the adhesin in the same vesicles. The results of studies of two strains are presented in Fig. 2. The antigens resolved were detected with the two homologous sera adjusted to the same titer. Lanes a show the OM antigenic profiles of each strain, and lanes b through e show the adhering antigens detected in twofold serial dilutions of the lysate of HeLa cells bearing adherent bacterial components. For strain 85H, two antigenic fractions (of 27 and 29 kDa) bound selectively to HeLa cells; other antigens including flagellin (FLA; 66 kDa) and the major OMP (43 kDa) did not bind. Spectrodensitometric recording of lanes a and b permitted calculation of the adhering proportion of each antigen. Normalization of the data in this way allows the results to be independent of the antigenicity of the different antigens. For strain 85H, which is adherent, P29 and P27 are 3.5 times more adherent than the major OMP and 28 times more adherent than FLA. For strain 79AH, which is nonadherent, each fraction adhered to HeLa cell membranes poorly and to the same degree. These results have been confirmed with four other adhering strains (4), and similar results have been obtained by other authors (2, 11). The OMPs between 26 and 30 kDa, which preferentially adhere to HeLa cells, have been designated as the cell-binding fractions (CBF).

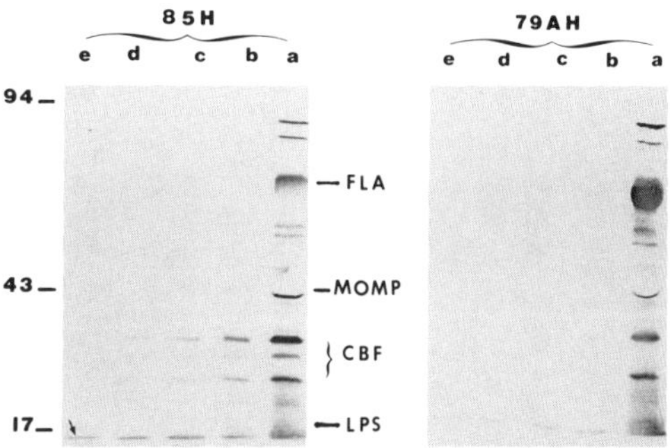

FIGURE 2. Adherence of OM fractions from two *Campylobacter* strains to HeLa cell monolayers. Lanes a show antigenic profiles of OM extracts; lanes b through e show antigenic profiles of twofold dilutions (from 1:1 [lanes b] to 1:8 [lanes e]) of the lysate of the HeLa cell monolayer bearing bacterial adhering components. SDS-PAGE was performed in 11% acrylamide gels. The immunoblot was resolved with homologous anti-whole-bacterial-cell sera previously absorbed on HeLa cells and found to recognize only *Campylobacter* antigens. Strain 85H, which has a high association index, was isolated from a febrile patient with bloody diarrhea. Strain 79AH, which has a low association index, was isolated from an asymptomatic patient. The arrow indicates the front of migration (pink dye). Abbreviations: MOMP, major OMP; LPS, lipopolysaccharide.

Evidence that CBF Are Involved In *Campylobacter* Adherence to Epithelial Cells

Rabbit antisera were raised against 26- to 30-kDa OMPs (anti-CBF) and against a 92-kDa OMP which does not adhere to HeLa cells. The antigens were obtained by preparative SDS-PAGE. The anti-CBF antisera reduced the adhesion of strain 85H to HeLa cells (100% inhibition when diluted 1/10, 80% inhibition when diluted 1/100, 60% inhibition when diluted 1/1,000, and 20% inhibition when diluted 1/10,000). In contrast, the anti-92 rabbit serum and a nonimmune rabbit serum did not inhibit *Campylobacter* adherence at any dilution. Likewise, a serum sample obtained from a patient early in infection did not inhibit adherence of the infecting strain, whereas a serum sample obtained 3 weeks later showed a strong antibody response against CBF and led to a dose-related adherence inhibition. Serum diluted 1/10 showed 100% inhibition; even at dilution of 1/10,000, there was 10% inhibition.

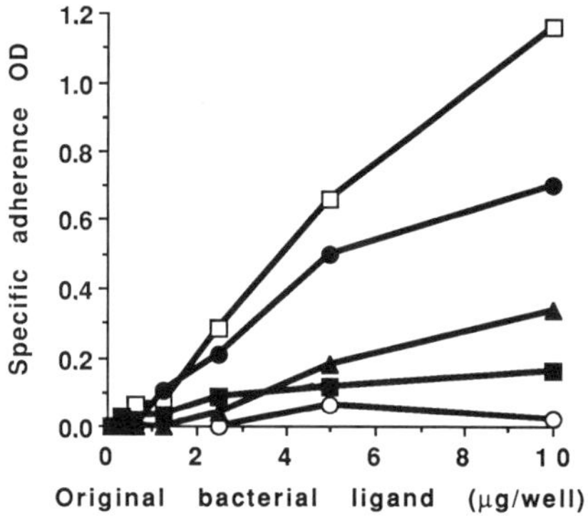

FIGURE 4. Adherence of purified OMPs from *Campylobacter* strain 85H compared with adherence of glycine extracts. A HeLa cell-membrane-enriched preparation was immobilized on a microtiter plate (10 μg per well) and incubated with various quantities of bacterial preparations. After washing, bacterial adhering material was revealed by an ELISA with an anti-whole-bacterial-cell serum. OD, optical density. Symbols: □, glycine extract from adherent strain; ○, glycine extract from nonadherent strain; ▲, purified FLA; ■, purified P29; ●, purified P27.

Purification of CBF

P27 and P29 were obtained from a glycine extract of strain 85H by subsequent preparative SDS-PAGE (12% acrylamide). The two fractions were electroeluted from the gel and electrodialyzed against Tris-glycine buffer (pH 8.3) to remove the SDS. We obtained about 200 μg of P27 and 500 μg of P29. As a control, we also gel purified the FLA. The purity of these three preparations was tested by SDS-PAGE (11% acrylamide), and bands resolved by silver stain (Fig. 3) show that each preparation contained only a single band at the expected position.

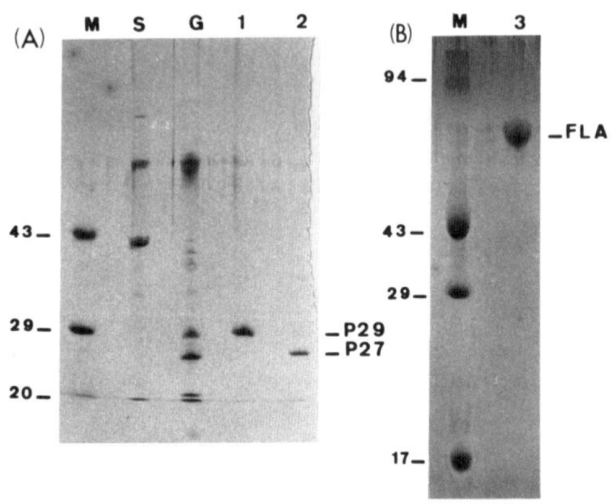

FIGURE 3. SDS-PAGE of purified OMPs from *Campylobacter* strain 85H. SDS-PAGE was performed with 11% acrylamide gels, double stained with Coomassie blue and silver. (A) Lanes: M, molecular weight standards (in thousands); S, Sarkosyl-extracted OMPs; G, glycine extract; 1 and 2, P29 and P27, respectively, purified from the glycine extract. (B) Lanes: M, molecular weight standards; 3, FLA purified from glycine extract.

Adherence of Purified CBF to HeLa Cell Membranes

The method of purification we used yielded small quantities of bacterial protein resolved in the presence of SDS and thus expected to contain a single subunit. However, this method could lead to partial or total denaturation of OMPs and to loss of adhering properties.

Using an adherence microassay previously described (3), we studied the adherence of P29, P27, and FLA to a HeLa cell membrane-enriched preparation immobilized on a microtiter plate. By this method, bacterial adhering material can be detected by an enzyme-linked immunosorbent assay (ELISA) with either anti-whole-bacterial-cell serum or monospecific sera; as such, the adherence of a particular bacterial component can be quantitatively studied. In addition, by this method the nonadherent material can be removed from the epithelial-cell membranes by washing in the presence of detergent (Tween 20). By this procedure, the bacterial material adhering nonspecifically or linked to the true adhesin by hydrophobic interactions can be removed and the remaining adherent material may be considered to be strongly and specifically fixed on the host cell membranes. Figure 4 shows the adherence of purified P29, P27, FLA, and total OMP (glycine extract) from strain 85H, compared with adherence of the total glycine extract from a nonassociative strain (79AH), detected with homologous anti-whole-bacterial-cell sera. The glycine extract from strain 79AH showed a low adherence, whereas the glycine extract from strain 85H exhibited a strong adherence. Of the purified proteins, FLA and P29 adhered poorly while P27 exhibited similar adherence properties to those of the glycine extract from strain 85H. Similarly, when we detected the adhering material of the glycine extract from strain 85H with anti-P29, anti-P27, and anti-FLA monospecific sera, we found that P29 and FLA in their native configurations adhered poorly whereas P27 adhered strongly (Fig. 5). Thus, P27 seems to be the most strongly adherent protein among these three preparations. The use of rabbit antisera raised against these two purified antigens confirmed these results since anti-P27 inhibited adherence of strain 85H whereas anti-P29 did not. The P29 OMP coadheres with the P27 adhesin and thus probably associates with it in the native adhering material.

OMP Profiles of Adhering and Nonadhering *C. jejuni* Strains

The OMP profiles of associative and nonassociative strains were indistinguishable under the usual experimental conditions of SDS-PAGE. In an attempt to distinguish OMPs from these two types of strains, we performed an electrophoretic separation under strong denaturing conditions by using SDS-PAGE with 3% SDS and 7 M urea included in a 11% acrylamide gel. The gels were immunoblotted to sera raised against antigens from the 85H adherent strain or from both OMP C and OMP F of *Escherichia coli* (10). When we revealed the blots with anti-CBF serum, the results showed that the major OMP from an adherent *Campylobacter* strain migrates like OMP C from *E. coli* and shares common epitopes (anti-CBF recognized OMP C from *E. coli* [Fig. 6A, lanes 1 and 3]). Major OMP from a nonadherent *Campylobacter* strain migrates like OMP F from *E. coli* (Fig. 6A, lanes 2 and 4; Fig. 6B, lane 4). Likewise, anti-OMP C/OMP F from *E. coli* recognized major OMP from the adherent strain, 85H (Fig. 6B, lane 1). When we revealed the blots with monospecific anti-P27 and anti-P29 antisera, the results showed different antigenic patterns for adherent and nonadherent strains (Fig. 7). For four adhering strains, P29 and P27 antigens displayed bands at levels which were similar from strain to strain. On the other hand, for four nonadherent strains, P29 and P27 antigens migrated at a different level and exhibited a different pattern, with bands in a "mustache" shape.

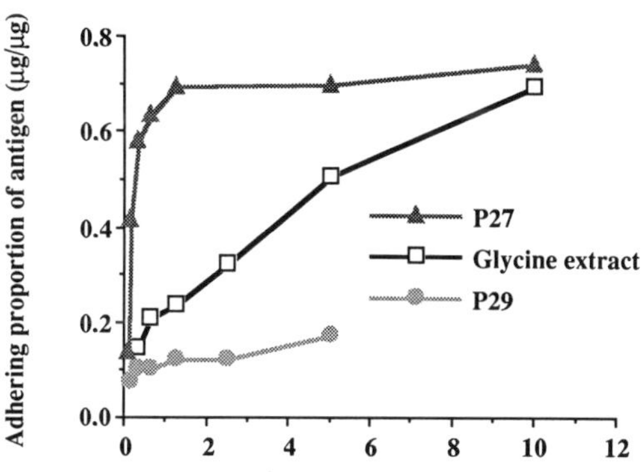

FIGURE 5. Adherence of glycine extract from strain 85H detected with monospecific sera. Adhering material of a crude glycine extract from strain 85H was detected by either (□) anti-whole-bacterial-cell serum or (▲) anti-P27 or (●) anti-P29 monospecific sera. The adhering proportion of each antigen was calculated by using the adherence ELISA previously described (3).

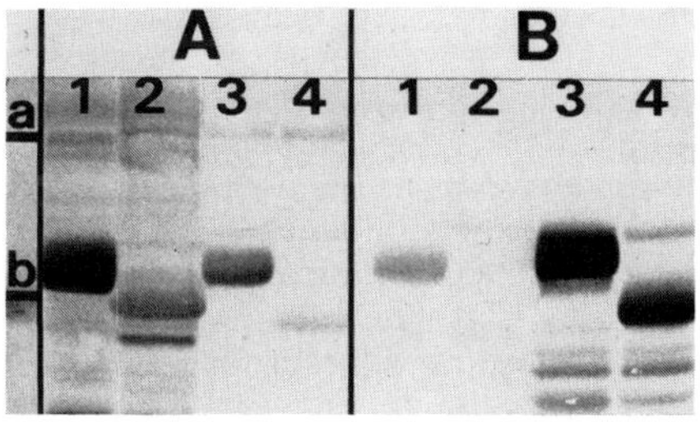

FIGURE 6. Electrophoretic migration of major OMP from two *Campylobacter* strains in SDS-PAGE (11% acrylamide, 7 M urea, 3% SDS). (A) Immunoblot revealed with *Campylobacter* anti-CBF. Lanes: 1, bacterial extract from *Campylobacter* strain 85H; 2, bacterial extract from *Campylobacter* strain 79AH; 3, bacterial extract from *E. coli* exhibiting OMP C only; 4, bacterial extract from *E. coli* exhibiting OMP F only. (B) Immunoblot revealed with a rabbit serum raised against OMP C and OMP F of *E. coli*. Lanes: 1, bacterial extract from *Campylobacter* strain 85H; 2, extract from *Campylobacter* strain 79AH; 3, extract from *E. coli* exhibiting OMP C only; 4, extract from *E. coli* exhibiting OMP F only.

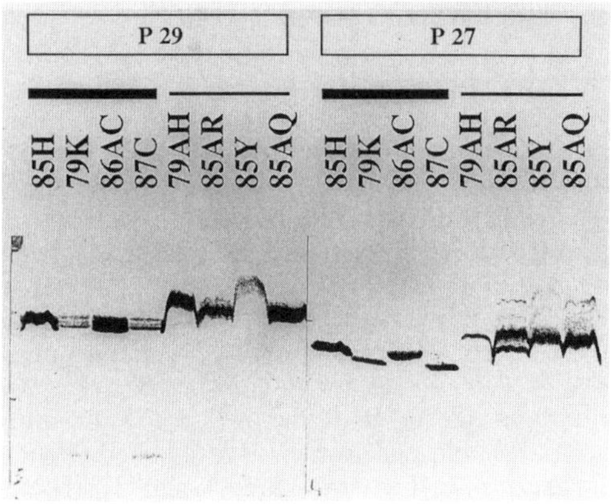

FIGURE 7. Western immunoblot of whole bacterial antigens revealed with monospecific anti-P29 and anti-P27 sera. Whole-cell antigens were separated on an 11% acrylamide–3% SDS–7 M urea gel and immunoblotted to anti-P27 (P27) or anti-P29 (P29) sera. The antigens were from four adherent and pathogenic strains (85H, 79K, 86G, and 87C [bold top line]), or from four nonadherent and nonpathogenic strains (79AH, 85R, 85G and 85Q [light top line]).

CONCLUSIONS

Pathogenic strains of enteric *Campylobacter* species adhere to epithelial cells. This property is related to an OMP of 27 kDa which preferentially binds to the host cell membrane. The nature of the cellular receptor of this bacterial ligand is still unknown, but it would be of interest to know whether it is present on human enterocytes. A 29-kDa antigen coadheres with P27. P27 and P29 are also present in nonadherent nonpathogenic strains, but they are nonadherent and migrate differently in SDS-PAGE under strong denaturing conditions. It may be hypothesized that the structures of the P27 and P29 *Campylobacter* adhesins are partially conserved among all strains and are partially specific for the adhesion function. Further work is needed to identify the specific domains required for adhesion. In any case, the associative phenotype is related to pathogenicity and may represent an important virulence marker. The major OMPs are different in adherent and nonadherent strains. The major OMP from an adherent strain exhibits the same motility and shares common epitopes with *E. coli* OMP C, whereas the major OMP from a nonadherent strain resembles *E. coli* OMP F. Studies are under way to determine the structures of these different *Campylobacter* OMPs.

ACKNOWLEDGMENTS. The studies described in this chapter were supported by grants from University Paris V, INSERM, Philippe, and IPSEN Foundations. We thank M. Veron for advice and M. J. Blaser for reviewing the manuscript.

REFERENCES

1. **Caprioli, A., V. Falbo, L. G. Roda, F. M. Ruggeri, and C. Zona.** 1983. Partial purification and characterization of an *Escherichia coli* toxic factor that induces morphological cell alterations. *Infect. Immun.* **39:**1300–1306.
2. **De Melo, M. A., G. Gabbiani, and J. C. Pechere.** 1989. Cellular events and intracellular survival of *Campylobacter jejuni* during infection of HEp-2 cells. *Infect. Immun.* **57:**2214–2222.
3. **Fauchère, J. L., and M. J. Blaser.** 1990. Adherence of Helicobacter pylori cells and superficial components to HeLa cell membranes. *Microb. Pathog.* **9:**427–439.
4. **Fauchère, J. L., M. Kervella, A. Rosenau, K. Mohanna, and M. Veron.** 1989. Adhesion to HeLa cells of Campylobacter jejuni and C. coli outer membrane components. *Res. Microbiol.* **140:**379–392.
5. **Fauchère, J. L., A. Rosenau, M. Veron, E. N. Moyen, S. Richard, and A. Pfister.** 1986. Association with HeLa cells of *Campylobacter jejuni* and *C. coli* isolated from human feces. *Infect. Immun.* **54:**283–287.
6. **Fauchère, J. L., M. Veron, A. Lellouch-Tubiana, and A. Pfister.** 1985. Experimental infection of gnotobiotic mice with Campylobacter jejuni: colonisation of intestine and spread to lymphoid and reticulo-endothelial organs. *J. Med. Microbiol.* **20:**215–224.
7. **Fendri, C., A. Rosenau, E. N. Moyen, and J. L. Fauchère.** 1991. Prevalence of virulence markers of enteric Campylobacter in France and Tunisia. *Res. Microbiol.* **142:**591–596.
8. **Field, L. H., J. L. Underwood, L. M. Pope, and L. J. Berry.** 1981. Intestinal colonization of neonatal animals by *Campylobacter fetus* subsp. *jejuni. Infect. Immun.* **33:**884–892.
9. **Johnson, W. M., and H. Lior.** 1984. Toxins produced by Campylobacter jejuni and C. coli. *Lancet* **i:**229–230.
10. **Kawaiji, H., T. Mizuno, and S. Mizushima.** 1979. Influence of molecular size and osmolarity of sugars and dextrans on the synthesis of outer membrane proteins O-8 and O-9 of *Escherichia coli* K-12. *J. Bacteriol.* **140:**843–847.
11. **Konkel, M. E., and L. A. Joens.** 1989. Adhesion to and invasion of HEp-2 cells by *Campylobacter* spp. *Infect. Immun.* **57:**2984–2990.
12. **Lee, A., J. L. O'Rourke, P. J. Barrington, and T. J. Trust.** 1986. Mucus colonization as a determinant of pathogenicity in intestinal infection by *Campylobacter jejuni:* a mouse cecal model. *Infect. Immun.* **51:**536–546.
13. **Rosenau, A., J. L. Fauchère, E. N. Moyen, A.**

Pouchelet, and S. Richard. 1987. Cellular factors influencing the association of Campylobacter jejuni with epithelial cells. Bacteriologic, cytologic and microcinematographic studies, p. 207. *In* B. Kaijser and E. Falsen (ed.), *Campylobacter IV.* University of Göteborg, Göteborg, Sweden.

14. **Ruiz-Palacios, G. M., E. Escamilla, and N. Torres.** 1981. Experimental *Campylobacter* diarrhea in chickens. *Infect. Immun.* **34:**250–255.
15. **Ruiz-Palacios, G. M., J. Torres, N. I. Torres, E. Escamilla, B. R. Ruiz-Palacios, and J. Tamayo.** 1983. Cholera like enterotoxin produced by C. jejuni. *Lancet* i:250–253.
16. **Walker, R. I., M. B. Caldwell, E. C. Lee, P. Guerry, T. J. Trust, and G. M. Ruiz-Palacios.** 1986. Pathophysiology of *Campylobacter* enteritis. *Microbiol. Rev.* **50:**81–94.
17. **Walker, R. I., E. A. Schmauder-Chock, J. L. Parker, and D. Burr.** 1988. Selective association and transport of Campylobacter jejuni through M cells of rabbit Peyer's patches. *Can. J. Microbiol.* **34:**1143–1147.

CHAPTER 19

In Vitro Models for Studying *Campylobacter* Infections

GUILLERMO M. RUIZ-PALACIOS, LUZ ELENA CERVANTES, DAVID S. NEWBURG, YOLANDA LOPEZ-VIDAL, AND JUAN J. CALVA

INTRODUCTION

The mechanisms by which *Campylobacter* species induce disease are not well understood. On the basis of the clinical presentation of inflammatory diarrhea (1, 7, 14, 34) or sepsis (17) described in patients seen in a hospital setting, it was initially thought that the illnesses produced and the mechanisms involved were those of an invasive pathogen such as *Shigella* species or possibly *Yersinia* and *Salmonella* species. It was not realized until later, when studies were done in developing countries and in the community (4, 16), that most *Campylobacter* infections were associated with loose stools or watery diarrhea, whereas only one-fifth presented with bloody diarrhea with fecal leukocytes. In vitro studies have demonstrated the ability of *Campylobacter* organisms to invade eukaryotic cells (12, 15, 28) and to produce a cytotoxin (18, 24) and an enterotoxin that increases intracellular cyclic AMP levels and cross-reacts with cholera toxin (11, 20, 32). Although this assortment of putative virulence factors has been found by several investigators, there is insufficient evidence to support a clinical significance in the pathogenesis of diarrhea.

It has been demonstrated that symptomatic *Campylobacter* infections occurring early in life protect against subsequent infections (4) and that this immunity is age related (2). On the other hand, it has been shown that human milk has a protective effect against *Campylobacter* diarrhea (30) and that antibodies present in milk play an important role in protection. Nevertheless, it is possible that nonimmunoglobulin factors in the milk contribute to this protective effect, as has been demonstrated for other pathogens (10, 27).

From previous longitudinal studies of *Campylobacter* infections carried out by our group with cohorts of children under 5 years of age (4), we have obtained isolates from patients with inflammatory and noninflammatory diarrhea and from asymptomatic patients. In these studies, in vitro assays to detect *Campylobacter* adherence, invasion, and toxin production were developed to investigate the clinical importance of these putative virulence factors in well-characterized *Campylobacter* isolates and to characterize receptor analogs present in human milk that interact with the pathogen.

CORRELATION BETWEEN CLINICAL PARAMETERS AND IN VITRO ASSAYS OF VIRULENCE

To study clinical correlation with in vitro assay results, we used *Campylobacter* isolates from stools of children under 5 years of age participating in a cohort study to determine the incidence of asymptomatic infection and illness-to-infection ratio in the community (4). A total of 90 isolates were studied; 39 were obtained from symptom-free children who had not had diarrhea in the previous month or within 7 days of isolation, 10 were obtained from children with inflammatory diarrhea, and 41 were obtained from children with noninflammatory diarrhea. Enterotoxin was detected in culture supernatants of *Campylobacter* species grown in 25 ml of Trypticase broth plus 1% IsoVitaleX, 1 g of starch per liter, and 1 g of potassium monophosphate per liter for 24 h at 42°C in a mi-

Guillermo M. Ruiz-Palacios, Luz Elena Cervantes, Yolanda Lopez-Vidal, and Juan J. Calva, Department of Infectious Diseases, National Institute of Nutrition, Mexico City 14000 D. F., Mexico. **David S. Newburg,** Department of Biochemistry, E. K. Shriver Center for Mental Retardation, Waltham, Massachusetts 02154.

croaerophilic atmosphere. Polymyxin B (1 mg/ml) was added for an additional 1 h, and the mixture was centrifuged at 20,000 × *g* for 20 min at 4°C. Supernatants for enterotoxin were filter sterilized and stored at −70°C until tested. A monoclonal antibody GM_1 enzyme-linked immunosorbent assay (ELISA) for detection of choleralike enterotoxin was performed as previously described (23). Cytotoxin was produced by the method of Guerrant et al. (18). To assess cell-associated bacteria, the method of HEp-2 cell monolayer culture in slides, reported by Cravioto et al. for enteropathogenic *Escherichia coli* (9), was used with some modifications (5). Slides were stained by the Warthin-Starry method (19) and examined under oil immersion by light microscopy. Results were expressed as the percentage of cells with associated *Campylobacter* organisms. To assess cell invasion, a method involving HEp-2 cells grown to confluence on Sephadex beads (Cytodex-II beads; Pharmacia Fine Chemicals, Uppsala, Sweden) was developed (5, 22) in which *Campylobacter* isolates radiolabeled with [^{3}H]alanine and [^{3}H]leucine were used. The results of this assay were presented as an invasiveness index.

To study nonimmunoglobulin milk factors in the role of protection, oligosaccharide fractions were obtained from pooled human milk as previously described (30). All fractions were tested for their ability to inhibit association of campylobacters with HEp-2 cells. Three *Campylobacter jejuni* strains, one invasive (INN-383IP), one adherent (INN-10SP), and one nonpathogenic (INN-57SP), were used to assess cell association (5). Briefly, 100 μl of a suspension of 9 × 10^8 bacteria of each of the strains, previously incubated with the test milk fractions, was added to monolayers of HEp-2 cells in an eight-chamber tissue culture slide. Slides were incubated at 37°C for 5 h, and cells were washed and stained with Warthin-Starry stain. Assays were done in triplicate, and results were given as mean ± standard deviation. Results were expressed as percent inhibition of *Campylobacter* association with cells, as compared with a positive control to which no milk fractions were added. Inhibition by milk fractions was considered significant when at least a 20% reduction from control values was observed. Differences between medians were tested by using the nonparametric Mann-Whitney U test (8). The association between each of the virulence markers (independent variables) and the likelihood of having secretory or inflammatory diarrhea (dependent variable) was assessed by estimating the odds ratio, the 95% confidence interval, and the *P* value through a univariate logistic regression analysis (33). Cal-

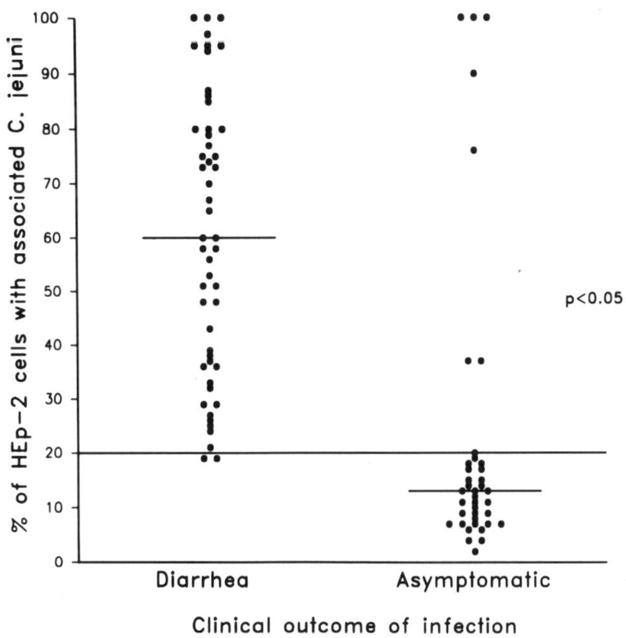

FIGURE 1. Association of HEp-2 cells and *Campylobacter* isolates obtained from children with diarrhea and asymptomatic children.

culations were made with the EGRET statistical program (PECAN analysis module, Version 0.22.10, 1987; SERC).

Cell Association and Invasiveness

There was a strong association between the type of isolate and clinical outcome. By the chamber slide assay for cell association, the median percentage of HEp-2 cells with associated bacteria was 60% for isolates from diarrhea cases, compared with 13% for isolates from asymptomatic children ($P < 0.05$) (Fig. 1). The median percentage of cells with associated bacteria was 79% for isolates from inflammatory diarrhea cases, compared with 56% for isolates from noninflammatory diarrhea cases ($P < 0.05$). The median of the invasiveness index of *Campylobacter* isolates as determined by the Sepharose bead assay was significantly different among isolates from patients with inflammatory and noninflammatory diarrhea and asymptomatic patients (78, 55, and 43, respectively; $P < 0.05$) (Fig. 2).

When results of the chamber slide and Sepharose bead assays were combined for analysis, strains could be grouped into three types: (i) nonadherent (strains that had <20% of cells with associated bacteria and with an invasiveness index of <60%), (ii) adherent (strains with >20% cell association and an invasiveness index of <60%), and (iii) invasive (strains with >20% cell association and an invasiveness index of >60%). According to this classification, a strong association was observed between the type of isolate and the clinical presentation. Sixty-eight percent of isolates from patients with secretory diarrhea were adherent, 70% of isolates from patients with inflammatory diarrhea were invasive, and 83% of isolates from asymptomatic individuals were nonadherent (Table 1).

Enterotoxin Production

Enterotoxin production was significantly higher in isolates from children with noninflammatory diarrhea than in those from asymptomatic children ($P < 0.05$) (Fig. 3). Enterotoxin levels were higher in isolates from patients with noninflammatory diarrhea than in those from patients with inflammatory diarrhea, although they did not reach statistical significance. Iso-

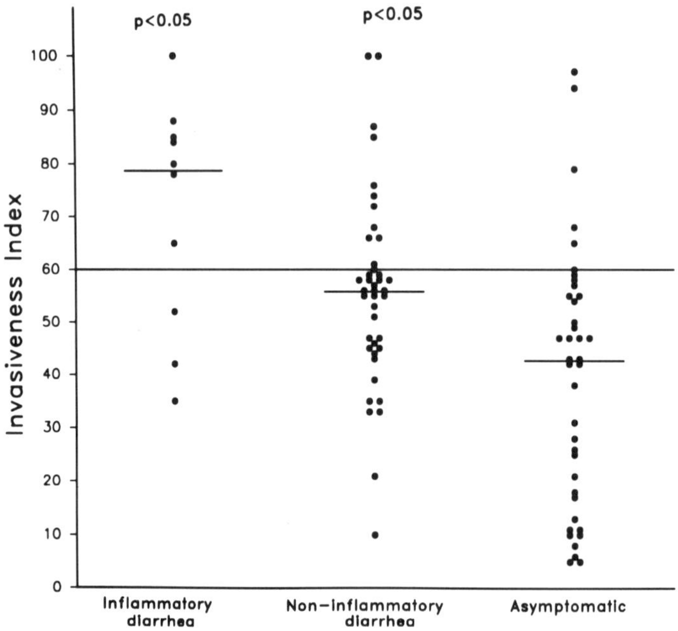

FIGURE 2. Results of a Sepharose bead assay for invasion of cells by *Campylobacter* isolates obtained from children with inflammatory and noninflammatory diarrhea and asymptomatic children. There was a statistically significant difference between the median invasiveness index for isolates from children with inflammatory and noninflammatory diarrhea ($P < 0.05$) and from asymptomatic children ($P < 0.05$) (a strain was considered invasive when the invasiveness index was >60%).

TABLE 1. Virulence traits of *C. jejuni* isolates and their association with clinical outcome

Source of isolate	No. (%) of isolate type: Adherent	Invasive	Nonadherent
Patients with diarrhea			
Noninflammatory	28 (68)	7 (17)	6 (14)
Inflammatory	3 (30)	7 (70)	0
Asymptomatic children	4 (10)	3 (7)	32 (83)

lation of adherent enterotoxigenic *Campylobacter* organisms was a significant risk factor for secretory diarrhea (Table 2), whereas only the isolation of invasive *Campylobacter* organisms was a significant risk for inflammatory diarrhea (Table 3). There was no greater risk for inflammatory diarrhea if the isolate produced cytotoxin or enterotoxin.

Milk Factors

The crude oligosaccharide fraction obtained from skimmed deproteinated milk inhibited the ability of *Campylobacter* strains to infect HEp-2 cells at its normal concentration in milk (2 mg/ml) (Table 4), although this inhibition was seen only with the invasive (not the adherent) strain. No inhibition of the association of *Campylobacter* organisms with HEp-2 cells was observed with the lactose, lipid, or nonimmunoglobulin protein fractions. Inhibition by crude oligosaccharide was still detected when it was present at only 0.2 mg/ml (1/10 its normal concentration in milk). When the crude oligosaccharide fraction was further separated into neutral and acidic fractions, only neutral oligosaccharide inhibited the association of the invasive *Campylobacter* strains with the cells but had no effect on the adherent strains (Fig. 4). To further define the active components, the neutral inhibitory

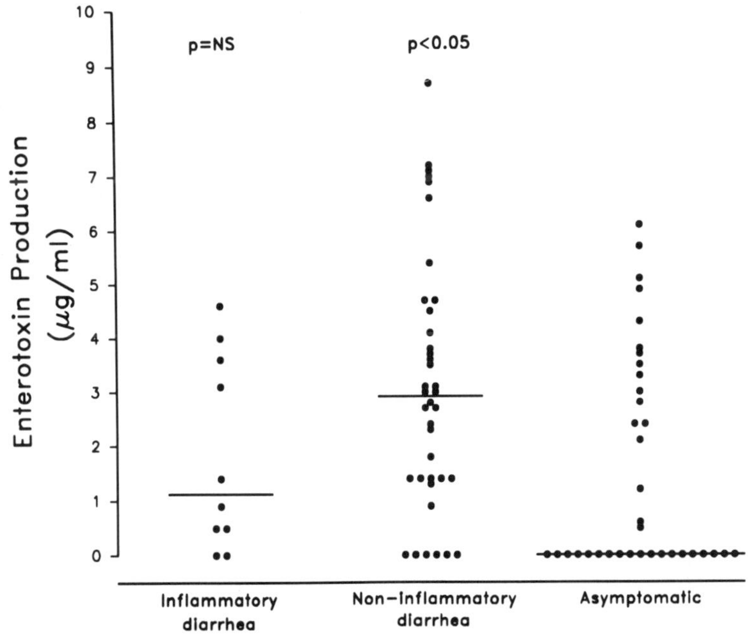

FIGURE 3. Enterotoxin production by *Campylobacter* isolates detected by the monoclonal antibody GM_1 ELISA. NS, not significant.

TABLE 2. Putative virulence factors of *C. jejuni* as risk factors for noninflammatory diarrhea

Virulence markers	Odds ratio	95% confidence interval	*P*
Cell adherence	224.0	29.58, 1,696	<0.001
Invasion	2.5	0.77, 8.00	NS[a]
Enterotoxin	6.2	2.16, 17.80	<0.001
Cytotoxin	0.8	0.31, 2.18	NS

[a] NS, not significant.

fraction was passed through a *U. europaeus* lectin affinity column. No inhibitory activity was seen with the unretained nonfucosylated oligosaccharide fraction, whereas most of the inhibitory activity was found in the fucosylated fraction eluted from the lectin column with a high-salt buffer. This inhibitory activity was still detected at concentrations lower than (0.1 mg/ml) or equal to (0.2 mg/ml) the normal concentration in milk (Fig. 5).

PERSPECTIVE

The pathogenesis of *Campylobacter* diarrhea involves a complexity of events in which, as could be seen in our studies, adherence to and invasion of gut mucosa are of primary importance. Using isolates from children participating in a cohort study in which the clinical outcome of infection was well characterized, and using novel in vitro techniques, we were able to define three types of strains: adherent, invasive, and nonadherent.

There are several in vitro studies which demonstrate the ability of *C. jejuni* to adhere to and invade epithelial cells (12, 15, 28). Also, outer membrane proteins and glycoprotein residues from invasive strains have been identified; these attach to intact host cell membranes (13, 21), suggesting that the binding of these surface-exposed glycoproteins may play a role in *C. jejuni*-host cell interaction and invasion. However, this interaction has been studied mainly with reference strains and with few isolates from patients with inflammatory diarrhea, and not with isolates from patients with other types of diarrhea or from asymptomatic individuals.

Clinical and epidemiologic studies on the natural history of *Campylobacter* infection have shown three clinical presentations: inflammatory and noninflammatory diarrhea and asymptomatic carriage (1, 4, 7, 14, 16, 17). To explain this, it has been postulated that the previous immune status of the host and the presence of putative virulence factors in the bacteria, such as adherence, enterotoxin production, and invasion, may determine the clinical outcome of infection (35). In our studies, we confirmed the existence of invasive strains and demonstrated a strong association with illness, especially with inflammatory diarrhea. Interestingly, we found that a considerable number of isolates were able to attach to but not penetrate epithelial cells, at least not in the proportion of the invasive strains. Furthermore, this property of sole attachment was strongly associated with illness, and particularly with noninflammatory diarrhea, and was very rarely seen in isolates from asymptomatic children. On the other hand, symptom-free children carrying *Campylobacter* species were more likely to have a nonadherent strain. Confirmation of these findings in other populations is important to determine whether, as in *E. coli,* there are strains with different virulence patterns and whether the mere isolation of a *Campylobacter* strain indicates that it is indeed the responsible pathogen.

By using a sensitive and specific monoclonal antibody-based GM_1 ELISA, we were also

TABLE 3. Putative virulence factors of *C. jejuni* as risk factors for inflammatory diarrhea

Virulence marker	Odds ratio	95% confidence interval	*P*
Invasion	15.9	3.05, 82.32	0.001
Enterotoxin	1.4	0.34, 5.70	NS[a]
Cytotoxin	0.5	0.1, 2.94	NS

[a] NS, not significant.

TABLE 4. In vitro effect of oligosaccharide from human milk in the interaction of adherent and invasive *Campylobacter* strains with HEp-2 cells

Oligosaccharide (concn)	Effect on *Campylobacter* association with HEp-2 cells[a]: Invasive strain (INN-383IP)	Adherent strain (INN 10SP)
Hanks PBS	65 ± 3.3	70.9 ± 5.7
Crude (3 mg/ml)	25 ± 4.5 (62)	72 ± 5.2 (0)
Neutral (3 mg/ml)	19 ± 2.6 (70)	60 ± 4.5 (14)
Acid (1 mg/ml)	65 ± 5.5 (0)	78 ± 6.2 (0)
Nonfucosylated (2.3 mg/ml)	62 ± 2.1 (4)	69 ± 5.8 (1.5)
Fucosylated (0.2 mg/ml)	30 ± 8.1 (54)	79 ± 2.0 (0)

[a] Data are expressed as percentage of infected cells. Each value represents the mean ± standard deviation of three experiments. The percent inhibition by oligosaccharide fractions is given.

able to identify enterotoxin-producing *Campylobacter* strains and to quantify toxin production. One of the first putative virulence factors identified in *Campylobacter* species was a choleralike enterotoxin (32), which is chromosome regulated (3) and induces intraluminal fluid accumulation by the same mechanisms as do cholera toxin and the heat-labile toxin of enterotoxigenic *E. coli.* A specific antitoxin-antibody response has been observed in patients with watery diarrhea who are carrying an enterotoxigenic *Campylobacter* strain (31). In spite of these findings, it is still unclear whether toxin production alone is responsible for the clinical manifestations. In studies done in India (25) no difference was found in the rates of isolation of toxigenic *Campylobacter* strains between children with diarrhea and symptom-free carriers. In a study of adults with acute inflammatory diarrhea in the United States, the enterotoxin could not be detected in any of the isolates (29). In the present study, in which isolates from patients with different clinical presentations of *Campylobacter* infection were tested, and with the use of a specific method for identification of *Campylobacter* choleralike enterotoxin with monoclonal antibodies, we were able to demonstrate a strong association between enterotoxin production and illness. The isolates from symptomatic children produced significantly larger quantities of the enterotoxin than did isolates from symptom-free children. Therefore, there may be a threshold in the amount of released enterotoxin to induce illness in susceptible individuals. With the availability of these new highly specific and quantitative methods, it will be important to analyze other *Campylobacter* isolates and to determine whether highly enterotoxigenic strains are also found in other geographic areas.

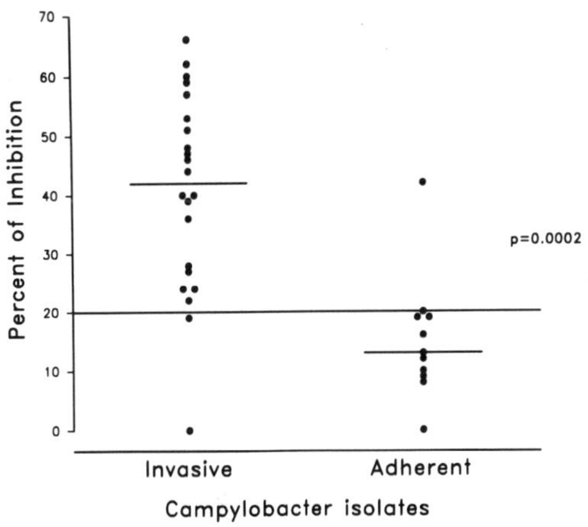

FIGURE 4. Inhibition of the association of *Campylobacter* isolates and HEp-2 cells by the neutral oligosaccharide from human milk.

Finally, we were not able to find an association between cytotoxin production and diarrhea. Although we do not have an explanation for this, the bioassay used may not be the most appropriate and the number of cytotoxin-producing strains might have been underestimated. The cytotoxin has recently been purified (24), so it seems possible that more sensitive and quantitative methods that provide a better characterization of strains will soon be developed.

We have also demonstrated the presence in human milk of receptor analogs for *Campylobacter* species. These analogs are fucosylated oligosaccharides which probably act by competing with the receptors present in epithelial cells for invasive, but not adherent, *Campylobacter*

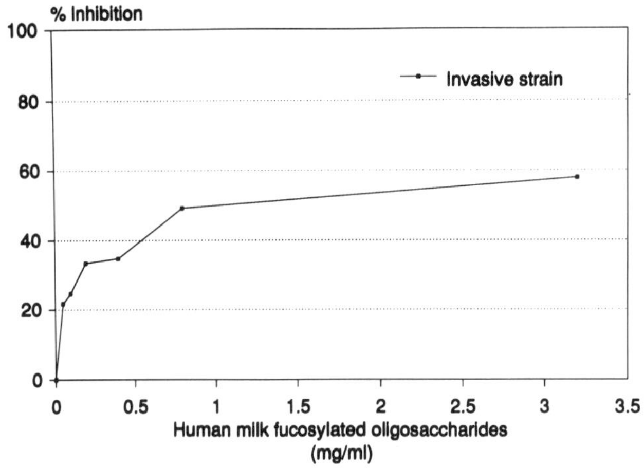

FIGURE 5. Inhibition of the association of *Campylobacter* isolates and HEp-2 cells by the fucosylated oligosaccharide fraction from human milk.

strains, suggesting that the mechanisms of interaction and the membrane receptors may be different for adherent and invasive strains. These findings also support the existence of strains with different pathogenic mechanisms. Interestingly, inhibition of *Campylobacter*-cell association by L-fucose has been previously demonstrated (6, 26), and it is possible that strains tested in those studies were of the invasive type. We are now further characterizing the oligosaccharides that are directly responsible for attachment to the surface components of invasive *Campylobacter* strains. In vivo studies are necessary to confirm the inhibitory activity of oligosaccharides against *Campylobacter* infection.

ACKNOWLEDGMENTS. We thank Beatriz R. Ruiz-Palacios for her contribution. The work described in this chapter was supported by grants from the National Institutes of Health (HD-13021) and Consejo Nacional de Ciencia y Technologia, Mexico (PCS BNA-021739).

REFERENCES

1. **Blaser, M. J., I. D. Berkowitz, F. M. LaForce, J. Cravens, L. B. Reller, and W. L. Wang.** 1979. *Campylobacter* enteritis: clinical and epidemiologic features. *Ann. Intern. Med.* **91**:179–185.
2. **Blaser, M. J., and D. N. Taylor.** 1986. Immune response to *Campylobacter jejuni* in a rural community in Thailand. *J. Infect. Dis.* **153**:249–254.
3. **Calva, E., J. Torres, M. Vasquez, V. Angeles, H. De la Vega, and G. M. Ruiz-Palacios.** 1989. *Campylobacter jejuni* chromosomal sequences that hybridize to *Vibrio cholerae* and *Escherichia coli* LT enterotoxin genes. *Gene* **75**:243–251.
4. **Calva, J. J., G. M. Ruiz-Palacios, A. B. Lopez-Vidal, A. Ramos, and R. Bojalil.** 1988. Cohort study of intestinal infection with campylobacter in Mexican children. *Lancet* **i**:503–506.
5. **Cervantes, L. E., J. J. Calva, and G. M. Ruiz-Palacios.** 1991. Assessment of virulence factors for definition of pathogenic strains in *Campylobacter* diarrhea, p. 206–208. *In* G. M. Ruiz-Palacios, E. Calva, and B. R. Ruiz-Palacios (ed.), *Campylobacter V.* National Institute of Nutrition, Mexico City, Mexico.
6. **Cinco, M., E. Banfi, E. Ruaro, D. Crevatin, and D. Crott.** 1984. Evidence for L-fucose (6-deoxyl-L-galatopyranose)-mediated adherence of *Campylobacter* spp. to epithelial cells. *FEMS Microbiol. Lett.* **21**:347–351.
7. **Colgan, T., J. R. Lambert, A. Newman, and S. C. Luk.** 1980. *Campylobacter jejuni* enterocolitis—a clinicopathologic study. *Arch. Pathol. Lab. Med.* **104**:571–574.
8. **Cotton, T.** 1974. *Statistics in Medicine.* Little, Brown, Boston.
9. **Cravioto, A., R. J. Gross, S. M. Scotland, and B. Rowe.** 1979. An adhesive factor found in strains of Escherichia coli belonging to the traditional infantile enteropathogenic serotypes. *Curr. Microbiol.* **3**:95–99.
10. **Cravioto, A., A. Tello, H. Villafan, J. Ruiz, S. Del Vedovo, and J. R. Neeser.** 1991. Inhibition of localized adhesion of enteropathogenic Escherichia coli to HEp-2 cells by immunoglobulin and oligosaccharide fractions of human colostrum and breast milk. *J. Infect. Dis.* **163**:1247–1255.
11. **Daikoku, T., M. Kawaguchi, K. Takama, and S. Suzuki.** 1990. Partial purification and characterization of the enterotoxin produced by *Campylobacter jejuni. Infect. Immun.* **58**:2414–2419.
12. **De Melo, M. A., G. Gabbiani, and J.-C. Pechere.** 1989. Cellular events and intracellular survival of

Campylobacter jejuni during infection of HEp-2 cells. *Infect. Immun.* **57**:2214–2222.

13. **De Melo, M. A., and J. C. Pechere.** 1990. Identification of *Campylobacter jejuni* surface proteins that bind to eucaryotic cells in vitro. *Infect. Immun.* **58**:1749–1756.
14. **Drake, A. A., M. J. R. Gilchrist, J. A. Washington, K. A. Huizenga, and R. E. Van Scoy.** 1981. Diarrhea due to *Campylobacter fetus* subsp. *jejuni.* A clinical review of 63 cases. *Mayo Clin. Proc.* **56**:414–423.
15. **Fauchère, J. L., A. Rosenau, M. Veron, E. N. Moyen, S. Richard, and A. Pfister.** 1986. Association with HeLa cells of *Campylobacter jejuni* and *Campylobacter coli* isolated from human feces. *Infect. Immun.* **54**:283–287.
16. **Glass, R. I., B. J. Stoll, M. I. Huq, M. J. Struelens, M. Blaser, and A. K. M. G. Kibriya.** 1983. Epidemiologic and clinical features of endemic *Campylobacter jejuni* infection in Bangladesh. *J. Infect. Dis.* **148**:292–296.
17. **Goossens, H., G. Henocque, L. Kremp, J. Rocque, R. Boury, G. Alanio, L. Vlaes, W. Hemelhof, C. V. Borre, M. Macart, and J. P. Butzler.** 1986. Nosocomial outbreak of *Campylobacter jejuni* meningitis in newborn infants. *Lancet* **ii**:146–149.
18. **Guerrant, R. L., C. A. Wanke, R. A. Pennie, L. A. Barrett, A. A. M. Linva, and A. D. O'Brien.** 1987. Production of a unique cytotoxin by *Campylobacter jejuni. Infect. Immun.* **55**:2526–2530.
19. **Kerr, D. A.** 1938. Warthin-Starry method for staining spirochetes. *Am. J. Clin. Pathol. Tech. Suppl.* **8**:63.
20. **Klipstein, F. A., and R. F. Engert.** 1984. Properties of crude *Campylobacter jejuni* heat-labile enterotoxin. *Infect. Immun.* **45**:314–319.
21. **Konkel, M. E., F. Babakhani, and L. A. Joens.** 1990. Invasion-related antigens of *Campylobacter jejuni. J. Infect. Dis.* **162**:888–895.
22. **Lindblom, G. B., L. E. Cervantes, E. Sjogren, B. Kaijser, and G. M. Ruiz-Palacios.** 1990. Adherence, enterotoxigenicity, invasiveness, and serogroups in *Campylobacter jejuni* and *Campylobacter coli* strains from adult humans with acute enterocolitis. *APMIS* **98**:179–184.
23. **Lopez-Vidal, Y., V. Angeles, D. Mass, and G. M. Ruiz-Palacios.** 1991. Monoclonal antibodies against *Campylobacter jejuni* enterotoxin, p. 206–208. *In* G. M. Ruiz-Palacios, E. Calva, and B. R. Ruiz-Palacios (ed.), *Campylobacter V.* National Institute of Nutrition, Mexico City, Mexico.
24. **Mahajan, S., and F. G. Rodgers.** 1990. Isolation, characterization, and host-cell-binding properties of a cytotoxin from *Campylobacter jejuni. J. Clin. Microbiol.* **28**:1314–1320.
25. **Mathan, V. I., D. P. Rajan, F. A. Klipstein, and R. F. Engert.** 1986. Prevalence of enterotoxigenic *Campylobacter jejuni* among children in South India. *Lancet* **ii**:981.
26. **McSweegan, E., and R. I. Walker.** 1986. Identification and characterization of two *Campylobacter jejuni* adhesins for cellular and mucous substrates. *Infect. Immun.* **53**:141–148.
27. **Newberg, D. S., L. K. Pickering, R. H. McClear, and T. G. Cleary.** 1990. Fucosylated oligosaccharide of human milk protect suckling mice from heat-stable enterotoxins of Escherichia coli. *J. Infect. Dis.* **162**:1075–1080.
28. **Newell, D. G., and A. Pearson.** 1984. The invasion of epithelial cell lines and the intestinal epithelium of infant mice by *Campylobacter jejuni/coli. J. Diarrhoeal Dis. Res.* **1**:19–26.
29. **Perez-Perez, G. I., D. L. Cohn, R. L. Guerrant, C. M. Patton, L. B. Reller, and M. J. Blaser.** 1989. Clinical and immunologic significance of cholera-like toxin and cytotoxin production by *Campylobacter* species in patients with acute inflammatory diarrhea in the U.S.A. *J. Infect. Dis.* **160**:460–468.
30. **Ruiz-Palacios, G. M., J. J. Calva, and L. K. Pickering.** 1990. Protection of breast fed infants against *Campylobacter* diarrhea by antibodies in human milk. *J. Pediatr.* **116**:707–713.
31. **Ruiz-Palacios, G. M., Y. Lopez-Vidal, J. Torres, and N. Torres.** 1985. Serum antibodies to heat-labile enterotoxin of *Campylobacter jejuni. J. Infect. Dis.* **152**:413–416.
32. **Ruiz-Palacios, G. M., J. Torres, N. I. Torres, E. Escamilla, B. R. Ruiz-Palacios, and J. Tamayo.** 1983. Cholera-like enterotoxin produced by *Campylobacter jejuni. Lancet* **i**:250–253.
33. **Schlesselman, J. J.** 1982. *Case Control Studies. Design, Conduct, Analysis.* Oxford University Press, Oxford.
34. **Skirrow, M. B.** 1977. *Campylobacter* enteritis: a new disease. *Br. Med. J.* **2**:9–11.
35. **Walker, R. I., M. B. Caldwell, E. C. Lee, P. Guerry, T. J. Trust, and G. M. Ruiz-Palacios.** 1986. Pathophysiology of *Campylobacter* enteritis. *Microbiol. Rev.* **50**:81–94.

CHAPTER 20

Lack of Evidence of Enterotoxin Involvement in Pathogenesis of *Campylobacter* Diarrhea

GUILLERMO I. PEREZ-PEREZ, DAVID N. TAYLOR, PETER D. ECHEVERRIA, AND MARTIN J. BLASER

INTRODUCTION

Several *Campylobacter* species are now recognized as important pathogens causing human diarrheal disease (7, 8), but specific virulence mechanisms are not yet well defined. *Campylobacter jejuni* and *C. coli* infection may result in classical dysentery with fever and the presence of blood and leukocytes in the stools, suggestive of an invasive process or cytotoxin production (3, 27, 37, 38). *Campylobacter* diarrhea may also be associated with episodes of loose or watery stools and the absence of fever, consistent with the effect of a choleralike enterotoxin (14, 33). Inflammatory diarrhea is the most common presentation in developed countries, whereas watery diarrhea is more often observed in developing countries (3, 6, 14). However, *Campylobacter* isolates from patients in both developed and developing countries have been reported to be enterotoxigenic (15, 19, 24).

Although toxin production is only one aspect of the total virulence potential of enteric pathogens, for many organisms, including *Vibrio cholerae* and *Clostridium difficile,* toxins play the major role in the pathogenesis of diarrhea (2). *Campylobacter* strains have been reported to produce an enterotoxin similar in structure, receptor, mechanism of action, and antigenic characteristics to cholera toxin (CT) and the heat-labile toxin (LT) of *Escherichia coli* (15, 19, 22, 23, 26, 33).

However, the following observations have raised questions about the biological role of *Campylobacter* enterotoxin: (i) there is no homology with *E. coli* or *V. cholerae* genes encoding enterotoxin production (29); (ii) several investigators have been unable to find toxin production by *Campylobacter* strains (17, 37); (iii) enterotoxin production, when present, is at low levels (20 to 2,000 times lower than for LT or CT) (19, 20); (iv) dehydration in *Campylobacter* enteritis is not a common clinical feature, in contrast to the secretory diarrhea caused by enterotoxigenic *E. coli* or *V. cholerae* (21); and (v) the typical *Campylobacter* clinical illness in developed countries is an inflammatory enteritis, but inflammation is not characteristically a response to enterotoxins.

To verify the role of enterotoxin in the pathogenicity of *C. jejuni* and *C. coli* diarrhea, useful approaches are to ascertain in vivo expression of the toxin or to demonstrate the presence of a host response to the toxin. If present, these findings would indicate that toxinogenesis has occurred in vivo. Either of these findings, if present, can be used as an indicator of the biological significance of toxin production.

In this chapter, we review previous data and present new observations on (i) whether patients from a developed and a developing country with sporadic cases of *Campylobacter* enteritis developed serologic responses to CT, as well as to

Guillermo I. Perez-Perez, Division of Infectious Diseases, Department of Medicine, Vanderbilt University School of Medicine, Nashville, Tennessee 37232–2605. **David N. Taylor,** Enteric Infections Branch, Walter Reed Army Institute of Research, Washington, D.C. 20307–5100. **Peter D. Echeverria,** U.S. Medical Component, Armed Forces Research Institute of Medical Sciences, Bangkok, Thailand. **Martin J. Blaser,** Division of Infectious Diseases, Department of Medicine, Vanderbilt University School of Medicine, Nashville, Tennessee 37232–2605, and Infectious Disease Section, Department of Veterans Affairs Medical Center, Nashville, Tennessee 37203.

Campylobacter common cellular antigens; and (ii) whether the isolated *Campylobacter* strains were toxigenic.

SURVEY OF PATIENTS WITH DIARRHEA IN THE UNITED STATES AND THAILAND

Populations Studied

For this survey, we sought to include persons with acute diarrheal illnesses in both developed and developing countries. An important part of our study design was the inclusion of appropriate controls. First, we used serum samples obtained between August 1982 and October 1984 from patients in Denver with sporadic acute inflammatory diarrheal illnesses (31). Entry criteria included an acute inflammatory enteritis, defined as abdominal pain, watery or loose stools, and either the presence of fecal leukocytes or a positive stool culture for a bacterial enteric pathogen, if fecal leukocytes were not present. Patients were classified into three groups as follows: 24 patients had confirmed *C. jejuni* or *C. coli* enteritis, 13 patients had enteritis due to other identified enteric pathogens, and 27 patients had enteritis of unknown cause. Serum samples also were obtained from July to December 1987 from children in Bangkok, Thailand, with acute diarrheal illnesses. Entry criteria included acute enteritis, defined as abdominal pain, watery or loose stools, and the isolation of *Campylobacter* or *Shigella* species (as a control group) as the sole pathogen. Children were classified into two groups as follows: 29 children (mean age, 13.5 months) had confirmed *C. jejuni* or *C. coli* enteritis, and 26 (mean age, 23.1 months) had *Shigella* enteritis. For both the U.S. and Thai patients, serum specimens were obtained during the initial visit to the outpatient department when the acute diarrheal illness was diagnosed (acute phase). For the Thai children, a second sample was obtained 14 days later. For all cases a convalescent-phase serum sample was obtained approximately 4 weeks after the onset of symptoms. Acute- and convalescent-phase serum samples collected from 12 Peace Corps volunteers infected with LT-producing *E. coli* (36), 12 single serum samples from healthy adults in Denver, and 100 serum samples from healthy children in Bangkok, Thailand, were used as controls in the assays for antibodies to enterotoxin. Serum samples had been stored at −20°C prior to testing.

Serologic Response to Enterotoxin

We first asked whether the infected persons and controls showed seroconversion to enterotoxin antigens. The ganglioside GM_1 enzyme-linked immunosorbent assay (ELISA) to detect anti-enterotoxin antibodies was performed essentially as described previously (31). In brief, polystyrene microtiter plates were coated with 0.15 μg of ganglioside GM_1, after which remaining binding sites were blocked with 0.1% gelatin in phosphate-buffered saline (PBS), with thimerosal and Tween 20 (PBS-T-T). The wells were then incubated with 0.1 ml of purified CT, the B subunit of CT, or LT (provided by R. A. Finkelstein) (1.0 μg/ml) in PBS-T-T containing 0.5% bovine gammaglobulin and 0.1% gelatin (PGG). After the plates were washed, a 1:100 dilution of the serum samples in PGG was added to duplicate wells and incubated. Peroxidase-conjugated goat antibody to human immunoglobulin G (IgG) diluted 1:2,000 was used, and

TABLE 1. Serum IgG response to CT in healthy controls and in patients in the United States with acute diarrhea[a]

Group	No. of persons studied	Mean ± SEM OD of serum in IgG ELISA	
		Acute phase	Convalescent phase
Healthy adults	12	0.12 ± 0.04	NA[b]
Infected with *E. coli* LT	12	0.14 ± 0.02	0.85 ± 0.13[c]
Infected with *Campylobacter* spp.	24	0.07 ± 0.10	0.07 ± 0.01
Not infected with *Campylobacter* spp.	13	0.12 ± 0.03	0.19 ± 0.09
No pathogen identified	27	0.12 ± 0.03	0.13 ± 0.03

[a] Adapted from reference 31.
[b] NA, not applicable.
[c] $P < 0.01$ by the paired t test.

antibody binding was measured as previously described (4).

Results of the ELISA determinations are presented in Table 1. These results were nearly identical to the results of the studies with the B subunit of CT or LT (data not shown). Acute-phase serum from all patients showed low optical density (OD) values. The positive control group (12 Peace Corps workers), known to be infected with *E. coli* LT, all seroconverted to the CT; OD values were significantly elevated in their convalescent-phase serum ($P < 0.01$). In contrast, none of the 24 U.S. patients with culture-confirmed *Campylobacter* infection showed seroconversion to CT. Identical results were noted in serum samples from 39 of the 40 other patients with diarrheal illnesses who were not infected with *Campylobacter* strains. The only seroconversion occurred in a *Shigella*-infected woman who had developed diarrhea in Mexico and who was probably coinfected with an LT-producing *E. coli* strain.

We then investigated the serologic response to enterotoxin in children with diarrhea and healthy control children in Thailand (Table 2). Of interest, the mean OD values of the acute-phase serum in the three groups of Thai children all were significantly higher than the value for the Peace Corps workers. The OD values of the convalescent-phase (28-day) serum samples from the *Shigella*-infected children were no higher than those of the acute-phase serum samples. None of the 23 *Campylobacter*-infected children seroconverted to CT, even though 12 (41.3%) children had watery diarrhea without fecal leukocytes or blood. Serum samples obtained 14 days after the onset of infection had OD values that were not significantly different from those of the acute- and convalescent (28-day)-phase serum samples.

Antibody Response to *C. jejuni* Surface Protein Antigens

The lack of serologic response to CT prompted us to investigate whether the patients from whom *Campylobacter* species were isolated had acute infection. To do this, we determined whether they showed serological responses to known cellular antigens. The antigen used in the *C. jejuni* surface protein ELISA was prepared as previously described (4). In brief, cells of three *C. jejuni* strains were extracted in glycine buffer (pH 2.2), and the supernatant was dialyzed against water, pooled, and used as the antigen at a final protein concentration of 5.0 μg/ml in 0.05 M carbonate buffer (pH 9.6). A 0.1-ml sample of this solution was added to each well of a flat-bottomed Immulon 2 plate. The screening-serum dilutions were 1:200 for IgM, 1:100 for IgG, and 1:50 for IgA determinations. Peroxidase conjugates of goat antibody to human IgG, IgA, and IgM were diluted 1:1,000. Assays were done in duplicate, results were read blindly, and reference sera were included in each ELISA run. For each patient, the OD value for each Ig class in the acute-phase sample was compared with that in the corresponding convalescent-phase sample. We defined seroconversion as occurring when a convalescent-phase serum sample showed a ≥100% increase from the OD value of the acute-phase serum sample. A threshold of 0.050 in the OD for the acute-phase sample was selected to eliminate low-level reactions that might meet the above criteria but were within the day-to-day variability of the assay. We investigated seroconversion to *C. jejuni* cellular antigens in children with diarrhea in Thailand (Table 3). Of the 29 children with *Campylobacter* infection, 22 (75.8%) showed seroconversion in at least one Ig class by day 14, and 19 (65.4%)

TABLE 2. Serum Ig response to CT in healthy controls and in patients with acute diarrhea in Thailand

Group	No. of persons studied	Mean ± SEM OD in IgG ELISA: Acute phase	Mean ± SEM OD in IgG ELISA: Convalescent phase
Asymptomatic children	100	0.30 ± 0.05	NA[a]
Shigella-infected children	13	0.28 ± 0.07	0.25 ± 0.10
Campylobacter-infected children	23	0.34 ± 0.10	0.30 ± 0.05
Infected with *E. coli* LT[b]	12	0.11 ± 0.04	0.98 ± 0.10[c]

[a] NA, not applicable.
[b] This is the same group as shown in Table 1. Serum samples were reexamined simultaneously with the other serum samples shown in this table to provide a positive control group.
[c] $P = 0.006$ by the paired t test.

TABLE 3. Seroconversion to *C. jejuni* cell surface antigens in patients with sporadic diarrhea in Denver and Bangkok

Seroconversion by Ig class	No. of patients showing seroconversion					
	Campylobacter infected			Non-*Campylobacter* infected		
	Day 14, Bangkok (*n* = 29)	Day 28, Bangkok (*n* = 29)	Day 28, Denver (*n* = 24)	Day 14, Bangkok (*n* = 26)	Day 28, Bangkok (*n* = 26)	Day 28, Denver (*n* = 40)
IgA only	1	0	0	2	1	1
IgG only	2	4	4	0	0	4
IgM only	3	3	0	1	3	0
IgA and IgG	1	0	0	0	2	0
IgG and IgM	0	0	6	0	0	0
All three classes	9	10	10	0	1	2
Any class	22	19	21	3	7	7
None of the classes	7	10	3	23	19	33

showed seroconversion by day 28. Of 26 children who had acute *Shigella* diarrhea, only 3 (11.5%) seroconverted in any Ig class by day 14, but 7 (26.9%) seroconverted by day 28. This may have been due to intercurrent *Campylobacter* infection. In contrast to the *Campylobacter*-infected patients, only one (3.8%) patient showed seroconversion in all three Ig classes by day 28. Among the 24 U.S. patients with culture-confirmed *Campylobacter* infection, 21 (87.5%) seroconverted to the cellular antigens in at least one Ig class, 20 (83.3%) showed IgG seroconversion, 17 (70.8%) showed seroconversion in more than one Ig class, and 10 (42%) showed seroconversion in all three Ig classes (Table 3). For persons who had acute diarrhea due to enteropathogens other than *Campylobacter* species, 7 (17.5%) of 40 paired serum samples showed seroconversion to *C. jejuni* antigens in at least one Ig class, but only 2 (5%) patients with acute diarrhea from whom no enteropathogen was isolated showed seroconversion in all three Ig classes.

When the serologic results were analyzed on the basis of clinical information, no correlations were found for any group between the ELISA results and the presence of blood in feces, a history of fever, the presence of fecal leukocytes, or watery diarrhea. Moreover, no relationship was found between the ELISA results and the presence of a particular *Campylobacter* species.

Height of Antibody Response to *Campylobacter* Cellular Antigens

For the Denver population, for the acute-phase serum samples the distribution of levels of IgG and IgM *C. jejuni* antibody was not significantly different between patients with and without *Campylobacter* infection (Table 4); however, the IgA levels were higher in the patients with *Campylobacter* infection ($P = 0.03$), suggesting that the specific IgA level already had risen. Levels of IgA, IgG, and IgM to *C. jejuni* antigens among the *Campylobacter*-infected group were significantly higher in the convalescent-phase serum samples than in the acute-phase samples and were higher than in convalescent-phase serum samples from the non-*Campylobacter*-infected group.

Similar analysis for the Thai children showed that IgA and IgM antibody levels were not significantly different in the acute-phase serum samples taken from children with or without *Campylobacter* infection (Table 5). However, levels of IgG to *C. jejuni* antigens were higher in the *Shigella*-infected children than in the *Campylobacter*-infected group ($P = 0.04$). By 14 days, levels of serum IgA and IgM to *C. jejuni* antigens in the *Campylobacter*-infected group were significantly higher than in the *Shigella*-infected group. By 28 days, no differences in the levels of IgA and IgG were observed between children with or without culture-confirmed *Campylobacter* infection (Table 5), but IgM levels were significantly higher in the children with *Campylobacter* infection. OD values in the IgG and IgM assays of the *Campylobacter*-infected group were significantly higher in both of the postinfection samples than in the acute-phase samples (Table 5). However, IgA OD values in the 28-day samples were similar to the acute-phase values, indicating that the IgA immune response in those children was transient, whereas IgG values remained elevated.

TABLE 4. *C. jejuni* ELISA determination for serum samples of patients with acute diarrheal illnesses in Denver[a]

Group (no. of patients)	Mean OD ± SEM for: Acute-phase serum	Convalescent-phase serum (21–32 days)	P^b
Campylobacter enteritis (24)			
IgA	0.29 ± 0.08	0.49 ± 0.10	0.024
IgG	0.34 ± 0.06	1.62 ± 0.31	0.0003
IgM	0.71 ± 0.15	2.02 ± 0.33	0.0005
No *Campylobacter* enteritis (40)			
IgA	0.16 ± 0.03	0.17 ± 0.03	NS[c]
IgG	0.33 ± 0.04	0.40 ± 0.05	NS
IgM	0.60 ± 0.07	0.85 ± 0.18	NS

[a] Adapted from reference 31.
[b] By paired *t* test.
[c] NS, not significant ($P > 0.05$).

Enterotoxin Production and Gene Probing in *Campylobacter* Isolates

Twenty-two *Campylobacter* isolates from the United States were incubated overnight at 37°C in an atmosphere of 85% N, 10% CO_2, and 5% O_2 in Casamino Acids-yeast extract (CAYE) broth supplemented with 1.0 μg of ferric chloride per ml, with shaking (100 rpm) in a water bath shaker, as previously described (31). Culture supernatants were examined in a GM_1 ganglioside ELISA to detect CT-like toxin (Table 6). CT at 25 ng/ml and uninoculated growth media were used as controls. All samples were added in 100-μl amounts in triplicate to a 96-well microtiter plate precoated with 1.5 μg of GM_1 ganglioside per ml, as previously described (34). After overnight incubation at room temperature, 0.1 ml of goat antibody to LT (provided by R. A. Finkelstein) diluted 1:500 was added to each well, and the plate was incubated overnight at 4°C. Peroxidase-conjugated goat antibody to human IgG was added and assayed as previously described (4). All the controls showed the expected reactions, but none of the *Campylobacter* isolates synthesized products recognized by antibodies to CT at any level approaching our threshold for positivity.

Because the lack of recognition of CT-like toxin by antibodies to CT in the culture supernatant did not rule out the possibility of CT-like toxin production in *Campylobacter* strains, we

TABLE 5. *C. jejuni* ELISA determination for serum samples of patients with sporadic diarrhea in Thailand

Group (no. of patients)	Mean OD ± SEM for: Acute-phase serum	Convalescent-phase serum (14 days)	Convalescent-phase serum (28 days)
Campylobacter enteritis (29)			
IgA	0.80 ± 0.29	1.14 ± 0.18	0.70 ± 0.11[a]
IgG	0.46 ± 0.06[b]	0.80 ± 0.10	0.81 ± 0.10
IgM	0.48 ± 0.12	1.40 ± 0.31[c]	0.77 ± 0.16
Shigella enteritis (26)			
IgA	0.76 ± 0.10	0.80 ± 0.15	0.69 ± 0.11
IgG	0.68 ± 0.11	0.67 ± 0.11	0.66 ± 0.10
IgM	0.31 ± 0.04	0.34 ± 0.06	0.45 ± 0.11

[a] Compared with day 14 ($P = 0.004$).
[b] Compared with day 14 ($P = 0.0002$) and day 28 ($P = 0.0001$).
[c] Compared with acute phase ($P = 0.005$) and day 28 ($P = 0.0005$).

TABLE 6. Production of *Campylobacter* choleralike toxin by 22 *Campylobacter* isolates from patients with inflammatory diarrhea in Denver

Strain designation	ELISA antibodies to CT[a]	Enterotoxin titer in CHO cell assay
85-308	0.07	<1:2
85-309	0.03	<1:2
85-314	0.08	<1:2
85-316	0.08	<1:2
85-318	0.18	<1:2
85-322	0.24	<1:2
85-323	0.11	<1:2
85-328	0.10	<1:2
85-329	0.14	<1:2
85-331	0.12	<1:2
85-334	0.04	<1:2
85-337	0.12	<1:2
85-343	0.14	<1:2
85-352	0.02	<1:2
85-356	0.06	<1:2
85-360	0.17	<1:2
85-361	0.02	<1:2
85-365	0.10	<1:2
85-367	0.06	<1:2
85-370	0.12	<1:2
85-371	0.10	<1:2
85-374	0.02	<1:2
E. coli H 10407[b]	1.97	>1:256
Broth alone[c]	0	<1:2

[a] The ELISA results are the mean of triplicate determinations from at least two experiments. Results represent OD values. An enterotoxin titer of ≥0.3 is considered positive.
[b] *E. coli* H 10407 is a control strain known to be a high-level producer of LT.
[c] Broth represents uninoculated growth medium.

examined the cytotonic activity present in culture supernatant for these 22 *Campylobacter* strains in the Chinese hamster ovary (CHO) cell assay, performed by the technique described by Guerrant et al. (16). *Campylobacter* strains were grown in various media including brucella broth (1), brucella broth with the addition of amino acids (15), and CAYE (11), and the supernatants were harvested. Culture supernatants of *V. cholerae,* enterotoxigenic *E. coli,* and an *E. coli* strain known not to produce LT were used as controls. Criteria used to define a positive supernatant were as previously described (31). The positive control showed clear cytotonic activity (titer, >256) but none of the 22 *Campylobacter* culture supernatants tested showed any activity in the CHO cell assay (Table 6).

The 29 *Campylobacter* strains from children in Thailand were tested for the presence of the *E. coli* LT gene by using a hybridization assay with the LT DNA probe as previously described (13). A cloned DNA fragment described by Dallas (12) and an oligonucleotide described by Murray et al. (28) were both used. *E. coli* strains known to be LT producers or nonproducers were used as controls. Examination of the 29 *Campylobacter* isolates from Thailand under low-stringency conditions showed that none of the *Campylobacter* strains apparently possessed the gene encoding an LT- or CT-like toxin (Table 7).

SUMMARY

In the United States and other developed countries most cases of *Campylobacter* enteritis occur in the young adult population (18 to 45 years of age) and most cases are characterized by an inflammatory process with fever and fecal leukocytes (3, 6, 16). In contrast, in developing countries most cases of *Campylobacter* enteritis occur during the first 2 years of life (5) and symptomatic infection is rare in adults. In developing countries the spectrum of illness may include severe inflammatory illness, a mild secretory diarrhea, or an asymptomatic carrier state (5, 9, 14). Two explanations may be offered for the differences between the clinical and epidemiologic features of *Campylobacter* enteritis in developed and developing countries. First, *Campylobacter* strains in the United States and other developed countries may differ in virulence characteristics. Second, *Campylobacter* infection is far more common among children in developing countries than in children in developed countries, and repeated exposure to the organism may produce immunity.

We first examined whether *Campylobacter*-infected hosts from developed and developing countries seroconverted to CT, which is immunologically related to the *Campylobacter* enterotoxin (23, 26, 32). None of the 47 *Campylobacter*-infected patients studied showed seroconversion to CT. In contrast, Ruiz-Palacios et al. (33) in Mexico and Martin et al. (25) in the Central African Republic frequently found seroconversion to CT among children with *Campylobacter* infection. One explanation for these discrepant results is that *Campylobacter* strains in the United States may not be enterotoxigenic whereas those from developing countries are. However, in this study 23 (48.9%) of the 47 *Campylobacter*-infected patients were from Thailand, a developing country, and 25.5% of

TABLE 7. Hybridization assay with LT probe of *Campylobacter* strains isolated from children with diarrhea in Bangkok[a]

Bacterial type	No. of strains tested	No. of strains showing hybridization
E. coli LT[+b]	2	2
E. coli K-12 LT[-]	1	0
C. jejuni	25	0
Other *Campylobacter* species	4	0

[a] Hybridizations were conducted under low-stringency conditions as described previously (13).
[b] Control strain carrying LT-encoding plasmids.

these children did not have leukocytes or blood in their stools. Similar clinical characteristics have been reported in the Mexican and Central African Republic studies (25, 33). Coincident infection with LT-producing *E. coli* strains is common among children in developing countries (19, 36). Immunologic memory from prior LT-producing *E. coli* infections may have primed the response to *Campylobacter* enterotoxin in the other studies. In our study, acute-phase serum OD values to CT were two- to threefold higher in Thai children than in persons from developed countries, further indicating the high-level exposure of this group to enterotoxins.

In contrast, most of the *Campylobacter*-infected patients seroconverted to *C. jejuni* cell surface antigens. Overall, only 3 of 66 non-*Campylobacter*-infected persons seroconverted in all three Ig classes. However, two of those "non-*Campylobacter*-infected" persons probably had false-negative cultures, as occurs when enrichment or more sensitive culture methods are not used (30, 35). Another piece of evidence that those two patients may have been infected with *Campylobacter* species is that they also showed clear seroconversion to homologous and heterologous *Campylobacter* lipopolysaccharide, as described by Blaser and Perez-Perez (this volume). Among the *Campylobacter*-infected Thai children, the increase in IgA and IgM levels was transient, in contrast to a more prolonged response in the U.S. patients. All these results suggested that it is unlikely that *Campylobacter* strains isolated in developed countries differ in virulence from strains isolated in developing countries. Further evidence is the fact that travelers from developed to developing countries develop acute illness, as seen in developed countries (36).

Despite several reports that *Campylobacter* strains produce a CT-like toxin (22, 26, 33), we were unable to demonstrate production of toxin in the *Campylobacter* strains examined in this study by either ELISA or cell culture assay (16, 34). The lack of significant toxin production in the GM_1-binding assay was demonstrated by using three different antibody preparations that cross-react with *Campylobacter* CT-like toxin (23, 26). A parallel lack of enterotoxic activity was observed in the cell culture assay, despite our testing of several growth conditions and media to improve enterotoxin production, as suggested by other investigators (15, 18, 19, 26).

The discrepancies reported by different laboratories regarding the presence (10, 26, 33) or absence (17, 29, 31) of enterotoxin in *Campylobacter* strains may be related to the growth of the organism under in vitro conditions that are not optimal for toxin expression. Therefore, we investigated whether the 29 *Campylobacter* strains isolated in Thailand hybridized with the gene encoding *E. coli* LT or with an oligonucleotide probe for *E. coli* LT. The lack of hybridization at low stringency is consistent with the negative results from our other assays. In sum, we have found no evidence that supports a role for enterotoxin production in the pathogenesis of *Campylobacter* diarrhea in those areas of developed and developing countries.

ACKNOWLEDGMENTS. The work described in this chapter was supported in part by the Thrasher Research Fund and by an interagency agreement between the U.S. Army Medical Research and Development Command and the Department of Veterans Affairs. We thank David L. Cohen and L. Barth Reller for providing clinical specimens used in these studies.

REFERENCES

1. **Akhtar, S. Q., and F. Hug.** 1989. Effect of *Campylobacter jejuni* extracts and culture supernatants on cell culture. *J. Trop. Med. Hyg.* **92:**80–85.
2. **Balakrish, G. N., and S. C. Pal.** 1989. Enterotoxin induced diarrhoea—an update. *Trop. Gastroenterol.* **10:**133–141.
3. **Blaser, M. J., I. D. Berkowitz, F. M. LaForce, J. Cravens, L. B. Reller, and W.-L. L. Wang.** 1979.

Campylobacter enteritis: clinical and epidemiological features. *Ann. Intern. Med.* **91**:179–185.
4. **Blaser, M. J., and D. J. Duncan.** 1984. Human serum antibody response to *Campylobacter jejuni* infection as measured in an enzyme-linked immunosorbent assay. *Infect. Immun.* **44**:292–298.
5. **Blaser, M. J., R. I. Glass, M. I. Huq, B. Stoll, G. M. Kibriya, and A. R. M. A. Alim.** 1980. Isolation of *Campylobacter fetus* subsp. *jejuni* from Bangladeshi children. *J. Clin. Microbiol.* **12**:744–747.
6. **Blaser, M. J., D. N. Taylor, and R. A. Feldman.** 1983. Epidemiology of *Campylobacter jejuni* infections. *Epidemiol. Rev.* **5**:157–176.
7. **Blaser, M. J., J. G. Wells, R. A. Feldman, R. A. Pollard, and J. R. Allen.** 1983. *Campylobacter* enteritis in the United States: a multicenter study. *Ann. Intern. Med.* **98**:360–365.
8. **Butzler, J. P., and M. B. Skirrow.** 1979. *Campylobacter* enteritis. *Clin. Gastroenterol.* **8**:737–765.
9. **Calva, E., J. Torres, M. Vazquez, V. Angeles, H. delaVega, and G. M. Ruiz-Palacios.** 1989. *Campylobacter jejuni* chromosomal sequences that hybridize to *Vibrio cholerae* and *Escherichia coli* LT enterotoxin genes. *Gene* **75**:243–251.
10. **Daikoku, T., M. Kawaguchi, K. Takama, and S. Suzuki.** 1990. Partial purification and characterization of the enterotoxin produced by *Campylobacter jejuni. Infect. Immun.* **58**:2414–2419.
11. **Daikoku, T., S. Suzuki, S. Oka, and K. Takama.** 1989. Profiles of enterotoxin and cytotoxin production in *Campylobacter jejuni* and *C. coli. FEMS Microbiol. Lett.* **58**:33–36.
12. **Dallas, W. S.** 1983. Conformity between heat-labile toxin genes from human and porcine enterotoxigenic *Escherichia coli. Infect. Immun.* **40**:647–652.
13. **Echeverria, P. D., D. N. Taylor, J. Seriwatana, A. Chatkaeomorakot, V. Kungralert, T. Sakuldaipeara, and R. D. Smith.** 1986. A comparative study of enterotoxin gene probes and tests for toxin production to detect enterotoxigenic *Escherichia coli. J. Infect. Dis.* **153**:255–260.
14. **Glass, R. J., B. J. Stoll, M. I. Huq, M. J. Struelens, M. J. Blaser, and A. K. G. Kybriya.** 1983. Epidemiological and clinical features of endemic *Campylobacter* infection in Bangladesh. *J. Infect. Dis.* **148**:292–296.
15. **Goossens, H., J. P. Butzler, and Y. Takeda.** 1985. Demonstration of cholera-like enterotoxin production by *Campylobacter jejuni. FEMS Microbiol. Lett.* **29**:73–76.
16. **Guerrant, R. L., L. L. Brunton, T. C. Schnaitman, L. I. Rebhun, and A. C. Gilman.** 1974. Cyclic adenosine monophosphate and alteration of Chinese hamster ovary cell morphology: a rapid sensitive in vitro assay for the enterotoxins of *Vibrio cholerae* and *Escherichia coli. Infect. Immun.* **10**:320–327.
17. **Honda, T., T. Miwatani, S. Mizuno, and S. Maki.** 1986. Serum antibodies reacting with *Escherichia coli* heat-labile enterotoxin in sera of patients suffering from *Campylobacter jejuni* infection. *FEMS Microbiol. Lett.* **36**:53–55.
18. **Johnson, W. M., and H. Lior.** 1984. Toxins produced by *Campylobacter jejuni* and *Campylobacter coli. Lancet* **i**:229–230.
19. **Johnson, W. M., and H. Lior.** 1986. Cytotoxic and cytotonic factor produced by *Campylobacter jejuni, Campylobacter coli,* and *Campylobacter laridis. J. Clin. Microbiol.* **24**:275–281.
20. **Johnson, W. M., and H. Lior.** 1988. A new heat-labile cytolethal distending toxin (CLDT) produced by *Campylobacter* spp. *Microb. Pathogen.* **4**:115–126.
21. **Karmali, M. A., and P. C. Fleming.** 1979. *Campylobacter* enteritis in children. *J. Pediatr.* **94**:527–533.
22. **Klipstein, F. A., and R. F. Engert.** 1984. Properties of crude *Campylobacter jejuni* heat-labile enterotoxin. *Infect. Immun.* **45**:314–319.
23. **Klipstein, F. A., and R. F. Engert.** 1985. Immunological relationship of the B subunits of *Campylobacter jejuni* and *Escherichia coli* heat-labile enterotoxins. *Infect. Immun.* **48**:629–633.
24. **Lindblom, G. B., M. Johny, K. Khalil, K. Mazhar, G. M. Ruiz-Palacios, and B. Kaijser.** 1990. Enterotoxigenicity and frequency of *Campylobacter jejuni, C. coli* and *C. laridis* in human and animal stool isolates from different countries. *FEMS Microbiol. Lett.* **66**:163–168.
25. **Martin, P. M. V., J. Mathiot, J. Ipeio, A. J. Georges, and M. C. Georges-Courbot.** 1988. Antibody response to *Campylobacter coli* in children during intestinal infection and carriage. *J. Clin. Microbiol.* **26**:1421–1424.
26. **McCardell, B. A., J. M. Madden, and E. C. Lee.** 1986. *Campylobacter jejuni* and *Campylobacter coli*—production of a cytotoxic toxin immunologically similar to cholera toxin. *J. Food Prot.* **47**:943–949.
27. **Moore, M. A., M. J. Blaser, G. I. Perez-Perez, and A. D. O'Brien.** 1988. Production of a shiga-like cytotoxin by *Campylobacter. Microb. Pathogen.* **4**:455–462.
28. **Murray, B. E., J. J. Mathewson, H. L. Dupont, and W. E. Hill.** 1987. Utility of oligodeoxyribonucleotide probes for detecting enterotoxigenic *Escherichia coli. J. Infect. Dis.* **155**:809–811.
29. **Olsvik, O., K. Wachsmuth, G. Morris, and J. C. Feeley.** 1984. Genetic probing of *Campylobacter jejuni* for cholera toxin and *Escherichia coli* heat-labile enterotoxin. *Lancet* **i**:449.
30. **Paisley, J. N., S. Mirrett, B. A. Lauer, M. Roe, and L. B. Reller.** 1982. Dark-field microscopy of human feces for presumptive diagnosis of *Campylobacter fetus* subsp. *jejuni* enteritis. *J. Clin. Microbiol.* **15**:61–63.
31. **Perez-Perez, G. I., D. L. Cohn, R. L. Guerrant, C. M. Patton, L. B. Reller, and M. J. Blaser.** 1989. Clinical and immunologic significance of cholera-like toxin and cytotoxin production by *Campylobacter* species in patients with acute inflammatory diarrhea in the USA. *J. Infect. Dis.* **160**:460–468.
32. **Ruiz-Palacios, G. M., E. Escamilla, and N. Torres.** 1981. Experimental *Campylobacter* diarrhea in chickens. *Infect. Immun.* **34**:250–255.

33. **Ruiz-Palacios, G. M., Y. Lopez-Vidal, J. Torres, and N. I. Torres.** 1985. Serum antibodies to heat-labile enterotoxin of *Campylobacter jejuni*. *J. Infect. Dis.* **152**:413–416.
34. **Sack, D. A., S. Huda, P. K. B. Neogi, R. R. Daniel, and W. M. Spira.** 1980. Microtiter ganglioside enzyme-linked immunosorbent assay for *Vibrio* and *Escherichia coli* heat-labile enterotoxins and antitoxin. *J. Clin. Microbiol.* **11**:35–40.
35. **Taylor, D. N., M. J. Blaser, P. Echeverria, C. Pitarangsi, L. Bodhidatta, and W.-L. L. Wang.** 1987. Erythromycin-resistant *Campylobacter* infection in Thailand. *Antimicrob. Agents Chemother.* **31**:438–442.
36. **Taylor, D. N., P. Echeverria, M. J. Blaser, C. Pitarangsi, N. Blacklow, J. Cross, and B. G. Weniger.** 1985. Polymicrobial aetiology of traveller's diarrhoea. *Lancet* **i**:381–383.
37. **Wadstrom, T., S. B. Baloda, K. Krovacek, A. Faris, S. Bengtson, and M. Walder.** 1983. Swedish isolates of *Campylobacter jejuni/coli* do not produce cytotonic or cytotoxic enterotoxin. *Lancet* **ii**:911.
38. **Wong, P. Y., S. D. Puthcheary, and T. Pang.** 1983. Demonstration of a cytotoxin from *Campylobacter jejuni*. *J. Clin. Pathol.* **36**:1237–1240.

CHAPTER 21

Examination of Multiple Isolates of *Campylobacter jejuni* for Evidence of Cholera Toxin-Like Activity

MICHAEL E. KONKEL, YVES LOBET, AND WITOLD CIEPLAK, JR.

INTRODUCTION

The clinical presentation of certain cases of enteritis caused by *Campylobacter jejuni* suggests that this organism may produce a toxin that is capable of producing a diarrheal syndrome similar to those associated with enterotoxigenic *Escherichia coli* and *Vibrio cholerae* (27). Indeed, a number of reports from several laboratories have indicated that *C. jejuni* produces material that is immunologically cross-reactive with cholera toxin (CT) and/or *E. coli* heat-labile enterotoxin (LT), elicits a CT-like cytotonic cell response in vitro, and/or causes electrolyte imbalance as judged by fluid accumulation in ligated ileal loops (3, 5, 7, 8, 10–14, 17, 18, 22, 23, 25). For example, McCardell et al. (16) have reported the partial purification from *C. jejuni* culture filtrates of a M_r 70,000 protein which is immunologically cross-reactive with anti-CT serum, elicits a cytotonic response (rounding) by Y-1 adrenal cells, and promotes fluid accumulation in ligated ileal loops. More recently, Daikoku et al. (7) reported the partial purification of an M_r 68,000 protein that is reactive with anti-CT serum and appears to promote increases of cyclic AMP levels in HeLa cells. Finally, an oligonucleotide probe from a region encoding a peptide common to the proposed GM_1 ganglioside-binding site of the B subunits of LT and CT has been shown to hybridize to *C. jejuni* genomic DNA (5).

Despite the aforementioned studies, the existence of a *Campylobacter*-associated cholera-like enterotoxin remains in some doubt. The uncertainty concerning the production of enterotoxin stems largely from the fact that such activity has not been a reproducible finding among various laboratories (2, 20, 21, 26). Furthermore, the methods and criteria used to establish the presence of such activity have not been uniform. For example, the M_r 68,000 material described by Daikoku et al. (7) was not examined for such other direct activities of CT or LT as the ability to induce cytotonic effects on CHO or Y-1 adrenal cells, the presence of ADP-ribosyltransferase activity, or the ability to promote fluid accumulation in ligated ileal loops. As a result of the ambiguities surrounding the production of an enterotoxin-like substance in *C. jejuni*, we undertook to examine a number of *C. jejuni* isolates, collected by ourselves and others, for evidence of the production of cholera toxin-like enterotoxin as judged by several criteria, including elicitation of cytotonic effects on CHO-K1 cells, presence of ADP-ribosyltransferase activity, and immunologic cross-reactivity with anti-CT serum. In addition, we have attempted to find evidence for a *C. jejuni* structural gene that might encode a CT- or LT-like toxin by using specific oligonucleotide probes coupled with the polymerase chain reaction.

EXAMINATION OF ISOLATES FOR TOXIN

Description of Procedures

Four strains of *C. jejuni* that were initially isolated from patients with enteritis were obtained from Martin Blaser, Vanderbilt University, Nashville, Tenn. Eleven clinical isolates from the University of Arizona Medical Center were also examined. The various isolates used and their passage history are listed in Table 1. According to clinical records, many of the Ari-

Michael E. Konkel, Yves Lobet, and Witold Cieplak, Jr., Laboratory of Vectors and Pathogens, National Institute of Allergy and Infectious Diseases, Rocky Mountain Laboratories, Hamilton, Montana 59840.

zona strains were obtained from patients with watery diarrhea. The LT-producing *E. coli* strain, C600, was used as a positive control. Purified LT and CT were obtained from Richard A. Finkelstein, University of Missouri, Columbia, and List Biologicals, respectively. For most studies, *C. jejuni* and *E. coli* C600 were grown for 24 to 48 h at 37°C in G-C medium supplemented with 1% IsoVitaleX enrichment and 1 μg of ferric chloride per ml in a 10% CO_2 incubator with agitation. At 10 min prior to harvest, 2 mg of polymyxin B sulfate per ml was added to the cultures to promote the release of cell-associated material. These conditions have been reported to result in significant enterotoxin production by *C. jejuni* (7, 12, 13, 27). Intact cells were removed by centrifugation, and the supernatant fractions were clarified by passage through a 0.45-μm-pore-size membrane. The culture filtrates were then concentrated 20-fold by positive-pressure ultrafiltration on Amicon PM10 or YM10 membranes or by centrifugation in Centricon-10 microconcentrators. All manipulations were performed at 4°C or on ice and were carried out under nitrogen when appropriate.

Serial dilutions of the concentrated filtrates were examined for their ability to induce CT-like cytotonic effects on CHO-K1 cells (16, 21). None of the *C. jejuni*-derived filtrates contained detectable activity beyond that present in concentrated, uninoculated medium (Table 1). In some cases, toxic effects could be observed among some samples at lower dilutions (i.e., 1:1 and 1:2); however, such effects were also exhibited by samples of uninoculated medium concentrates and were probably due to residual polymyxin B. In contrast, filtrates from *E. coli* C600 induced readily observable cytotonic effects (elongation of more than 50% of cells) at dilutions greater than 1:512 when grown under the same conditions. Activities of less than 500 pg of purified CT per ml could be reliably detected under the conditions used. Similar findings were made by using purified LT preparations (results not shown).

We attempted to detect material in the concentrated filtrates that might be immunologically related to CT or LT by using both the GM_1 ganglioside enzyme-linked immunosorbent assay (ELISA) and sodium dodecyl sulfate-polyacrylamide gel electrophoresis (SDS-PAGE) coupled with immunoblotting. The former assay has been widely used for the reported detection of CT-like enterotoxin production by various *C. jejuni* isolates (21, 27). Goat antibodies directed against choleragenoid (List Laboratories) were used in the GM_1 ganglioside ELISA, and the assay was performed by using serial dilutions of the filtrates as described by Sack et al. (24). None of the *C. jejuni* culture filtrates yielded optical density values at 405 nm in the ELISA that were significantly greater than those associated with concentrated uninoculated medium (Table 1). It is noteworthy that the uninoculated medium concentrates yielded reactive absorbance values greater than most of the *C. jejuni* culture filtrates at lesser dilutions (i.e., undiluted through 1:4). Again, and in contrast, LT in the *E. coli* C600 filtrates could be readily detected at sizable di-

TABLE 1. GM_1 ELISA and CHO-K1 cytotonic activity of *C. jejuni* culture filtrates

		Activity measured by:	
Isolate[a]	Passage[b]	GM_1 ELISA[c]	CHO-K1 cell assay[d]
F38011	6	<2[e]	<2
H70100	5	<2	<2
M125	8	<2	<2
M129	15	<2	<2
M222	5	<2	<2
SJ	27	<2	<2
M3143	5	<2	<2
F1474	5	<2	<2
T6644	7	<2	<2
TG1971	5	<2	<2
T8531	5	<2	<2
82-16	>5	<2	<2
87-95	>5	<2	<2
78-42	>5	<2	<2
81-176	>5	<2	<2
E. coli C600	NA[f]	>1,024	>512

[a] Isolates designated 82-16, 87-95, 78-42, and 81-176 were obtained from Martin Blaser; the remainder of the isolates were obtained from the University of Arizona Medical Center.

[b] The number of times the isolate was subcultured after primary isolation.

[c] The ELISA was performed as described in the text and by Sack et al. (24). The values represent the reciprocal of the dilution which yielded an absorbance value greater than twice that associated with the identical dilution of uninoculated medium.

[d] Monolayers of CHO-K1 cells in 96-well plates (10^4 cells per well) were pulsed at 37°C in a 5% CO_2 incubator for 2 h with serial dilutions of concentrated culture filtrates from the isolates indicated. After incubation, the monolayers were washed and fresh culture medium was added. The assays were evaluated after 24 and 48 h of continued incubation. The values represent the reciprocal of the dilution which elicited the elongation of 50% of the CHO-K1 cells.

[e] A reciprocal titer of less than 2 (<2) indicates that no significant activity was detected at any dilution.

[f] NA, passage history not available.

lutions (Table 1). The *C. jejuni* culture filtrates were also examined by SDS-PAGE and immunoblotting. For these analyses, monoclonal antibodies directed against a peptide sequence that is conserved in the catalytic A subunits of CT, LT, and the S1 subunit of pertussis toxin (generously provided by James Kenimer, Food and Drug Administration, Bethesda, Md.) were also used. The analyses revealed no evidence of specifically immunoreactive material that resembled the subunit composition of CT or LT in any of the *C. jejuni* culture filtrates when using a mixture of polyvalent anti-choleragenoid and the monoclonal anti-A subunit antibodies as the detection reagent (Fig. 1). Nonspecific reactivity, as judged by the simultaneous appearance of bands on blots not exposed to primary antibodies, could frequently be observed at a position corresponding to M_r 60,000 to 70,000 and elsewhere in all of the *C. jejuni*- and *E. coli*-derived samples examined (data not shown). Parallel analyses of the filtrates by using SDS-PAGE and staining with Coomassie brilliant blue R-250 revealed that the most abundant *C. jejuni* proteins in the filtrates also migrated in the region corresponding to M_r 60,000 to 70,000.

Culture filtrates were also examined for the presence of specific ADP-ribosyltransferase activity characteristic of CT and LT. Both CT and LT are capable of ADP-ribosylating the M_r 39,000 alpha subunit of transducin (Tα) in bovine rod outer segment membranes (1, 15), and it has been presumed that a *C. jejuni* enterotoxin would exhibit a similar type of enzymatic activity (27). Assays of the *C. jejuni* culture filtrates, under conditions optimal for the transferase activity associated with CT and LT, failed to reveal the presence of any such activity as judged by the ability to catalyze the transfer of [^{32}P]ADP-ribose to acceptor proteins from [*adenylate*-^{32}P]NAD (Fig. 2). Filtrates prepared from *E. coli* C600 exhibited readily detectable activity as judged by the presence of both self-ADP-ribosylation of the A subunit of LT (M_r 30,000) and ADP-ribosylation of Tα (Fig. 2). Pretreatment of the *C. jejuni* culture filtrates with trypsin (1 μg/ml), which is known to enhance the activity of LT (19), did not change the results (not shown).

As noted above, Calva et al. (5) have reported hybridization to discrete *Sau*3A fragments of *C. jejuni* genomic DNA by an oligonucleotide probe containing the sequence which encodes the proposed GM_1 ganglioside-binding site of the B subunits of CT and LT. This finding was used to indicate the presence of a gene encoding a CT- or LT-like enterotoxin in *C. jejuni.* Using an identical oligonucleotide probe to that used by Calva et al. (5) and *Mbo*I-digested *C. jejuni* genomic DNA, we have also observed hybridization restricted to one or two

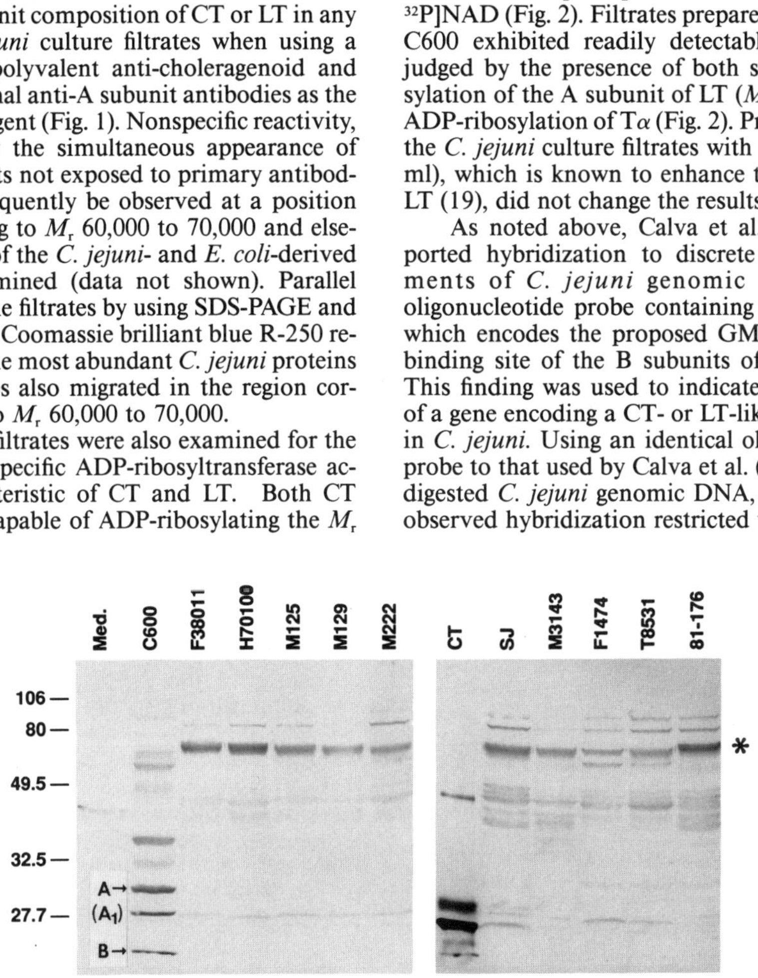

FIGURE 1. Representative immunoblot analyses of selected *C. jejuni* culture filtrates. Aliquots (15 μl) of the concentrated culture filtrates indicated were solubilized in double-strength electrophoresis sample buffer and electrophoresed in SDS–12.5% polyacrylamide gels. The proteins were then blotted onto polyvinylidene fluoride membranes. Bound proteins were reacted with anti-CT A subunit monoclonal antibodies and anti-choleragenoid followed by appropriate horseradish peroxidase-conjugated secondary antibodies. Bound antibodies were detected by using 4-chloro-1-naphthol as the chromogenic substrate. The positions of the A and B subunits of LT in the *E. coli* C600 culture filtrate, as well as the presumptive A1 fragment, are indicated. The corresponding fragments of CT can also be seen. Molecular masses of the standards (indicated at left) are given in kilodaltons. The asterisk indicates the position of the M_r 60,000 to 70,000 material in the *C. jejuni* filtrates that exhibits cross-reactivity with the antibodies.

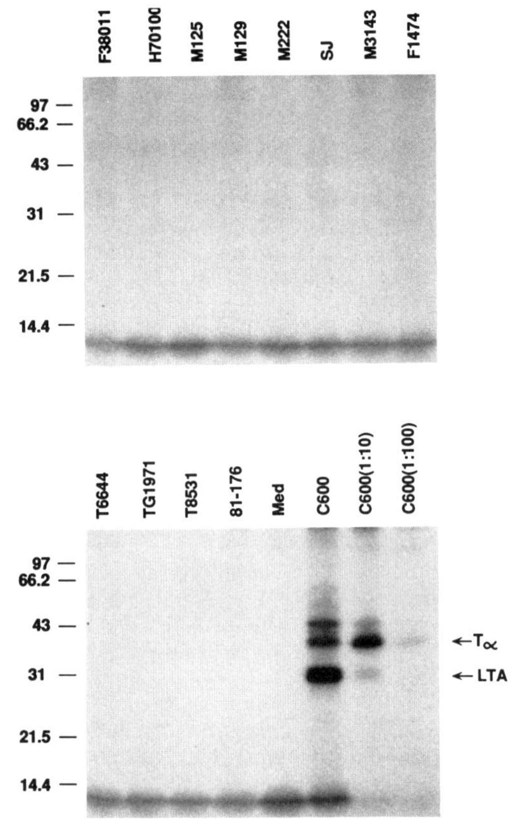

FIGURE 2. ADP-ribosyltransferase activity of concentrated culture filtrates. Aliquots (20 μl) of filtrates from the isolates indicated were incubated with 10 mM dithiothreitol prior to assay. Assays were initiated by the addition of [*adenylate*-^{32}P]NAD and bovine rod outer segment membranes in a total volume of 40 μl containing cofactors and buffers as described elsewhere (1,15). The assays were incubated at 30°C for 2 h and terminated by the addition of 0.2 ml of of 10% (wt/vol) trichloroacetic acid. The precipitated proteins were solubilized, and labeled material was analyzed by SDS-PAGE and autoradiography. The positions of the ADP-ribosylated forms of the M_r 39,000 Tα and the M_r 30,000 LT A subunit are indicated. Molecular masses of the standards (indicated at left) are given in kilodaltons.

bands under conditions of low to moderate stringency. Such a pattern was not observed when genomic DNA from nonenterotoxigenic *E. coli* was used. We attempted to extend these observations by using this probe and several others in polymerase chain reaction analysis of *C. jejuni* genomic DNA. Comparison of the sequences of the active or A subunits of CT, LT, and pertussis toxin reveals the presence of two octapeptide sequences which exhibit a high degree of similarity among all three subunits (residues 6 to 13 and 60 to 67 in the LT and CT A subunit sequences, respectively). A functional conservation of these residues is supported by the observations that site-specific mutations in the first of these two regions abrogate the enzymatic activities of pertussis toxin, LT, and CT (4, 6, 15). Using four sets of degenerate probes, designed to hybridize to all possible sequences encoding these apparently conserved regions, and the probe described by Calva et al. (5), we found that no combination of primers yielded a pattern of specifically amplified *C. jejuni* DNA fragments that was consistent with the presence of a single gene similar to those of LT or CT. However, DNA from the LT gene contained in plasmid EWD299 (9) yielded amplified fragments of the appropriate size with each set of primers used (data not shown).

Discussion

Using a number of primary clinical isolates of *C. jejuni* and several established strains, we have been unable to detect any material in concentrated culture filtrates that has properties similar to LT or CT as judged by several in vitro assays. These assays included measurement of cytotonic effects on CHO-K1 cells, detection of material immunologically cross-reactive with LT or CT, and assays for ADP-ribosyltransferase activity. Furthermore, we have been unable to detect proposed enterotoxin-encoding sequences in *C. jejuni* DNA by using various oligonucleotide primers and the polymerase chain reaction. Although our studies do not represent an exhaustive survey of all available *C. jejuni* strains or isolates, they have included strains that would be likely to possess the potential to produce enterotoxinlike molecules as judged by the clinical presentation of the patients from which the isolates were obtained. Our results appear to be in agreement with the recent findings of Perez-Perez et al. (21), who examined 22 clinical isolates of *C. jejuni* from sporadic cases and found no evidence of enterotoxin production as judged by either immunologic cross-reactivity with CT or the presence of cytotonic activity for CHO-K1 cells. However, we acknowledge the caveat that the current studies have not included those specific strains that have been reported by others to produce CT-like enterotoxins. The failure to detect enterotoxin activity might also be related to the fastidious nature of *C. jejuni,* which may render it difficult to find appropriate culture conditions for the production of such an enterotoxin. We have attempted to use conditions and cofactors which have been previously reported to result in the production of CT-like activity by *C. jejuni.* Nevertheless, the possibility exists that optimal culture conditions vary with the strain or isolate and will have to be established on an empirical basis. This possibility would indicate that the production of an enterotoxin by *C. jejuni* is highly variable and is unlike that associated with either *V. cholerae* or enterotoxigenic *E. coli,* which produce their respective enterotoxins under a variety of culture conditions. It is also possible that the enterotoxin produced by *C. jejuni* possesses unique properties that either render its activity extremely labile or make it otherwise difficult to detect by the means conventionally used for the detection of CT or LT. Such unique properties, if due to primary sequence differences in a putative A subunit, might also obviate the possibility of detecting amplified CT- or LT-related sequences in genomic DNA by the polymerase chain reaction. It is apparent that resolution of the discrepancies surrounding the production of enterotoxin by *C. jejuni* and its potential role in human disease will rely on further detailed description of the molecular and biological attributes of substances reported to possess enterotoxin activity and on the independent replication of positive results by using either shared strains or materials.

REFERENCES

1. **Abood, M. E., J. B. Hurley, M.-C. Pappone, H. R. Bourne, and L. Stryer.** 1982. Functional homology between signal coupling proteins. *J. Biol. Chem.* **257**:10540–10543.
2. **Baig, B. H., I. K. Wachsmuth, G. K. Morris, and W. E. Hill.** 1986. Probing *Campylobacter jejuni* with DNA coding for *Escherichia coli* heat-labile enterotoxin. *J. Infect. Dis.* **154**:542.
3. **Belbouri, A., and F. Migraud.** 1988. Enterotoxin-like activity produced by *Campylobacter jejuni* and *Campylobacter coli* isolated from patients and healthy controls in Algeria. *FEMS Microbiol. Lett.* **51**:25–28.
4. **Burnette, W. N., V. L. Mar, B. W. Plattler, J. D. Schlotterbeck, and H. R. Kaslow.** 1991. Site-specific mutagenesis of the catalytic subunit of cholera toxin: substituting lysine for arginine 7 causes loss of activity. *Infect. Immun.* **59**:4266–4270.
5. **Calva, E., J. Torres, M. Vasquez, V. Angeles, H. de la Vega, and G. M. Ruiz-Palacios.** 1989. *Campylobacter jejuni* chromosomal sequences that hybridize to *Vibrio cholerae* and *Escherichia coli* enterotoxin genes. *Gene* **75**:243–251.
6. **Cieplak, W., W. N. Burnette, V. L. Mar, K. T. Kaljot, C. F. Morris, K. K. Chen, H. Sato, and J. M. Keith.** 1988. Identification of a region of the S1 subunit of pertussis toxin that is required for enzymatic activity and contributes to the formation of a neutralizing antigenic determinant. *Proc. Natl. Acad. Sci. USA* **85**:4667–4671.
7. **Daikoku, T., M. Kawaguchi, K. Takama, and S. Suzuki.** 1990. Partial purification and characterization of the enterotoxin produced by *Campylobacter jejuni. Infect. Immun.* **58**:2414–2419.
8. **Daikoku, T., S. Suzuki, S. Oka, and K. Takama.** 1989. Profiles of enterotoxin and cytotoxin production in *Campylobacter jejuni* and *Campylobacter coli. FEMS Microbiol. Lett.* **58**:33–36.
9. **Dallas, W. S., D. M. Gill, and S. Falkow.** 1979. Cistrons encoding *Escherichia coli* heat-labile toxin. *J. Bacteriol.* **139**:850–858.
10. **Goossens, H., J. P. Butzler, and Y. Takeda.** 1985. Demonstration of cholera-like enterotoxin production by *Campylobacter jejuni. FEMS Microbiol. Lett.* **29**:73–79.
11. **Johnson, W. M., and H. Lior.** 1986. Cytotoxic and cytotonic factors produced by *Campylobacter jejuni, Campylobacter coli,* and *Campylobacter laridis. J. Clin. Microbiol.* **24**:275–281.
12. **Klipstein, F. A., and R. F. Engert.** 1984. Properties of crude *Campylobacter jejuni* heat-labile enterotoxin. *Infect. Immun.* **45**:314–319.
13. **Klipstein, F. A., and R. F. Engert.** 1985. Purification of *Campylobacter jejuni* enterotoxin. *Lancet* **i**:1123–1124.
14. **Klipstein, F. A., R. F. Engert, H. Short, and E. A. Schenk.** 1985. Pathogenic properties of *Campylobacter jejuni:* assay and correlation with clinical manifestations. *Infect. Immun.* **50**:43–49.
15. **Lobet, Y., C. W. Cluff, and W. Cieplak, Jr.** 1991. Effect of site-directed mutagenic alterations in ADP-ribosyltransferase activity of the A subunit of *Escherichia coli* heat-labile enterotoxin. *Infect. Immun.* **59**:2870–2879.
16. **McCardell, B. A., J. M. Madden, and E. C. Lee.** 1984. *Campylobacter jejuni* and *Campylobacter coli.* Production of a cytotonic toxin immunologically similar to cholera toxin. *J. Food Prot.* **47**:943–949.
17. **McCardell, B. A., J. M. Madden, and E. C. Lee.** 1984. Production of cholera-like toxin by *Campylobacter jejuni/coli. Lancet* **ii**:448–449.
18. **McCardell, B. A., J. M. Madden, and J. T. Stanfield.** 1986. Effect of iron concentration on toxin production in *Campylobacter jejuni* and *Campylobacter coli. Can. J. Microbiol.* **32**:395–401.
19. **Moss, J., J. C. Osborne, Jr., P. H. Fishman, S. Nakaya, and D. C. Robertson.** 1981. *Escherichia coli* heat-labile enterotoxin. *J. Biol. Chem.* **256**:12861–12865.
20. **Olswik, O., K. Wachsmuth, G. Morris, and J. C. Feeley.** 1984. Genetic probing of *Campylobacter jejuni* for cholera toxin and *Escherichia coli* heat-labile enterotoxin. *Lancet* **ii**:449.
21. **Perez-Perez, G. I., D. L. Cohn, R. L. Guerrant, C. M. Patton, L. B. Reller, and M. J. Blaser.** 1989. Clinical and immunologic significance of cholera-like toxin and cytotoxin production by *Campy-*

lobacter species in patients with acute inflammatory diarrhea in the USA. *J. Infect. Dis.* **160**:460–468.

22. **Ruiz-Palacios, G. M., Y. Lopez-Vidal, J. Torres, and N. Torres.** 1985. Serum antibodies to heat-labile enterotoxin of *Campylobacter jejuni. J. Infect. Dis.* **152**:413–416.
23. **Ruiz-Palacios, G. M., N. I. Torres, B. R. Ruiz-Palacios, J. Torres, E. Escamilla, and J. Tamayo.** 1983. Cholera-like enterotoxin produced by *Campylobacter jejuni. Lancet* **ii**:250–253.
24. **Sack, D. A., S. Huda, P. K. B. Neogi, R. R. Daniel, and W. M. Spira.** 1980. Microtiter ganglioside enzyme-linked immunosorbent assay for *Vibrio* and *Escherichia coli* heat-labile enterotoxin and antitoxin. *J. Clin. Microbiol.* **11**:35–40.
25. **Saha, S. K., N. P. Singh, and S. C. Sanyal.** 1988. Enterotoxigenicity of chicken isolates of *Campylobacter jejuni* in ligated ileal loops of rats. *J. Med. Microbiol.* **26**:87–91.
26. **Wadstrom, T., S. B. Baloda, K. Krovacek, A. Faris, S. Bengston, and M. Walder.** 1983. Swedish isolates of *C. jejuni/coli* do not produce cytotonic enterotoxins. *Lancet* **ii**:911.
27. **Walker, R. I., M. B. Caldwell, E. C. Lee, P. Guerry, T. J. Trust, and G. M. Ruiz-Palacios.** 1986. Pathophysiology of *Campylobacter* enteritis. *Microbiol. Rev.* **50**:81–94.

V. IMMUNE RESPONSES AND ANTIGENIC ANALYSIS

CHAPTER 22

Immune Responses Directed against *Campylobacter jejuni*

DIANE G. NEWELL AND IRVING NACHAMKIN

INTRODUCTION

Campylobacter jejuni appears to be a remarkably successful organism. It is ubiquitous in the environment and is able to repeatedly colonize susceptible hosts, surviving in the gastrointestinal tract long enough to replicate and be excreted in large numbers. Although *C. jejuni* is able to cause disease in humans and some animals, epidemiological studies indicate that the majority of human and animal infections involve asymptomatic infection and excretion. Moreover, even in the symptomatic host, disease is generally self-limiting. Both clinical and scientific studies suggest that the immunocompetent host can specifically respond to this infection to effectively terminate or minimize disease symptoms.

CIRCULATING HUMORAL RESPONSES DURING HUMAN INFECTIONS

The majority of patients with *Campylobacter* infection develop circulating antibodies directed against a number of *Campylobacter* cellular antigens. Such antibodies can be demonstrated by a wide variety of techniques, including complement fixation, bacterial agglutination, radioimmunoprecipitation, enzyme-linked immunosorbent assay, and Western immunoblotting. Experimental observations on human volunteers and primate animal models (32; Black et al., this volume) show that serum antibodies are first detectable 6 to 7 days after the onset of illness, probably 10 days after the initial infection (2, 10, 29). Immunoglobulin G (IgG), IgA, and IgM levels in serum rise rapidly during early infection; the specific IgA level generally peaks at about 7 to 10 days after the onset of symptoms and before the specific IgG peak at 3 to 4 weeks (10, 29; Black et al., this volume). IgM antibody levels peak earlier than those of the IgG class. Both IgM and IgA antibody levels decline rapidly, whereas the specific IgG level persists for several weeks. Which IgG subclasses are involved and whether they reflect the total IgG response, are unknown. IgA1 is detected in serum primarily during infection, mainly in the polymeric form, and is characteristic of a secretory IgA response (15). Monomeric IgA is also detected in serum and persists during convalescence. Thus, detection of monomeric IgA in serum may reflect persistent reexposure to *C. jejuni* (4). Detection of circulating IgM and polymeric IgA responses may be useful markers of acute infection, but additional studies are required to confirm their usefulness in diagnosis.

LOCAL IMMUNE RESPONSES DURING HUMAN INFECTIONS

Studies suggest that during *C. jejuni* infection the intestinal mucosa mobilizes a rapid local antibody response. Fecal and urinary antibodies are detectable during natural infections (13, 38; Nachamkin and Yang, this volume), and specific secretory IgA (sIgA) has been found in jejunal fluid during volunteer infections studies (Black et al., this volume). Far less is known about the isotype and time sequence of the local mucosal antibody responses to the infection. Furthermore, it is unclear whether there

Diane G. Newell, Central Veterinary Laboratory, Ministry of Agriculture, Fisheries and Food, New Haw, Weybridge, Surrey KT15 3NB, United Kingdom. **Irving Nachamkin,** Department of Pathology and Laboratory Medicine, University of Pennsylvania School of Medicine, Philadelphia, Pennsylvania 19104–4283.

is a serotype-specific local antibody responses during infection (Nachamkin and Yang, this volume) or whether antibodies directed against *Campylobacter* species are broadly cross-reactive. Immunoglobulin responses are also detectable at other sites of the common mucosal system, especially in breast milk (30; Nachamkin and Yang, this volume), which has important implications for the development of appropriate vaccines.

The cellular immune responses at the mucosal level have not yet been investigated. Nevertheless, the observation of persistent and recurrent *C. jejuni* infections in patients infected with human immunodeficiency virus (28) suggests that an effective T-cell response is essential for limiting the disease.

EFFECTIVENESS OF THE HUMAN IMMUNE RESPONSE

Effective antibody responses directed against bacterial infections of the gastrointestinal tract may act at several levels. During primary infections, developing antibodies could minimize disease symptoms, for example by neutralizing toxins, and/or eradicate infections via bactericidal activity. Effective memory responses during secondary infections in immune individuals are more likely to prevent, or significantly reduce, the extent of colonization by inhibiting adherence or motility. There is ample circumstantial, but little direct, evidence for the effectiveness of the antibodies in either preventing or eliminating *C. jejuni* infections in immunocompetent individuals. Under normal circumstances *C. jejuni* excretion lasts for 2 to 12 weeks whereas symptoms of campylobacteriosis last only 2 to 7 days. The self-limiting nature of this infection is concomitant with the detection of circulating antibodies (35). The presence of recurrent infections, frequently accompanied by bacteremia observed in agammaglobulinemic or immunocompromised patients (9, 17), also supports an antibacterial activity of the humoral immune response which acts to limit systemic infection.

Specific antibodies may also protect immune individuals from the consequences of infection. Human and animal studies (30; Black et al., this volume) indicate that primary infection with *C. jejuni* provides homologous protection against illness, but not necessarily colonization. Epidemiologic studies provide good evidence that immunological protection can be acquired. As discussed by Taylor (chapter 3 of this volume), infection in developed countries is relatively infrequent and is usually accompanied by illness. In developing nations, however, infection is common but is associated with a high rate of asymptomatic cases, particularly in adults. This decrease in the illness-to-infection ratio with age is concomitant with increasing levels of antibodies directed against *C. jejuni* (4). There is no indication that this is a reflection of geographical differences between strains. Such phenomena can more readily be explained by the immune status of the hosts allowing colonization but preventing illness. Under such conditions *C. jejuni* may have commensal-like properties. The widespread incidence of asymptomatic infection in the developing world suggests that persistent exposure to multiple strains allows the development of protective immune responses against common epitopes.

Antibodies have a variety of effector mechanisms which are dependent on their specificity, avidity, and affinity and are determined largely by class or subclass and site of action. *C. jejuni* is believed to be able to penetrate the intestinal epithelial barrier by invasion (25) and by translocation through the M cells of the Peyer's patches (36). As a consequence, a short-lived bacteremia and extraintestinal infections are not uncommon (35). The host appears to have evolved several mechanisms to limit this invasive potential. In vitro studies show that most *C. jejuni* strains are serum sensitive, and such a nonspecific defense mechanism may have an important role in preventing bacteremia (7). However, specific immune responses may also be involved. Such responses, mediated primarily by IgG1 and IgM antibodies, can both opsonize and participate in the complement-mediated killing of campylobacters (27; Black et al., this volume). This seems likely to be a significant limiting factor for extraintestinal infection. Experimental infections in primates induce a significant neutrophilic infiltration into areas of colonic mucosa adjacent to the presumed site of colonization (32; Black et al., this volume). The role of the bactericidal activity of phagocytic cells in restricting the dissemination of infection must therefore be important (7) and should be investigated further. However, the ability of phagocytic cells to inhibit colonization by campylobacters at the intestinal mucosal surface is questionable. The recent demonstration of bacterial surface antigens associated with invasion which could be inhibited by a monoclonal antibody (12) suggests that the invasive potential of some strains may also be limited by appropriate antibody responses.

Antibody effector mechanisms at the mucosal surface are mediated largely by secretory IgA; they include neutralization of toxins, inhibition of adherence, and blocking of bacterial adhesions and agglutinating properties (31). The relevance of both enterotoxins and cytotoxins in the pathogenesis of *Campylobacter* enteritis is still debatable and is discussed elsewhere in this volume. Nevertheless, cholera toxin-like and various cytotoxic activities have been detected in vitro. However, there are conflicting reports on the detection of antibodies directed against cholera toxin or its subunits, *Escherichia coli* heat-labile toxin, or *Shigella* toxin during *C. jejuni* infection. Therefore, the role of toxin-neutralizing antibody activity in protection from disease is uncertain. Antibody-mediated inhibition of colonization is potentially an effective host mechanism of limiting persistent *Campylobacter* infection of the gastrointestinal tract. Certainly, specific secretory IgA can inhibit adherence (16) and polyclonal antibodies can inhibit motility (22) in in vitro models. Both of these bacterial properties would appear to be essential for maintenance of infection.

C. JEJUNI SURFACE ANTIGENS AS POTENTIAL VACCINE CANDIDATES

Experimental studies suggest that immunization against *C. jejuni* infections is a realistic proposition, but the choice of immunogen will require considerable investigation. Identification and characterization of surface antigens will allow assessment of the potential of bacterial components as vaccine candidates. Although immunogenicity does not necessarily prove the presence of protective epitopes, it is a good indicator. There are remarkably few reports of the protective value of vaccination with defined *C. jejuni* antigens. However, immunization with heat-stable (5) antigens, presumably lipopolysaccharide (LPS), affords some protection from colonization. Although the importance of LPS in serotyping schemes has long been recognized, the role of this antigen in inducing effective antibody responses has not been extensively investigated. Investigations of naturally acquired and experimental human infections (Black et al., this volume; Blaser and Perez-Perez, this volume) have now confirmed that LPS is immunogenic during human infection and that it can induce cross-reacting as well as strain-specific responses, although to a lesser extent.

In naturally acquired immunity, heat-labile antigens, presumably surface proteins, also appear to confer some protection (32). Of the surface bacterial proteins identified to date, flagellin seems likely to be a potentially useful vaccine candidate. Flagella appear to be essential virulence factors in human (Black et al., this volume) and animal (18, 23; Nachamkin and Yang, this volume; Walker et al., this volume) infections, mediating motility and possibly adherence. In addition, the antigenicity and immunodominance of flagellins during infection are well established (37; Nachamkin and Yang, this volume) and anti-flagella antibodies are at least partly protective (20, 34; Nachamkin and Yang, this volume; Walker et al., this volume). Epidemiological studies also suggest that maternal anti-flagella secretory IgA antibodies protect infants from infection (Nachamkin and Yang, this volume). However, the flagellins of *C. jejuni* express both serotype-restricted and common epitopes (14, 21). Several human and animal studies indicate that there is type-specific protection against infection (Black et al., this volume; Walker et al., this volume) which may be associated with flagellin antigens. There is accumulating evidence that the serotype-restricted epitopes are immunodominant, particularly during immunization with intact flagella rather than flagellin subunits (22, 26). This serotype restriction of antibody responses to flagellin could be a significant problem in developing this protein as a vaccine candidate. Studies with human serum show, however, that patients elicit an antibody response against common flagellin epitopes. The flagellin gene products have recently been cloned and expressed in *E. coli* and partly epitope mapped (26), and so common epitopes can now be identified and the value of synthetic peptides as vaccines can be assessed.

The major outer membrane protein (MOMP) of *C. jejuni/C. coli* is surface exposed (24) and is also believed to be immunogenic during infection (6, 19). The MOMP, like flagellin, is presumed to have conserved epitopes (3). Unfortunately, monoclonal antibodies directed against this protein have not been produced, and the only available polyclonal monospecific antiserum is directed against the denatured polypeptide (33). Since MOMP is probably a porin, antibodies directed against it could interfere with a variety of bacterial metabolic processes, and therefore MOMP is an interesting potential vaccine candidate. However, it is difficult to analyze the antigenicity of MOMP, first because MOMP is an integral protein and therefore requires complex and denaturing isolation and purification procedures, which will destroy three-dimensional structures (33); and second because it appears to induce antibodies primarily against discontinuous epitopes, which probably accounts for inconsistent observations when using Western immunoblotting techniques. Fortunately MOMP can be radioiodinated in situ (24) so that radioimmunoprecipitation can be used to investigate its value as a vaccine component.

Finally, Pei et al. (this volume) have recently purified and partially characterized several surface proteins within a molecular mass range of 28 to 31 kDa. These proteins appear to be antigenic during infection. N-terminal sequence analysis indicates that at least one protein, PEB3, has homology with a meningococcal type I pilus. Further studies are needed to assess whether these proteins are involved in pathogenesis and whether they are suitable as vaccine candidates.

BACTERIAL MECHANISMS TO AVOID THE HOST IMMUNE RESPONSE

Human immune responses seem to be effective in limiting disease but not necessarily in protecting the immune host from colonization. There are number of potential explanations for this observation. Antibody responses may be directed primarily against virulence factors which cause disease rather than those which allow colonization, but such virulence factors remain to be defined. Immune responses are known to be directed against certain colonization factors such as flagella. The presence of repeated, albeit asymptomatic, infections in endemic regions indicates that these responses are ineffective. This lack of ability of the immune response to prevent colonization may be due to type-restricted protective immunity, poorly immunogenic protective antigens, or short life of the induced antibodies. Alternatively, campylobacters may have evolved some means of protection from the immune defense.

There are many mechanisms by which bacterial pathogens can avoid host immune defenses. To date the role of such mechanisms in *C. jejuni* infections has been only poorly investigated. Campylobacters do not appear to inactivate antibodies by producing IgG, IgM, or IgA1 proteases (8) or by expressing Fc-like bacterial surface receptors. There is no evidence for an antiphagocytic surface component, like that found in *C. fetus* subsp. *fetus*. Other mechanisms may involve the inhibition of antibody binding, for example the unusual sialylation of *C. jejuni* LPS (Mills et al., this volume). Bacteria may also evade the immune response by shifting their antigenic profile. The antigenic repertoire expressed by *C. jejuni* and *C. coli* is well illustrated by the large number of serotypes. Certainly the diversity of sugar sequences in the LPS structure allows the potential for antigenic variation (Mills et al., this volume). The antigenicity of the other major surface antigen, flagellin, is complex and is discussed elsewhere in this volume. Both phase variation and antigenic variation can occur in vivo. In addition, colonization of susceptible hosts can apply selection pressures to allow the predominance of different flagellin phenotypes (11) from mixed populations. For at least some *Campylobacter* surface antigens, therefore, the mechanisms are available for antigenic drift to prevent effective antibody activity.

ANIMAL MODELS OF IMMUNE RESPONSE

Several animal models have been used to study *Campylobacter* infection, but few models mimic human disease, as is discussed elsewhere in this volume. Animals appear to develop both local and systemic antibody responses after challenge with *C. jejuni.* Experimental infections of rabbits, for example, have shown that the level of specific IgA rises early after challenge and declines rapidly (Walker et al., this volume), similar to that observed in the human response. However, little information is known about the immunogenicity of purified bacterial antigens in inducing local or systemic immune responses. Studies by Walker et al. (this volume) suggest that administration of antigen with immunoadjuvants may potentiate the local immune response to defined antigens. To develop vaccines, particularly synthetic vaccines, it is necessary that animal models accurately mimic the human immune response, especially the epitope specificity. In addition, suitable animal models must have good immunological tools to detect immunoglobulin classes and subclasses and lymphocyte markers. Such tools are not currently available for several of the models (1).

CONCLUSION

The human host response is partly effective against *C. jejuni* infections. Experimental and epidemiological evidence indicates that there are good prospects for vaccination to prevent illness if not colonization. Future studies should focus on identifying the antigens involved in protection at the epitope level. If synthetic vaccines are to be developed in the future, T-cell as well as B-cell epitopes will have to be identified.

REFERENCES

1. **Bell, J. A., and D. O. Manning.** 1990. A domestic ferret model of immunity to *Campylobacter jejuni*-induced enteric disease. *Infect. Immun.* **58:**1848–1852.
2. **Blaser, M. J., D. J. Duncan, M. T. Osterholm, G. R. Istra, and W. L. Wang.** 1984. Serologic study of two clusters of infection due to *Campylobacter jejuni. J. Infect. Dis.* **147:**820–823.
3. **Blaser, M. J., J. A. Hopkins, and M. L. Vasil.** 1984. *Campylobacter jejuni* outer membrane proteins. *Infect. Immun.* **45:**986–993.
4. **Blaser, M. J., D. N. Taylor, and P. Echeverria.** 1986. Immune response to *Campylobacter jejuni* in a rural community in Thailand. *J. Infect. Dis.* **153:**249–254.
5. **Dolby, J. M., and D. G. Newell.** 1986. The protection of infant mice from colonization with *Campylobacter jejuni* by vaccination of the dams. *J. Hyg.* **96:**143–151.
6. **Dunn, B. E., M. J. Blaser, and E. L. Synder.** 1987. Two-dimensional gel electrophoresis and immunoblotting of *Campylobacter* outer membrane proteins. *Infect. Immun.* **55:**1564–1572.
7. **Field, L. H., J. L. Underwood, S. M. Payne, and J. L. Berry.** 1991. Virulence of *Campylobacter jejuni* for chicken embryos is associated with decreased bloodstream clearance and resistance to phagocytosis. *Infect. Immun.* **59:**1448–1456.
8. **Goossens, H., S. Frutiger, M. Loche, F. Mascart, J. P. Butzler, and C. Pecher.** 1985. Examination of Campylobacter for IgG, IgM and IgA1 proteases, p. 38. *In* A. D. Pearson, M. B. Skirrow, H. Lior, and B. Rowe (ed.), *Campylobacter III.* Public Health Laboratory Service, London.
9. **Johnson, L. J., C. Nolan, S. P. Wang, W. R. Shelton, and M. J. Blaser.** 1984. Persistent *Campylobacter jejuni* infection in an immunocompromised patient. *Ann. Intern. Med.* **100:**832–834.
10. **Kaldor, J., H. Pritchard, A. Serpell, and W. Metcalf.** 1983. Serum antibodies in *Campylobacter* enteritis. *J. Clin. Microbiol.* **18:**1–4.
11. **King, V., T. Wassenaar, B. A. M. van der Zeijst, and D. G. Newell.** 1991. Variations in *Campylobacter jejuni* flagellin and flagellin genes during in vivo and in vitro passage. *Microb. Ecol. Health Dis.* **4:**135–140.
12. **Konkel, M. E., F. Babakhani, and L. A. Joens.** 1980. Invasion-related antigens of *Campylobacter jejuni. J. Infect. Dis.* **162:**888–895.
13. **Lane, E. M., R. A. Batchelor, A. L. Bourgeois, D. H. Burr, and J. G. Olson.** 1987. Urine and fecal IgA response during naturally acquired infection with *Campylobacter jejuni. Lancet* **i:**1141.
14. **Lior, H.** 1984. Serotyping of *Campylobacter jejuni* and *Campylobacter coli* by slide agglutination based on heat-labile antigen factors, p. 61–76. *In* J. P. Butzler (ed.), *Campylobacter Infection in Man and Animals.* CRC Press, Inc., Boca Raton, Fla.
15. **Mascart-Lemone, F. O., J. R. Duhateau, J. Oosterom, J. P. Butzler, and D. L. DeLacroix.** 1987. Kinetics of anti-*Campylobacter jejuni* monomeric and polymeric immunoglobulin A1 and A2 responses in serum during acute enteritis. *J. Clin. Microbiol.* **25:**1253–1257.
16. **McSweegan, E., D. H. Burr, and R. T. Walker.** 1987. Intestinal mucus gel and secretory antibody are barriers to *Campylobacter jejuni* adherence to INT 407 cells. *Infect. Immun.* **55:**1431–1435.
17. **Melamed, J., Y. Bujanover, Y. S. Igra, D. Schwartz, V. Zakuth, and Z. Spirer.** 1983. *Campylobacter* enteritis in normal and immunodeficient children. *Am. J. Dis. Child.* **137:**752–753.
18. **Morooka, T., A. Umeda, and K. Amako.** 1985. Motility as an intestinal infection factor for *Campylobacter jejuni. J. Gen. Microbiol.* **131:**1973–1980.
19. **Nachamkin, I., and A. M. Hart.** 1985. Western blot analysis of the human antibody response to *Campylobacter jejuni* cellular antigens during gastrointestinal infection. *J. Clin. Microbiol.* **21:**33–38.
20. **Newell, D. G.** 1986. Monoclonal antibodies directed against the flagella of *Campylobacter jejuni:* production characterization and lack of effect on colonization of infant mice. *J. Hyg.* **96:**131–141.
21. **Newell, D. G.** 1986. Monoclonal antibodies directed against the flagella of *Campylobacter jejuni:* cross-reacting and serotypic specificity and potential use in diagnosis. *J. Hyg.* **96:**377–384.
22. **Newell, D. G.** Unpublished data.
23. **Newell, D. G., H. McBride, and J. M. Dolby.** 1985. Investigations on the role of flagella in the colonization of infant mice with *Campylobacter jejuni* and attachment of *Campylobacter jejuni* to human epithelial cell lines. *J. Hyg.* **95:**215–227.
24. **Newell, D. G., H. McBride, and A. D. Pearson.** 1984. The identification of outer membrane proteins and flagella of *Campylobacter jejuni. J. Gen. Microbiol.* **130:**1201–1208.
25. **Newell, D. G., and A. D. Pearson.** 1984. The invasion of epithelial cell lines and the intestinal epithelium of infant mice by *Campylobacter jejuni/coli. J. Diarrhoeal Dis. Res.* **2:**19–26.
26. **Nuijten, P. J. M., B. A. M. van der Zeijst, and D. G. Newell.** 1991. Localization of immunogenic regions of the flagellin proteins of *Campylobacter jejuni* 81116. *Infect. Immun.* **59:**1100–1105.
27. **Pennie, R. A., R. D. Pearson, L. J. Barrett, H. Lior, and R. L. Guerrant.** 1986. Susceptibility of *Campylobacter jejuni* to strain-specific bactericidal activity in sera of infected patients. *Infect. Immun.* **52:**702–706.
28. **Perlman, D. M., N. H. Ampel, R. B. Schifman, D. L. Cohn, C. M. Patton, M. L. Aguirre, W.-L. L. Wang, and M. J. Blaser.** 1988. Persistent *Campylobacter jejuni* infections in patients infected with human immunodeficiency virus (HIV). *Ann. Intern. Med.* **108:**540–546.

29. **Rautelin, H. I., and T. U. Kosunen.** 1987. *Campylobacter* etiology in human gastroenteritis demonstrated by antibodies to acid extract antigen. *J. Clin. Microbiol.* **25:**1944–1951.
30. **Ruiz-Palacios, G. M., J. J. Calva, L. K. Pickering, Y. Lopez-Vidal, P. Volkow, H. Pezzaross, and M. S. West.** 1990. Protection of breast-fed infants against *Campylobacter* diarrhea by antibodies in human milk. *J. Pediatr.* **116:**707–713.
31. **Russell, M. W., and J. Mestecky.** 1988. Induction of the mucosal immune response. *Rev. Infect. Dis.* **10:**S440–S446.
32. **Russell, R. G., M. J. Blaser, J. I. Sarmiento, and J. Fox.** 1989. Experimental *Campylobacter jejuni* infection in *Macaca nemestrina. Infect. Immun.* **57:**1438–1444.
33. **Taylor, D. E., and N. Chang.** 1987. Immunoblot and enzyme-linked immunosorbent assays of *Campylobacter* major outer-membrane protein and application to the differentiation of *Campylobacter* species. *Mol. Cell. Probes* **1:**261–274.
34. **Ukei, Y., A. Umeda, S. Fujimoto, M. Mitsuyama, and K. Amako.** 1987. Protection against *Campylobacter jejuni* infection in suckling mice by anti-flagellar antibody. *Microbiol. Immunol.* **31:**1161–1171.
35. **Walker, R. I., M. B. Caldwell, E. C. Lee, P. Guerry, T. J. Trust, and G. M. Ruiz-Palacios.** 1986. Pathophysiology of *Campylobacter* enteritis. *Microbiol. Rev.* **50:**81–94.
36. **Walker, R. I., E. A. Schauder-Chock, J. L. Parker, and D. Burr.** 1988. Selective association and transport of *Campylobacter jejuni* through M cells of rabbit Peyer's patches. *Can. J. Microbiol.* **34:**1142–1147.
37. **Wenman, W. M., J. Chai, T. J. Louie, C. Goudreau, H. Lior, D. G. Newell, A. D. Pearson, and D. E. Taylor.** 1985. Antigenic analysis of *Campylobacter* flagellar protein and other proteins. *J. Clin. Microbiol.* **21:**108–112.
38. **Winsor, D. K., J. J. Mathewson, and H. L. Dupont.** 1986. Western blot analysis of intestinal secretory immunoglobulin A response to *Campylobacter jejuni* antigens in patients with naturally acquired *Campylobacter* enteritis. *Gastroenterology* **90:**1217–1272.

CHAPTER 23

Human Volunteer Studies with *Campylobacter jejuni*

ROBERT E. BLACK, DANIEL PERLMAN, MARY LOU CLEMENTS, MYRON M. LEVINE, AND MARTIN J. BLASER

INTRODUCTION

Campylobacter jejuni and closely related organisms are established enteropathogens, resulting in diarrhea and often dysentery in susceptible children and adults (6). These organisms also cause asymptomatic infections, which are especially frequent in children residing in developing countries, who appear to be exposed frequently from an early age.

As has been found with other enteropathogens, volunteer studies in healthy adults can provide important insights into the pathogenesis of these illnesses, into the systemic and local immune responses to infection and illness, and into the extent and duration of protection afforded by prior exposure. They can also provide an efficient means of evaluating the reactogenicity, immunogenicity, and efficacy of candidate vaccines and of relating this efficacy to levels of natural protection demonstrated through volunteer rechallenge studies. Thus, studies were initiated to establish a volunteer model of *C. jejuni* diarrhea, including establishing the number of organisms needed to cause illness and the pathogenicity of different strains, and to use this model to evaluate the immune responses following infection and the extent of protective immunity.

ESTABLISHMENT OF THE VOLUNTEER MODEL

Volunteers for these studies were healthy, young adults from the Baltimore community. The methods of medical screening, informed consent, and therapy of illness have been published previously (8). The specific methods used for these studies at the Center for Vaccine Development have also been published (1). Briefly, volunteers were admitted to the isolation ward and challenged with *C. jejuni* suspended in 150 ml of milk (reconstituted from dry skim-milk powder). Four volunteers received the *C. jejuni* with 2 g of sodium bicarbonate instead of milk. After challenge, volunteers were interviewed daily for 12 days by a physician. All stools were collected, graded for consistency, and weighed. During the first 7 days after challenge, diarrhea was defined as the passage of two or more liquid stools, weighing in total at least 200 g, in a period of 48 h, or of a single liquid stool weighing at least 300 g or containing blood. Temperatures were taken every 6 h. Illness was defined as the presence of diarrhea or fever (temperature, >38°C). After the 7-day period of observation, all volunteers were treated with 250 mg of erythromycin stearate every 6 h for 5 days.

Two *C. jejuni* strains were used in these challenge studies. Strain A3249 (Penner serotype 27) was isolated from a 16-year-old boy with a sporadic infection after an outbreak at a camp in Connecticut. The patient had had a 2-day illness with several loose stools, headache, nausea, and a temperature of 38°C. Strain 81-176 (Penner serotype 23/36) was isolated from an ill 9-year-old girl in a milk-borne outbreak in Minnesota. Strain A4349 manifested two colony types, spreading and nonspreading, which were

---

Robert E. Black and Mary Lou Clements, Department of International Health, Johns Hopkins School of Hygiene and Public Health, Baltimore, Maryland 21205. **Daniel Perlman,** University Park Medical Clinic, Denver, Colorado. **Myron M. Levine,** Center for Vaccine Development, Division of Geographic Medicine, Department of Medicine, University of Maryland School of Medicine, Baltimore, Maryland 21201. **Martin J. Blaser,** Division of Infectious Diseases, Department of Medicine, Vanderbilt University School of Medicine, Nashville, Tennessee 37232-2605, and Infectious Disease Section, Department of Veterans Affairs Medical Center, Nashville, Tennessee 37203.

TABLE 1. Results of volunteer studies with *C. jejuni* A3249

C. jejuni challenge dose (CFU)	No. of volunteers	% Infected	% Ill	Mean no. of diarrheal stools	Mean diarrheal vol (ml)
8×10^2	10	50	10	2.0	106
8×10^3	10	60	10	4.0	158
9×10^4	13	85	46	5.3	533
8×10^5	11	73	9	4.0	302
1×10^6	19	79	11	16.0	1,574
1×10^8	5	100	0	2.5	388

subsequently demonstrated to represent flagellated and aflagellated variants, respectively (9). In total, each strain had been passaged 5 to 10 times on artificial media before being given to volunteers; stock cultures of *C. jejuni* for all volunteer studies were stored at −70°C in glycerol. Challenge inocula were prepared as previously described, and replicate pour plate quantitative cultures of the inocula were made before and after challenge to confirm the concentration of viable organisms. Because strain A3249 manifested both spreading and nonspreading colony types, separate challenge inocula were prepared to equally represent these two types in the final inoculum.

Cultures were made of samples of all stools passed after challenge until discharge from the study. If no stool was passed in a 24-h period, a rectal swab was obtained for culture. A wet mount of each stool sample was made on a glass slide and stained with methylene blue, and the number of leukocytes per high-power field was counted by an experienced technician who did not know the clinical status of the volunteers; stools were also tested for blood by using Hemoccult (SmithKline Beckman, Sunnyvale, Calif.). Cultures of blood were done for all volunteers at 0.5, 12, 24, 48, 72, 96, 120, and 144 h after challenge. Jejunal fluid for culture was collected by having volunteers ingest a gelatin string device (Entero-Test; Health Development, Palo Alto, Calif.) at intervals of 20 and 44 h after challenge and withdrawing the string for culture after 4 h. Stool specimens, rectal swabs, and fluid from Entero-Test strings were plated onto Campy-BAP (BBL Microbiology Systems, Cockeysville, Md.) as previously described. Blood cultures in thioglycolate broth were done by two methods, with subsequent incubation in an anaerobic jar with Campy Pak II (BBL Microbiology Systems) and in aerobic and anaerobic BACTEC bottles (BACTEC Systems; Johnson Laboratories, Cockeysville, Md.), and processed by standard methods.

Six studies were performed to establish the relationship between the ingested dose of *C. jejuni* A3249 and the rates of infection and illness (Table 1). At the lowest dose (800 total or 400 flagellated *C. jejuni* organisms), 5 of 10 volunteers became infected and one developed a mild illness. As the inoculum was raised to 10^8 CFU, the rate of infection increased to 100%. With higher doses, the attack rate did not increase consistently, nor did the severity of illness appear to differ. Overall, 11 (15%) of 68 persons given strain A3249 in milk became ill; 10 had diarrhea (4 also had fever), and 1 had fever without diarrhea. Of the four volunteers who received 10^8 CFU with 2 g of sodium bicarbonate, two developed diarrhea. For all volunteers, the incubation period until the onset of fever was 68 h, and the period to the onset of diarrhea was 88.5 h. In general, the diarrhea was mild with an average of approximately five liquid stools and 0.5 liter total stool volume. Anorexia, malaise, and abdominal cramps were reported by 52 to 60% of ill volunteers. All of the volunteers with diarrhea had fecal leukocytes, and the majority had

TABLE 2. Results of volunteer studies with *C. jejuni* 81-176

C. jejuni challenge dose (CFU)	No. of volunteers	% Infected	% Ill	Mean no. of diarrheal stools	Mean diarrheal vol (ml)
1×10^6	7	100	43	29.7	2,896
2×10^8	10	100	60	11.0	1,092
2×10^9	22	100	41	12.3	1,275

TABLE 3. Homologous rechallenge with *C. jejuni* A3249 and 81-176

C. jejuni strain	Volunteer status	Rechallenge dose (CFU)	No. of volunteers		
			Studied	Infected	Ill
A3249	Ill after challenge with 10^6 CFU of *C. jejuni* 1 mo earlier	10^8	2	0[a]	0
	Healthy (control)	10^8	5	5[a]	0
81-176	Ill after challenge with 10^8–10^9 CFU of *C. jejuni* 1 mo earlier	10^9	7	5	0[b]
	Healthy (control)	10^9	12	12	6[b]

[a] $P = 0.048$.
[b] $P = 0.034$.

fecal blood, at least by Hemoccult testing. Sigmoidoscopy in three ill volunteers showed normal rectal mucosa in two, whereas one demonstrated a diffusely abnormal mucosa with edema and loss of the normal vascular pattern. This person and one of those with a normal sigmoidoscopic examination had an abnormal mucosa visualized on a microscopic study of rectal biopsy specimens. These two biopsies showed a mixed population of inflammatory cells with neutrophils in the crypts and lymphocytes and plasma cells in the muscularis mucosa.

Three studies were done with *C. jejuni* 81-176 (Table 2). All volunteers who ingested inocula ranging from 10^6 to 10^9 CFU developed a positive stool culture. Overall, 18 (46%) of 39 volunteers challenged with strain 81-176 became ill with diarrhea (6 also had fever). No obvious dose-response relationship was noted, but the attack rate appeared to be higher than that after challenge with strain A3249, when only 2 (8%) of 24 volunteers receiving 10^6 to 10^8 CFU of *C. jejuni* in milk became ill. The incubation period to the onset of fever was 67 h, and the period to the onset of diarrhea was 53 h. Of the 18 persons who became ill after receiving strain 81-176, the average diarrhea consisted of 15 liquid stools and 1.5 liters of stool volume, illnesses that were substantially more severe than those caused by strain A3249. Anorexia, malaise, and abdominal cramps were reported in 67 to 78% of ill volunteers. All ill volunteers had fecal leukocytes, and 78% had blood in the stool.

In studies with both strains, stool cultures usually became positive by day 2 to 3 after challenge and stayed positive until 24 to 48 h after erythromycin treatment was begun. All infections were eliminated by erythromycin treatment, and no relapses were observed. Despite inoculation with equal numbers of organisms of the spreading and nonspreading colony types of strain A3249, stool cultures revealed only the spreading-colony type. At the high challenge inocula, string cultures of jejunal contents were often positive at 24 h, but rarely at 48 h (1). None of the blood cultures were positive.

These studies demonstrate that ingestion of even low doses of *C. jejuni* results in diarrhea with fecal leukocytes and blood, similar to naturally occurring illness caused by this enteropathogen. Of the two strains used, one produced a higher attack rate and more definite illness, making it a more suitable challenge strain for a volunteer model. The lack of bacteremia during infection and the ability to terminate illness and infection by antibiotic therapy are desirable characteristics in a volunteer model, indicating low risk of serious systemic infection and of relapse or transmission of infection upon return to the community.

PROTECTION INDUCED BY *C. JEJUNI* ILLNESS

Protective immunity by prior disease was evaluated in homologous rechallenge studies

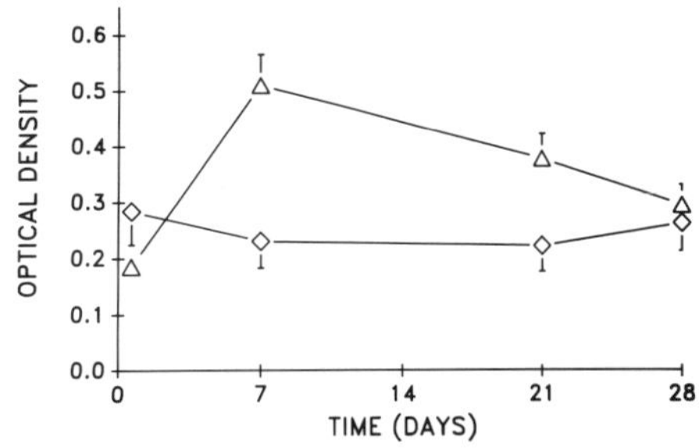

FIGURE 1. Serum IgA response to *C. jejuni* acid-extracted proteins in healthy volunteers. Symbols: △, infected; ◇, not infected.

with each of the strains (Table 3). Two volunteers, who had developed illness after challenge with 10^6 CFU of *C. jejuni* A3249, were rechallenged 28 days later with 10^8 CFU of the same strain, as were with five volunteers who had not participated in previous *C. jejuni* studies. Neither of the two rechallenged persons became infected, whereas all five controls became infected, although none became ill. Seven volunteers who had developed illness after receiving 10^8 to 10^9 CFU of *C. jejuni* 81-176 were rechallenged 28 days later with 10^9 CFU of the same strain, as were 12 controls. Infection occurred in five of the seven previously ill volunteers and in all of the controls. However, diarrheal illness was not observed in previously ill persons on rechallenge, but was observed in 6 of the 12 controls.

These studies indicate that homologous immunity can be induced, at least for the short term, by symptomatic *C. jejuni* infection. This confirms the suggestion from epidemiologic studies that natural infection confers protective immunity and may explain the age-related decrease in the case-to-infection ratio for *C. jejuni* in developing countries (7). The extent and mechanism of heterologous immunity remain to be determined.

IMMUNOLOGIC RESPONSE AFTER CHALLENGE WITH *C. JEJUNI*

Serum samples were collected before challenge and at 7, 21, and 28 days later. Among persons rechallenged on day 28, serum samples were also obtained on days 35, 49, and 56. Jejunal fluid was collected by intubation before and 11 days following challenge or rechallenge with *C. jejuni*. Jejunal aspirate specimens were standardized to 6 μg of total immunoglobulin A (IgA) per well.

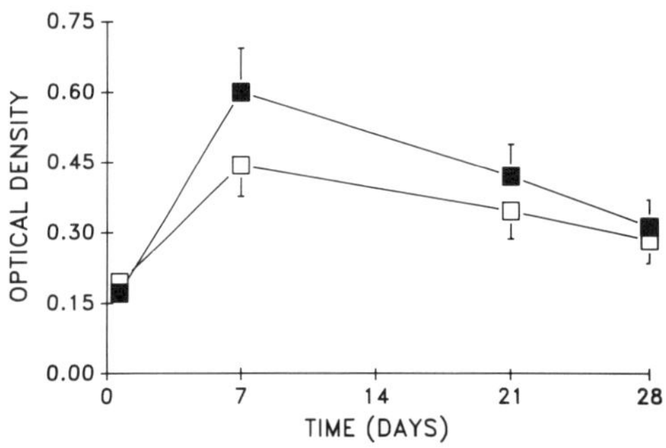

FIGURE 2. Serum IgA response to *C. jejuni* acid-extracted proteins in well (□) and ill (■) infected volunteers.

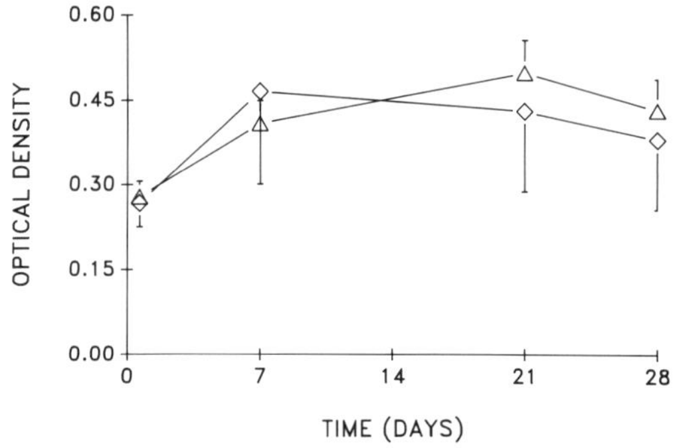

FIGURE 3. Serum IgM response to *C. jejuni* acid-extracted proteins in well (△) and ill (◇) infected volunteers.

Immune Responses to Acid-Extracted Proteins of *C. jejuni*

For the first set of immunologic studies, an enzyme-linked immunosorbent assay (ELISA) with *C. jejuni* group-specific proteins as the antigen was used. The antigen was prepared from Penner 1, 2, and 3 strains by using an acid extraction procedure as has been described previously (2). Goat anti-human Ig class-specific peroxidase conjugates were used in the assay. Because analysis of serially diluted test sera has shown a linear relation between the optical density value and the reciprocal titer, all sera were assayed at single screening dilutions: 1:50 for IgA and IgM and 1:100 for IgG.

Volunteers who were challenged but did not become infected had a higher preexisting IgA level in serum on the day of challenge than those who did become infected ($P = 0.04$) (Fig. 1). Volunteers who did not become infected showed no significant increase in IgA antibody levels following challenge. Infected volunteers had an IgA response that peaked at day 7 and declined to the baseline level by day 28. Rises in antibody levels of IgG and IgM were also noted, but did not differ in infected and noninfected volunteers.

Among volunteers who became infected, those who remained well and those who became ill were compared (Fig. 2). In both groups, the IgA level in serum peaked at day 7, but the ill group had a significantly higher peak IgA level. IgM (Fig. 3) and IgG (Fig. 4) levels peaked at day 21, but did not differ in ill and well volunteers.

Since the severity of illness differed with the two strains evaluated, the serum IgA response was evaluated separately for volunteers given each of the two strains. The serum IgA response was higher after ingestion of strain 81-176 than

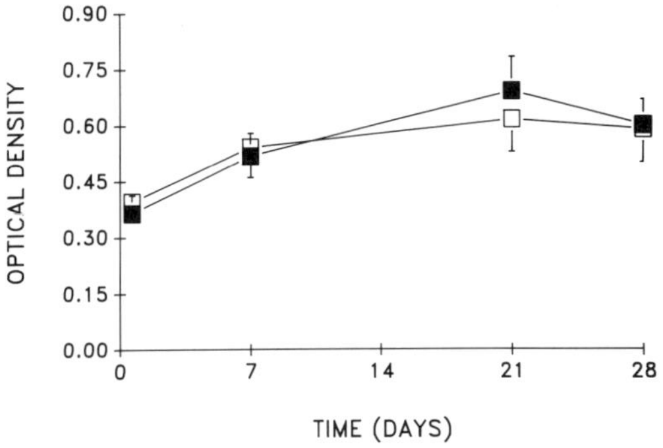

FIGURE 4. Serum IgG response to *C. jejuni* acid-extracted proteins in well (□) and ill (■) infected volunteers.

after exposure to strain A3249 (Fig. 5). Similar differences were seen in IgM and IgG responses.

The immunologic responses of the nine volunteers who became ill and were subsequently rechallenged with homologous strains were studied separately. During the initial illness in these nine volunteers, levels of all three Ig classes rose and had begun to fall by the day of rechallenge on day 28 (Fig. 6). However, the levels of all three Igs were significantly higher at day 28 than they had been prior to challenge. Following rechallenge, there were no additional rises in antibody levels in serum.

Jejunal fluid aspirates were also assessed for *C. jejuni*-specific IgA. The prechallenge levels of intestinal IgA were higher in the group that remained well after challenge than they were in the group that developed illness (Fig. 7), but this difference was not significant ($P > 0.05$). The groups of ill and well volunteers had comparable rises in intestinal IgA levels after challenge. Of the 32 ill volunteers, 9 were rechallenged with the homologous strain of *C. jejuni* on day 28 after the initial challenge. In these volunteers, the levels of intestinal IgA rose on day 11 after challenge and further by day 28. At that time, the IgA levels were similar to the prechallenge levels in the group of volunteers who remained well after the initial challenge. None of the nine rechallenged volunteers became ill, but they did have a further rise in intestinal IgA levels.

Immune Responses to *C. jejuni* LPS

ELISA was used to assay for antilipopolysaccharide (anti-LPS) antibody; serum specimens were evaluated for levels of IgA, IgG, and IgM, and jejunal fluid was evaluated for IgA. The antigen used was prepared from strain 81-176 as described by Blaser and Perez-Perez (this volume). The 2-keto-3-deoxyoctanoate concentration in the phenol-water-extracted LPS preparation was 5.7%, and the protein contamination was 0.87%. By sodium dodecyl sulfate-polyacrylamide gel electrophoresis with 15% acrylamide, silver stain resolved a single band for the LPS preparation. For the ELISA, 1.25 μg of the LPS preparation was used to coat each microtiter plate well. After blocking the plates, 100 μl of serum was placed in each well in triplicate in the following dilutions: IgA, 1:50; IgG, 1:100; IgM, 1:200. Peroxidase conjugates of class-specific goat anti-human Igs (Tago, Burlingame, Calif.) were used, and optical densities were assessed using a Titertek Multiscan (Dynatech Laboratories, Alexandria, Va.). Seroconversion was defined as a rise in optical density of >0.2 U from the prechallenge serum sample in any of the 7-, 21-, or 28-day serum samples. The optical density threshold value was defined to be more than 3 standard deviations from the mean optical density of 25 prechallenge serum samples.

Of the 111 volunteers, 39 were fed *C. jejuni* 81-176, from which the ELISA antigen was derived (homologous group), and 72 volunteers were fed strain A3249 (heterologous group). In 18 of the 39 volunteers in the homologous challenge group, there were 7 IgA, 10 IgG, and 8 IgM seroconversions (Table 4). Of the 18 volunteers who seroconverted in the homologous group, 8 (44%) seroconverted in two Ig classes. All of these eight double seroconverters had a rise in IgG levels, while four each had a rise in IgA and IgM levels. In 18 of the 72 volunteers challenged with A3249 and tested with the heterologous antigen, there were 11 IgA, 6 IgG, and 4 IgM seroconversions. Only 4 (22%) of the 18 volunteers who seroconverted in this group converted in two Ig classes. One of these four volunteers con-

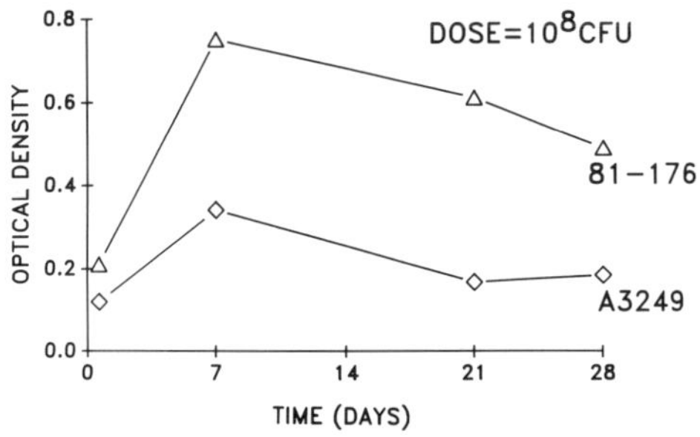

FIGURE 5. Serum IgA response to *C. jejuni* acid-extracted proteins in all volunteers ingesting strains A3249 and 81-176.

TABLE 4. Seroconversion to *Campylobacter* LPS[a] in 111 volunteers challenged with *C. jejuni* strains

Dose (CFU)	No. of volunteers	No. (%) of volunteers with seroconversion		
		IgA	IgG	IgM
Strain 81-176				
1 × 10⁶	7	2 (28.6)	4 (57.1)	2 (28.6)
1 × 10⁸	10	1 (10.0)	1 (10.0)	1 (10.0)
1 × 10⁹	22	4 (18.2)	5 (22.7)	5 (22.7)
Total	39	7 (17.9)	10 (25.6)	8 (20.5)
Strain A3249				
0.4–5.0 × 10⁴	33	5 (15.1)	5 (15.1)	2 (6.1)
0.8–1.0 × 10⁶	30	4 (13.3)	0 (0)	2 (6.7)
1.0 × 10⁸	9	2 (22.2)	1 (11.1)	0 (0)
Total	72	11 (15.3)	6 (8.3)	4 (5.5)

[a] Derived from strain 81-176.

verted in all three classes. The rate of seroconversion was significantly greater in the homologous group than in the heterologous group ($P < 0.05$), as was the rate of seroconversion to two Ig classes ($P < 0.05$). However, for both groups the seroconversion rates were not dose dependent.

The mean optical densities for the IgA (Fig. 8), IgG, and IgM assays were compared for the homologous and heterologous groups. For IgA, there were no significant differences between the mean optical densities at any sampling point for the two groups of volunteers; however, the homologous group had a consistently higher mean optical density at each datum point. In both groups, the IgA level peaked at day 7 postchallenge and declined to the baseline value by day 28. Neither group of volunteers demonstrated a serologic response assessed by mean optical density in IgM or IgG.

Volunteers who ingested strain 81-176 were divided into two groups: those who became ill and those who remained well (Fig. 9). The ill group had a significant increase in specific IgA levels which peaked at day 7 and dropped to baseline by day 28. The well group, all of whom were infected with *C. jejuni,* had a much smaller rise in IgA levels at day 7 ($P = 0.01$). Mean levels of their IgA antibody did not increase significantly. In volunteers fed the homologous strain, the severity of illness was rated on a scale of 0 to 5, based on the quantity and consistency of diarrheal stools, fever, and associated symptoms. The volunteers were stratified by serologic response to determine whether there was an association between disease severity and serologic

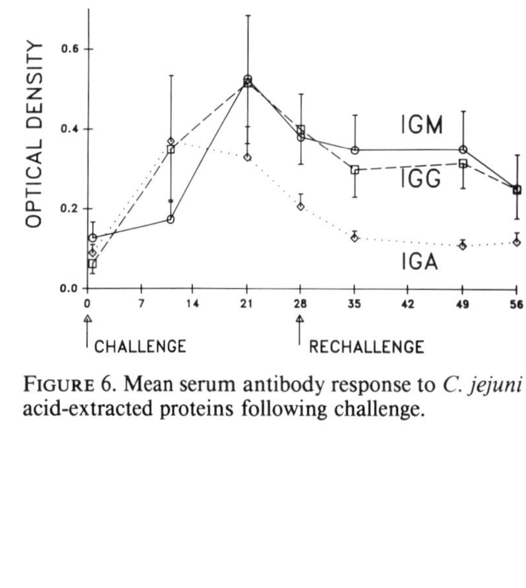

FIGURE 6. Mean serum antibody response to *C. jejuni* acid-extracted proteins following challenge.

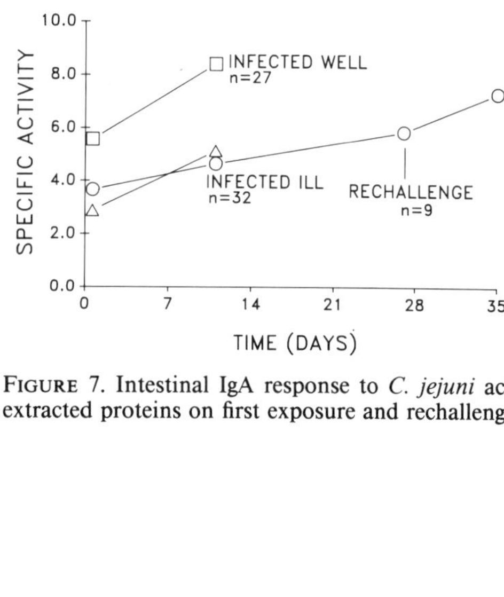

FIGURE 7. Intestinal IgA response to *C. jejuni* acid-extracted proteins on first exposure and rechallenge.

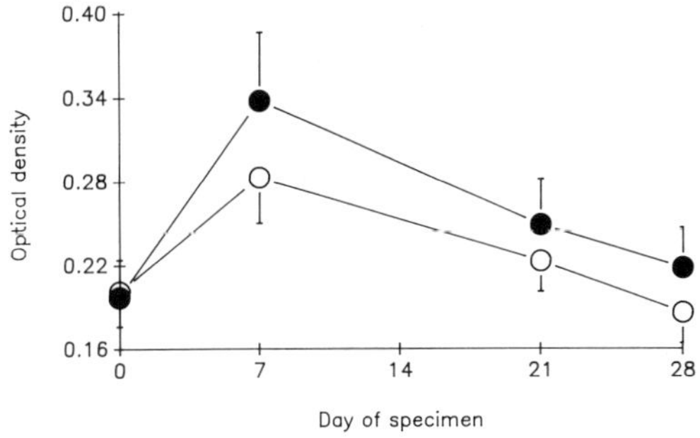

FIGURE 8. Serum IgA anti-LPS antibodies in 111 volunteers following challenge with *C. jejuni.* Symbols: ●, homologous challenge ($n = 39$); ○, heterologous challenge ($n = 72$).

response. There were no significant relationships between the severity of illness and the magnitude of the serologic response for any immunologic class.

Seven volunteers who became ill when fed strain 81-176 on initial challenge were rechallenged with the same strain 28 days later. Of these seven volunteers, five of whom became infected but none became ill, two had a rise in anti-LPS IgA and IgM levels after challenge; both of these persons had previously seroconverted after initial challenge.

OPSONIC ACTIVITY OF VOLUNTEER SERUM SAMPLES

To better understand the functional activity of the antibodies present in the serum samples from the volunteers, the ability of the sera to opsonize *C. jejuni* 81-176 was measured in a chemiluminescent (CL) assay (3, 4). To independently assess the effect of antibody and complement, serum samples were heated at 56°C for 30 min to inactivate complement, and a standard complement source from a hypogammaglobulinemic patient was added to each (Fig. 10). Normal human serum was a pool from three healthy persons uninfected with *C. jejuni* (2), and as a positive control, convalescent-phase serum from a volunteer infected with 81-176 who developed high IgG levels as measured by ELISA was used (1). All experiments were performed in triplicate on at least two separate days. The ratio of bacteria to neutrophils was 100:1.

In the absence of complement activity, antibodies present in normal human serum or in immune serum (data not shown) had no effect on CL response, and the complement source alone had a minimal effect. Adding back the complement source to the normal serum had little CL effect, but induced a strong CL response for the immune serum. In other experiments, the major activity of the immune serum was related to neutrophil ingestion of the organism, since pretreatment of the neutrophils with sodium fluoride blocked most of the CL response (data not shown).

Since homologous immune serum induced a strong response, the strain specificity of this response was assessed. Serum samples from the volunteers infected with strain A3249 (heterologous strain) were compared with those from the volunteers infected with strain 81-176 (homologous strain). In the presence of a complement source, as expected, the convalescent-phase serum to the homologous strain induced a strong

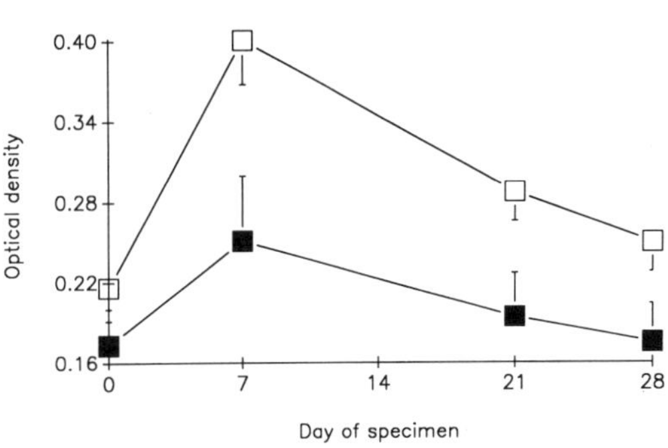

FIGURE 9. Serum IgA anti-LPS antibodies in well (■; $n = 17$) and ill (□; $n = 22$) volunteers infected with *C. jejuni* 81–176.

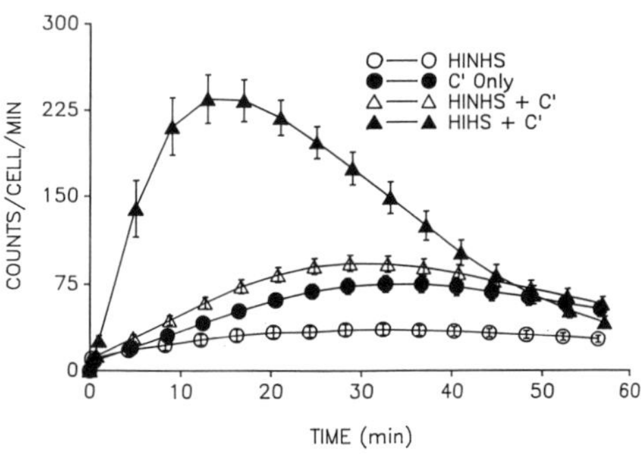

FIGURE 10. Polymorphonuclear cell CL response to *C. jejuni* 81-176 preopsonized with one of several serum sources. Abbreviations: HINHS, heat-inactivated normal human serum; C′, complement source (serum sample from a hypogammaglobulinemic patient); HIHS, heat-inactivated immune human serum (convalescent-phase serum from a patient infected with strain 81-176).

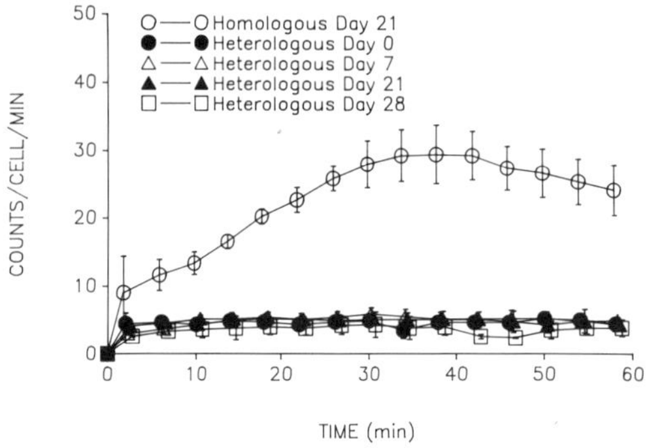

FIGURE 11. Polymorphonuclear cell CL response to *C. jejuni* 81-176 preopsonized with serum samples from volunteers challenged with strain 81-176 (homologous) or strain A3249 (heterologous). All serum samples were heat inactivated, and an exogenous complement source was added. Days refer to the number of days after *C. jejuni* challenge that serum samples were obtained.

response (Fig. 11), whereas serum samples from patients infected with the heterologous strain did not. These data suggest that infection induced strain-specific opsonizing activity.

To determine the kinetics of opsonizing activity in serum in the volunteers, serum samples from seven volunteers who were challenged (on day 0) and then rechallenged with strain 81-176 on day 28 were examined. Figure 12 shows the mean maximal values for the CL responses. Over the course of the first challenge, CL responses increased progressively until day 28. Upon rechallenge, which induced infection but not illness, CL responses declined. Therefore, homologous rechallenge did not boost the level of opsonizing activity in serum.

The data from the CL experiments indicate that the antibodies induced after *C. jejuni* infection not only recognize specific *C. jejuni* antigens, but also have opsonic activity. Such antibodies may play a role in vivo in permitting the elimination of extracellular *C. jejuni* within tissue. Normal serum apparently has little opsonizing activity, as does immune serum directed against the heterologous strain. The antigenic determinants inducing opsonizing activity are not known but are apparently strain specific. That homologous opsonizing activity rose progressively after *C. jejuni* challenge is not surprising; however, the lack of a booster response after rechallenge must be explained. One possibility is that the opsonizing antibodies are chiefly IgG and IgM, as they are after other infections. The development of effective gut immunity as measured by specific serum and intestinal IgA responses (as shown in Fig. 1 through 9) may have precluded tissue involvement that would lead to stimulation of IgG- or IgM-producing cells. Such a hypothesis has been proposed to explain the development of immunity to *C. jejuni* and falling specific IgG levels among children who are recurrently exposed to the organism under hyperendemic conditions in developing countries (2, 5).

CONCLUSIONS

Volunteer studies in healthy adults demonstrated that diarrheal (usually dysenteric) illnesses can be induced by ingestion of *C. jejuni.* With doses ranging from 8×10^2 to 2×10^9 CFU of two strains of *C. jejuni,* the rates of infection increased with the dose, but development of illness did not show a clear dose relationship. The resulting illness was more severe with strain 81-176 than with strain A3249. The dysenteric illness and presence of fecal leukocytes indicate that the pathogenesis of *C. jejuni* illness includes inflammation.

Protective immunity from prior disease was found when volunteers were rechallenged with the same strain 28 days later. Immunologic responses to acid-extracted proteins and to LPS after challenge with *C. jejuni* were assessed, and the opsonic activity of serum samples from the volunteers was evaluated by a CL assay, to better understand the functional activity of antibodies. Volunteers who became infected, but not those who remained uninfected, had a rise by day 7

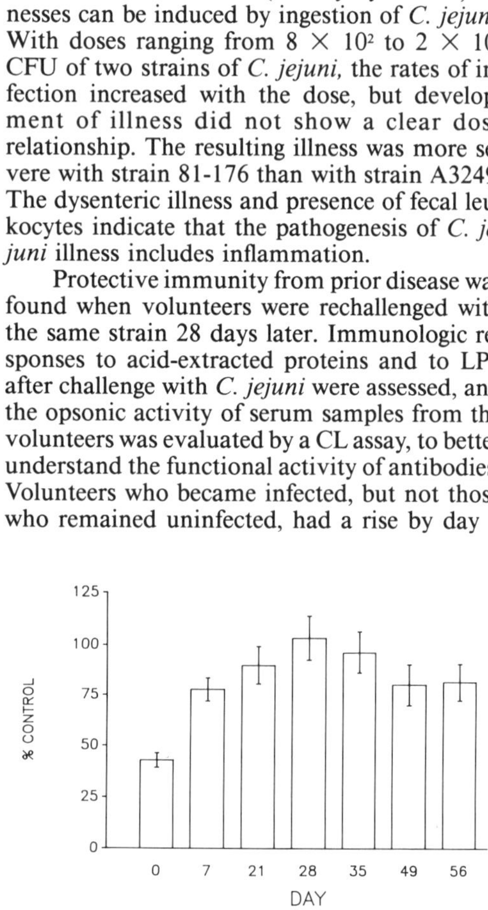

FIGURE 12. Polymorphonuclear cell CL response to *C. jejuni* 81-176 preopsonized with serum samples obtained from volunteers who were both challenged (day 0) and rechallenged (day 28) with strain 81-176. Data shown are mean (± standard error of the mean) maximal CL responses (counts per cell per minute) in comparison with a standard positive control.

in levels of serum IgA to acid-extracted proteins, and volunteers who became ill had higher peak levels. The serum immune response was greater for volunteers receiving strain 81-176. Infected volunteers also had a rise in intestinal *C. jejuni*-specific IgA levels. Volunteers with a high preexisting serum IgA level to acid-extracted proteins were less likely to become infected after challenge, and those with higher preexisting levels of intestinal IgA tended to remain well upon challenge. Volunteers who became infected had a rise in levels of serum IgA to LPS by day 7, and ill volunteers had higher peak levels. The serum immune response was greater against the homologous LPS (antigen from 81-176 used) than against the heterologous LPS. Postchallenge serum samples from volunteers induced a strong opsonizing activity, which appeared to be strain specific. It is likely that the antibodies induced by *C. jejuni* infection play a role by means of this opsonizing activity in eliminating the organism from tissue. Volunteer studies can be very useful for studying the serum and intestinal immune responses to *C. jejuni* infection and illness and can provide important insights into the extent and possible mechanisms of protection from prior exposure to *C. jejuni* or to artificial immunogens, such as candidate vaccines.

ACKNOWLEDGMENTS. We thank Paul F. Smith for technical assistance and John Repine for assistance with the CL studies. The work described in this chapter was supported in part by an interagency agreement between the U.S. Army Medical Research and Development Command and the Department of Veterans Affairs, by the Thrasher Research Fund, and by contract AI-12666 from the National Institute of Allergy and Infectious Diseases.

REFERENCES

1. **Black, R. E., M. M. Levine, M. L. Clements, T. P. Hughes, and M. J. Blaser.** 1988. Experimental *Campylobacter jejuni* infection in humans. *J. Infect Dis.* **157**:472–479.
2. **Blaser, M. J., R. E. Black, D. J. Duncan, and J. Amer.** 1985. *Campylobacter jejuni*-specific serum antibodies are elevated in healthy Bangladeshi children. *J. Clin. Microbiol.* **21**:164–167.
3. **Blaser, M. J., P. A. Smith, J. E. Repine, and K. A. Joiner.** 1988. Pathogenesis of *Campylobacter fetus* infections. Failure to bind C3b explains serum and phagocytosis resistance. *J. Clin. Invest.* **81**:1434–1444.
4. **Blaser, M. J., P. F. Smith, and P. A. Kohler.** 1985. Susceptibility of *Campylobacter* isolates to the bacterial activity in human serum. *J. Infect. Dis.* **151**:227–235.
5. **Blaser, M. J., D. N. Taylor, and P. Echeverria.** 1986. Immune response to *Campylobacter jejuni* in a rural community in Thailand. *J. Infect. Dis.* **153**:249–254.
6. **Blaser, M. J., D. N. Taylor, and R. A. Feldman.** 1983. Epidemiology of *Campylobacter jejuni* infections. *Epidemiol. Rev.* **5**:157–176.
7. **Calva, J. J., G. M. Ruiz-Palacios, A. B. Lopez-Vidal, A. Ramos, and R. Bojalil.** 1988. Cohort study of intestinal infection with *Campylobacter* in Mexican children. *Lancet* **i**:503–506.
8. **Levine, M. M., R. E. Black, M. L. Clements, C. Lanata, S. Sears, T. Honda, C. R. Young, and R. A. Finkelstein.** 1984. Evaluation in humans of attenuated *Vibrio cholerae* El Tor Ogawa strain Texas Star-SR as a live oral vaccine. *Infect. Immun.* **43**:515–522.
9. **Lior, H.** Personal communication.

CHAPTER 24

Immune Response to *Campylobacter* Flagellin

IRVING NACHAMKIN AND XIAO-HE YANG

INTRODUCTION

A number of studies have suggested that the flagellum of *Campylobacter jejuni* may be an important determinant in the ability of the organism to cause gastrointestinal infection. Flagella/motility variants have a reduced ability to infect a number of different animals (2, 6, 25, 34, 37). Flagella may, in part, play some role in adhesion to the gut surface (22–34), although motility may be the major determinant in the ability of *C. jejuni* to colonize intestinal mucus (14, 17, 34). Patients with *Campylobacter* infection develop serum and intestinal antibodies to several antigens (4, 13, 15, 38) including flagellin; flagellin is a major immunodominant protein during infection (19, 20, 28, 31). Several studies have shown that there is immunity after *Campylobacter* infection, and a few studies suggest that this protection may involve flagella (1, 2, 20, 27, 37). Thus, understanding the role of flagellin in the pathogenesis of infection and whether immune responses to flagellin are protective is crucial to developing strategies for preventing *Campylobacter* infections.

EXPERIMENTAL EVIDENCE

Animal Models

A number of studies have examined the role of *Campylobacter* flagella in experimental infections. Morooka et al. (25) mutagenized *C. jejuni* with *N*-methyl-*N'*-nitro-*N*-nitrosoguanidine or methyl methanesulfonate to produce flagella/motility variants that could be assessed for biologic activity in a mouse model of infection. Whereas the wild-type strains and mutants with intact flagella with altered mobility could colonize the mouse intestinal tract, mutants without flagella or with intact flagella but with loss of mobility were not able to do so.

In a study of motility variants by Caldwell et al. (6), using a rabbit model of infection, no differences were observed in the ability of Fla^+ and Fla^- organisms to cause illness in the animals. However, Fla^+ organisms were always excreted by rabbits inoculated with Fla^- organisms. These authors found that flagellin expression was reversible with a high frequency in vitro.

Work in our laboratory with a hamster model of infection (2) has also shown that the presence of intact flagella is important in infection. Aguero-Rosenfeld et al. (2) showed that 35 of 43 hamsters inoculated with a Fla^+ Mot^+ *C. jejuni* strain developed gastrointestinal infection whereas only 1 of 42 hamsters inoculated with a Fla^- Mot^- *C. jejuni* strain, derived from the wild type, developed infection. Although in vitro reversion from Fla^- to Fla^+ was not observed, reversion from Fla^- to Fla^+ occurred in vivo in eight animals challenged with up to 5×10^{10} CFU. Reversible expression of flagella in these studies was associated with antigenic variation of the flagellin protein.

Newell et al. (34) found that wild-type Fla^+ Mot^+ *C. jejuni* 81116 colonized the intestinal tract of mice whereas a Fla^- variant did not colonize as well as the parental strain. In contrast, a Fla^+ Mot^- variant colonized the gut as well as the wild-type strain did, suggesting that motility was the essential determinant in establishing colonization. Pavlovskis et al. (37) also found that an aflagellate mutant of *C. coli,* VC167, essentially did not colonize the rabbit gastrointestinal tract.

Human Infection

The role of flagella in pathogenesis in humans has not been studied directly. Black et al.

Irving Nachamkin and Xiao-He Yang, Department of Pathology and Laboratory Medicine, University of Pennsylvania School of Medicine, Philadelphia, Pennsylvania 19104–4283.

(3) found that human volunteers challenged with a mixture of motile and nonmotile colonies of *C. jejuni* A3249 excreted only colonies of the motile phenotype. This suggested that there was, at the very least, some selective advantage for the motile phenotype in human infection.

IMMUNE RESPONSES

Several studies of the immune response to flagellin indicate that the humoral response is important during infection and that antibodies directed against flagellin may have a protective effect.

Human Infection

Campylobacter flagellin appears to be an immunodominant protein during human infection. Western immunoblot analysis of serum samples from patients with *Campylobacter* infection show that flagellin is a major immunodominant protein in acute- and convalescent-phase sera (24, 28, 41). Work in our laboratory showed that different patterns of reactivity were found when different serum samples were tested (28). In most serum samples, antiflagellin antibodies were detected in acute- and convalescent-phase sera, and flagellin was immunodominant in the latter. Antibodies to other outer membrane proteins were clearly detected, especially in convalescent-phase serum samples; however, these proteins did not appear as immunogenic as flagellin. In another study, we measured the isotype-specific human antibody response to *Campylobacter* flagellin (31). Serum samples from patients with gastrointestinal infection caused by *C. jejuni* ($n = 20$) and controls ($n = 40$) including healthy individuals and patients with diarrheal illness due to other causes were tested by an enzyme-linked immunosorbent assay (ELISA). Patients with *Campylobacter* infection had significantly higher serum levels of immunoglobulin G (IgG), IgA, and IgM to flagellin than did controls ($P < 0.001$) for all isotypes.

Martin et al. (19) studied the antibody response to *C. coli* in children from the Central African Republic. By Western immunoblot, flagellin was also found to be immunodominant in patients. In patients with *Campylobacter* infection (symptomatic or asymptomatic), antibody responses to flagellin were detected in most patients. Children with diarrheal illness had higher levels of anti-flagellin antibodies than did asymptomatic children. In a study of the immune response in a cohort of children in the Central African Republic studied by Martin et al. (20), levels of antiflagellin antibodies decreased between birth and 3 months of age, with a subsequent increase between 6 and 9 months of age. This effect was also seen when acid-glycine extracts, which also contain considerable amounts of flagellin antigen, were used as the antigen. There was an inverse relationship between antibody responses to flagellin and diarrheal disease in infants during the first 6 months of life, suggesting that flagellin antibodies had a protective effect on intestinal infection. Children who did not have *Campylobacter* infection in the first 6 months of life had higher levels of antiflagellin antibodies at birth than did those who became infected.

A recent study by Ruiz-Palacios et al. (39) showed that breast-feeding had a protective effect on preventing *Campylobacter* infections in newborns living in an urban Mexican city. This protection was associated with breast milk antibodies to acid-glycine, of which flagellin is a major component. We recently studied the role of breast-feeding and specific antibodies against *Campylobacter* flagellin in preventing infection in newborns (27). We studied the relationship between the presence of IgA anti-*Campylobacter* flagellin antibodies in breast milk samples and protection from *Campylobacter* infection of breast-fed infants living in a rural Mexican village. The details of this cohort study have recently been published by Cravioto et al. (7). Thirty-five infants (from a cohort of 75) who were breast-fed during the first year of life were compared with 10 control infants from the same cohort, who were not breast-fed or were weaned during the first month of life. Approximately 15 breast milk samples collected from each infant's mother during the first year were analyzed for IgA content and anti-*Campylobacter* flagellin antibody activity. There were fewer episodes of *Campylobacter* infection in breast-fed infants than in controls ($P = 0.007$), and protection was associated with antibody activity. Fewer episodes of *Campylobacter* infection occurred in infants whose mothers' breast milk showed antiflagellin antibody activity than occurred in controls ($P = 0.005$). There was no difference in episodes of *Campylobacter* infection in infants whose mothers' breast milk did not have antibody activity and control infants ($P = 0.082$). We concluded from this study that breast-feeding is an important deterrent to *Campylobacter* infection and that antiflagellin antibodies may be important in passive protection against infections in breast-fed infants.

Local Immunity

Few studies have been performed to examine the specific intestinal antibody response to *Campylobacter* infection. In a brief study by Lane et al. (16), the time course of intestinal IgA response in acute *Campylobacter* enteritis was examined. The peak IgA levels as determined by ELISA occurred 6 to 10 days postinfection. Most patients had detectable antibody 1 to 5 days after the acute onset of disease; the level of antibody declined rapidly after 6 to 10 days. Patients with *Campylobacter* infection also exhibited rapid rises in IgA levels in serum after infection. Similar results were reported by Burr et al. (5) using a rabbit model of infection. Mascart-Lemone et al. (21) showed that IgA levels in serum peaked approximately 2 weeks after infection, that polymeric IgA accounted for the majority of the IgA response in serum in early infection, and that the level of polymeric IgA decreased over several weeks.

Windsor et al. (42) examined the secretory IgA response to *Campylobacter* antigens by using Western blot analysis. Stool samples from eight patients with diarrhea due to *Campylobacter* infection and five healthy individuals were tested. Antibodies to flagellin were observed in five of eight patients. Other reactions to outer membrane proteins were also observed in most of the stool samples tested.

We recently studied the local IgA antibody response to flagellin in patients with culture-documented *Campylobacter* infection and in patients with infection due to other pathogens (32). We used an ELISA to measure the level of IgA antiflagellin antibodies as previously described (31), except that stool filtrates were tested at a concentration of 6.7 μg of IgA per ml and diluted in buffer containing 100 μg of phenylmethylsulfonyl fluoride per ml as a protease inhibitor. Patients with *Campylobacter* infection (n = 29) had similar mean IgA concentrations in their stools (61.6 mg/dl; 95% confidence interval, 50.4 to 72.8) to those for control subjects (n = 11) (mean, 48.2 mg/dl; 95% confidence interval, 22.6 to 73.8). This is not statistically significant. When the specific IgA antibody activity directly against flagellin was measured, the mean ELISA optical density (OD) was significantly higher in patients (0.338, 95% confidence interval, 0.109 to 0.567) than in controls (0.051; 95% confidence interval, 0.004 to 0.098) (P = 0.020). Only 12 of 29 patients (41.4%) with *Campylobacter* infection had specific IgA antibodies against flagellin (OD, ≥0.100), with a mean value of 0.755 (95% confidence interval, 0.265 to 1.25). It was possible that in patients who did not exhibit an antibody response, the lack of reactivity was due to a type-specific antibody response. Since our ELISA uses an antigen preparation from a single strain (Lior 7), we decided to test different filtrate samples from patients against their homologous and heterologous flagellins. Filtrates from 10 patients with *Campylobacter* infection were tested against a panel of 10 homologous and heterologous flagellins (Table 1). In only one instance was the ELISA OD highest for the homologous flagellin compared with the heterologous proteins, suggesting type specificity. Several samples that did not exhibit detectable IgA antiflagellin antibodies in the initial ELISA also lacked detectable antibody when the homologous and heterologous flagellins were used. Since the samples were obtained during the first week after the onset of symptoms, it was likely that the lack of reactivity was due to the timing of specimen collection in the early phase of infection before the patients had mounted a local immune response. However, of the other positive samples, cross-reactivity was not seen with all heterologous proteins. Interestingly, we did not find a correlation between the Lior serotype of the strain and cross-reactivity of the flagellin antigens. These data suggest that in acute infection, the local response may be type specific or restricted in cross-reactivity with flagellin epitopes. Additional studies are needed with a larger number of patients with acute infection to better assess the nature of local immune responses.

Animals

Ueki et al. (40) pretreated suspensions of *C. jejuni* with different monoclonal antibodies directed against the flagellum and examined the ability of antibody-treated organisms to colonize the suckling ddY mouse intestinal tract. Mice inoculated with 1.9×10^4 CFU of *C. jejuni* pretreated with an IgM monoclonal antiflagellin antibody were protected from colonization, but the protective effect could be overcome by using a higher concentration of treated bacteria such that up to 100% of mice became colonized when 1.9×10^6 CFU per mouse was used. An IgA monoclonal antibody against flagellin also had a protective effect, but to a lesser degree than the IgM antibody did. Of 20 mice inoculated with 1.9×10^4 CFU of treated bacteria per ml, 6 became colonized. In contrast, mice inoculated with untreated bacteria were easily colonized at 35 to 50 CFU/ml. Rabbit polyclonal antiflagella antisera only weakly inhibited colonization, with 8 of 20 animals colonized at 35 CFU of

TABLE 1. Intestinal IgA anti-*Campylobacter* flagellin antibody reactivity directed against homologous and heterologous flagellin antigens in patients with *Campylobacter* infection[a]

Antigen (Lior type)	ELISA OD of stool sample from patient no:									
	1	2	3	4	5	6	7	8	9	10
1 (36)	<u>0.10</u>[b]	0.03	0.24	0.00	0.16	2.00	1.69	0.37	0.46	2.00
2 (8)	0.06	<u>0.03</u>	0.19	0.01	0.23	2.00	1.66	0.72	0.37	2.00
3 (36)	0.08	0.04	<u>0.19</u>	0.06	0.16	2.00	1.49	0.23	0.66	2.00
4 (36)	0.11	0.04	0.29	<u>0.00</u>	0.16	2.00	2.00	0.63	0.65	2.00
5 (36)	0.09	0.02	0.12	0.02	<u>0.10</u>	0.69	0.29	0.09	0.21	0.46
6 (36)	0.01	0.00	0.06	0.00	0.00	<u>0.30</u>	0.12	0.04	0.03	0.26
7 (NT)[c]	0.11	0.01	0.11	0.02	0.08	0.95	<u>0.60</u>	0.16	0.14	0.79
8 (36, 4)	0.24	0.07	0.18	0.04	0.27	1.64	0.31	<u>0.30</u>	0.31	1.33
9 (8)	0.09	0.06	0.36	0.01	0.38	2.00	1.67	0.92	<u>1.00</u>	2.00
10 (NT)	0.07	0.02	0.13	0.00	0.09	1.12	0.64	0.16	0.22	<u>1.20</u>

[a] From reference 32.
[b] Underline indicates ELISA OD with the patient's homologous antigen.
[c] NT, nontypable (Lior serotyping kindly performed by Charlotte Patton, Centers for Disease Control).

treated bacteria per ml and 100% colonization at 6.0 × 10³ CFU/ml.

Abimiku and Dolby (1) studied the role of heat-labile antigens detected by the Lior serotyping scheme in protection of infant mice against gut colonization. Although the determinants of this scheme have not been clearly defined, flagellin is a determinant in some serotypes (41). Adult female mice were immunized with live *C. jejuni* cells and were mated after vaccination. Their infant mice were challenged with live *C. jejuni* cells of either the homologous or heterologous strain, matched for heat-labile (Lior) or heat-stable (Penner) antigens. None of the infants were protected from oral challenge when the challenge strain matched the vaccine strain for the Penner serotype but not for the Lior type. However, when matched for the Lior type but not the Penner type, 43 to 77% protection was observed. More recently, Pavlovskis et al. (37) have shown similar results in cross-protection studies with a rabbit model of infection and have implicated the flagellum as the cross-strain protective component.

Aguero-Rosenfeld et al. (2) studied the serum antibody response of hamsters infected with flagellar variants of *C. jejuni.* All animals infected with the Fla⁺ strain developed serum antibodies to flagellin as well as to other outer membrane proteins. Animals infected with a variant that produced flagellin intracellularly but did not assemble into an intact flagellum did not develop antibodies after infection. In a preliminary study reported by Aguero-Rosenfeld et al. (2) and a subsequent experiment performed in our laboratory on protection (Nachamkin and Yang, unpublished data), seven of eight hamsters challenged with *C. jejuni* IN1 were protected from rechallenge by the homologous strain (Lior 7) but were not protected against rechallenge by a heterologous strain (Lior 2). Local IgA antibodies to flagellin were detected in three of four animals tested by ELISA compared with none of five age-matched uninfected controls (unpublished data).

Several studies have shown that coadministration of cholera toxin with antigen can stimulate stronger IgA responses to that antigen than if the antigen were administered alone. Cholera toxin acts as an immunoadjuvant and selectively stimulates IgA-producing antibody cells at the mucosal surface (10). To examine flagellin as a mucosal immunogen, we have performed some preliminary immunization experiments comparing flagellin alone and in combination with cholera toxin as an immunoadjuvant (Nachamkin and Yang, unpublished data). Hamsters were immunized with either flagellin (100 μg, intraduodenal) (n = 3), flagellin (100 μg) plus cholera toxin (10 μg) (n = 5), or CT alone (10 μg) (n = 5), using three immunizations. After the third immunization, intestinal contents were collected by the method of Elson et al. (8) and IgA antiflagellin levels were measured by ELISA. One of three animals immunized with flagellin alone developed detectable IgA levels compared with all five animals immunized with flagellin plus CT. None of the five animals immunized with CT alone developed detectable antiflagellin antibodies. Therefore, these experiments suggest that coadministration of CT with flagellin may be a useful strategy for mucosal immunization for assessing the protective effect of *Campylobacter* proteins.

EPITOPES OF FLAGELLIN

Flagellin is the subunit protein of the flagellar filament; it has an approximate molecular mass of 62 kDa and varies in molecular mass and charge depending upon the strain analyzed (26, 30). In wild-type strains, flagellin appears to be the product primarily of the gene *flaA* in both *C. jejuni* and *C. coli* (12, 18, 35). The nucleotide sequence for *flaA* has been determined for three different serotypes including *C. jejuni* 81116 (Lior 6) (35), *C. jejuni* IN1 (Lior 7) (9), and *C. coli* VC167 (Lior 8) (18). Based on analysis of the deduced amino acid sequence from all three flagellins, the common regions, C1 and C2, which make up the N terminus (residues 1 to 170) and C terminus (residues 477 to 576), respectively, are highly conserved, showing 94 and 96% conserved amino acid sequences, respectively. The internal variable sequence, V1 (residues 171 to 476), shows only a 61% conserved sequence (9). Computer analysis of predicted antigenic determinants shows that potentially surface-exposed regions are located in both the C and V regions, with the majority in the V1 region. Both serotype-specific and cross-reactive epitopes of flagellin have been described (29, 33, 36). Many of the type-specific epitopes are located within the V1 region, as recently described by Nuijten et al. (36) using monoclonal antibodies.

In a previous investigation we studied the immune response of infected patients to several synthetic peptides corresponding to flagellin sequences, one of which was reported previously (31). Two peptides within the N-terminal conserved region of *C. jejuni* IN1 are antigenic in some infected patients. To begin to identify potential protective epitopes of *Campylobacter* flagellin, we have used the strategy of Geysen et al. (11) to examine antigenic regions of FlaA by using synthetic peptide technology (I. Nachamkin, unpublished data). By synthesizing overlapping peptides that make up the amino acid sequence of flagellin, peptides can be screened with dif-

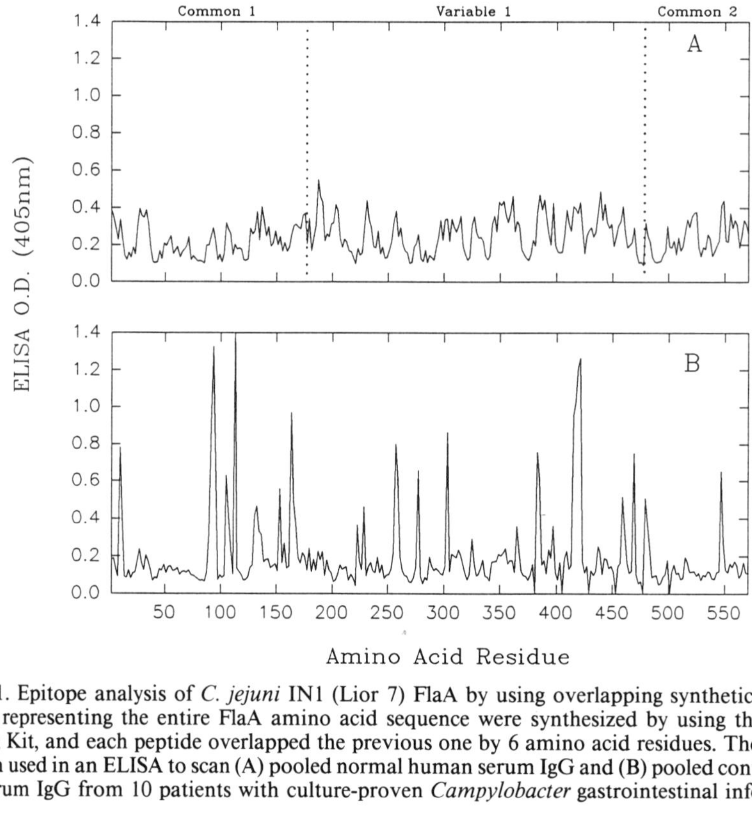

FIGURE 1. Epitope analysis of *C. jejuni* IN1 (Lior 7) FlaA by using overlapping synthetic peptides. Peptides representing the entire FlaA amino acid sequence were synthesized by using the Epitope Scanning Kit, and each peptide overlapped the previous one by 6 amino acid residues. The peptides were then used in an ELISA to scan (A) pooled normal human serum IgG and (B) pooled convalescent-phase serum IgG from 10 patients with culture-proven *Campylobacter* gastrointestinal infection.

ferent antibody preparations to identify sequences that may form some of the important protein epitopes. We prepared synthetic octapeptides that overlap by 6 amino acids, corresponding to the deduced amino acid sequence of *C. jejuni* IN1 (Lior 7) (9), by using the Epitope Scanning Kit (Cambridge Research Biochemicals, Wilmington, Del.) as specified by the manufacturer. Using this strategy, we prepared 285 overlapping peptides representing 570 amino acids of the FlaA from this strain. We used these peptides in an ELISA to measure the IgG activity in pooled human sera from 10 patients with documented *Campylobacter* infection and compared this with results for pooled normal human serum (Fig. 1). Specific sequences that reacted with polyclonal antiserum could be identified, whereas in normal human serum no specific sequences were identified. Further analysis of each individual serum sample should help to identify common and specific antigenic regions.

CONCLUSIONS

Campylobacter flagellin appears to be an important cell surface component involved in the pathogenesis of *Campylobacter* infection. Studies with humans and experimental animals show that gastrointestinal infection leads to immunity; however, this immunity is type specific. Patients with *Campylobacter* infection develop local IgA antibodies in response to infection; however, these responses must be better characterized. Strategies directed at vaccine development and immunoprophylaxis should include flagellin as a vaccine candidate, but protective epitopes of flagellin must be identified in future research activities.

ACKNOWLEDGMENT. Studies performed in our laboratory were supported in part by Public Health Service grant RO1-AI24122 from the National Institutes of Health.

REFERENCES

1. **Abimiku, A. G., and J. M. Dolby.** 1988. Cross-protection of infant mice against intestinal colonization by *Campylobacter jejuni:* importance of heat-labile serotyping (Lior) antigens. *J. Med. Microbiol.* **26:**265–268.
2. **Aguero-Rosenfeld, M. E., X.-H. Yang, and I. Nachamkin.** 1990. Infection of adult Syrian hamsters with flagellar variants of *Campylobacter jejuni. Infect. Immun.* **58:**2214–2219.
3. **Black, R. E., M. M. Levine, M. L. Clements, T. P. Hughes, and M. J. Blaser.** 1988. Experimental *Campylobacter jejuni* infections in humans. *J. Infect. Dis.* **157:**472–479.
4. **Blaser, M. J., and D. J. Duncan.** 1984. Human serum antibody response to *Campylobacter jejuni* infection as measured in an enzyme-linked immunosorbent assay. *Infect. Immun.* **44:**292–298.
5. **Burr, D. H., D. T. Kerner, C. S. Blanco, A. L. Bourgeois, and R. Wistar.** 1987. Gastric lavage: a simple method to obtain IgA rich intestinal secretions from the rabbit. *J. Immunol. Methods* **99:**277–281.
6. **Caldwell, M. B., P. Guerry, E. C. Lee, J. P. Burans, and R. I. Walker.** 1985. Reversible expression of flagella in *Campylobacter jejuni. Infect. Immun.* **50:**941–943.
7. **Cravioto, A., R. E. Reyes, F. Trujillo, F. Uribe, A. Navarro, J. M. De La Roca, J. M. Hernandez, G. Perez, and V. Vaszquez.** 1990. Risk of diarrhea during the first year of life associated with initial and subsequent colonization by specific enteropathogens. *Am. J. Epidemiol.* **131:**886–904.
8. **Elson, C. O., W. Ealding, and J. Lefkowitz.** 1984. A lavage technique allowing repeated measurement of IgA antibody in mouse intestinal secretions. *J. Immunol. Methods* **67:**101–108.
9. **Fischer, S. H., and I. Nachamkin.** 1991. Common and variable domains of the flagellin gene, flaA, in *Campylobacter jejuni. Mol. Microbiol.* **5:**1151–1158.
10. **Fuhrman, J. A., and J. J. Cebra.** 1981. Special features of the priming process for a secretory IgA response: B cell priming with cholera toxin. *J. Exp. Med.* **153:**534–544.
11. **Geysen, H. M., S. J. Rodda, T. J. Mason, G. Tribbick, and P. G. Schoofs.** 1987. Strategies for epitope analysis using peptide synthesis. *J. Immunol. Methods* **102:**259–274.
12. **Guerry, P., S. M. Logan, S. Thornton, and T. J. Trust.** 1990. Genomic organization and expression of *Campylobacter* flagellin genes. *J. Bacteriol.* **172:**1853–1860.
13. **Herbrink, P., H. A. M. van den Munckhof, M. Bumkens, J. Lindeman, and W. C. van Dijk.** 1988. Human serum antibody response to *Campylobacter jejuni* enteritis as measured by enzyme-linked immunosorbent assay. *Eur. J. Clin. Microbiol. Infect. Dis.* **7:**388–393.
14. **Hugdahl, M. B., J. T. Beery, and M. P. Doyle.** 1988. Chemotactic behavior of *Campylobacter jejuni. Infect. Immun.* **56:**1560–1566.
15. **Kaldor, J., H. Pritchard, A. Serpell, and W. Metcalf.** 1983. Serum antibodies in *Campylobacter* enteritis. *J. Clin. Microbiol.* **18:**1–4.
16. **Lane, E. M., R. A. Batchelor, A. L. Bourgeois, D. H. Burr, and J. G. Olson.** 1987. Urine and faecal IgA response during naturally acquired infection with *Campylobacter jejuni. Lancet* **i:**1141. (Letter.)
17. **Lee, A., J. L. O'Rourke, P. J. Barrington, and T. J. Trust.** 1986. Mucus colonization as a determinant of pathogenicity in intestinal infection by *Campylobacter jejuni:* a mouse cecal model. *Infect. Immun.* **51:**536–546.
18. **Logan, S. M., L. A. Harris, and T. J. Trust.** 1989. Evidence for posttranslational modification and

gene duplication of *Campylobacter* flagellin. *J. Bacteriol.* **171**:3031–3038.
19. **Martin, P. M. V., J. Mathiot, J. Ipero, A. J. Georges, and M. C. Georges-Courbot.** 1988. Antibody response to *Campylobacter coli* in children during intestinal infection and carriage. *J. Clin. Microbiol.* **26**:1421–1424.
20. **Martin, P. M. V., J. Mathiot, J. Ipero, M. Kirimat, A. J. Georges, and M.-C. Georges-Courbot.** 1989. Immune response to *Campylobacter jejuni* and *Campylobacter coli* in a cohort of children from birth to 2 years of age. *Infect. Immun.* **57**:2542–2546.
21. **Mascart-Lemone, F. O., J. R. Duchateau, J. Oosterom, J. P. Butzler, and D. L. Delacroix.** 1987. Kinetics of anti-*Campylobacter jejuni* monomeric and polymeric immunoglobulin A1 and A2 responses in serum during acute enteritis. *J. Clin. Microbiol.* **25**:1253–1257.
22. **McSweegan, E., D. H. Burr, and R. I. Walker.** 1987. Intestinal mucus gel and secretory antibody are barriers to *Campylobacter jejuni* adherence to INT407 cells. *Infect. Immun.* **55**:1431–1435.
23. **McSweegan, E., and R. I. Walker.** 1986. Identification and characterization of two *Campylobacter jejuni* adhesins for cellular and mucous substrates. *Infect. Immun.* **53**:141–148.
24. **Mills, S. D., and W. C. Bradbury.** 1984. Human antibody response to outer membrane proteins of *Campylobacter jejuni* during infection. *Infect. Immun.* **43**:739–743.
25. **Morooka, T., A. Umeda, and K. Amako.** 1985. Motility as an intestinal colonization factor for *Campylobacter jejuni. J. Gen. Microbiol.* **131**:1973–1980.
26. **Nachamkin, I., R.-H. Angeletti, and M. B. Prystowsky.** 1988. Biochemical similarity among serologically distinct flagellins of *Campylobacter jejuni. FEMS Microbiol. Lett.* **51**:149–152.
27. **Nachamkin, I., S. H. Fischer, X.-H. Yang, O. Benitez, and A. Cravioto.** 1990. Protective effect of breast milk immunoglobulin A anti-*Campylobacter* flagellin antibodies against *Campylobacter* infection in infants, abstr. B-50, p. 35. *Abstr. 90th Annu. Meet. Am. Soc. Microbiol. 1990.* American Society for Microbiology, Washington, D.C.
28. **Nachamkin, I., and A. M. Hart.** 1985. Western blot analysis of the human antibody response to *Campylobacter jejuni* cellular antigens during gastrointestinal infection. *J. Clin. Microbiol.* **21**:33–38.
29. **Nachamkin, I., and A. M. Hart.** 1986. Common and specific epitopes of *Campylobacter* flagellin recognized by monoclonal antibodies. *Infect. Immun.* **53**:438–440.
30. **Nachamkin, I., and X.-H. Yang.** 1988. Isoelectric focusing of *Campylobacter jejuni* flagellin: microheterogeneity and restricted antigenicity of charged species with a monoclonal antibody. *FEMS Microbiol. Lett.* **49**:235–238.
31. **Nachamkin, I., and X.-H. Yang.** 1989. Human antibody response to *Campylobacter jejuni* flagellin protein and a synthetic N-terminal flagellin peptide. *J. Clin. Microbiol.* **27**:2195–2198.
32. **Nachamkin, I., and X.-H. Yang.** 1992. Local immune responses to the *Campylobacter* flagellin in acute *Campylobacter* gastrointestinal infection. *J. Clin. Microbiol.* **30**:509–511.
33. **Newell, D. G.** 1986. Monoclonal antibodies directed against flagella of *Campylobacter jejuni:* cross-reacting and serotypic specificity and potential use in diagnosis. *J. Hyg.* **96**:377–384.
34. **Newell, D. G., H. McBride, and J. M. Dolby.** 1985. Investigations on the role of flagella in the colonization of infant mice with *Campylobacter jejuni* and attachment of *Campylobacter jejuni* to human epithelial cell lines. *J. Hyg.* **95**:217–227.
35. **Nuijten, P. J. M, F. J. Van-Asten, W. Gaastra, and B. A. M. van der Zeijst.** 1990. Structural and functional analysis of two *Campylobacter jejuni* flagellin genes. *J. Biol. Chem.* **265**:17798–17804.
36. **Nuijten, P. J. M., B. A. M. van der Zeijst, and D. G. Newell.** 1991. Localization of immunogenic regions of the flagellin proteins of *Campylobacter jejuni* 81116. *Infect. Immun.* **59**:1100–1105.
37. **Pavlovskis, O. R., D. M. Rollins, R. L. Haberberger, A. E. Green, L. Habash, S. Strocko, and R. I. Walker.** 1991. Significance of flagella in colonization resistance of rabbits immunized with *Campylobacter* spp. *Infect. Immun.* **59**:2259–2264.
38. **Rautelin, H. I., and T. U. Kosunen.** 1987. *Campylobacter* etiology in human gastroenteritis demonstrated by antibodies to acid extract antigens. *J. Clin. Microbiol.* **25**:1944–1951.
39. **Ruiz-Palacios, G. M., J. J. Calva, L. K. Pickering, Y. Lopez-Vidal, P. Volkow, H. Pezzarossi, and M. S. West.** 1990. Protection of breast fed infants against *Campylobacter* diarrhea by antibodies in human milk. *J. Pediatr.* **116**:707–713.
40. **Ueki, Y., A. Umeda, S. Fujimoto, M. Mitsuyama, and K. Amako.** 1987. Protection against *Campylobacter jejuni* infection in suckling mice by antiflagellar antibody. *Microbiol. Immunol.* **31**:1161–1171.
41. **Wenman, W. M., J. Chai, T. J. Louie, C. Goudreau, H. Lior, D. G. Newell, A. D. Pearson, and D. E. Taylor.** 1985. Antigenic analysis of *Campylobacter* flagellar protein and other proteins. *J. Clin. Microbiol.* **21**:108–112.
42. **Windsor, D. K., J. J. Mathewson, and H. L. DuPont.** 1986. Western blot analysis of intestinal secretory immunoglobulin A response to *Campylobacter jejuni* antigens in patients with naturally acquired *Campylobacter* enteritis. *Gastroenterology* **90**:1217–1222.

CHAPTER 25

Lipopolysaccharide Antigens of *Campylobacter jejuni*

S. D. MILLS, G. O. ASPINALL, A. G. McDONALD, T. S. RAJU, L. A. KURJANCZYK, AND J. L. PENNER

INTRODUCTION

Lipopolysaccharides (LPSs), also known as endotoxins, are well-recognized molecules in the outer membranes of gram-negative bacteria. They are important factors in enhancing the virulence of infectious bacteria, and they exert numerous deleterious effects on various physiological systems of the mammalian host. Interest in *Campylobacter jejuni* LPSs has centered mostly on their use in serotyping schemes as the serotypic markers for differentiating isolates in epidemiological studies (32, 33). Progress in determining the role of *C. jejuni* LPS in the pathogenic process has been hindered by a lack of information on the biological nature and chemical structure of the molecules. Recently fundamental work in addressing this deficiency has been forthcoming, but studies of the molecular biology of LPS have revealed unexpected features that suggest an LPS of a unique kind with hitherto unknown complexities. It was to gain insight into these complexities that collaborative projects were arranged to investigate the composition and detailed molecular structure of *C. jejuni* LPS. The results of preliminary research in this new area and a brief review of earlier work are the subject of this chapter.

PASSIVE HEMAGGLUTINATION TECHNIQUE FOR DETERMINING *CAMPYLOBACTER* O ANTIGENIC SPECIFICITIES

In attempts to O-serotype *C. jejuni* by the classical method, using the slide agglutination procedure, it was found that the heated cell suspensions tended to autoagglutinate and give nonspecific reactions (32). However, the passive (indirect) hemagglutination (PHA) technique was found to be very effective in differentiating isolates of *Campylobacter* species when antigenic extracts obtained from heated bacterial cell suspensions were used to sensitize the erythrocyte carrier (4, 10, 15, 29, 32). The PHA technique has been known since the 1950s to be highly sensitive and specific for the somatic O LPS antigens of gram-negative bacteria (6, 30). The erythrocytes may be sensitized with LPS extracted by the simple method of heating cell suspensions (15, 30, 32), by the method of Leive et al. (16, 32) with EDTA, or by the standard phenol-water method of Westphal and Jann (22, 42). The efficiency of the sensitization of mammalian erythrocytes with LPS is attributable to a lipoglycoprotein receptor on the erythrocyte which binds LPS (40). Washing of the LPS-sensitized erythrocytes removes less firmly bound or unbound proteins that may be present as impurities in the LPS preparation, further enhancing the specificity of PHA for LPS.

Since PHA utilizes extracted antigenic material rather than the suspensions of whole cells that are required in the classical slide agglutination technique, the extracted antigens from isolates to be serotyped, instead of the live bacteria, may be sent to the reference laboratory (14). PHA is a titration procedure, and the results of antigen-antibody reactions are expressed as titers, permitting the antigenic determinants (epitopes, O factors) of an isolate to be characterized by titer profiles. High titers identify major determinants, and low titers are interpreted to signify minor or cross-reacting determinants.

S. D. Mills, L. A. Kurjanczyk, and J. L. Penner, Department of Microbiology, University of Toronto, Toronto, Ontario, Canada M5G 1L5. **G. O. Aspinall, A. G. McDonald, and T. S. Raju,** Department of Chemistry, York University, North York, Toronto, Ontario, Canada M3J 1P3.

The PHA technique is considerably more labor intensive than is the classical slide agglutination test. However, it does not require the use of costly cross-absorbed typing antisera because routine serotyping is performed with unabsorbed antisera. In a simplified PHA procedure the titration step is omitted and the sensitized erythrocytes are typed by slide agglutination (34). The results obtained by the simplified technique are the same as those obtained by the complete PHA procedure for approximately 80% of the isolates. Both methods identify the major determinants, but discrepancies occur in the identification of minor cross-reacting determinants (unpublished observation). The simplified version is useful for discriminating among isolates in epidemiological studies in which the primary interest is to identify epidemic strains and for separating them from unrelated isolates. The complete PHA serotyping procedure is advocated for use in reference laboratories for infrasubspecific classification and comparison of isolates from different sources.

PROGRESS IN DEVELOPMENT OF A SEROTYPING SCHEME

Following the discovery in 1980 that serotyping of *C. fetus* subsp. *jejuni* by the PHA technique was feasible (32), the scheme was expanded to include new serotypes and later divided into separate schemes for *C. jejuni* and *C. coli* when evidence for the existence of the two species became available (33). Currently 48 antisera for *C. jejuni* and 19 for *C. coli* are used for serotyping in our laboratory. Altogether, 2,590 *C. jejuni* isolates and 332 *C. coli* isolates have been serotyped. Of the 2,590 *C. jejuni* isolates, 1,837 (71%) reacted in only one or another of the antisera and 653 (29%) reacted in two or more antisera. The most frequently occurring serovars that were characterized by a single determinant are O:2 (12%), O:4 (10%), O:1 (7.6%), and O:3 (7.1%), and the most frequently observed serovars that were identified by reactions in two or more antisera are O:6,7 (3.1%), O:23,36 (2.7%), O:13,16,50 (2.5%), O:13,16 (2.3%), and O:1,44 (2.2%). It was found that 79% of the *C. coli* isolates were identified by one antiserum, and for the 21% that were defined by two or more antisera the most common serovar was O:46,47 (3.3%). The most common serovars of *C. coli*, in decreasing frequency of isolation, are O:48 (10%), O:49 (8%), O:34 (7.8%), O:28 (7.5%), O:30 (7.5%), O:46 (6.9%), O:51 (6.3%), and O:39 (6.0%). There are 179 different serovars among the 2,590 *C. jejuni* isolates; 36 serovars have been identified among the 332 *C. coli* isolates.

APPLICATION OF SEROTYPING IN EPIDEMIOLOGICAL INVESTIGATIONS

The use of the serotyping schemes in epidemiological studies served the purpose of determining the sources and routes of transmission of *C. jejuni* and *C. coli* to humans (3, 5, 7, 20, 21, 35, 36). In this way it was established that a number of the serovars isolated from patients occurred also in farm animals, family pets, and environmental sources (25). Outbreaks of diarrhea were demonstrated to be due to epidemic strains (21) or to contact with animals (7). It was shown that some patients could be infected with two or more strains at the same time (13). Serovar distributions among isolates from patients in North America and the United Kingdom were similar, but were different from the distributions seen among isolates from individuals in developing nations (11, 12, 21). From untypable isolates recovered from patients in developing nations, new serovars that have not yet been shown to be present in patients from the United States and Canada were identified (unpublished observation).

Serotyping of isolates has also provided evidence for the occurrence of antigenic variation during maintenance of strains in the laboratory (23) and during the course of an infection (unpublished data).

MOLECULAR BIOLOGY OF LPS

In initial studies on the thermostable antigens of *C. jejuni* (32) it was believed that they were O antigens characteristic of gram-negative bacteria because they could be extracted by procedures commonly used to extract LPS and because they were capable of sensitizing sheep erythrocytes to render them agglutinable in specific antisera by PHA. However, more convincing evidence became available through a series of studies from a number of laboratories including our own. Jones et al. (10) and Mills et al. (22) showed that LPSs extracted from serotype reference strains (serostrains) possess the same serological specificities as the extracts that are obtained by heat treatment and used in the PHA technique for serotyping. Naess and Hofstad produced antisera against *C. jejuni* strains and showed that they had antibodies specific for the

LPS from the homologous strains (29). Logan and Trust demonstrated the presence of low-M_r LPS in *C. jejuni* strains by sodium dodecyl sulfate-polyacrylamide gel electrophoresis (SDS-PAGE) and immunoblotting and concluded that this material conferred the serological specificity (17). In a systematic examination of the *C. jejuni* serostrains, Preston and Penner found that approximately one-third possessed high-M_r bands characteristic of LPS with O side chains in addition to low-M_r LPS (37). Interestingly, the low-M_r LPS could be visualized in SDS-PAGE by the silver stain of Tsai and Frasch (41) and by immunoblotting with specific antisera, but the high-M_r molecules were visualized only by immunoblotting. The demonstration of the high-M_r LPS precluded the conclusion that *C. jejuni* possessed only the short-chain molecules characteristic of the lipooligosaccharides (LOSs) of *Neisseria* species (8, 19) and *Haemophilus* species (9). In immunoblotting experiments to investigate the basis of cross-reactions that occur between two serostrains (O:23 and O:36) of *C. jejuni* it was found that determinants common to both strains appeared to be located on the high-M_r LPS molecules (38).

In contrast to *C. jejuni,* the LPSs of the 18 serostrains of *C. coli* that were examined by Mandatori and Penner (18) all had both low- and high-M_r LPSs consistent with LPS that has O side chains. As with *C. jejuni,* the high-M_r LPS molecules were not demonstrable with the silver stain after SDS-PAGE but could be seen in immunoblots on treatment with homologous antisera. The chemical basis for the inability to silver stain the high-M_r LPS molecules of *C. jejuni* and *C. coli* is not known.

CHEMICAL COMPOSITION AND MOLECULAR STRUCTURE OF *C. JEJUNI* LOW-M_r LPS

As described above, investigations of the biological nature of *C. jejuni* LPS revealed the presence of silver-stainable low-M_r LPS in all strains of *C. jejuni,* but high-M_r LPS characteristic of LPS with O side chains occurred in only one-third of the *C. jejuni* serostrains (38). However, all strains, whether they possessed only low-M_r LPS or both low- and high-M_r LPS, were distinctly different in their antigenic specificities (37). The nature of the low-M_r LPSs and the basis for their serotypic specificities remained unclear.

To account for a large number of serovars with low-M_r LPS, each with recognizably different structure, it has been proposed that the core regions of relatively invariant structure might be terminated by a single O-antigen repeating unit, as in the semirough form of LPS (37). Alternatively, there could be an unusual degree of structural variation with short oligosaccharide chains in the core region of low-M_r LPS, as already shown for LPS of the known serotypes of some nonenterobacterial species. This type of low-M_r LPS has been referred to as lipooligosaccharide (LOS) and is reported to occur in *Neisseria meningitidis, N. gonorrhoeae,* and *Haemophilus influenzae* (8, 9, 19).

Attempts to find supporting evidence for the semirough structure by means of SDS-PAGE and immunoblotting were inconclusive (38), and it became evident that determination of the chemical structure at the molecular level was necessary to reveal the basis of the serotypic specificities of low-M_r LPS. To meet this objective, the phenol-water method of Westphal and Jann (42) was used to extract LPS from the O:1 serostrain, which does not possess high-M_r LPS, and from serostrains O:4, O:23, and O:36, which have been shown to possess both high- and low-M_r LPS (37, 38). The latter two serostrains were selected because they have been shown to cross-react by PHA and by immunoblotting (38). The extracted LPS was dialyzed and lyophilized in preparation for compositional and structural studies.

After further ultracentrifugation to purify the LPS, it was cleaved by controlled hydrolysis with acetic acid to produce oligosaccharides terminated with 2-keto-3-deoxyoctulosonic acid. Compositional analysis for sugars, 2-keto-3-deoxyoctulosonic acid, and noncarbohydrate substituents such as ethanolamine and phosphate was supported by the results of nondestructive ^{1}H, ^{31}P, and ^{13}C nuclear magnetic resonance spectroscopic examination. Enantiomeric configurations (D or L) of individual sugars were confirmed by analysis of chiral glycosides.

Structural studies of the core oligosaccharides, although not completed, have proceeded furthest with those of serovars O:1 and O:4. A very surprising observation at the outset of the investigations was the discovery of sialic acid (*N*-acetylneuraminic acid) as a frequent LPS constituent (1). Similar results had been obtained independently by Moran et al. (24). Since ketosidic linkages are acid sensitive, it was expected that some loss of sialic acid would occur during the process of liberating the core oligosaccharide from lipid A by heating the LPS in acetic acid. Further treatment of the isolated core oligosaccharide with acetic acid resulted in selective removal of the remaining sialic acid residues. In common with other LPSs, those from O:1 and O:4 carry attached phosphorylethanolamine.

Although the structures of O:1 and O:4 LPS remain less than fully defined with respect to fine-structure details, it is clear that both similarities and differences exist. They both have linked phosphorylethanolamine and sialic acid, but the latter differs in its location on the oligosaccharide. The terminal sugar for O:1 LPS is *N*-acetylgalactosamine, but for O:4 it is a nonacetylated hexose. The most marked difference, however, is in the sequences of the sugars. This, in combination with the modifying effects of the sialic acid on conformation of different sites, clearly indicates distinct tertiary structures for each oligosaccharide. It would appear, therefore, that sufficient variations in composition and structure are present to account for serotypic differences. In addition, serotypic diversity would be further augmented if variations in hexose side branches are shown to occur in future studies. In neither of these oligosaccharides was there evidence of an O repeating unit as would be expected if the structure was that of LPS in the semirough form.

Investigation of low-M_r LPS from the O:23 and O:36 serostrains revealed the unexpected occurrence of two different oligosaccharides in each of the LPS preparations. A unique oligosaccharide constituted 65% of the low-M_r LPS from the O:23 strain, and similarly a unique structure constituted 90% of the O:36 serostrain low-M_r LPS, but the unusual feature was the presence of an oligosaccharide that was common to both serostrains. It constituted the remaining 35% of the low-M_r LPS from the O:23 serostrain and 10% of the O:36 low-M_r LPS. The quoted percentages are approximate, since possible batch-to-batch variation has not yet been investigated.

In comparing the common oligosaccharide with the one exclusive to O:23, it would appear that the latter is an incomplete version of the common oligosaccharide because it lacks both sialic acid and phosphorylethanolamine and a proportion of the chains lack the terminal *N*-acetylglucosamine. In other respects, such as composition and sequence of sugars, they are indistinguishable. The oligosaccharide characteristic of low-M_r LPS from O:36 has a sequence of heptoses and hexoses different from those of the common oligosaccharide and from the one unique to O:23.

The three oligosaccharides liberated from the low-M_r LPS of O:23 and O:36 serostrains each contained glucose as internal and external units, but this sugar was present only as an external unit in the oligosaccharides of O:1 and O:4. For the oligosaccharides from O:23 and O:36, no evidence was obtained for the presence of the *N*-acetylglucosamine–galactose–heptose O repeating unit found in O:23 and O:36 high-M_r LPS (described below). Hence it is reasonable to conclude that, as with the O:1 and O:4 strains, low-M_r LPS does not have semirough-type LPS molecules.

Despite the similarities in sugar compositions that have been shown in this study and in earlier studies by others (2, 26–28), the detailed structures at the molecular level have revealed marked differences. There is a wide diversity not only in sequences, particularly in the sequences of the heptoses, but also in the types of linkages and in the presence or absence of glucose and *N*-acetylglucosamine. Moieties with this type of structural and antigenic diversity have been referred to as LOS (8, 19). However, the species that are recognized for their possession of LOS (8, 9, 19) do not have a counterpart to the high-M_r LPS seen in approximately one-third of the *C. jejuni* serostrains (37, 38).

COMPOSITION AND STRUCTURE OF THE HIGH-M_r LPS OF THE O:23 AND O:36 SEROSTRAINS

Detailed structural studies on the high-M_r LPS from serotypes O:23 and O:36 have shown that generally similar O-antigen chains are present. The situation is complicated by the fact that there is batch-to-batch variation in the structure of the repeat unit. Each O polysaccharide contains a trisaccharide repeating unit in which two of the three sugar residues (*N*-acetylglucosamine and galactose) are always the same but the third sugar residue is one of four similarly linked and stereochemically related heptose sugars. At this time only the O-antigen chain that contains 6-deoxy-D-*altro*-heptose as the third sugar residue has been firmly established. The absolute configurations of the other three heptose sugars have not yet been established unambiguously and are provisionally assigned by analogy. O-antigen chains carrying D-*glycero*-D-*altro* heptose as the heptose residue in the repeat unit have been found only in the LPS from O:36, and those carrying 6-deoxy-D-*altro*-heptose, 6-deoxy-3-*O*-methyl-D-*altro*-heptose, or 3-*O*-methyl-D-*glycero*-D-*altro*-heptose have been found in both O:23 and O:36. Studies have been initiated to determine whether the variety of repeat units is due to colony variation or to the ability of the organisms to synthesize more than one type of repeating unit. Preliminary results of composition studies appear to support the latter process.

In previously reported experiments by Preston and Penner (37) it was shown by PHA and immunoblotting that determinants located on the high-M_r LPS were the basis of the cross-reaction between O:23 and O:36 serostrains. Although the shared determinants have not been precisely identified, it is expected that the presence of polysaccharides with identical repeating units in LPS from both serotypes will constitute a major factor in contributing to the cross-reaction.

LINKAGE OF THE O-SIDE CHAIN TO CORE LPS

At present it is unknown which of the oligosaccharide moieties found in low-M_r LPS serve as the receptors for the O side chain. The polysaccharides found in the high-M_r LPS would be expected to be terminated at the end proximal to the bacterial surface by an oligosaccharide-lipid A moiety. The situation is complicated by the fact that this moiety would constitute such a very small proportion of the total mass of the polysaccharide that an analysis of its chemical structure would be very difficult. A final resolution may require the use of monoclonal antibodies prepared against the individual oligosaccharides found in the low-M_r LPSs of both the O:23 and O:36 serostrains. This may also shed light on the nature and function of the oligosaccharides. It is important to determine whether some strains of *C. jejuni* synthesize oligosaccharides of only the LOS type and others synthesize not only the LOS-type oligosaccharides but also oligosaccharides that have a primary role as receptors for the O polysaccharides. Another possibility that can be anticipated is that the O antigen is linked to both types of oligosaccharides.

Although it is well known that bacteria such as those of the family *Enterobacteriaceae* have LPS molecules varying in length from those of the rough Re form (lipid A and 2-keto-3-deoxyoctulosonic acid only) to the smooth form (lipid A, oligosaccharide, and O side chain) whereas *Neisseria* and *Haemophilus* species have only LOS, we are unaware of bacteria other than the *C. jejuni* strains under study that elaborate both classes of lipid-associated molecules. If these findings prove to be general throughout the species as more strains are studied, *C. jejuni* would be the first species to be characterized by this unusual complex of molecules.

SIGNIFICANCE OF SIALIC ACID

The importance of sialic acid, which is commonly present in mammalian glycoproteins and glycolipids and against which antibodies are not normally produced, is that it is likely to be a major virulence factor for this species. It has been shown that sialylation of gonococcal LPS causes inhibition of the reaction with serum bactericidal antibodies (39). A similar role may be anticipated for the sialylated LPS of *C. jejuni* whether or not this sugar is host generated, as in *N. gonorrhoeae* (39).

Cell suspensions of *C. jejuni,* whether live, heated, or unheated, do not agglutinate specifically in hyperimmune antisera used in serotyping (32). An advance in the field of serotyping would be an understanding of the nonspecificity of the slide test, and thus the possible role of sialic acid residues in masking the epitopes and creating steric hindrance to antibody binding must be investigated. Indeed, the presence of sialic acid may prove to be a contributing factor in other unexplained biological and immunological complexities.

CONCLUSIONS AND CHALLENGES FOR THE FUTURE

It has been observed previously that *Campylobacter* species have offered microbiologists many surprises and challenges (31). This also continues to be the experience of workers interested in *Campylobacter* LPSs. It appears that the bacteria are as much a treasure of novel and unexpected phenomena for the carbohydrate chemist as they are for the microbiologist.

Although much of the work is preliminary, the unanticipated discovery of sialic acid linked to the LPS is bound to attract investments of effort in determining the role of this material in virulence and pathogenesis. The biosynthesis of a variety of repeat units by the same strain suggests a hypervariability that may also be investigated as a possible factor in mediating its ability to evade the immune defenses of the host. The demonstration that the structure and composition of the low-M_r LPS resembles LOS more than it does the rough type of LPS characteristic of the family *Enterobacteriaceae* is a novel finding. Particularly puzzling is the observation that some strains possess the more typical high-M_r LPS with O side chains in addition to the LOS-like molecules. What is the genetic basis that enables the bacterium to synthesize both LOS-like molecules and typical LPS? Is the LOS-type molecule the receptor for the O side chains, or is the receptor an LPS core of different composition and structure? Although there is still much uncertainty about the nature of the LPS, one fact that does remain clear is that *C. jejuni* has again proved to reveal new and unexpected biological phenomena and, no doubt, will continue to do so.

ACKNOWLEDGMENTS. We are grateful to Trudy Carroll for typing the manuscript. The research described in this chapter is supported by separate strategic grants from the Natural Sciences and Engineering Research Council of Canada to G.O.A. and J.L.P.

REFERENCES

1. **Aspinall, G. O., A. G. McDonald, and T. S. Raju.** 1990. Lipopolysaccharides from *Campylobacter jejuni,* abstr. CO52, p. 354. *XVth Int. Carbohydr. Symp.* Yokohama, Japan.
2. **Beer, W., M. Adam, and G. Seltmann.** 1986. Monosaccharide composition of lipopolysaccharides from *Campylobacter jejuni* and *Campylobacter coli. J. Basic Microbiol.* **26:**201–204.
3. **Blaser, M. J., J. L. Penner, and J. G. Wells.** 1982. Diversity of serotypes in outbreaks of *Campylobacter* enteritis. *J. Infect. Dis.* **146:**826.
4. **Bokkenheuser, V.** 1972. *Vibrio fetus* infection in man: a serological test. *Infect. Immun.* **5:**222–226.
5. **Chan, F. T. H., A. M. R. MacKenzie, J. L. Penner, and J. N. Hennessy.** 1984. Usefulness of serotyping in the epidemiology of *Campylobacter jejuni* in family outbreaks. *J. Infect. Dis.* **150:**790.
6. **Eskenazy, M., and R. Cohen.** 1974. *Salmonella* O antigen-coated red blood cells as a stable reagent for passive hemagglutination tests. *J. Immunol. Methods* **6:**129–131.
7. **Fox, J. G., N. S. Taylor, J. L. Penner, B. Shames, R. V. Gurgis, and F. N. Tomson.** 1989. Investigation of zoonotically acquired *Campylobacter jejuni* enteritis with serotyping and restriction endonuclease DNA analysis. *J. Clin. Microbiol.* **27:**2423–2425.
8. **Griffiss, J. M., J. P. O'Brien, R. Yamasaki, G. D. Williams, P. A. Rice, and H. Schneider.** 1987. Physical heterogeneity of neisserial lipooligosaccharide reflects oligosaccharides that differ in apparent molecular weight, chemical composition, and antigenic expression. *Infect. Immun.* **55:**1792–1800.
9. **Inzana, T. J., W. E. Seifert, Jr., and R. P. Williams.** 1985. Composition and antigenic activity of the oligosaccharide moiety of *Haemophilus influenzae* type b lipooligosaccharide. *Infect. Immun.* **48:**324–330.
10. **Jones, D. M., A. J. Fox, and J. Eldridge.** 1984. Characterization of the antigens involved in serotyping strains of *Campylobacter jejuni* by passive hemagglutination. *Curr. Microbiol.* **10:**105–110.
11. **Karmali, M. A., J. L. Penner, P. C. Fleming, A. Williams, and J. N. Hennessy.** 1983. The serotype and biotype distribution of clinical isolates of *Campylobacter jejuni* and *Campylobacter coli* over a three year period. *J. Infect. Dis.* **147:**243–246.
12. **Lastovica, A. J., E. Le Roux, R. V. Congi, and J. L. Penner.** 1986. Distribution of serobiotypes of *Campylobacter jejuni* and *coli* isolated from paediatric patients. *J. Med. Microbiol.* **21:**1–5.
13. **Lastovica, A. J., E. Le Roux, and J. L. Penner.** 1986. Mixed infections with different species and serotypes of *Campylobacter. J. Infect. Dis.* **154:**375.
14. **Lastovica, A. J., R. L. Marshall, and J. L. Penner.** 1986. Campylobacter serotyping on shipped antigen extracts. *Lancet* **i:**320. (Letter.)
15. **Lauwers, S., L. Vlaes, and J. P. Butzler.** 1981. Campylobacter serotyping and epidemiology. *Lancet* **i:**158–159. (Letter.)
16. **Leive, L., V. K. Shovlin, and S. E. Mergenhagen.** 1968. Physical, chemical and immunological properties of lipopolysaccharide released from *Escherichia coli* by ethylenediaminetetraacetate. *J. Biol. Chem.* **243:**6384–6391.
17. **Logan, S. M., and T. J. Trust.** 1984. Structural and antigenic heterogeneity of lipopolysaccharides of *Campylobacter jejuni* and *Campylobacter coli. Infect. Immun.* **45:**210–216.
18. **Mandatori, R., and J. L. Penner.** 1989. Structural and antigenic properties of *Campylobacter coli* lipopolysaccharides. *Infect. Immun.* **57:**3506–3511.
19. **Mandrell, R., H. Schneider, M. Apicella, W. Zollinger, P. A. Rice, and J. M. Griffiss.** 1986. Antigenic and physical diversity of *Neisseria gonorrhoeae* lipooligosaccharides. *Infect. Immun.* **54:**63–69.
20. **McMyne, P. M. S., J. L. Penner, R. G. Mathias, W. A. Black, and J. N. Hennessy.** 1982. Serotyping of *Campylobacter jejuni* isolated from sporadic and outbreak cases in British Columbia. *J. Clin. Microbiol.* **16:**281–285.
21. **Melby, K., G. Storvold, R. V. Congi, and J. L. Penner.** 1985. Serotyping of *Campylobacter jejuni* isolated from sporadic cases and outbreaks in Northern Norway. *Acta Pathol. Microbiol. Immunol. Scand. Sect. B* **93:**83–86.
22. **Mills, S. D., W. C. Bradbury, and J. L. Penner.** 1985. Basis for serological heterogeneity of thermostable antigens of *Campylobacter jejuni. Infect. Immun.* **50:**284–291.
23. **Mills, S. D., L. A. Kurjanczyk, B. Shames, J. N. Hennessy, and J. L. Penner.** 1991. Antigenic shifts in serotypic determinants of *Campylobacter coli* are accompanied by changes in the chromosomal DNA restriction endonuclease digest pattern. *J. Med. Microbiol.* **35:**168–173.

24. **Moran, A. P., E. T. Rietschel, T. U. Kosunen, and U. Zahringer.** 1991. Chemical characterization of *Campylobacter jejuni* lipopolysaccharides containing *N*-acetylneuraminic acid and 2,3-diamino-2,3-dideoxy-*o*-glucose. *J. Bacteriol.* **173:**618–626.
25. **Munroe, D. L., J. F. Prescott, and J. L. Penner.** 1983. Serotypes of *Campylobacter jejuni* and *Campylobacter coli* isolated from chickens, cattle, and pigs. *J. Clin. Microbiol.* **18:**877–881.
26. **Naess, V., and T. Hofstad.** 1982. Isolation and chemical composition of lipopolysaccharide from *Campylobacter jejuni. Acta Pathol. Microbiol. Scand. Sect. B* **90:**135–139.
27. **Naess, V., and T. Hofstad.** 1984. Chemical composition and biological activity of lipopolysaccharides prepared from type strains of *Campylobacter jejuni* and *Campylobacter coli. Acta Pathol. Microbiol. Immunol. Scand. Sect. B* **92:**217–222.
28. **Naess, V., and T. Hofstad.** 1984. Chemical studies of partially hydrolysed lipopolysaccharides from four strains of *Campylobacter jejuni* and two strains of *Campylobacter coli. J. Gen. Microbiol.* **130:**2783–2789.
29. **Naess, V., and T. Hofstad.** 1985. Antigenicity of lipopolysaccharides from *Campylobacter jejuni* and *Campylobacter coli* in passive hemagglutination tests and enzyme-linked immunosorbent assays. *Acta Pathol. Microbiol. Immunol. Scand. Sect. C* **93:**97–104.
30. **Neter, E., L. F. Bertram, and C. E. Arbesman.** 1952. Demonstration of *Escherichia coli* O55 and O111 antigens by means of hemagglutination test. *Proc. Soc. Exp. Biol. Med.* **79:**255–257.
31. **Penner, J. L.** 1988. The genus *Campylobacter:* a decade of progress. *Clin. Microbiol. Rev.* **1:**157–172.
32. **Penner, J. L., and J. N. Hennessy.** 1980. Passive hemagglutination technique for serotyping *Campylobacter fetus* subsp. *jejuni* on the basis of heat-stable antigens. *J. Clin. Microbiol.* **12:**732–737.
33. **Penner, J. L., J. N. Hennessy, and R. V. Congi.** 1983. Serotyping of *Campylobacter jejuni* and *Campylobacter coli* on the basis of thermostable antigens. *Eur. J. Clin. Microbiol.* **2:**378–383.
34. **Penner, J. L., J. N. Hennessy, and R. V. Congi.** 1984. A simplified procedure for serotyping *Campylobacter jejuni* and *Campylobacter coli,* abstr. C-52, p. 245. *Abstr. 84th Annu. Meet. Am. Soc. Microbiol. 1984.* American Society for Microbiology, Washington, D.C.
35. **Penner, J. L., J. N. Hennessy, S. D. Mills, and W. C. Bradbury.** 1983. Application of serotyping and chromosomal restriction endonuclease digest analysis in investigating a laboratory-acquired case of *Campylobacter jejuni* enteritis. *J. Clin. Microbiol.* **18:**1427–1428.
36. **Penner, J. L., A. D. Pearson, and J. N. Hennessy.** 1983. Investigation of a waterborne outbreak of *Campylobacter jejuni* using a serotyping scheme based on the thermostable antigens. *J. Clin. Microbiol.* **18:**1362–1365.
37. **Preston, M. A., and J. L. Penner.** 1987. Structural and antigenic properties of lipopolysaccharides from serotype reference strains of *Campylobacter jejuni. Infect. Immun.* **55:**1806–1812.
38. **Preston, M. A., and J. L. Penner.** 1989. Characterization of cross reacting serotypes of *Campylobacter jejuni. Can. J. Microbiol.* **35:**265–273.
39. **Smith, H.** 1990. Pathogenicity and the microbe *in vivo. J. Gen. Microbiol.* **136:**377–383.
40. **Springer, G. F., J. C. Adye, A. Bezkorouainy, and J. R. Murthy.** 1973. Functional aspects and nature of the lipopolysaccharide receptor of human erythrocytes, p. 194–204. *In* E. W. Kass and S. H. Wolff (ed.), *Bacterial Lipopolysaccharides. The Chemistry, Biology and Clinical Significance of Endotoxins.* The University of Chicago Press, Chicago.
41. **Tsai, C.-M., and C. E. Frasch.** 1982. A sensitive silver stain for detecting lipopolysaccharides in polyacrylamide gels. *Anal. Biochem.* **119:**115–119.
42. **Westphal, O., and K. Jann.** 1965. Bacterial lipopolysaccharides: extraction with phenol-water and further applications of the procedure. *Methods Carbohydr. Chem.* **5:**83–91.

CHAPTER 26

Humoral Immune Response to Lipopolysaccharide Antigens of *Campylobacter jejuni*

MARTIN J. BLASER AND GUILLERMO I. PEREZ-PEREZ

INTRODUCTION

Campylobacter jejuni and the closely related organism *Campylobacter coli* have been established as among the most common bacterial causes of acute diarrheal disease of humans in developed and developing countries (5, 8). A wide variety of mammalian and avian species also are infected by those organisms and thus represent an important reservoir for transmission to humans. Development of vaccines against these organisms would therefore be worthwhile, but knowledge of their antigens is rudimentary (11, 12).

Epidemiologic and experimental data indicate that immunity to *C. jejuni* may be acquired following one or more infections (1, 6, 26). However, because these organisms are serologically diverse (19, 20), the nature of the protective antigens has not been immediately obvious. One approach to defining protective antigens is to determine which bacterial components are recognized by the host during infection (4, 23). Although such antigens are not necessarily protective, this approach nevertheless provides a first approximation of potential vaccine candidates.

We have been studying the humoral immune response to *Campylobacter* antigens in persons with acute diarrheal illnesses in the United States (22) in our search to define group-specific antigens which may have potential as vaccine candidates. One group of antigens studied, the proteins that are extracted from *C. jejuni* at low pH, are the subjects of several other reports (3, 6, 22). In the present chapter, we will describe humoral responses to the lipopolysaccharide (LPS) molecules of *C. jejuni*.

The LPS molecules of *C. jejuni* and *C. coli* are sufficiently diverse that typing schemes which rely on their heterogeneity have been developed (19); more than 50 different O types have been described (19, 20). However, our previous work has shown that *C. jejuni* LPS molecules possess both strain-specific epitopes and epitopes that are shared among campylobacters (23). LPS molecules of gram-negative bacteria are often immunodominant, and therefore their components have the potential to be used for serodiagnosis of infection (9) or to be considered for inclusion in vaccine formulations. Although *C. jejuni* LPS molecules contain epitopes conserved in other gram-negative organisms (24), other antigenic (23) and structural (10, 21) features suggest that they may be useful for serodiagnosis. Therefore, it is reasonable to question whether persons who are naturally infected with *Campylobacter* species show humoral immune responses to the LPS from homologous organisms (same O type) or from heterologous organisms (different O type). The response to heterologous organisms can be considered to be a response to group antigens.

DISTRIBUTION OF THE O ANTIGENS AMONG THE *CAMPYLOBACTER* ISOLATES

We first sought to determine whether *C. jejuni* and *C. coli* strains isolated from patients with sporadic cases of diarrhea (22) represented

Martin J. Blaser, Division of Infectious Diseases, Department of Medicine, Vanderbilt University School of Medicine, Nashville, Tennessee 37232–2605, and Infectious Disease Section, Department of Veterans Affairs Medical Center, Nashville, Tennessee 37203. **Guillermo I. Perez-Perez,** Division of Infectious Diseases, Department of Medicine, Vanderbilt University School of Medicine, Nashville, Tennessee 37232–2605.

a broad distribution of O antigens (heat stable) so that we could study immune response to both homologous and heterologous LPSs. The 22 strains which had been studied were phenotypically characterized by using standard criteria (18). Ten different heat-labile antigens were represented, and five strains were nontypable (22). The *Campylobacter* isolates were then serotyped for heat-stable antigens by the Penner method as previously described (19, 20), and 12 different O types were found. For 10 strains, two or more O types were identified. Thus, in total, 37 O-type antigens were represented among these 22 strains. Six (27.2%) strains each had O:4 or O:5 antigenic determinants, and one strain had both group antigens. Other antigens identified (and the number of strains carrying them) were as follows: O:13 (n = 5); O:21 (n = 4); O:16 (n = 3); O:29, O:18, O:2, and O:3 (n = 2); O:38, O:41, and O:54 (n = 1). To study responses to both homologous and heterologous LPS antigens, we then prepared LPS from *C. jejuni* strains with O:4 and O:5 antigens, which were the antigens most commonly identified in the patient isolates. For comparison, we studied responses to O:1 and O:NT antigens, which represented unrelated *C. jejuni* LPS antigens.

CHARACTERISTICS OF THE LPS PREPARATIONS

These LPS molecules were prepared from each of four *C. jejuni* strains by the hot phenol-water method of Westphal and Jann (27), with subsequent purification steps performed as described by Hanson and Phillips (14). Each LPS preparation underwent a second phenolic extraction so that protein contamination was minimized, as previously described. Protein concentrations were measured by the method of Markwell et al. (17). For determination of the 2-keto-3-deoxyoctonate (KDO) concentration of the fractions, the thiobarbituric acid method described by Keleti and Lederer (16) was used, as previously described (21). Polyacrylamide gel electrophoresis (PAGE) was performed with slab gels as previously described (21). After electrophoresis, gels were fixed and LPS was resolved with a silver stain by the method of Hitchcock and Brown (15).

We found that for whole cells of all four strains, the ratio of KDO to protein (ratio A) was similar (Table 1). The ratio of KDO to protein in the LPS preparations (ratio B) ranged from 2.27 to 4.27. The ratio B/A ranged from 349.2 to 574.1, indicating that there had been a substantial decrease in the level of protein contamination of the preparations. In each case, protein contamination of the LPS preparation was <3%. By PAGE, each preparation appeared characteristic for *C. jejuni* LPS, with a core component migrating at less than 14,000 molecular weight and no bands greater than 20,000 (Fig. 1). Since LPS O type is heterogeneous (20), these four preparations afforded an opportunity to examine the antigenicity of strain-specific features of *Campylobacter* species.

SEROCONVERSION TO *C. JEJUNI* LPS

We then asked whether seroconversion to any of the LPS antigens differentiated the *Campylobacter*-infected and uninfected persons. The enzyme-linked immunosorbent assay (ELISA) used in this study was a modification of one described previously (3). In brief, a purified LPS preparation from each of the four strains was diluted in carbonate buffer to 100 μg/ml and used as antigen to coat wells of polystyrene microtiter plates. The screening serum dilutions were 1:200 for immunoglobulin M (IgM), 1:100 for IgG, and 1:50 for IgA measurements as de-

TABLE 1. Characteristics of LPS preparations extracted from four *C. jejuni* strains

Strain	O type[a]	Content (% of dry cell wt) of: KDO	Content (% of dry cell wt) of: Protein	Ratio A[b]	Content (% of dry LPS wt) of: KDO	Content (% of dry LPS wt) of: Protein	Ratio B[b]	Ratio B/A
85-329	4	0.13	20	0.0065	5.9	2.6	2.27	349.2
85-360	5	0.14	22	0.0064	6.8	2.9	2.34	365.6
81-93	1	0.17	21	0.0081	4.7	1.1	4.27	527.2
79-193	NT[c]	0.15	26	0.0058	5.0	1.5	3.33	574.1

[a] By serotyping based on heat-stable antigens, as developed by Penner and Hennessy (20).
[b] Ratios A and B are defined in the text.
[c] NT, nontypable.

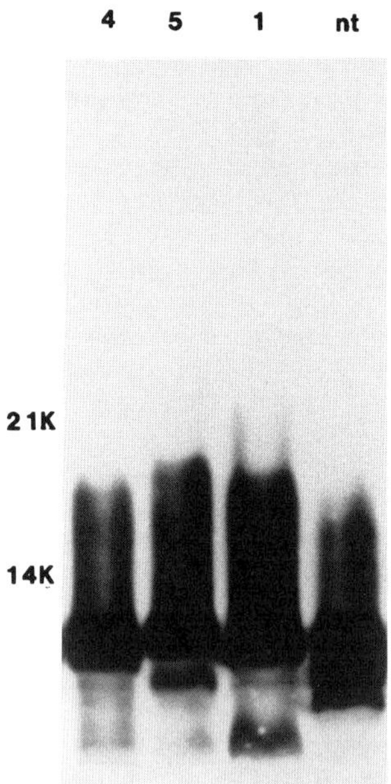

FIGURE 1. PAGE (15% acrylamide) of purified LPS preparations from four *C. jejuni* strains as resolved by silver stain. Preparations are as described in the text and represent LPS of types O:4, O:5, O:1, and O:NT (nontypable). Numbers at left refer to protein molecular weight standards simultaneously electrophoresed on the same gel.

termined by checkerboard titrations. Peroxidase conjugates of goat anti-human IgG diluted 1:4,000, IgA diluted 1:1,000, and IgM diluted 1:500 were used. Twenty-nine patients who were diagnosed as having acute (less than 1 week) inflammatory enteritis, based on an appropriate clinical history and the finding of fecal leukocytes in stool specimens, were included in the main study, as originally described (22). Twenty-two of these patients had enteritis due to *Campylobacter* species (17 *C. jejuni* and 5 *C. coli*). Another seven patients were infected with other enteric pathogens (two each with *Salmonella* or *Shigella* species) or no pathogen was identified (22); these seven represented the control group of persons with acute enteritis who were not infected with *Campylobacter* species. From each of the 29 patients we examined both an acute-phase serum sample obtained at the time of presentation of acute diarrheal illness and a convalescent-phase serum sample obtained 3 to 4 weeks later. Seroconversion was defined as a 50% increase in optical density between the acute- and convalescent-phase serum samples, as previously described (22). Of the seven persons who were not infected with *Campylobacter* species, none seroconverted to any of the four LPS preparations in any Ig class. In contrast, among the 22 persons infected with a *Campylobacter* species, seroconversion in one or more Ig classes occurred in 11, 12, 7, and 11 when the O-type 4, 5, 1, or NT LPS preparations, respectively, were used. In total, 17 (77.3%) of the 22 persons seroconverted to at least one LPS preparation in any Ig class. Compared with the response of the persons known to be uninfected, each of these differences was significant ($P < 0.02$; Fisher's exact test).

Because of the central role of IgA in mucosal immunity, the results of the studies of the IgA response in serum are highlighted (Fig. 2). There was essentially no serologic response among the persons without *Campylobacter* infection to any of the four *C. jejuni* LPS preparations. In contrast, among the infected persons, there was a significant ($P < 0.05$) rise in IgA levels directed toward each of the four LPS preparations.

Next, we focused on only a single LPS preparation, O:4, to examine the role of strain-specific and group-specific responses. The samples from the *Campylobacter*-infected persons showed significant increases in optical density values in the IgA, IgG, and IgM ELISAs toward the O:4 antigen (Fig. 3). As a group, the persons not infected with *Campylobacter* also had high antibody levels to the preparation, although the differences between acute- and convalescent-phase serum samples were not statistically significant.

Among the *Campylobacter*-infected persons, paired serum samples were available from 7 who were infected with an O:4-bearing strain and from 15 who were infected with heterologous *Campylobacter* strains. For the IgA and IgG classes, the optical density rose to an almost identical extent in the paired serum samples from the patients infected with homologous (O:4) and heterologous strains. However, patients infected with homologous strains showed a significant increase in the IgM response ($P < 0.01$), whereas those infected with heterologous strains did not (Fig. 4). A similar analysis of the data when the O:5 LPS (7 persons with homologous strains, 15 persons with heterologous strains) was used showed significant increases in IgG ($P = 0.02$) and IgM ($P = 0.05$) responses in persons infected with homologous strains; however, among persons infected with heterologous strains, only the IgA response was significant ($P < 0.008$).

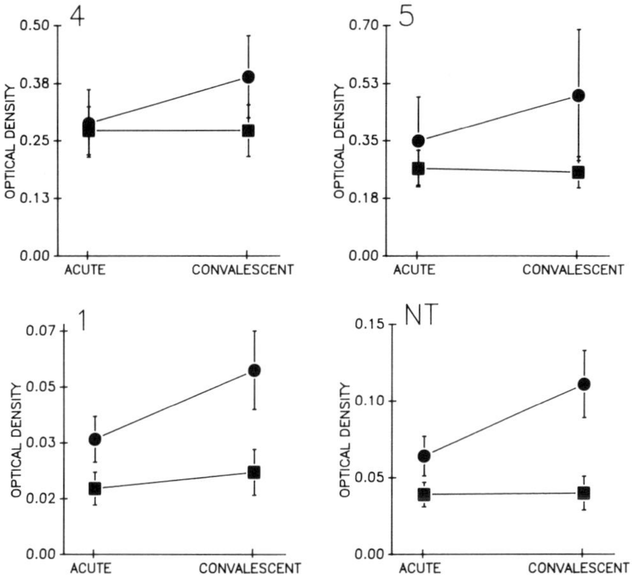

FIGURE 2. Serum IgA response to each of four *C. jejuni* LPS preparations by persons with inflammatory diarrhea infected (●; $n = 22$) or not infected (■; $n = 7$) with *Campylobacter* species. Optical densities in ELISAs directed against each LPS preparation were determined for both acute- and convalescent-phase serum samples.

SEROCONVERSION IN PATIENTS FROM WHOM NO PATHOGEN WAS IDENTIFIED

As part of this project, we examined serum from five patients from whom no pathogen was identified. Two of these patients had seroconverted to the group-specific *C. jejuni* protein antigens in each of the three Ig classes and were suspected of having been infected with *C. jejuni* (22). For comparison, serum was examined from three persons from whom no pathogen was identified and who had not responded to the protein antigens, suggesting that they had not been infected by a *Campylobacter* species. Assessing seroconversion to each of the four LPS preparations in each of the three Ig classes showed that serum samples from the two persons who recognized the protein antigens were positive in 11 (45.8%) of 24 assays, whereas none of 36 assays was positive for the three persons whose serum did not recognize the protein antigens ($P = 0.0001$; Fisher's exact test). These results further suggest that the two persons had been infected by a *Campylobacter* strain and that serology was probably more sensitive than culture for diagnosing this infection.

PERSPECTIVES

The presence of a serum antibody response to a particular antigen does not imply that that antigen elicits protective responses, nor that the serum antibody response measured is the mechanism of protection from reinfection. Nevertheless, the fact that naturally infected persons develop specific serum antibody responses to particular antigens suggests that such structures

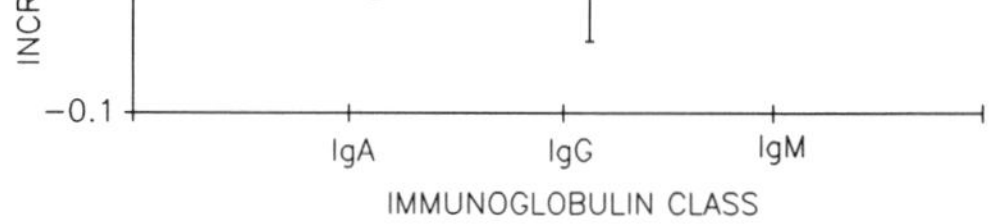

FIGURE 3. Serum antibody response to *C. jejuni* O:4 LPS in patients infected with *Campylobacter* species (open bars) or other pathogens (hatched bars). Differences in optical densities for acute- and convalescent-phase serum samples are compared for responses in the IgA, IgG, and IgM classes. For each Ig class, there was a significant difference ($P < 0.05$) between the *Campylobacter*-infected and noninfected persons.

could play a role in virulence or could have immunogenic potential.

We found that persons with natural *Campylobacter* infections showed serum antibody responses to purified *C. jejuni* LPS in each of the IgA, IgG, and IgM classes, whereas persons infected with other gram-negative pathogens or with acute diarrheal illness of unknown cause did not. Similarly, among persons experimentally infected with *C. jejuni,* a response to *C. jejuni* LPS also was observed (25). Although we examined preparations of *C. jejuni* LPS of four different O types, the responses to each of these were similar and there was little difference in response between persons infected with the homologous and heterologous LPS types. These phenomena suggest that the immunodominant *Campylobacter* LPS antigens are conserved among the four O types studied. In previous studies, we showed that by immunoblot *C. jejuni* LPS contained strain-specific antigens (23), as well as conserved antigens to which persons with heterologous infections respond. Alternatively, it is possible that the method of preparing the *C. jejuni* LPS altered or removed important distinguishing antigenic determinants; nevertheless, the PAGE profiles indicate that clear differences are apparent. However, under the assay conditions, no more than about half of the patients responded to any one preparation. Whether the difference in IgM and IgG response between those infected with strains of the homologous or heterologous LPS type is biologically significant must await further study.

Epidemiologic studies indicate that immunity to *C. jejuni* is acquired in areas in which infection is hyperendemic (2, 7, 13). Development of immunity implies that common immunogenic epitopes exist. Our studies suggest that some of these epitopes may be related to LPS-specific antigens. One implication of these investigations is that if an LPS constituent of a *Campylobacter* vaccine is considered, it may not be necessary to include a wide diversity of types. The results from our studies suggest that a single type might suffice. Similarly, an LPS preparation might be useful for serologic detection of *Campylobacter* infection. In fact, the results of this study are very similar to those from our previous work in which a *C. jejuni* surface protein-based preparation was used (22) and confirm that serology may be more sensitive than culture. It appears paradoxical that the LPS type can be used to differentiate *C. jejuni* and *C. coli* strains (19, 20) but that infected persons respond similarly to homologous and heterologous preparations. However, serotyping involves parenteral hyperimmunization of rabbits and absorption of the sera produced with heterologous strains. In contrast, since *Campylobacter* enteritis is a mucosal infection, antigen processing may be fundamentally different.

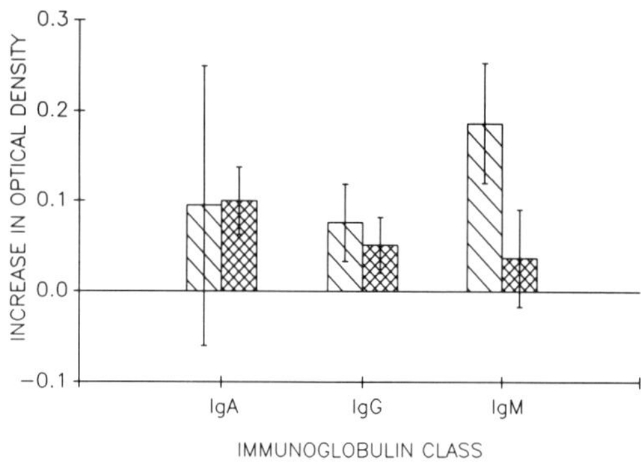

FIGURE 4. Serum antibody response to *C. jejuni* O:4 LPS among 7 persons infected with a *Campylobacter* strain bearing the O:4 antigen (homologous strain) (hatched bars) and 15 persons infected with a *Campylobacter* strain bearing heterologous LPS determinants (cross-hatched bars). Differences in optical densities for acute- and convalescent-phase serum samples are compared in the IgA, IgG, and IgM classes. For the IgM assay, there was a significant ($P = 0.01$) difference in response between the persons infected with homologous and heterologous strains.

ACKNOWLEDGMENT. The studies described in this chapter were supported in part by an interagency agreement between the U.S. Army Medical Research and Development Command and the Department of Veterans Affairs and by the Thrasher Research Fund.

REFERENCES

1. **Black, R. E., M. M. Levine, M. L. Clements, T. P. Hughes, and M. J. Blaser.** 1988. Experimental *Campylobacter jejuni* infection in humans. *J. Infect. Dis.* **157:**472–479.
2. **Blaser, M. J., R. E. Black, D. J. Duncan, and J. Amer.** 1985. *Campylobacter jejuni*-specific serum antibodies are elevated in healthy Bangladeshi children. *J. Clin. Microbiol.* **21:**164–167.
3. **Blaser, M. J., and D. J. Duncan.** 1984. Human serum antibody response to *Campylobacter jejuni* as measured in an enzyme-linked immunosorbent assay. *Infect. Immun.* **44:**292–298.
4. **Blaser, M. J., J. A. Hopkins, and M. L. Vasil.** 1984. *Campylobacter jejuni* outer membrane proteins are antigenic for humans. *Infect. Immun.* **43:**986–993.
5. **Blaser, M. J., and L. B. Reller.** 1981. *Campylobacter* enteritis. *N. Engl. J. Med.* **305:**1444–1452.
6. **Blaser, M. J., E. Sazie, and L. P. Williams.** 1987. The influence of immunity on raw milk-associated *Campylobacter* infection. *JAMA* **257:**43–46.

7. **Blaser, M. J., D. N. Taylor, and P. Echeverria.** 1986. Immune response to *Campylobacter jejuni* in a rural community in Thailand. *J. Infect. Dis.* **153**:249–254.
8. **Blaser, M. J., D. N. Taylor, and R. A. Feldman.** 1983. Epidemiology of *Campylobacter jejuni* infections. *Epidemiol. Rev.* **5**:157–176.
9. **Cohen, D., M. S. Green, C. Block, R. Slepon, and I. Ofek.** 1991. Prospective study of the association between serum antibodies to lipopolysaccharide O antigen and the attack rate of shigellosis. *J. Clin. Microbiol.* **29**:386–389.
10. **Conrad, R. S., and C. Galanos.** 1990. Characterization of *Campylobacter jejuni* lipopolysaccharide. *Curr. Microbiol.* **21**:377–379.
11. **Cover, T. J., and M. J. Blaser.** 1989. Pathobiology of *Campylobacter* infections in humans. *Annu. Rev. Med.* **40**:269–285.
12. **Dunn, B. E., M. J. Blaser, and E. L. Snyder.** 1987. Two-dimensional electrophoresis and immunoblotting of *Campylobacter* outer membrane proteins. *Infect. Immun.* **55**:1564–1572.
13. **Glass, R., B. J. Stoll, M. I. Huq, M. Struelens, M. J. Blaser, and A. K. M. Kibriya.** 1983. Epidemiological and clinical features of endemic *Campylobacter jejuni* infection in Bangladesh. *J. Infect. Dis.* **148**:292–296.
14. **Hanson, R. S., and J. A. Phillips.** 1981. Chemical composition, p. 328–364. *In* P. Gerhardt, R. G. E. Murray, R. N. Costilow, E. W. Nester, W. A. Wood, N. R. Krieg, and G. B. Phillips (ed.), *Manual of Methods for General Bacteriology*. American Society for Microbiology, Washington, D.C.
15. **Hitchcock, P. J., and T. M. Brown.** 1983. Morphological heterogeneity among *Salmonella* lipopolysaccharide chemotypes in silver-stained polyacrylamide gels. *J. Bacteriol.* **154**:269–277.
16. **Keleti, G., and W. H. Lederer (ed.).** 1974. *Handbook of Micromethods for the Biological Sciences*, p. 74–75. Van Nostrand Reinhold Co., New York.
17. **Markwell, M. A. K., S. M. Haar, L. L. Bieber, and N. E. Tolbert.** 1978. A modification of the Lowry procedure to simplify protein determinations in membrane and lipoprotein samples. *Anal. Biochem.* **87**:206–210.
18. **Morris, G. K., and C. M. Patton.** 1985. *Campylobacter*, p. 302–308. *In* E. Lennette, A. Balows, W. J. Hausler, Jr., and H. J. Shadomy (ed.), *Manual of Clinical Microbiology*, 4th ed. American Society for Microbiology, Washington, D.C.
19. **Patton, C. M., T. J. Barrett, and G. K. Morris.** 1985. Comparison of the Penner and Lior methods for serotyping *Campylobacter* spp. *J. Clin. Microbiol.* **22**:558–565.
20. **Penner, J. L., and J. N. Hennessy.** 1980. Passive hemagglutation technique for serotyping *Campylobacter fetus* susp. *jejuni* on the basis of soluble heat-stable antigens. *J. Clin. Microbiol.* **12**:732–737.
21. **Perez-Perez, G. I., and M. J. Blaser.** 1985. Lipopolysaccharide characteristics of pathogenic campylobacters. *Infect. Immun.* **47**:353–359.
22. **Perez-Perez, G. I., D. L. Cohn, R. L. Guerrant, C. Patton, L. B. Reller, and M. J. Blaser.** 1989. Clinical and immunological significance of cholera-like toxin and cytotoxin production by *Campylobacter* species in patients with acute inflammatory diarrhea. *J. Infect. Dis.* **160**:460–468.
23. **Perez-Perez, G. I., J. A. Hopkins, and M. J. Blaser.** 1985. Antigenic heterogeneity of lipopolysaccharides from *Campylobacter jejuni* and *Campylobacter fetus. Infect. Immun.* **48**:528–533.
24. **Perez-Perez, G. I., J. A. Hopkins, and M. J. Blaser.** 1986. Lipopolysaccharide structures in *Enterobacteriaceae, Pseudomonas,* and *Vibrio* related to those in *Campylobacter. Infect. Immun.* **51**:204–208.
25. **Perlman, D. M., M. M. Levine, R. E. Black, and M. J. Blaser.** May 1988. Anti-lipopolysaccharide antibody response to *Campylobacter jejuni* infection following challenge in volunteers, abstr. E-81, p. 122. *Abstr. 88th Annu. Meet. Am. Soc. Microbiol. 1988.* American Society for Microbiology, Washington, D.C.
26. **Taylor, D. N., P. Echeverria, C. Pitarangsi, J. Seriwatana, L. Bodhidatta, and M. J. Blaser.** 1988. Influence of strain characteristics and immunity on the epidemiology of *Campylobacter* infections in Thailand. *J. Clin. Microbiol.* **26**:863–868.
27. **Westphal, O., and K. Jann.** 1965. Bacterial lipopolysaccharides. *Methods Carbohydr. Chem.* **5**:83–91.

CHAPTER 27

Identification and Characterization of Major Common Antigens from *Campylobacter jejuni*

ZHIHENG PEI, RICHARD T. ELLISON III, AND MARTIN J. BLASER

Campylobacter jejuni and the closely related species *Campylobacter coli* are now recognized as important causes of acute diarrheal disease in humans throughout the world (3). Several lines of evidence suggest that protective immunity can be developed against these pathogens during natural infections (2, 5), in long-term drinkers of raw milk (4), and in human volunteers (1), but the antigenic basis for this protection is poorly defined. We have purified to homogeneity from the acid extract of an epidemic *C. jejuni* strain (81-176; ATCC 55026) four proteins with molecular masses of 28 kDa (PEB1), 29 kDa (PEB2), 30 kDa (PEB3), and 31 kDa (PEB4) by using sequential ion-exchange, hydrophobic interaction, and gel filtration chromatography. The full report of this work has recently been published (8).

The purified proteins were compared with the acid extract to assess their utility as antigens in an immunoglobulin G enzyme-linked immunosorbent assay to detect antibody responses in patients with sporadic cases of diarrhea. Acute- and convalescent-phase serum samples were available from 29 patients. Of 19 patients with *C. jejuni* or *C. coli* diarrhea, 14 seroconverted to the acid extract mixture, 15 to PEB1 or PEB3, 2 to PEB2, and 6 to PEB4. None of 10 patients without *Campylobacter* diarrhea seroconverted to any of these antigens.

We next examined the potential application of antibodies to *C. jejuni* proteins for identification and diagnosis of *Campylobacter* and/or *Helicobacter* species. Antiserum to the acid extract from *C. jejuni* 81-176 recognized all 35 *C. jejuni*, all 15 *C. coli*, 9 of 10 *C. fetus*, all 5 *C. lari*, and 3 of 5 *Helicobacter pylori* strains. In contrast, antiserum to PEB1 recognized all 35 *C. jejuni* and all 15 *C. coli* isolates but none of the isolates of the other three bacterial species. We then performed a Western immunoblotting experiment to determine the bands recognized by anti-PEB1 in preparations of whole cells of various *Campylobacter* and *Helicobacter* species. A 28-kDa band was found in all 18 *C. jejuni* and all 14 *C. coli* strains, but was not present in any of the *C. fetus, C. lari,* or *H. pylori* strains tested. This Western blot experiment provided physical evidence that PEB1 from various *C. jejuni* and *C. coli* strains are all conserved in size and were antigenically related.

We next tested whether the common antigen PEB1 is a protein by using V8 protease or proteinase K to digest whole cells of *C. jejuni* and *C. coli*. Rabbit antiserum to PEB1 was used in Western blots to monitor the sensitivity of PEB1 to the protease digestion. The 28-kDa band disappeared after proteinase K digestion but not after sham digestion, indicating that the major antigenic component of PEB1 is a protein. Protease V8 partially hydrolyzed PEB1 into two antigenic fragments, which migrated at 16 and 12 kDa.

We then determined the native molecular mass of PEB1 by using a Superose 12 gel filtration column. PEB1 extracted in water or low-pH glycine buffer from either *C. jejuni* or *C. coli* strains had a molecular mass of 28.9 ± 1 kDa.

Zhiheng Pei, Division of Infectious Diseases, Department of Medicine, and Department of Microbiology and Immunology, Vanderbilt University School of Medicine, Nashville, Tennessee 37232–2605. **Richard T. Ellison III,** Medical and Research Services, Department of Veterans Affairs Medical Center, and Division of Infectious Diseases, Department of Medicine, University of Colorado School of Medicine, Denver, Colorado 80220. **Martin J. Blaser,** Division of Infectious Diseases, Department of Medicine, Vanderbilt University School of Medicine, Nashville, Tennessee 37232–2605, and Infectious Disease Section, Department of Veterans Affairs Medical Center, Nashville, Tennessee 37203.

The similarity in the molecular mass of PEB1 as defined by sodium dodecyl sulfate-polyacrylamide gel electrophoresis and gel filtration chromatography, compared with the findings obtained using Superose 12, indicates that the native form of PEB1 is a monomer. Isoelectric focusing showed that all four PEBs are basic proteins with pI 8.5 for PEB1 protein and pI > 9.3 for the other three proteins. The amino acid composition of the four proteins was found to be similar. Basic amino acids (Lys, His, and Arg) predominate, ranging from 26.4 to 33.6%. Cysteine was not found in any of the four proteins. Treatment with dithiothreitol did not change the electrophoretic migration of the four proteins, confirming the absence of intermolecular disulfide bands.

A comparison of the (amino) N-terminal amino acid sequences of the four proteins indicated that each is unique, although there is 51.4% homology in the N-terminal 35 amino acids of PEB2 and PEB3. None of the N termini of these mature proteins starts with methionine, suggesting that a leader sequence was cleaved during maturation. The four amino acid sequences were compared with several gene bank databases. The N termini of PEB1 and PEB2 had no significant in-frame homology with other known proteins. For PEB3, we identified a potential in-frame homology with class I pili from *Neisseria meningitidis* (9) and *Escherichia coli* heat-labile enterotoxin B subunit (11). PEB4 exhibits partial homology with two proteins related to the serine protease inhibitor superfamily, including human corticosteroid-binding protein (7) and serine proteinase inhibitor I of vaccinia virus (10), and with the human major histocompatibility complex class II lymphocyte antigen Dpw4-β-1 (6).

In summary, we have purified four basic proteins from *C. jejuni*. Two of the four proteins, PEB1 and PEB3, are targets for the human immune system during natural infection and appear to be candidate antigens for both a *Campylobacter* vaccine and serological assays for the pathogen. Antibodies to these proteins may be useful for diagnosis of infection by antigen detection or for passive immunization.

REFERENCES

1. **Black, R. E., M. M. Levine, M. L. Clements, T. P. Hughes, and M. J. Blaser.** 1988. Experimental *Campylobacter jejuni* infection in humans. *J. Infect. Dis.* **157**:472–479.
2. **Blaser, M. J., R. E. Black, D. J. Duncan, and J. Amer.** 1985. *Campylobacter jejuni*-specific serum antibodies are elevated in healthy Bangladeshi children. *J. Clin. Microbiol.* **21**:164–167.
3. **Blaser, M. J., and L. B. Reller.** 1981. *Campylobacter* enteritis. *N. Engl. J. Med.* **305**:1444–1452.
4. **Blaser, M. J., E. Sazie, and L. P. Williams, Jr.** 1987. The influence of immunity on raw milk-associated *Campylobacter* infection. *JAMA* **257**:43–46.
5. **Blaser, M. J., D. N. Taylor, and P. Echeverria.** 1986. Immune response to *Campylobacter jejuni* in a rural community in Thailand. *J. Infect. Dis.* **153**:249–254.
6. **Gustafsson, K., E. Widmark, A. K. Jonsson, B. Servenius, D. H. Sachs, D. Larhammar, L. Rask, and P. A. Peterson.** 1987. Class II genes of the human major histocompatibility complex: evolution of the DP region as deduced from nucleotide sequences of the four genes. *J. Biol. Chem.* **262**:8776–8786.
7. **Harley, M. G., J. Reventos, N. A. Musto, G. L. Gunsalus, and C. W. Bardin.** 1987. Primary structure of human corticosteroid binding globulin deduced from hepatic and pulmonary cDNAs exhibits homology with serine protease inhibitors. *Proc. Natl. Acad. Sci. USA* **84**:5153–5157.
8. **Pei, Z., R. T. Ellison III, and M. J. Blaser.** 1991. Identification, purification and characterization of major antigenic proteins of *Campylobacter jejuni. J. Biol. Chem.* **266**:16363–16369.
9. **Potts, W. J., and J. R. Saunders.** 1988. Nucleotide sequences of the structural gene for class I pili from *Neisseria meningitidis:* homologies with the pilE locus of *Neisseria gonorrhoeae. Mol. Microbiol.* **2**:647–653.
10. **Smith, G. L., S. T. Howard, and Y. S. Chan.** 1989. Vaccinia virus encodes a family of genes with homology to serine proteinase inhibitors. *J. Gen. Virol.* **70**:2333–2343.
11. **Yamamoto, T., T. Gojobori, and T. Yokota.** 1987. Evolutionary origin of pathogenic determinants in enterotoxigenic *Escherichia coli* and *Vibrio cholerae. J. Bacteriol.* **169**:1352–1357.

VI. MOLECULAR PATHOGENESIS

CHAPTER 28

Genetic and Molecular Approach to *Campylobacter* Pathogenesis

LUCY S. TOMPKINS

GENETIC VERSUS MOLECULAR BIOLOGICAL APPROACH TO PATHOGENESIS

The strategies that geneticists use to investigate determinants of pathogenicity differ from the molecular biologist's approach. Even though contemporary genetic studies require molecular tools in most instances, the basis of microbial genetics has not changed in the modern era of recombinant DNA. When first studying a putative gene encoding a known phenotype, the first and most basic genetic requirement is to find (or make) a mutant. The second is to create a selective environment in which to isolate the mutant. The third requirement is to map the gene by analysis of genetic recombinants, scoring for linked traits to create a genetic map. If the genetic map position of other linked genes is known, these data can then be used to localize the putative gene in relation to its neighbors. A fourth step is to determine whether the gene encodes a structural protein or is a regulatory gene. If a structural product is made, the fifth step is to find whether the gene is part of an operon. For example, the gene encoding pilin (the basic subunit of pili) in *Escherichia coli* is part of a large operon containing genes that promote secretion, assembly, stabilization, and adhesion.

As compared with the genetic approach, the molecular biologist's approach is more often directed toward isolation of a genetic sequence, cloning of the gene, and sequencing it, thereby constructing a physical map versus a genetic map. At this point one may proceed directly to the cloning of a gene encoding a structural protein, bypassing mutant construction or selection. Cloning involves the construction of a library of genomic DNA in a vector, either a plasmid, cosmid, or bacteriophage, and the introduction of this library into a suitable recipient, usually *E. coli* K-12. The next step is to search the library for the clone containing the desired sequence. If expression (protein synthesis, secretion) can occur in the foreign recipient, the library can be screened by using specific antibody (Western immunoblots, etc.). However, expression of foreign DNA may not occur; in this case, the library can be screened by using oligonucleotide probes derived from the amino acid sequence of the protein.

Having cloned the gene, which is usually incorporated into a larger fragment, subclones are constructed, thereby reducing the fragment to a manageable size. To further define the limits of the structural gene, transposon mutations can be placed throughout the cloned fragment, as shown in Fig. 1. By screening the clones containing transposon insertions for phenotypic expression and by locating each insert by restriction digestion mapping, the physical limits of the functional gene can be more precisely defined, since each transposon insertion into the structural gene will produce a "knockout" of the phenotype, whereas transposon insertions outside the gene will have minimal effects on expression. Often the next phase of the process is to examine the behavior of *E. coli* K-12 clones containing the recombinant plasmid in a model system. Cloning the gene in a foreign background may provide clues to the effect of gene expression in the natural host. For example, *E. coli* K-12 clones containing the *Yersinia inv* gene are able to enter eukaryotic epithelial cells, whereas *E. coli* K-12 cannot. Although these kinds of experiments can be helpful in elucidating the pos-

Lucy S. Tompkins, Department of Medicine (Infectious Diseases) and Department of Microbiology and Immunology, Stanford University Medical Center, Stanford, California 94305.

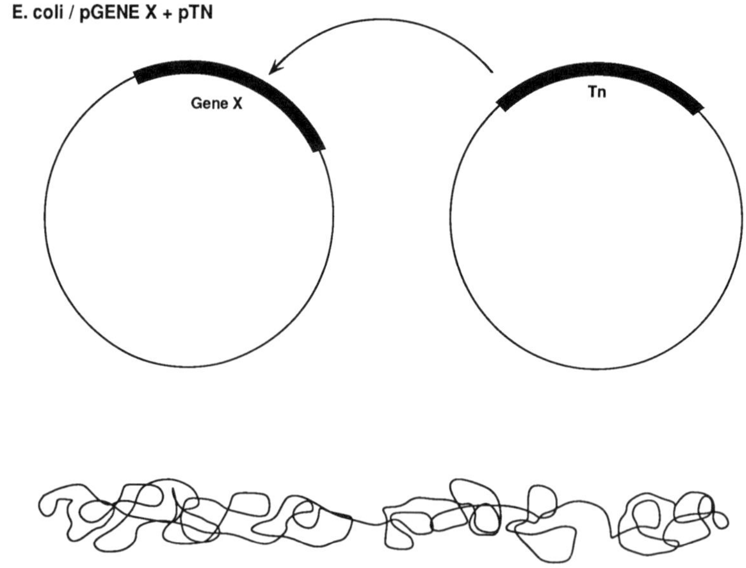

FIGURE 1. Schematic depiction of transposon mutagenesis of a plasmid-mediated gene (X) in which a suicide plasmid is used to deliver the transposon.

sible function of the gene in the natural host, in many instances the results can be misleading, or at least not definitive. As an example, the *Bordetella pertussis* toxin gene expressed in *E. coli* does not respond to the same environmental signals that affect coordinate regulation in *B. pertussis.* Therefore, one must look beyond cloning *E. coli* to gain an understanding of the role of the gene in pathogenesis in nature. Here, construction of a mutant by transposon mutagenesis of the chromosome or by introduction of an inactivated gene which may replace the wild-type copy by homologous recombination is often required to implicate a particular determinant. There is a theoretical disadvantage to the straight molecular approach to pathogenesis in which the initial impetus is to identify a particular protein expressed by wild-type strains which is not expressed by a mutant or variant. In this approach, the focus is on a phenotypic marker but not necessarily on the biological behavior of the organism. For example, without ever observing the interaction of motile *Campylobacter* spp. in the gastrointestinal tract, one could directly identify and clone the genes encoding *Campylobacter* flagellin by screening a library with oligonucleotides derived from the N-terminal amino acid sequence. However, this information alone is not likely to reveal very much about the role of flagella and motility in pathogenesis.

GENETIC EXCHANGE IN *CAMPYLOBACTER* SPP.

Shuttle Plasmids

Molecular techniques are required to accomplish one essential step in the assessment of gene function: to return the cloned gene to the natural host. A system to exchange genes between the natural host and the foreign recipient is essential to discern the specific contribution of a single genetic determinant to pathogenesis. One means of obtaining gene transfer employs shuttle vectors to carry genes between species during bacterial conjugation. Shuttle plasmids must be capable of replicating in both the host and the recipient and must be capable of overcoming restriction barriers to entry. These plasmids have been particularly useful as vectors to introduce transposons into the chromosome or into plasmids containing DNA inserts, as a means of producing mutations in the gene (Fig. 1 and 2). Shuttle vectors can also be used to introduce a cloned determinant into a mutant lacking in the phenotype. For example, it should be possible to complement a deficiency in an essential *Campylobacter* enzyme by transferring the gene encoding the enzyme which has been cloned into a shuttle plasmid into a *Campylobacter* mutant lacking this ability; the enzyme, produced in *trans* from the plasmid, could then

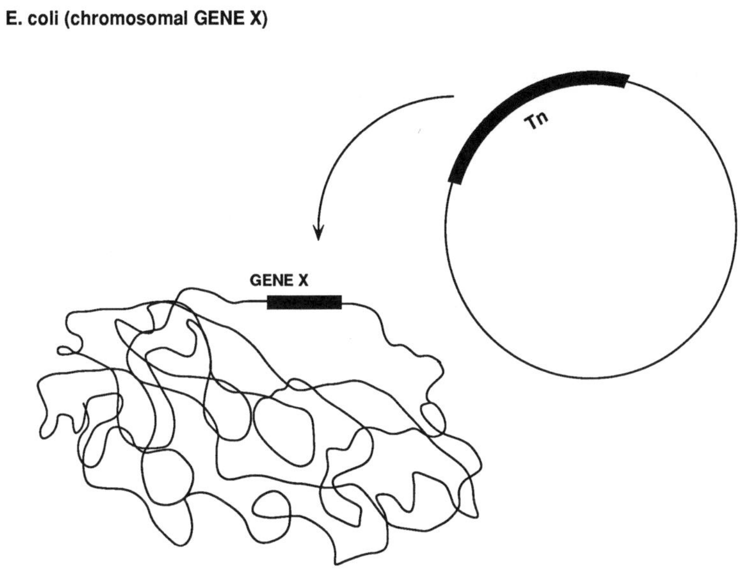

FIGURE 2. Transposon mutagenesis of a chromosomal gene (X) in which a suicide plasmid containing the transposon is used.

functionally restore this capacity. One could also screen genetic libraries constructed in the shuttle plasmid by using this system to clone complementing genes.

Another type of shuttle plasmid, a suicide vector, can also serve to shuttle DNA from a host into a recipient. Like the shuttle vector, suicide vectors must be able to replicate inside the donor cells and must have the genetic functions which permit them to be mobilized in conjugation or to be transformed; however, the essential difference is that suicide vectors cannot replicate inside the recipient cells. Following introduction of the suicide plasmid carrying a transposon or a cloned DNA sequence, the only way for the incoming transposon or DNA fragment sequence to be rescued is to be incorporated into the recipient chromosome or resident plasmid. Therefore, suicide plasmids are especially useful in constructing chromosomal mutants and in promoting homologous recombination between incoming recombinant sequences and the chromosomal homolog.

In the early years of *Campylobacter* genetics, the greatest obstacle preventing the construction of mutants and the cloning of *Campylobacter* genes was the absence of genetic exchange systems. Although plasmids could be transferred between two different *Campylobacter* species via bacterial conjugation, attempts to transfer *Campylobacter* plasmids to *E. coli* were unsuccessful, but, more importantly, even broad-host-range plasmids did not appear to be maintained in *Campylobacter* species. Part of the difficulty in assessing the ability of broad-host-range plasmids to transfer to *Campylobacter* species was that antibiotic resistance markers that were expressed in *E. coli* were not expressed in *Campylobacter* species; therefore, even if transfer had been achieved, it might not have been possible to detect the event because of lack of expression. None of the conventional broad-host-range plasmids could be mobilized into *Campylobacter* species by conjugation, and there were no known transducing phages for *Campylobacter* species. Additionally, attempts to transform viable *Campylobacter* cells by conventional methods were unsuccessful.

Our laboratory began studies on *Campylobacter* pathogenesis by developing means of accomplishing genetic exchange. Labigne designed a shuttle plasmid having the following elements: (i) it could replicate in both *E. coli* and *Campylobacter* species by virtue of containing the replication functions of an *E. coli* plasmid and those encoded in a *Campylobacter* cryptic plasmid; (ii) it contained a kanamycin resistance gene isolated from a *Campylobacter coli* strain that expressed resistance in both *E. coli* and *Campylobacter* species; and (iii) it could be mobilized from *E. coli* donors into *Campylobacter* recipients by virtue of containing the *oriT* sequence (*mob* function) isolated from a broad-host-range plasmid. After introducing the shuttle plasmid into *E. coli* which also contained the transfer (*tra*) function on a second broad-host-range plasmid, Labigne et al. were able to successfully mobilize the recombinant shuttle plasmid from *E. coli* into *Campylobacter* cells by mating (9).

A suicide plasmid was then constructed by deleting the sequence encoding the entire cryptic plasmid that had been originally ligated into the *Campylobacter* shuttle plasmid (8). This vector could replicate in *E. coli* cells but was unable to replicate in *Campylobacter* cells. A variety of transposons were ligated into the *Campylobacter* suicide vector and tested to see whether transposition to the chromosome might occur after mating. However, none of the common transposons tested seemed to be able to transpose at a high enough frequency to be detected; some of these also may not have been expressed.

Labigne subsequently used the suicide vector to introduce a modified *Campylobacter* gene into *Campylobacter* recipients to test whether the suicide plasmid could shuttle modified genes into *Campylobacter* cells and then permit recombination with chromosomal homologs. This process has been termed "shuttle mutagenesis" by Seifert et al. (18). We used the gene encoding 16S rRNA for these experiments because there are multiple copies of 16S rDNA genes in the chromosome, and therefore the knockout of one of these would not be lethal. The gene was modified by inserting a block of DNA which promoted kanamycin resistance (kanamycin cassette) into the center of the 16S rDNA gene by in vitro ligation; this is an effective strategy to disrupt gene transcription. The modified gene cloned into the suicide vector was then returned to a wild-type *Campylobacter* recipient, and mutants that were produced by homologous recombination via double crossover were selected by plating onto kanamycin. The results clearly demonstrated that the suicide vector could promote replacement of the wild-type gene with a modified gene, thereby creating a stable mutation (Fig. 3).

Labigne has continued to develop *Campylobacter* mutants via shuttle mutagenesis, and very recently she has succeeded in constructing a leucine synthetase mutant by shuttle transposon mutagenesis (7). The experimental design is as follows. First, a kanamycin transposable element was constructed by replacing the ampicillin resistance gene of Tn*3* with the *Campylobacter* kanamycin gene, creating a kanamycin transposon. A plasmid containing the MiniTn:Km was introduced into *E. coli* cells containing a suicide shuttle vector into which a library of *Campylobacter* DNA fragments had been inserted, thereby producing mutations in each cloned random sequence. *E. coli* donors containing the mutagenized library and a mobilization plasmid were mated with kanamycin-susceptible *Campylobacter* recipient cells, and transconjugants expressing kanamycin resistance were selected. Of these, some had lost the plasmid and were also deficient in the ability to synthesize leucine, showing that the wild-type copy of the gene had been exchanged for the modified gene. These experiments demonstrate that it is possible to construct a *Campylobacter* mutant by using a recombinant transposon to introduce mutations into a cloned gene in *E. coli,* thereby circumventing the requirement that a transposable element must directly transpose in *Campylobacter* species.

Transformation

A second system of exchanging genetic information is via transformation, a process in which naked DNA molecules are taken up by recipient cells. Plasmid transformation is followed by replication in the cytoplasm, while transformation of linear DNA fragments may lead to recombination and incorporation into the chromosome. Transformation of plasmid DNA offers an alternative to conjugation, which requires accessory genetic determinants. As another means of exchanging genes, our laboratory developed a transformation system by using electroporation to introduce recombinant plasmids into *Campylobacter* cells (14). Under appropriate conditions, we achieved a reasonable degree of transformation efficiency (10^4 cells per μg of DNA) while maintaining viability (a 50% reduction in viable count). During the course of these experiments, we were also able to confirm a previous observation made by Labigne et al., who noted that restriction digests of recombinant shuttle plasmids extracted from *E. coli* had somewhat different patterns if the plasmid DNA was extracted from *Campylobacter* cells, indicating that a specific change in cleavage sites for *Eco*RI and *Mbo*I had occurred (9). These data suggested that *C. jejuni* DNA was modified at certain sites in *Campylobacter* cells and hence modified plasmids transformed into the natural host resisted cleavage. We subsequently showed that shuttle plasmids grown in *E. coli* could not be electroporated into *Campylobacter* cells, whereas those grown in *Campylobacter* cells were transformed via electroporation at a rela-

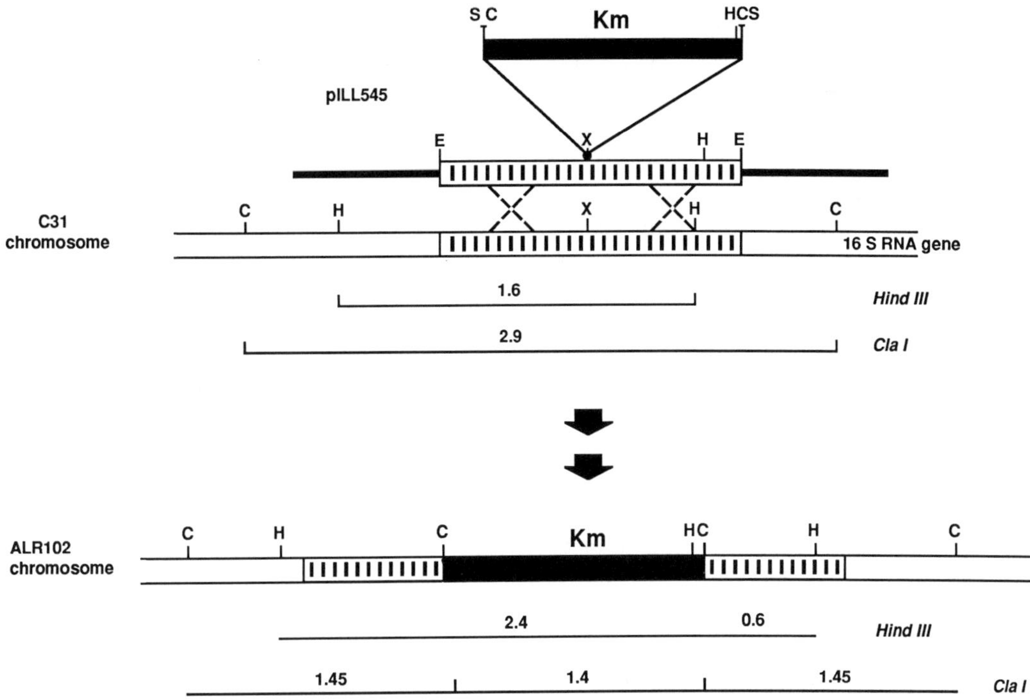

FIGURE 3. Incorporation of the disrupted 16S rRNA allele carried on the suicide vector into the chromosomal 16S rRNA-encoding region. The double-crossover event promotes the incorporation of the allele containing the kanamycin cassette into the chromosome, thereby replacing it. Reprinted from reference 8 with permission.

tively high frequency, suggesting that *Campylobacter* cells probably restricted incoming *E. coli* DNA that was not specifically modified (14). This *Campylobacter*-specific restriction-modification system could explain the basis of the lack of stability and of expression of foreign DNA in *Campylobacter* cells.

The use of electroporation to transform *Campylobacter* cells was necessitated by the absence of a system to achieve natural transformation. Wang and Taylor have recently demonstrated that some strains of *C. jejuni* could be transformed by shuttle plasmids via natural transformation (19), although the efficiency was not as great as that obtained with electroporation. Transformation efficiency was found to be much greater with chromosomal linear fragments than with plasmids. However, when recipients contained a homologous plasmid, the transformation efficiency of plasmid DNA was increased 100-fold. This was thought to be due to rescue of the incoming plasmid by recombination with the homologous element. The evidence suggested that *Campylobacter* DNA contains a specific sequence necessary for binding to and uptake into *Campylobacter* cells, in a fashion analogous to the situation for *Haemophilus* and *Neisseria* species. Of interest to our laboratory was that the Taylor laboratory found that strain C31, which we initially tried to transform by $CaCl_2$ treatment, could not be transformed by natural transformation (19).

PROBLEMS ENCOUNTERED IN *CAMPYLOBACTER* MOLECULAR GENETICS

Our laboratory embarked upon the genetic approach to *Campylobacter* species in 1985 by attempting to produce genetic libraries of *C. jejuni* DNA in *E. coli* K-12. Several different vectors were tried, including plasmids and cosmids, with little success. The first problem we encountered was the instability of *Campylobacter* DNA sequences cloned in *E. coli*. For example, the cosmid pHC79 packages large DNA fragments, ranging in size from 38 to 45 kb. In the absence of selection, *E. coli* recipients transfected with pHC79 cosmids containing large *Campylobacter* fragments quickly deleted the foreign DNA, leaving only plasmids that contained very small or no inserts. Other investigators have also noted problems in maintaining large inserts in *E. coli*. However, we and others have found that genes could be maintained in *E. coli* by providing selective pressure. Using the cosmid pHC79, Labigne et al. were able to select clones containing a *Campylobacter* gene encoding leucine biosynthesis in an *E. coli* auxotroph by plating cells containing the cosmid library onto minimal media. Only *E. coli* cells that inherited a *Campylobacter* synthetase gene could grow on this medium (7). These experiments showed us that it was possible to develop libraries in *E. coli* if positive selection could be applied and the problem of insert stability could be overcome. The inability to detect expression of *Campylobacter* genes by using specific antibody (Western blots or enzyme-linked immunosorbent assays) has been another stumbling block to cloning in *E. coli*. Although it is now apparent that not all of the early problems were due to a lack of transcription, there are few published data to suggest that *E. coli* recipients can express *Campylobacter* proteins sufficiently well to be readily detected by antibody screening methods. Another hurdle to attempts to construct *Campylobacter* mutants has been the difficulty in finding a suitable transposon that could transpose in *Campylobacter* cells and could express in both *E. coli* donors and recipients. Again, most of the widely used transposons are not suitable for *Campylobacter* mutagenesis. The molecular construction of a mini-kanamycin transposon by Labigne et al. (7) has provided a satisfactory alternative.

GENETIC AND MOLECULAR APPROACH TO *CAMPYLOBACTER* PATHOGENESIS

Background

Although many investigators have been able to clone *Campylobacter* sequences and genes in *E. coli*, the only genes encoding pathogenic factors that have been cloned and sequenced to date are those encoding flagellin. In large part the focus on flagella was the result of the strong experimental data demonstrating the important contribution of flagella in other enteric infections, the in vivo results suggesting a role for *Campylobacter* flagella in establishing infection in animals, and the immunodominance of flagellar protein. Although some data suggest that *C. jejuni* may produce adherence factors, enterotoxin, and cytotoxin and is capable of invasion, the data are not sufficiently convincing to demonstrate conclusively that discrete genes are responsible for these effects, which have been measured only in bioassays. Until such factors can be purified and extensively characterized to the extent that oligonucleotide probes and specific antibody probes can be produced, it is the general consensus that it would be premature to clone these putative "virulence" genes. However, chemical mutagenesis to create mutations in chromosomal determinants would be a valid approach toward determining whether mutants deficient in one of these activities might behave differently in bioassays or model infection. This approach has been used in studying the contribution of determinants in other enteric species, primarily as a way to gain an initial understanding of the possible contribution of a specific factor. After these experiments had been carried out, the search for the gene and the construction of isogenic mutants could proceed.

Current Progress

Chromosomal mapping

Chang and Taylor (1) and Nuijten et al. (15) have physically mapped several chromosomal genes by using rare-cutting restriction endonucleases and pulsed-field gel electrophoresis (PFGE). These genes include those encoding 16S rRNA, flagellar structural protein, ribosomal proteins, and antibiotic resistance. The genome size of *Campylobacter* species has also been determined and is only ca. 36% that of *E. coli*. These studies lay an important foundation for future research to place new genes on the map and will permit us to compare the genetic organization of the *Campylobacter* genome with that of *E. coli*.

Genetic and molecular studies of flagella and flagellin

Earlier studies by a variety of investigators strongly suggested that *Campylobacter* flagella were involved in the pathogenesis of infection; however, their precise role was not clear. Some investigators had postulated that motility was most important to establish colonization by propelling the bacteria through the highly viscous mucous layer of the intestine (10a), and others had suggested that the flagella might serve as an adhesin to intestinal epithelial cells (13a).

Previous studies showing that *Campylobacter* flagellar proteins contained regions which were homologous to the flagellar proteins of *E.*

coli and *Salmonella* species provided a basis to identify the *Campylobacter* structural genes (6, 10, 12). Logan and Trust had already established that *Campylobacter* flagellar filaments possessed a number of serospecific surface-exposed epitopes (13). The serospecificity of flagella was confirmed by the observation that the loss of flagella was accompanied by the loss of ability to serotype by the heat-labile typing method of Lior (21). The work of Trust and coworkers further investigated the presence of flagellin molecules of different subunit molecular weights, suggesting that some strains of *C. coli* produced two different flagellin species (T1 and T2), providing a theoretical basis for antigenic variation (5). Their previous findings suggested that the flagellar filament of *C. coli* VC167 was composed of multiple copies of a single species of flagellin and that the antigenic difference between the two flagellar filaments produced by this strain might be related to the difference in the subunit molecular weights of the species making up the filament. They found that T1 cells could be selected over T2 cells by growth in vitro in the presence of specific antibody and also in vivo during infection in the rabbit, where a gradual transition occurred from the production of T1 to T2 cells (11). During conversion between T1 and T2 flagellins, Guerry et al. noticed a genomic rearrangement at a locus adjacent to one of the rRNA genes, as well as sequence variation within the flagellin genes (3, 4).

Guerry et al. have now succeeded in cloning the structural flagellin genes from a strain of *C. coli* and have elucidated the molecular structure of *C. coli* flagellin and the mechanism of antigenic variation (2). Two copies of the flagellar structural gene, *flaA* and *flaB,* are present in *C. coli* VC167 in tandem orientation; these are highly homologous, each encoding an open reading frame of 572 amino acids. These investigators have also constructed isogenic mutants of *C. coli* by exchanging a *flaA* gene modified by the insertion of a kanamycin cassette with the wild-type copy (3), by using the vector and gene replacement mutagenesis scheme developed by Labigne-Roussel et al. (8). Three classes of mutants were noted: (i) *flaA flaB* (bald, nonmotile); (ii) *flaA*$^{+}$ *flaB* (flagella, decreased motility); and (iii) *flaA flaB*$^{+}$ (truncated filament, partially motile) (3). By Western blot analysis of the mutants, FlaA and FlaB flagellins of T1 cells both run at an apparent M_r of 61,500 while the T2 flagellins both run at an apparent M_r of 59,500. For both *flaA* and *flaB* genes, T1 and T2 cells contained nucleotide sequence variations. Amino acid sequencing of FlaA flagellin suggested that certain residues were posttranslationally modified by phosphorylation of some of the serine residues. These changes might contribute to the molecular weight discrepancy on sodium dodecyl sulfate-polyacrylamide gel electrophoresis (SDS-PAGE) and the predicted M_r and may be involved in the antigenic properties. Northern (RNA) blot analysis indicated that both structural genes were expressed in both T1 and T2 cells. More *flaA* mRNA was present than *flaB* transcript, although other data indicated that the flagellar filament of VC167 might be composed of *flaA* and *flaB* gene products. These results suggest that the native filament represents a complex flagellum composed of both *flaA* and *flaB* gene products, and even though filaments composed of either gene product are functional, the *flaA* filament confers the greater motility whereas a composite flagellum consisting of both gene products confers maximum motility. Mapping by immunogold electron microscopy showed that FlaB may be distributed throughout the length of the wild-type filament. The overall physical organization of the flagellin appeared to be most similar to that found in *Helicobacter pylori.* Even though Nuijten et al. were unable to find mRNA transcribed from the *flaB* gene in *C. jejuni* (17; see below), Guerry et al. (this volume) found that A^{-} B^{+} *C. jejuni* and *C. coli* mutants display a truncated flagellar filament composed of FlaB.

Nuijten et al. have investigated the molecular structure of the flagellar operon of *C. jejuni* 81116 (16, 17). As has been demonstrated for *C. coli,* there are two structural genes, *flaA* and *flaB,* organized in tandem with an intervening short stretch of DNA. These genes encode very similar but not identical proteins of 576 residues, with 32 amino acid changes which are clustered in both termini and in the middle. *C. jejuni* flagellin migrates at approximately 62 kDa in SDS-PAGE, although two bands (at 60 and 62 kDa) can be seen by high-resolution gel electrophoresis. However, these do not represent the protein products of *flaA* and *flaB* but, rather, are due to posttranslational modification of *flaA* protein.

Nuijten et al. have also presented a model of the filament assembly of *Campylobacter* flagellin in comparison with other bacterial flagellins (17). Alignment of termini showed that nonpolar residues appeared to be conserved in some locations. In this model, nonpolar backbones of two alpha-helices were postulated to interact during assembly to stabilize the filament. By analogy with *Salmonella typhi,* a direct repeat separated by 30 residues was present in

Campylobacter flagellin; this could provide for a recombinational event to create new flagellar antigens, although no such recombination has been observed.

To study the antigenic regions on flagellin, Nuijten et al. (this volume) mapped conformation-independent epitopes by expressing flagellar gene segments in the vector pEX, which produces temperature-regulated fusion proteins. Three immunogenic regions were found in fusion proteins encoded by portions of *flaA* and *flaB*. The central part of the flagellin genes appear to encode serotype- and species-specific sequences, similar to the H-antigen regions of *Salmonella* species.

Nuijten et al. (this volume) also studied the control of transcription and expression of flagellin. FlaA is the major protein produced by *C. jejuni* 81116, although FlaB flagellin was found in minor amounts in $A^- B^+$ and Fla^- variants. The *flaA* gene is transcribed from a typical σ^{28} promoter, while the *flaB* gene is preceded by a σ^{54} promoter, similar to the results obtained by Guerry et al. (2). Transcription studies demonstrated that only FlaA mRNA could be detected during in vitro growth and that only σ^{28} holoenzyme activated the *flaA* promoter.

The mechanism of flagellar phase variation in *C. jejuni* has also been examined. Aflagellate spontaneous mutants (Fla^-) produced small amounts of flagellin mRNA from *flaA* and *flaB* genes, suggesting that flagellar gene expression is regulated at the transcriptional level (17). No DNA rearrangements or mutations in the flagellin locus were responsible for switching off flagellin gene expression.

To construct isogenic mutants, Nuijten et al. (this volume) used a pBR322-type suicide plasmid and a kanamycin cassette inserted into the structural genes to accomplish homologous recombination in the *C. jejuni* 81116, Lior serotype 6, chromosome. Three classes of mutants were observed: (i) $A^+ B^-$ (motile, normal flagella); (ii) $A^- B^+$ (nonmotile, truncated flagella consisting of FlaB; reacts with Lior type 6 antiserum); and $A^- B^-$ (nonmotile; bald). The last of these mutants resulted from recombination of the construct with the 5′ region of *flaA* and the 3′ region of *flaB*. As reported by Nuijten et al. (this volume), Wassenaar et al. recently showed (20) that *C. jejuni* 81116 was adherent and invasive, while mutants lacking a functional *flaA* gene and the variant had a highly reduced capacity to enter into INT 407 cells whereas centrifugation of bacteria onto the monolayer restored their capacity to invade (20). These results were interpreted as confirming the direct involvement of flagella per se in infection.

Grant and Tompkins (1a) have also constructed flagellar mutations in *C. jejuni* 81116 by shuttle mutagenesis with a suicide vector (8) containing a kanamycin cassette-modified flagellar gene insert. The overall scheme to construct the mutants by genetic recombination is shown in Fig. 4 and 5. Three classes of mutants were observed: (i) bald (nonmotile), (ii) stubby (truncated, nonmotile), and (iii) motile Fla^+ mutants, all containing the kanamycin cassette (1a). Preliminary data suggest that mutations occurred in the *flaA* structural gene sequence to produce the bald and stubby mutants, while the molecular rearrangement in the third mutant is not yet characterized. In collaboration with Cieplak and Konkel, we examined the mutants for changes in hydrophobicity and for surface charge differences by using a laser Doppler apparatus. All mutants containing the kanamycin cassette gave a slightly higher hydrophobicity index than did the parent strain 81116, which had a highly hydrophobic surface; therefore, we concluded that the absence of flagella on the surface does not affect the surface hydrophobicity to any significant extent. We discovered that, unlike most other bacterial species, *C. jejuni* 81116 had an overall negative surface charge, which was not significantly different in the isogenic mutants, again suggesting that the absence of flagella does not change the surface charge. Preliminary evidence also suggested that the insertion of the kanamycin cassette might have pleiotropic effects as demonstrated by the appearance of new surface-labeled proteins in the mutants, including those in the third class, which were still motile.

The parent strain 81116 and mutants were also examined for the ability to adhere to and enter eukaryotic cells. In contrast to the results of Wassenaar et al. (20), we found that strain 81116 adhered rather poorly to INT 407 and to HEp-2 cells in comparison with other wild-type *C. jejuni* strains tested. The flagellar mutants were also poorly adherent (fewer than 1.0% adhered), and since the adherence values for the wild-type parent were so low, we could not draw any conclusions about the effect of flagella on adherence per se. We also compared the ability of the wild-type strain and the mutants to enter INT 407 and HEp-2 cells. In contrast to Wassenaar et al. (20), we found that strain 81116 did not enter cells to any measurable extent, and therefore no difference between the wild-type parent strain and mutants was detected.

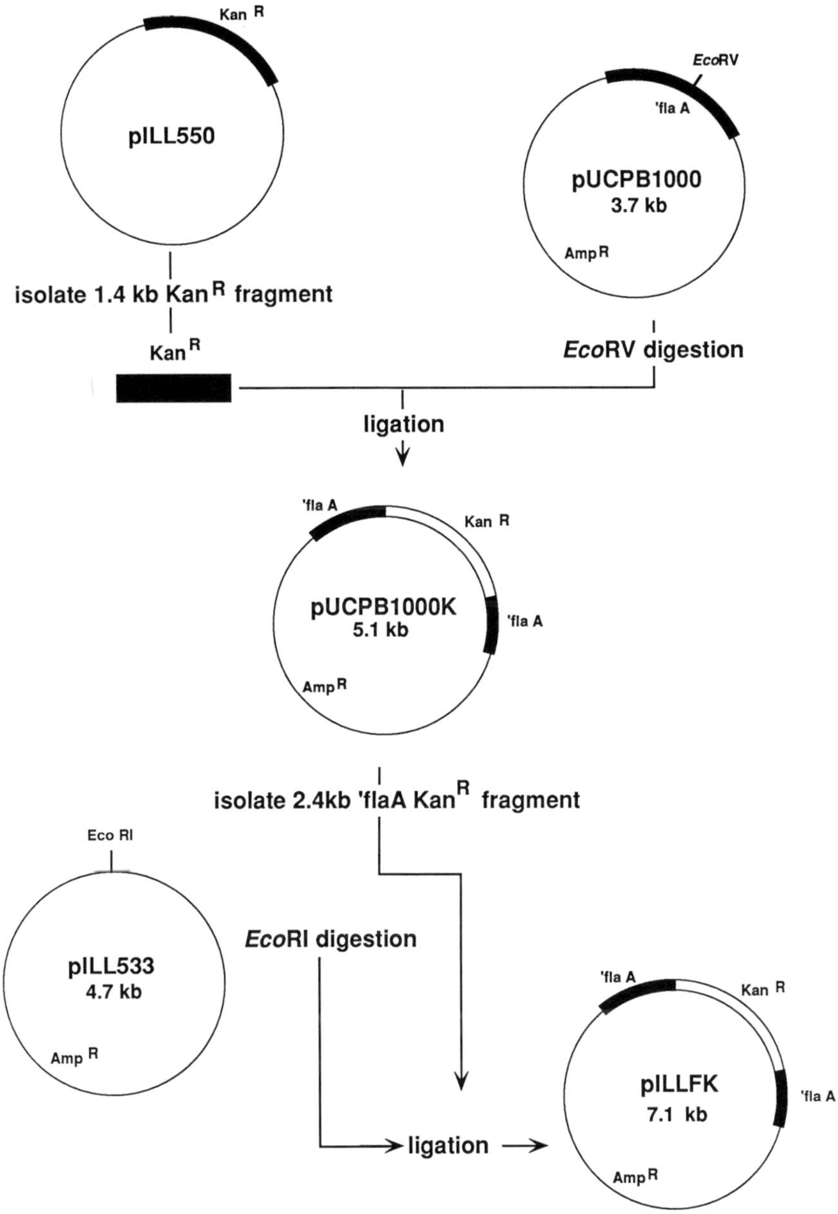

FIGURE 4. Construction of a mutation in the *flaA* gene by ligation with a kanamycin cassette, followed by introduction into the suicide plasmid pILL533, to form pILLFK.

Discussion

All of the groups reporting on *Campylobacter* flagella have confirmed that there is duplication of flagellar genes on the chromosome and that mutations in the *flaA* gene produced nonmotile, bald cells, while mutations in the *flaB* locus produced cells with decreased motility containing a truncated flagellar structure. In *C. coli,* flagellin products of *flaA* and *flaB* have identical molecular weights, whereas antigenic variants produce two distinct flagellin products with apparent M_r of 61,500 and 59,500. Both T1 and T2 cells produce flagella composed of FlaA and FlaB in a complex arrangement; in the wild-type strain, FlaA is the predominant moiety. The

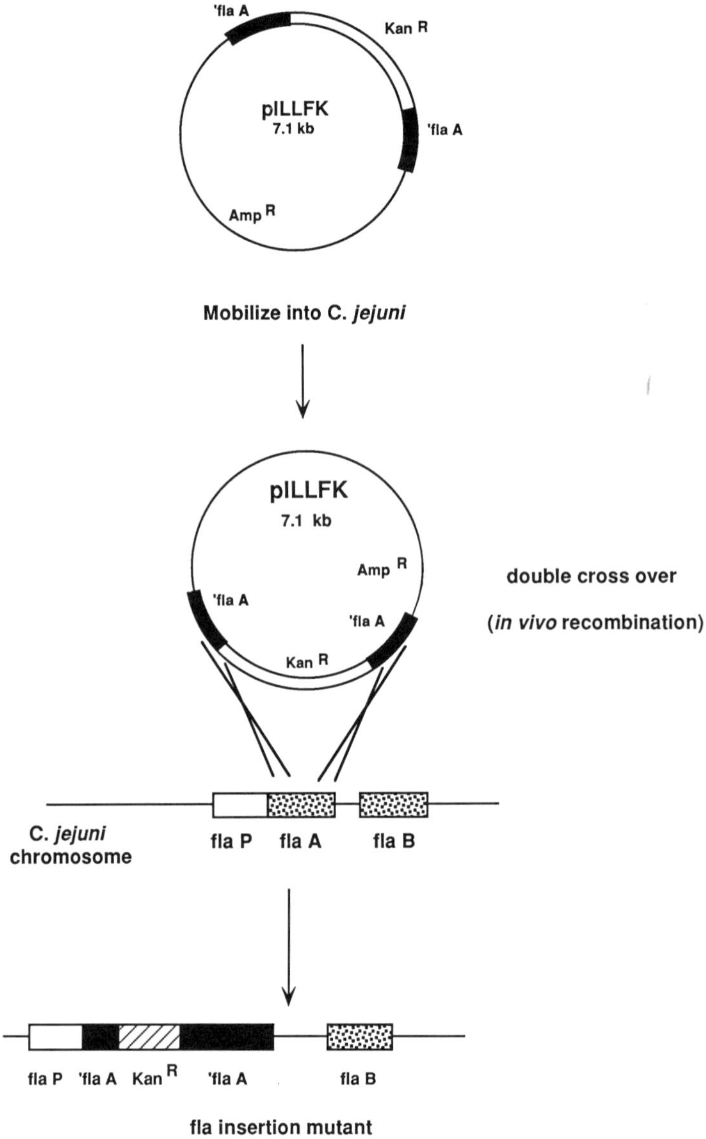

FIGURE 5. Introduction of the *flaA* mutation into the *C. jejuni* 81116 chromosome by homologous recombination. A double-crossover event in *C. jejuni* containing pILLFK (Fig. 4) would promote the formation of a modified *flaA* gene in the chromosome.

basis for antigenic variation in *C. coli* and *C. jejuni* is apparently not related to nucleotide changes in *flaA* and *flaB* genes but is more likely to be due to posttranslational modification of FlaA or FlaB, although differences in the degree of posttranslational phosphorylation may not account for all modifications seen in the variants. The association of antigenic variation with genomic rearrangement was reexamined, and it was discovered that none of the antigenic variants that had not been exposed to selective pressure showed genomic rearrangements, confirming that antigenic variation occurred beyond the level of transcription. Phase variation of *C. jejuni* (conversion from Mot^+ to Mot^-) was correlated with transcriptional regulation of *flaA* expression. Although Nuijten et al. (17) found that *C. jejuni* 81116 could attach to and enter eukaryotic cells, our laboratory was unable to confirm these results.

Guerry et al. (this volume) have confirmed their previous hypothesis that the Lior heat-labile serotyping scheme does not necessarily depend on flagellar antigens, as had been presumed. In a series of clever experiments to transform *C. jejuni* and *C. coli* strains with DNA from mutant *C. coli* VC167, they were able to obtain recombinants that no longer expressed flagellar antigens and had a bald, nonmotile phenotype. Of seven serotypes in which flagellin mutations were constructed, only in Lior serogroup 4 did flagellin seem to be involved in serospecificity, whereas the bald mutants in Lior serogroups 1, 6, 8, 17, 19, and 20 still serotyped as the parental wild type. In conjunction with immunogold-labeling experiments, these data strongly suggest that other cell surface antigens are responsible for most of the heat-labile serospecificity of most serotypes.

The theoretical basis for gene duplication could involve a selective advantage since motility in the highly viscous environment of intestinal mucus is apparently quite important in colonization. Although tandem duplication could lead to recombination between *flaA* and *flaB* and subsequent mutations or deletions, the fact that both genes are stably maintained suggests that this arrangement is advantageous. One reason may be that cells expressing filaments containing both subunits have greater motility than mutants lacking FlaB. The duplication also provides the organism with a backup copy to overcome possible mutations via recombination. Also, bacteria that contain duplicated genes often engage in natural transformation to ensure antigenic diversity.

FUTURE STUDIES ON THE ROLE OF FLAGELLA IN PATHOGENESIS

Birds are among the primary reservoirs of *Campylobacter* spp. However, even though consumption of contaminated poultry is the major mode of transmission of disease to humans, *Campylobacter* infections may also occur as a result of ingestion of contaminated water or milk, demonstrating the ability of *Campylobacter* cells to survive and perhaps replicate under different conditions. The diverse environments of the chicken gut, the human gastrointestinal tract, milk, and water pose a challenge to *Campylobacter* cells to be able to modulate the expression of factors that might be needed for each unique niche. Although there is little information about the possible effects of pH, temperature, oxygen tension, nutrients, and other factors on the expression of any *Campylobacter* genes, the lifestyle of *Campylobacter* species suggests that differential gene expression might be necessary to enable them to modulate factors governing growth in these unique niches. How do *Campylobacter* species survive and replicate in such diverse environments? Which genes are needed to establish colonization in chickens? What niche in the chicken gut is preferentially infected? Where in the human gastrointestinal tract do *Campylobacter* cells express their pathogenic determinants, such as motility or chemotaxis, and where do they replicate? These important questions should be addressed with respect to the role of flagella in pathogenesis. Nuijten et al. have already shown that nonmotile variants do not synthesize flagellin mRNA, and therefore flagellin expression seems to be regulated at the transcriptional level. However, the environmental factors that influence transcription have not yet been elucidated.

By analogy with some other bacterial pathogens, investigators in my laboratory are interested in finding whether expression of flagella and motility is modified at different temperatures, under different atmospheric conditions, in the presence of specific nutrients, etc. Although it is quite straightforward to examine the effect of these during growth in vitro, how can we reveal the response of the organism to different in vivo conditions? Examination of the behavior of mutants that have been genetically modified such that factors which modulate expression of flagellar genes would also induce synthesis of a marker protein, such as β-galactosidase, in experimentally infected animals might help to reveal in vivo factors that operate to control expression, thereby providing further clues to the role of flagella and motility in pathogenesis. Our strategy is to examine the expression of flagellin in vivo by fusing the promoter region of the *flaA* structural genes to *lacZ*, whose expression can be readily detected. Grant has constructed such fusion genes (unpublished data). First, a fragment containing the *flaA* promoter region and the initial portion of the *flaA* structural gene was ligated to the *lacZ* gene of *E. coli*, thereby placing the expression of β-galactosidase under the control of the *flaA* promoter. The fusion gene has been cloned into a lambda vector and introduced as a lambda lysogen into the *E. coli* chromosome. The regulation of expression of the structural flagellin gene during growth under different conditions of oxygen concentration, temperature, pH, etc., can now be monitored by measuring β-galactosidase production by *E. coli* cells containing the recombinant plasmid. Although the regulation of flagellin in *E. coli* may be instructive, we plan to mobilize the *lacZ* fusions into the *Campylobacter* chromosome, by using a scheme outlined in Fig. 6, to obtain genetic recombination. Factors that affect the promoter region should theoretically up- or down-regulate expression. We may find that factors which influence *E. coli* expression will differ from those that regulate *Campylobacter* genes. For *C. coli* and *C. jejuni,* both copies of flagellin genes were transcribed during in vitro growth under one set of conditions, although the FlaA

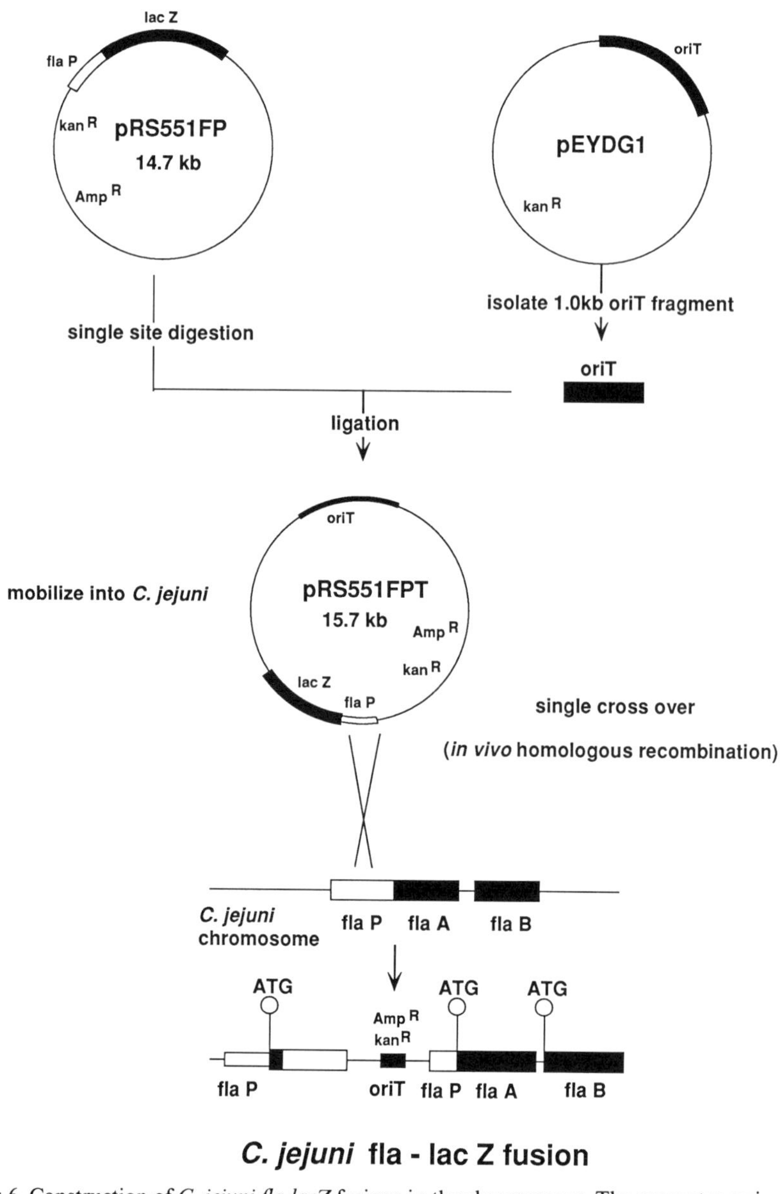

FIGURE 6. Construction of *C. jejuni fla-lacZ* fusions in the chromosome. The promoter region of *flaA* (*flaP*) has been linked to *lacZ,* upstream of the structural gene. Environmental signals that operate on the promoter of flagellin would be expressed in fusion proteins that can be monitored by measuring β-galactosidase synthesis.

product predominated (Guerry et al. and Nuijten et al., this volume). Using fusion constructs of *flaA* and *flaB,* we can now monitor the effect of environmental conditions that might activate the promoters of *flaA* in preference to those of *flaB* by measuring β-galactosidase activity. We may find that both copies are transcribed in vivo, perhaps under different conditions, or that growth of a *flaA* mutant in vivo unmasks expression of *flaB.* In addition to these experiments, genetic fusions of *flaA* and *flaB* could be useful to assess the purpose of gene duplication in *Campylobacter* species.

SUMMARY

Investigation of the molecular pathogenesis of *Campylobacter* species usually involves a genetic or molecular approach to provide genetic and physical maps of the chromosome and to study the role of putative determinants of pathogenicity. This often focuses on flagella and/or motility because a sufficient body of experimental data exists to indicate that these are important factors that function during in vivo infection. The greatest impediment in applying this approach to other putative determinants currently is the lack of convincing data showing that other factors, such as enterotoxins, cytotoxins, adhesins, or invasins, are important in the biology of *Campylobacter* species. In my view, bcforc addrcssing thcsc wc should rccxaminc thc behavior of *Campylobacter* cells in the human gut and in the gut of naturally and experimentally infected animals. Relevant questions which should be answered before proceeding to clone other genes or to identify new proteins are as follows. Where does *C. jejuni* live and replicate in the chicken versus the human gut? Are the organisms motile in the mucous layer in humans? Is there any pathologic evidence in vivo for cytotoxins, enterotoxins, etc.? What natural function would such factors play in *Campylobacter* adaptation to diverse environments? Until we know the answers to these basic questions about the biology of *Campylobacter* species, a strictly molecular approach or factor isolation strategy is not likely to produce useful information about the role of putative pathogenic determinants. Once sufficient biological and clinical information is known, the following sort of molecular genetic approach would be more useful in discerning relevant virulence or pathogenic determinants: (i) make a mutant, e.g., knock out the gene, and compare the mutant with the wild type; (ii) clone the gene; (iii) return the modified gene to the chromosome and compare the behavior of the isogenic mutant with that of the wild-type parent; (iv) clone the wild-type copy into the mutant to restore wild-type function; and (v) examine mutants and wild-type parent strains in relevant models of infection.

It should now be possible, given suitable models of infection, to test the contribution of motility versus the structural flagellar filament to the pathogenesis of infection by using isogenic mutants. Similar strategies could be used to develop isogenic mutants lacking other putative pathogenic determinants. It is clear that all investigators working on the molecular basis of pathogenicity depend upon relevant models of infection, and in this regard further work should be done to develop new animal models in which mutants can be tested.

REFERENCES

1. **Chang, N., and D. E. Taylor.** 1990. Use of pulsed-field agarose gel electrophoresis to size *Campylobacter* spp. genomes and to construct a *Sal*I map of *Campylobacter jejuni. J. Bacteriol.* **172:**4206–4213.

1a. **Grant, C., and L. S. Tompkins.** Unpublished results.

2. **Guerry, P., R. A. Alm, M. E. Power, S. M. Logan, and T. J. Trust.** 1991. Role of two flagellin genes in *Campylobacter* motility. *J. Bacteriol.* **173:**4757–4764.

3. **Guerry, P., S. M. Logan, S. Thornton, and T. J. Trust.** 1990. Genomic organization and expression of *Campylobacter* flagellin genes. *J. Bacteriol.* **172:**1853–1860.

4. **Guerry, P., S. M. Logan, and T. J. Trust.** 1988. Genomic rearrangements associated with antigenic variation in *Campylobacter coli. J. Bacteriol.* **170:**316–319.

5. **Harris, L. A., S. M. Logan, P. Guerry, and T. J. Trust.** 1987. Antigenic variation of *Campylobacter* flagella. *J. Bacteriol.* **169:**5066–5071.

6. **Kostryznska, M., J. D. Betts, J. W. Austin, and T. J. Trust.** 1991. Identification, characterization, and spacial localization of two flagellin species of *Helicobacter pylori* flagella. *J. Bacteriol.* **173:**937–946.

7. **Labigne, A., P. Courcoux, and L. Tompkins.** Submitted for publication.

8. **Labigne-Roussel, A., P. Courcoux, and L. S. Tompkins.** 1988. Gene disruption and replacement as a feasible approach for mutagenesis of *Campylobacter jejuni. J. Bacteriol.* **170:**1704–1708.

9. **Labigne-Roussel, A., J. Harel, and L. S. Tompkins.** 1987. Gene transfer from *Escherichia coli* to *Campylobacter* species: development of shuttle vectors for genetic analysis of *Campylobacter jejuni. J. Bacteriol.* **169:**5320–5323.

10. **Lee, A, S. M. Logan, and T. J. Trust.** 1987. Demonstration of a flagella antigen shared by a diverse group of spiral-shaped bacteria that colonize intestinal mucus. *Infect. Immun.* **55:**828–831.
10a. **Lee, A., J. L. O'Rourke, P. J. Barrington, and T. Trust.** 1986. Mucus colonization as a determinant of pathogenicity in intestinal infection by *Campylobacter jejuni*: a mouse cecal model. *Infect. Immun.* **51:**536–546.
11. **Logan, S. M., P. Guerry, D. M. Rollins, D. H. Burr, and T. J. Trust.** 1989. In vivo antigenic variation of *Campylobacter* flagellin. *Infect. Immun.* **57:**2583–2585.
12. **Logan, S. M., L. A. Harris, and T. J. Trust.** 1987. Isolation and characterization of *Campylobacter* flagellins. *J. Bacteriol.* **169:**5072–5077.
13a. **McSweegan, E., and R. I. Walker.** 1986. Identification and characterization of two *Campylobacter jejuni* adhesins for cellular and mucous substrates. *Infect. Immun.* **53:**141–148.
13. **Logan, S. M., and T. J. Trust.** 1982. Molecular identification of surface protein antigens of *Campylobacter jejuni*. *Infect. Immun.* **42:**675–682.
14. **Miller, J. F., W. Dower, and L. S. Tompkins.** 1988. High-voltage electroporation of bacteria: genetic transformation of *Campylobacter jejuni* with plasmid DNA. *Proc. Natl. Acad. Sci. USA* **85:**856–860.
15. **Nuijten, P. J. M., C. Bartels, N. M. C. Bleumink-Pluym, W. Gaastra, and B. A. M. van der Zeijst.** 1990. Size and physical map of the *Campylobacter jejuni* chromosome. *Nucleic Acids Res.* **18:**6211–6214.
16. **Nuijten, P. J. M., N. M. C. Bleumink-Pluym, W. Gaastra, and B. A. M. van der Zeijst.** 1989. Flagellin expression in *Campylobacter jejuni* is regulated at the transcriptional level. *Infect. Immun.* **57:**1084–1088.
17. **Nuijten, P. J. M., F. J. A. M. van Asten, W. Gaastra, and B. A. M. van der Zeijst.** 1990. Structural and functional analysis of two *Campylobacter jejuni* flagellin genes. *J. Biol. Chem.* **265:**17798–17804.
18. **Seifert, H. S., E. Y. Chen, M. So, and F. Heffron.** 1986. Shuttle mutagenesis: a method of transposon mutagenesis for *Saccharomyces cerevisiae*. *Proc. Natl. Acad. Sci. USA* **83:**735–739.
19. **Wang, Y., and D. E. Taylor.** 1990. Natural transformation of *Campylobacter* species. *J. Bacteriol.* **172:**949–955.
20. **Wassenaar, T. M., N. M. C. Bleumink-Pluym, and B. A. M. van der Zeijst.** 1991. Inactivation of *Campylobacter jejuni* flagellin genes by homologous recombination demonstrates that *fla*A but not *fla*B is required for invasion. *EMBO J.* **10:**2055–2061.
21. **Wenman, W. M., D. E. Taylor, and H. Lior.** 1985. The flagellar protein determines *Campylobacter jejuni* heat labile serotype, p. 212. *In* A. D. Pearson, M. B. Skirrow, H. Lior, and B. Rowe (ed.), *Campylobacter III*. Public Health Laboratory Service, London.

CHAPTER 29

Genetic Analysis of *Campylobacter* spp.

DIANE E. TAYLOR

INTRODUCTION

The appreciation of *Campylobacter jejuni* as a major pathogen and the recognition of its role in previously undiagnosed cases of gastroenteritis occurred in 1977 (53). Three years later the first simple genetic studies were published with the visualization of plasmids in *C. jejuni* and *C. coli* (2) and the demonstration of plasmid and concomitant antibiotic resistance transfer within the genus *Campylobacter* (60). During the next 10 years research on plasmid-mediated antibiotic resistance mechanisms continued apace. These topics are covered in this volume by Tenover et al. (chapter 8) and Taylor (chapter 9).

This chapter will review the current state of genetic analysis in *Campylobacter* species including descriptions of cloning vectors designed for use in *Campylobacter* species. Our current knowledge of genetic exchange in *Campylobacter* species will be discussed. Within the past year significant headway has been made in constructing genetic maps of the *C. jejuni* and *C. coli* chromosomes by using pulsed-field gel electrophoresis (PFGE). The application of PFGE to *C. jejuni* and *C. coli* will be described, and some preliminary genetic maps will be presented.

GENES CLONED FROM *CAMPYLOBACTER* SPECIES

Few genes have been cloned from *Campylobacter* species. Published studies of genes cloned from *C. jejuni* or *C. coli* are shown in Table 1. Genes encoding three enzymes, γ-glutamyl kinase (31), γ-glutamylphosphate reductase (31), and serine hydroxymethyltransferase (9), were cloned in *Escherichia coli* from gene libraries constructed from *C. jejuni* DNA by selection for complementation in a *proA proB* mutant of *E. coli* (for the proline biosynthesis genes) and in an *E. coli glyA* mutant (for the serine hydroxymethyltransferase gene). Unfortunately, confirmatory DNA sequencing data on the *proA proB* and *glyA* genes have yet to be published.

Significant amounts of time and energy have been expended on cloning flagellin genes from *C. coli* and *C. jejuni* (Table 1). These elegant studies are described in detail in reviews in this volume by Guerry et al. and Nuijten et al. and will not be considered here.

A polyclonal antibody directed against the major outer membrane protein from *C. jejuni* UA580 was used to screen λgt11 libraries for genes specifying such a protein(s) (57). Two different DNA fragments were identified (63). One fragment hybridized only with *C. jejuni* DNA and can be used as a *C. jejuni*-specific probe, whereas the other hybridized with all *C. jejuni* and *C. coli* strains tested and some *C. lari* strains (63). DNA sequencing (64) demonstrated that both of these fragments lacked the complete open reading frame for the major outer membrane protein, which is believed to be a porin (21). Work is in progress to complete the sequence of these putative major outer membrane protein genes and to compare the deduced protein sequences with those of porins from other species.

rRNA genes (16S and 23S) have been cloned by Rashtchian et al. (45) and Kim and Chan (26). These genes, of which there appear to be three copies in *C. jejuni* and *C. coli* strains, are proving useful in genome-mapping studies (see the section on PFGE). Two tRNA genes (Table 1) were cloned by their close physical association with 16S rRNA (46).

Diane E. Taylor, Department of Medical Microbiology and Infectious Diseases and Canadian Bacterial Diseases Network, University of Alberta, Edmonton, Alberta, Canada T6G 2H7.

TABLE 1. Genes cloned from *C. jejuni* and *C. coli*

Genetic property	Cloning strategy	Reference(s)
γ-Glutamyl kinase[a] γ-Glutamylphosphate reductase[a]	Reverse genetics[b]	31
Serine hydroxymethyltransferase[c]	Reverse genetics	9
Flagellin	λgt11 plus antibody[d]	40, 41
Flagellin	Oligonucleotide probes	19, 34
Major outer membrane protein[e]	λgt11 plus antibody	63, 64
rRNA (16S, 23S)	Hybridization of rRNA[f]	26, 45
tRNA (Ala)	Located next to 16S rRNA gene	46
tRNA (Leu)	Located next to 16S rRNA gene	46

[a] Complementation of *proA* and *proB* mutations in *E. coli*.
[b] Reverse genetics refers to complementation of an *E. coli* mutant by a cloned gene(s) from *Campylobacter* species.
[c] Complementation of *glyA* mutation in *E. coli*.
[d] Refers to the procedure of constructing gene libraries in phage λgt11 and subsequent screening with an antibody to the protein of interest (22).
[e] The complete open reading frame of the major outer membrane protein has not yet been cloned.
[f] Clones were detected by hybridization of labeled rRNA from *C. jejuni*.

The small number of genes cloned from *Campylobacter* species has led to the conclusion that *Campylobacter* genes are difficult to clone and that problems are encountered in the expression of *Campylobacter* genes in *E. coli.* This has been noted previously by Walker et al. in their review of the pathophysiology of *Campylobacter* species (71). General housekeeping genes such as *glyA* and *proA proB,* however, would appear to be more easily cloned and expressed in *E. coli* than genes encoding more specialized proteins such as flagellins or porins.

CLONING VECTORS FOR *CAMPYLOBACTER* SPP.

Shuttle Vectors

Several cloning vectors have now been constructed for use in *C. jejuni* and *C. coli,* including shuttle vectors which can be transferred from *E. coli* to *Campylobacter* species. Labigne-Roussel et al. constructed pILL550, which represents the first generation of *E. coli*-to-*Campylobacter* shuttle vectors (30). Unfortunately, pILL550 has

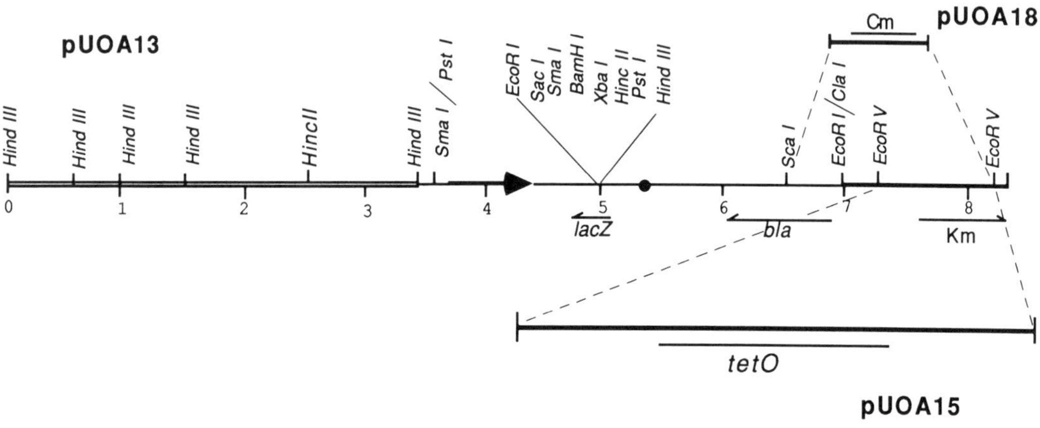

FIGURE 1. Restriction maps of the shuttle vectors pUOA13, pUOA15, and pUOA18. Positions of resistance determinants are indicated: Km (kanamycin resistance), Cm (chloramphenicol resistance), *tetO* (tetracycline resistance) (all of which are expressed in both *E. coli* and *Campylobacter* species), *bla,* and ampicillin resistance (β-lactamase production) (which is expressed only in *E. coli*). Double lines represent DNA sequence from the *Campylobacter* plasmid pIP1445; arrow represents *oriT* DNA; thin line represents pUC13 DNA. Numbers represent kilobase pairs. (Reprinted with permission from D. E. Taylor, *Annu. Rev. Microbiol.*, Vol. **46**, in press.)

been lost (28) and the only vector that has survived is pILL550A, which contains additional *Pst*I and *Sma*I sites, making it less useful than its predecessor for cloning (72).

Wang and Taylor (72) have constructed a series of shuttle vectors (Fig. 1; Table 2) based on the same strategy used by Labigne et al. (30). However, in addition, our vectors contain the *lacZ'* determinant, which can complement a defective β-galactosidase in *E. coli* and is useful for selection of clones by their blue or white appearance on plates containing 5-bromo-4-chloro-3-indolyl-β-D-galactopyranoside (X-Gal) (70). An origin of replication derived from the *C. coli* plasmid pIP1445 (30), which functions in *Campylobacter* species, is included, as well as an origin of replication from plasmid pUC13 (70), which functions in *E. coli.* The investigator can then choose up to three antibiotic resistance markers which function in *E. coli, C. jejuni,* and *C. coli.* The pUOA13 and pUOA17 plasmids encode kanamycin resistance specified by an aminoglycoside phosphotransferase (Tenover et al., this volume), whereas pUOA15 encodes tetracycline resistance specified by the TetO determinant and pUOA18 encodes chloramphenicol resistance specified by a chloramphenicol acetyltransferase (Taylor, chapter 9 of this volume). All plasmids contain an *oriT* sequence from the IncPα plasmid RK2 (68), which can be used to mobilize the plasmids when transfer functions are supplied in *trans* from a transfer-competent P-group plasmid.

Other Vectors

Vectors for the study of transformation in *Campylobacter* spp. have also been constructed (74). They consist of the origin of replication from a *C. coli* plasmid, a resistance determinant which functions in *Campylobacter* spp., and a multiple cloning site (Table 2). The uptake of these vectors into both plasmid-free strains of *C. jejuni* and *C. coli* and strains containing homologous rescue plasmids is currently being analyzed (74). DNA fragments from *Campylobacter* spp. can be cloned into the multiple cloning site and used to search for sequences which enhance uptake by the natural transformation process (72).

Suicide vectors which are able to be introduced into *Campylobacter* spp. by conjugation, transformation, or electroporation but are unable to replicate in these species have also been constructed (29, 74). So far only one successful study has been reported involving shuttle mutagenesis of 16S rRNA genes (29). In the absence of effective transposon mutagenesis for *Campylobacter* spp., shuttle mutagenesis holds the greatest promise for the construction of mutants and for improvements in genetic analysis.

GENETIC EXCHANGE MECHANISMS

Plasmid Transfer

Conjugative plasmids encoding resistance to tetracycline, kanamycin, and chloramphenicol, either separately or in combination, have been found in *Campylobacter* spp. (59). We examined several tetracycline resistance (Tc^r) plasmids from *C. coli* and *C. jejuni* and constructed restriction endonuclease maps of the plasmids and their Tc^r regions (58, 66). Most of these plasmids are from 45 to 50 kb in size, with a G+C content of 31.0 to 33.0 mol%, which is approximately equivalent to that of the *C. jejuni* chromosome (32.5 mol%) (62). Plasmid transfer frequencies ranged from about 10^{-5} to 10^{-3} transconjugants per recipient cell in a 24-h mating period. All plasmids tested transferred more efficiently on a solid surface than in liquid medium (61, 62). No evidence of sex pili has been noted in plasmid-containing *C. jejuni* cells (65). The host range of these plasmids is entirely restricted to closely related *Campylobacter* species (59, 61).

Nothing is known about the arrangement of genes involved in conjugative transfer or replication in *Campylobacter* plasmids. Unfortunately, transposon mutagenesis has not been successful in *Campylobacter* spp. (29). Neither Tn*5* (4), a typical gram-negative transposon, nor Tn*917* (52), a gram-positive transposable element, has been found to insert into *Campylobacter* DNA (29). Therefore, this technique, so useful for mapping transfer genes in conjugative plasmids from members of the family *Enterobacteriaceae* (56), has not been successfully applied to analysis of *Campylobacter* plasmids. These studies must await the development of better genetic tools for *Campylobacter* spp.

Natural Transformation

Wang and Taylor (72) observed that both *C. coli* and *C. jejuni* could take up DNA without the requirement for any special treatment, such as $CaCl_2$ or heat shock. Natural transformation frequencies for homologous chromosomal DNA markers, streptomycin resistance (Str^r) and nalidixic acid resistance (Nal^r), were approximately 1×10^{-3} transformant per recipient cell for *C. coli* and 1×10^{-4} transformant per recipient cell

TABLE 2. *Campylobacter* cloning vectors

Plasmid	Resistance marker(s)	Size (kb)	Replication origin			Reference
			E. coli	*Campylobacter* spp.	*oriT*[a]	
pUOA13	Ap^r Km^r	8.3	+	+	+	72
pUOA14	Ap^r Cm^r Km^r	8.2	+	+	+	73
pUOA15	Ap^r Tc^r	11.7	+	+	+	72
pUOA17	Km^r	8.2	+	+	+	72
pUOA18	Cm^r	7.4	+	+	+	73
pUOA19	Km^r	4.9	−	+	−	72
pUOA20	Cm^r	4.8	−	+	−	73

[a] *oriT* is the transfer origin from an IncPα plasmid (68).

for *C. jejuni*. Cotransformation frequencies for Str^r and Nal^r are 2×10^{-7}, indicating that these markers are not closely linked. Transformation was prevented by incubation with DNase I. Some campylobacters produce extracellular DNase; however, there was no correlation between the DNase-producing ability of the recipient and its ability to take up endogenous DNA. Of five *C. coli* strains tested, all were naturally competent, whereas only three of six *C. jejuni* strains appeared to be competent.

The competence process in *Campylobacter* spp. is not understood but is almost completely independent of the growth phase of the cells (72). Early-log-phase bacteria were found to be very slightly more competent than were late-log-phase cells. The maximum transformation frequency obtained with *C. coli* UA585, when 0.01 μg of DNA per ml was added, was 4×10^5 transformants per μg of DNA (72).

Transformation of plasmid DNA in *Campylobacter* spp. is much less efficient than that of chromosomal DNA. The frequency of transformation of plasmid pUOA17 (Table 2) into plasmid-free *C. coli* UA585 was about 1,000 times lower than that of chromosomal DNA markers. However, when UA585 contained a homologous plasmid, such as pUOA15, transformation frequencies were increased 100-fold. The plasmid present in the recipient acts as a rescue plasmid by recombining with the incoming plasmid (72).

The uptake of both *Campylobacter* chromosomal DNA and plasmid DNA has been monitored by examining the uptake of ^{32}P-labeled DNA into *C. coli* UA585 (72). *C. coli* chromosomal DNA was taken up efficiently, whereas plasmid pUOA13 and *E. coli* DNA were taken up in barely detectable amounts. Competition experiments were also used to examine chromosomal DNA uptake. Both *C. jejuni* and *C. coli* unlabeled DNA could compete for uptake of ^{32}P-labeled *C. coli* DNA with approximately equal efficiency, whereas *E. coli* DNA could not (72).

The available evidence suggests that *Campylobacter* DNAs contain a specific sequence necessary for binding to and uptake into *Campylobacter* cells. An uptake sequence of 11 bp has been identified in *Haemophilus* spp. (13), and one of 10 bp has been reported in *Neisseria gonorrhoeae* (17). The presence of the required sequences periodically throughout the *Campylobacter* genome DNA may then ensure efficient uptake. Plasmids may not carry these sequences or may not carry them in large enough numbers to trigger uptake, particularly if part of the plasmid has come from a different organism.

Natural transformation is being used successfully in chromosome mapping (see below) and in analysis of chromosomal genes such as those encoding flagellin (Guerry et al., this volume; Nuijten et al., this volume). Even though the process is presently poorly understood, natural transformation is proving to be a useful technique for *Campylobacter* genetic analysis.

Electroporation

Miller et al. reported electrotransformation of a shuttle vector, pILL512, into *C. jejuni* C31 at frequencies as high as 1.2×10^6 transformants per μg of DNA (36). We have used both pILL550A and pUOA13 in plasmid electroporation studies. Using the commercially available Gene Pulsar apparatus (Bio-Rad), a field strength of 12.5 kV/cm, and a time constant of 2 ms, we obtained maximum transformation frequencies of 5×10^3 transformants per μg of DNA (or approximately 1×10^{-6} transformant per viable cell) (74). *Campylobacter* spp. appear to tolerate exposure to high-voltage electric fields

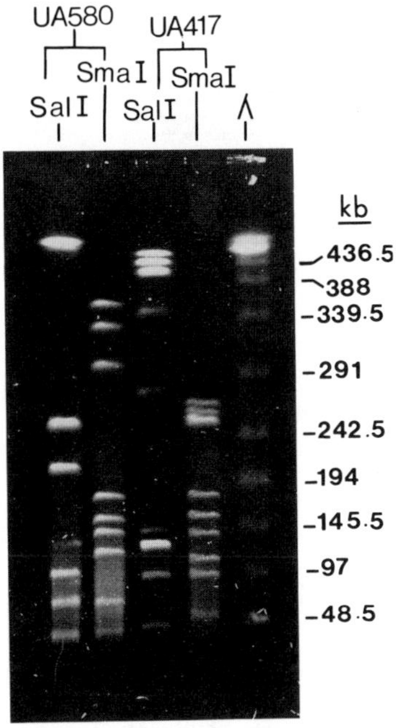

FIGURE 2. PFGE of *C. jejuni* UA580 and *C. coli* UA417 digested with *Sal*I and *Sma*I. The lanes contain (from left to right) *C. jejuni* UA580 digested with *Sal*I and *Sma*I, *C. coli* UA417 digested with *Sal*I and *Sma*I, and a phage lambda DNA ladder, the sizes of which are shown on the right-hand side of the figure. Conditions for PFGE were 1% agarose at 175 V with a 25-s switching pulse for 25 h in 0.05 M TBE as described previously (10). The sizes of the *Sal*I and *Sma*I fragments are given in Table 3.

without difficulty (36, 74). We found that pulsing at a maximum voltage of 12.5 kV/cm for five cycles of 2 ms did not reduce cell viability (74). *C. jejuni* C31 has been used successfully in electroporation studies (36, 76), although, for unknown reasons, some other strains of *C. jejuni* and *C. coli* appear to take up DNA poorly by this technique.

Bacteriophages for *Campylobacter* spp.

Bacteriophages specific for *C. jejuni* and *C. coli* have been described by Ritchie et al. (47), Grajewski et al. (18), and Salama et al. (49, 50). These studies have been aimed primarily at developing bacteriophage typing schemes for epidemiological purposes. None of the phages obtained by Salama et al. were lysogenic, and induction with mitomycin C was not useful for phage selection (49). Although the *Campylobacter* phages identified so far are lytic, it is possible that genetic information could be disseminated by bacteriophage transduction in this genus. However, bacteriophage transduction of *Campylobacter* genetic markers has yet to be reported.

GENETIC MAPPING OF *CAMPYLOBACTER* SPP.

Genome Sizes of *Campylobacter* spp.

PFGE has facilitated the determination of genome sizes and the construction of physical maps of the chromosomes of a number of different bacterial species (see reference 27 for a review). Bacterial genome sizes vary from *Mycoplasma genitalium* (55), with a size of only 585 kb, to *Myxococcus xanthus* (11), the largest, with a size of 9,454 kb (9.45 Mb).

The genome sizes of both *C. jejuni* and *C. coli* are approximately equal at 1.7 Mb (10). Restriction endonucleases found to be most useful for PFGE analysis of *C. jejuni* and *C. coli* genomes were *Sal*I and *Sma*I. These enzymes generate a manageable number of well-separated DNA fragments (Fig. 2). Fragment sizes of *C. jejuni* UA580 (NCTC 11168) and *C. coli* UA417 are shown in Table 3 along with their total genome sizes. Both the *C. jejuni* UA580 and *C. coli* UA417 genomes have been shown to be circular by analysis of partial digest patterns (10, 77). Genome sizes of *C. jejuni* UA501 (which is equivalent to *C. jejuni* 81116) and *C. coli* UA578 (NCTC 11353) were also determined by us to be 1.7 Mb (10, 77). Nuijten et al. have also determined that *C. jejuni* 81116 has a genome size of 1.7 Mb by PFGE studies (39).

C. jejuni and *C. coli* genomes are the same size as that of *Streptococcus thermophilus* (5) and slightly smaller than those of *Haemophilus influenzae* Rd (1.9 Mb) (32, 33), *Streptococcus sanguis* (2.3 Mb) (5), or *Haemophilus parainfluenzae* (2.3 Mb) (25). They are only 36% of the size of the *E. coli* chromosome (54). Campylobacters are small and delicate, require supplemented medium for growth, and are biochemically inert. Their small genome size is also consistent with their failure to ferment carbohydrates or degrade complex substances (24).

Construction of Genome Maps

A preliminary *Sal*I genome map of *C. jejuni* UA580 was constructed by analysis of fragments

TABLE 3. Restriction fragments of *C. jejuni* UA580 and *C. coli* UA417 generated by *Sal*I and *Sma*I digestion

	Fragment size (kb)[a]			
	C. jejuni UA580		*C. coli* UA417	
Fragment no.	*Sal*I	*Sma*I	*Sal*I	*Sma*I
1	980	371	430	255
2	280	345	400	250
3	220	316	344	240
4	110	191	276	238
5	80	161	125	163
6	48.5	141	97	143
7		107	25	124
8		55		97
9		39		85
10				42
11				23
12				13
13				6
Total	1,718.5	1,726	1,697	1,679

[a] Average sizes were based on at least three independent estimates obtained by PFGE as described in reference 10.

obtained from incomplete *Sal*I digestion (10). This map has been expanded to include *Sma*I restriction sites (Fig. 3). Following PFGE, DNA fragments were transferred to nitrocellulose filters as described previously (56). The filters were hybridized to individual DNA fragments which had been labeled with [α-^{32}P]dATP by nick translation after extraction from low-melting-point agarose (77). The relative positions of some overlapping fragments were determined by hybridization with a series of DNA probes (see below). A similar strategy was used to construct a genome map of *C. coli* UA417 (Fig. 4).

Gene Mapping with DNA Probes

Location of genes on genome maps of other species has been based on hybridization of both homologous and heterologous DNA probes (6, 8). Some genes, such as those required for routine housekeeping, are highly conserved between species (8, 27). DNA probes specific for conserved genes are very useful for mapping genes in species from which few genes have been cloned (8).

For mapping *Campylobacter* genes we used two probes from *C. jejuni*, a flagellar gene probe (41) and a 16S rRNA gene probe (45), as well as a series of heterologous probes (shown in Table 4). The heterologous probes which did not hybridize to *Campylobacter* DNA are also listed in Table 4. The positions of the various genes were localized as far as possible on the *C. jejuni* UA580 and *C. coli* UA417 maps (Fig. 3 and 4) (67).

Gene Mapping by Using Natural Transformation

Natural transformation can also be used to map genetic determinants in *Campylobacter* spp. (76, 77). *Sma*I DNA fragments extracted from low-melting-point agarose after separation by PFGE were used to transform *C. coli* UA417. Only *Sma*I fragment 3 was able to transform erythromycin resistance, whereas only *Sma*I fragment 6 was able to transform streptomycin resistance to *C. coli* UA417. Thus the genes specifying erythromycin resistance and streptomycin resistance in *C. coli* UA417 could be mapped to *Sma*I fragment 3 and *Sma*I fragment 6, respectively (Fig. 4).

Conclusions and Questions Arising from Gene-Mapping Studies

We are continuing to refine the maps of the *C. jejuni* UA580 and *C. coli* UA417 genomes.

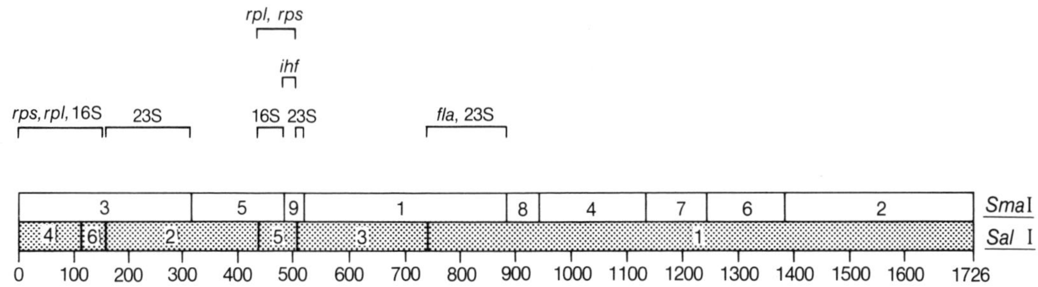

FIGURE 3. Genomic map of *C. jejuni* UA580. The physical map was constructed on the basis of analysis of partially digested DNA fragments and DNA hybridization studies. The circular chromosome has been linearized to aid in presentation. The positions of 16S and 23S rRNA genes were determined by hybridization of DNA probes (see Table 4). The positions of other markers were also determined by DNA hybridization with the probes listed in Table 4. Abbreviations: *fla, C. jejuni flaA, flaB; ihf, E. coli hip himA; rpl, E. coli rplJ rplL; rps, E. coli rpsG rpsL.* The positions are in kilobase pairs.

Analysis of cloned genomic fragments of UA580 and UA417 in progress in our laboratory will enable us to more precisely map genes which have been as yet imprecisely located. However, some conclusions can be drawn from our work so far.

Arrangement of flagellar genes

The two flagellar genes in *C. jejuni* 81116 are located together approximately 300 kb from one 16S rRNA gene and 700 kb from another (39). Similarly, the flagella genes in *C. jejuni* UA580 as judged by hybridization are located about 700 and 170 kb away from the two closest 16S rRNA genes (Fig. 2) (67). These results suggest that the relative locations of flagellar genes and 16S rRNA genes are conserved in two different *C. jejuni* strains.

Arrangement of rRNA genes

Our results confirm work by Kim and Chan (26), Labigne-Roussel et al. (29), and Nuijten et al. (39; see also reference 15) that there are three copies of 16S and 23S rRNA genes in *C. jejuni* and *C. coli.* However, we cannot confirm that 16S and 23S rRNA genes are always located in the same operon, as suggested by Kim and Chan (26). Our results demonstrate that in several instances in both *C. jejuni* and *C. coli* strains the 16S and 23S rRNA genes appear to be separate (Fig. 3 and 4). In *C. jejuni* 81116, at least one of the 16S and 23S rRNA genes is located separately (39, 67). This arrangement is characteristic of rRNA genes in organisms such as *Mycoplasma gallisepticum* (12), *Leptospira in-*

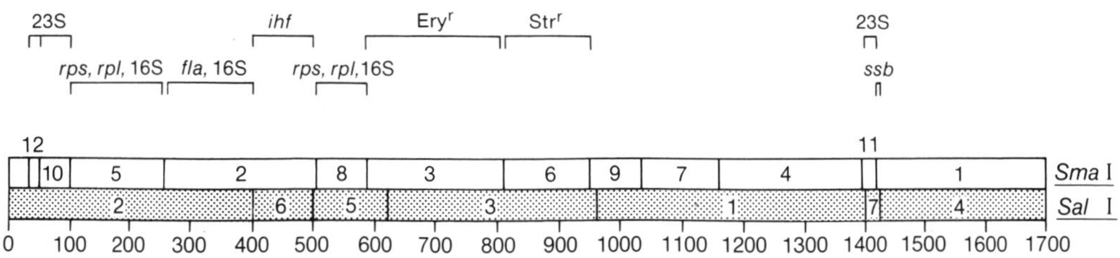

FIGURE 4. Genomic map of *C. coli* UA417. The physical map was constructed on the basis of analysis of partially digested DNA fragments and DNA hybridization studies. The circular chromosome has been linearized to aid in presentation. The positions of 16S and 23S rRNA genes were determined by hybridization of DNA probes (see Table 4). The positions of other markers were also determined by DNA hybridization with the probes listed in Table 4. The positions of Ery^r and Str^r markers were determined by natural transformation of genomic DNA fragments (77). Abbreviations: *fla, C. jejuni flaA flaB; ihf, E. coli hip himA; rpl, E. coli rplJ rplL; rps, E. coli rpsG rpsL; ssb, E. coli ssb.* The positions are in kilobase pairs.

TABLE 4. DNA probes used in mapping *Campylobacter* genes

Gene(s)	Plasmid	Species[a]	Homology[b] with campylobacters	Source	Reference
16S rRNA	pAR140	*C. jejuni*	+	A. Rashtchian	45
flaA flaB	pIVB-300	*C. jejuni*	+	B. A. M. van der Zeijst	41
23S rRNA[c]	pCW1	*E. coli*	+	J. Ofengand and C. Weitzmann	75
rplJ rplL[d]	pNO2016	*E. coli*	+	M. Nomura	44
rpsG rpsL[d]	pNO2005	*E. coli*	+	M. Nomura	43
ssb[e]	pTL119A-5	*E. coli*	+	C. Radding	35
hip himA[f]	pPLhip.himA-5	*E. coli*	+	M. Dubow	38
dnaK[g]	pCG1	*E. coli*	−	C. Georgopoulos	23
grpE[g]	pOF39	*E. coli*	−	C. Georgopoulos	1
groES and *groEL*[g]	pDA1	*E. coli*	−	C. Georgopoulos	14
katE[h]	pAMlkatE6	*E. coli*	−	P. C. Loewen	37
katG[i]	pBT22	*E. coli*	−	P. C. Loewen	69
LT-A and LT-B	pJM17	*V. cholerae*	−	J. Mekalanos	42
recA	pDR1453	*E. coli*	−	C. Radding	51

[a] Species from which the cloned fragment originated.
[b] Homology was determined by hybridization under conditions of moderate stringency to Southern blots prepared from agarose gels after PFGE.
[c] 23S rRNA gene is from the *rrnB* operon.
[d] *rplJ* encodes the L10 ribosomal protein; *rplL* encodes the L7/L12 ribosomal protein; *rpsG* encodes the S7 ribosomal protein; *rpsL* enclodes the S12 ribosomal protein.
[e] *ssb* encodes the single-stranded binding protein that hybridized only with *C. coli* DNA.
[f] *hip himA* encodes integration host factor.
[g] Heat shock proteins.
[h] *katE* encodes the structural gene for HPII, a bifunctional catalase-peroxidase.
[i] *katG* encodes the bifunctional catalase-peroxidase HPI.

terrogans (16), and *Thermus thermophilus* (20) but not of rRNA genes in *E. coli* or *H. influenzae* (27, 33).

Arrangement of ribosomal protein genes and other conserved genes

Ribosomal protein genes (*rplJ* and *rplL*), which encode the large ribosomal subunit proteins L10 and L7/L12, respectively, are located together at 90 min on the *E. coli* map (3, 44). A probe carrying these genes (Table 4) hybridized to two regions located within the *Sal*I 5 and 8 fragments separated by 250 kb in *C. coli* UA417 (*rpl* in Fig. 4). Similarly in *C. jejuni* UA580 the L7/L12 and L10 probe hybridized to two regions separated by at least 250 kb. Therefore, the arrangement of L7/L12 and L10 ribosomal protein genes is not conserved between *Campylobacter* spp. and *E. coli*. Also, the same two *Sal*I fragments in *C. coli* UA417 hybridized to a probe for two *E. coli* genes, *rpsG* and *rpsL*, which encode two small-subunit ribosomal proteins, S7 and S12 (43). In *C. jejuni* a similar arrangement is seen with the *rpsG* and *rpsL* probe hybridizing to the same fragments as the *rplJ* and *rplL* probe did. In *E. coli rpsG* and *rpsL* are located at 73 min on the genetic map (3), quite a distance from *rplJ* and *rplL* at 90 min. In both *C. jejuni* and *C. coli*, however, there appear to be two separate clusters making up one 16S rRNA gene and both large and small ribosomal protein genes together in two different regions of the genome.

The StrA mutation, which results in streptomycin resistance, maps to the *rpsL* gene (3). Streptomycin resistance in *C. coli* UA417R was mapped by natural transformation of genomic DNA fragments (see Taylor, chapter 9 of this volume). The location of the Str^r marker in UA417R did not correspond to the fragment which hybridized to the *rpsL* gene probe. Therefore, the mutation responsible for streptomycin resistance in *C. coli* appears to result from a different mutation from that seen in *E. coli* StrA mutants.

In another region of the *C. coli* UA417 genome a single 23S rRNA gene is located close to a locus which hybridized to a probe for the single-stranded binding-protein gene *(ssb)*. In *E. coli* K-12 the *ssb* gene is located at 92 min on the map (3). The position of an *ssb* gene on *C. jejuni* has not yet been identified (67). However, a probe for the *E. coli* integration host factor genes *(hip himA)* appeared to hybridize to both

C. jejuni and *C. coli* genomes at a single position. The genes within this probe are located at different positions on the *E. coli* map and have been spliced in this vector (38). The gene encoding the α subunit of the integration host factor *(himA)* is located at 37 min, whereas the β-subunit gene *(hip)* is located at 20 min (3).

There is no sound reason to expect that the gene organization of campylobacters and that of *E. coli* K-12 would be similar. Comparisons are made simply because so much information is available for *E. coli* K-12 and so little for most other bacteria. Although there is conservation of gene arrangement at the origins and termini of replication in many bacteria (27), these regions have yet to be identified in *Campylobacter* spp.

Heterologous probes that are nonhomologous with Campylobacter spp.

One of the heterologous gene probes that did not hybridize with *C. jejuni* and *C. coli* genome DNA carries the *Vibrio cholerae* LT-A and LT-B genes (42). This result agrees with results of previous hybridization studies by Calva et al. (7) and also with results of studies discussed in reference 71, in which workers failed to demonstrate nucleic acid homology between *C. jejuni* chromosomal DNA and gene probes for the A and B subunits of cholera toxin.

Two *E. coli* genes (*katE* and *katG*), which encode catalase-peroxidases (37, 69), hybridized to neither *C. jejuni* nor *C. coli*. Even though both species produce catalase (24), the enzymes involved are presumably quite distinct from the *E. coli* enzymes.

None of the heat shock gene probes (*dnaK, grpE,* or *groES* and *groEL*) (1, 14, 23) from *E. coli* were able to hybridize with *C. jejuni* or *C. coli* DNA, even though these genes are considered to be well conserved throughout evolution. Similarly, *recA,* which is highly conserved across numerous species boundaries (48), showed no homology with *Campylobacter* DNA.

General arrangement of Campylobacter genes

Other questions also arise from our results. Are campylobacters constantly undergoing chromosomal rearrangements which have separated the 16S and 23S rRNA genes in some strains (*C. jejuni* UA580) but not in others (*C. jejuni* TGH9001 [26])? Have different gene arrangements evolved to fulfill different growth needs: facultative *(E. coli)* versus microaerobic (*C. jejuni* and *C. coli*)? As genome maps of other microorganisms become available, it will be fascinating to compare their gene locations with those of *Campylobacter* spp. to try to understand whether gene organization is purely random, resulting from previous homologous recombination events, or whether there is indeed a higher degree of organization, perhaps related to the regulation of functionally related genes (27).

PERSPECTIVES

It is 5 years since the review article on the pathophysiology of *Campylobacter* enteritis was published (71). Genetic studies of *Campylobacter* spp. were considered then to be in their infancy, with only two genes (γ-glutamyl kinase and γ-glutamylphosphate reductase) cloned in *E. coli* (31). Since that time several more genes have been cloned from *Campylobacter* spp., and their sequences are being completed. Considerable progress has been made since 1986 in the genetic analysis of *Campylobacter* spp., with the determination of the genome sizes of *C. jejuni* and *C. coli,* the construction of genome maps of some strains, and the location of a number of genes on the maps. Much more work remains to be done, but a good start has been made.

There are now quite a lot of useful vectors available for *C. jejuni* and *C. coli.* Plasmid DNA can be introduced into *Campylobacter* spp. by conjugation using P-group plasmid mobilization, by natural transformation, or by electroporation. The identification of a transposon for mutagenesis still eludes us, but a method for gene replacement mutagenesis is now available. Over the next 5 years, we can expect to see an increase in both the number and the level of sophistication of genetic studies of *Campylobacter* spp.

ACKNOWLEDGMENTS. I thank N. Chang, K. Hiratsuka, M. Eaton, Y. Wang, and W. Yan for their help in the preparation of this chapter, D. Maher for comments on the manuscript, and H. Mitchell for excellent secretarial assistance. The contribution of all those listed in Table 4 who supplied DNA probes is acknowledged. Work on PFGE described in this chapter has been financially supported by the National Centre of Excellence Program as part of the Canadian Bacterial Diseases Network.

REFERENCES

1. **Ang, D., and C. Georgopoulos.** 1989. The heat-shock-regulated *grpE* gene of *Escherichia coli* is required for bacterial growth at all temperatures but is dispensable in certain mutant backgrounds. *J. Bacteriol.* **171:**2748–2755.

2. **Austen, R. A., and T. J. Trust.** 1980. Detection of plasmids in the related group of the genus *Campylobacter*. *FEMS Microbiol. Lett.* **8:**201–204.
3. **Bachmann, B. J.** 1987. Linkage map of *Escherichia coli* K-12, edition 7, p. 807–876. *In* F. C. Neidhardt, J. L. Ingraham, K. B. Low, B. Magasanik, M. Schaechter, and H. E. Umbarger (ed.), *Escherichia coli and Salmonella typhimurium: Cellular and Molecular Biology*. American Society for Microbiology, Washington, D.C.
4. **Berg, D.** 1989. Transposon Tn*5*, p. 185–210. *In* D. E. Berg and M. M. Howe (ed.), *Mobile DNA*. American Society for Microbiology, Washington, D.C.
5. **Bourgeois, P. L., M. Mata, and P. Ritzenthaler.** 1989. Genome comparison of Lactococcus strains by pulsed-field gel electrophoresis. *FEMS Microbiol. Lett.* **59:**65–70.
6. **Butler, P. D., and E. R. Moxon.** 1990. A physical map of the genome of *Haemophilus influenzae* type b. *J. Gen. Microbiol.* **136:**2333–2342.
7. **Calva, E., J. Torres, M. Vazquez, V. Angeles, H. de la Vega, and G. M. Ruiz-Palacios.** 1989. *Campylobacter jejuni* chromosomal sequences that hybridize to *Vibrio cholerae* and *Escherichia coli* LT enterotoxin genes. *Gene* **75:**243–251.
8. **Canard, B., and S. T. Cole.** 1989. Genome organization of the anaerobic pathogen *Clostridium perfringens*. *Proc. Natl. Acad. Sci. USA* **86:**6676–6680.
9. **Chan, V. L., H. Bingham, A. Kibue, P. R. V. Nayudu, and J. L. Penner.** 1988. Cloning and expression of the *Campylobacter jejuni glyA* gene in *Escherichia coli*. *Gene* **73:**185–191.
10. **Chang, N., and D. E. Taylor.** 1990. Use of pulsed-field agarose gel electrophoresis to size *Campylobacter* spp. genomes and to construct a *Sal*I map of *Campylobacter jejuni* UA580. *J. Bacteriol.* **172:**5211–5217.
11. **Chen, H., I. M. Keseler, and L. J. Shimkets.** 1990. The genome size of *Myxococcus xanthus* determined by pulsed-field gel electrophoresis. *J. Bacteriol.* **172:**4206–4213.
12. **Chen, X., and E. R. Finch.** 1989. Novel arrangement of rRNA genes in *Mycoplasma gallisepticum*. *J. Bacteriol.* **171:**2876–2878.
13. **Danner, D. B., R. A. Deich, K. L. Sisco, and H. O. Smith.** 1980. An eleven-base-pair sequence determines the specificity of DNA uptake in *Haemophilus* transformation. *Gene* **11:**311–318.
14. **Fayet, O., J.-M. Louarn, and C. Georgopoulos.** 1986. Suppression of the *Escherichia coli dnaA46* mutation by amplification of the *groES* and *groEL* genes. *Mol. Gen. Genet.* **202:**434–445.
15. **Frydenberg, J., and C. Christiansen.** 1985. The sequence of 16S rRNA from *Mycoplasma* strain PG50. *DNA* **4:**127–137.
16. **Fukunaga, M., and I. Mifuchi.** 1989. Organization of *Leptospira interrogans* rRNA genes. *J. Bacteriol.* **171:**5763–5767.
17. **Goodman, S. D., and J. J. Scocca.** 1988. Identification and arrangement of the DNA sequence recognized in specific transformation of *Neisseria gonorrhoeae*. *Proc. Natl. Acad. Sci. USA* **85:**6982–6986.
18. **Grajewski, B. A., J. W. Kusek, and H. M. Gelfand.** 1985. Development of a bacteriophage typing system for *Campylobacter jejuni* and *Campylobacter coli*. *J. Clin. Microbiol.* **22:**13–18.
19. **Guerry, P., S. M. Logan, S. Thornton, and T. J. Trust.** 1990. Genomic organization and expression of *Campylobacter* flagellin genes. *J. Bacteriol.* **172:**185–1860.
20. **Hartmann, R. K., and V. A. Erdmann.** 1989. *Thermus thermophilus* 16S rRNA is transcribed from an isolated transcription unit. *J. Bacteriol.* **171:**2933–2941.
21. **Huyer, M., T. R. Parr, Jr., R. E. W. Hancock, and W. J. Page.** 1986. Outer membrane porin protein of *Campylobacter jejuni*. *FEMS Microbiol. Lett.* **37:**247–250.
22. **Huynh, T. V., R. A. Young, and R. W. Davis.** 1985. Construction and screening cDNA libraries in lambda gt10 and lambda gt11, 49–78. *In* D. Glover (ed.), *DNA Cloning Techniques: A Practical Approach*, vol. 2. IRL Press, Eynsham, England.
23. **Johnson, C., G. N. Chandrasekhar, and C. Georgopoulos.** 1989. *Escherichia coli* DnaK and GrpE heat shock proteins interact both in vivo and in vitro. *J. Bacteriol.* **171:**1590–1596.
24. **Karmali, M. A., and M. B. Skirrow.** 1984. Taxonomy of the genus Campylobacter, p. 1–20. *In* J. Butzler (ed.), *Campylobacter Infection in Man and Animals*. CRC Press, Inc., Boca Raton, Fla.
25. **Kauc, L., and S. H. Goodgal.** 1989. The size and physical map of the chromosome of *Haemophilus parainfluenzae*. *Gene* **83:**377–380.
26. **Kim, N. W., and V. L. Chan.** 1989. Isolation and characterization of the ribosomal RNA genes of *Campylobacter jejuni*. *Curr. Microbiol.* **19:**247–252.
27. **Krawiec, S., and M. Riley.** 1990. Organization of the bacterial chromosome. *Microbiol. Rev.* **54:**502–539.
28. **Labigne, A.** Personal communication.
29. **Labigne-Roussel, A., P. Courcoux, and L. Tompkins.** 1988. Gene disruption and replacement as a feasible approach for mutagenesis of *Campylobacter jejuni*. *J. Bacteriol.* **170:**1704–1708.
30. **Labigne-Roussel, A., J. Harel, and L. Tompkins.** 1987. Gene transfer from *Escherichia coli* to *Campylobacter* species: development of shuttle vectors for genetic analysis of *Campylobacter jejuni*. *J. Bacteriol.* **169:**5320–5323.
31. **Lee, E. C., R. I. Walker, and P. Guerry.** 1985. Expressions of *Campylobacter* genes for proline biosynthesis in *Escherichia coli*. *Can. J. Microbiol.* **31:**1064–1067.
32. **Lee, J. J., and H. O. Smith.** 1988. Sizing of the *Haemophilus influenzae* Rd genome by pulsed-field agarose gel electrophoresis. *J. Bacteriol.* **170:**4402–4405.
33. **Lee, J. J., H. O. Smith, and R. J. Redfield.** 1989. Organization of the *Haemophilus influenzae* Rd genome. *J. Bacteriol.* **171:**3016–3024.
34. **Logan, S. M., T. J. Trust, and P. Guerry.** 1989. Evidence for posttranslational modification and

gene duplication of *Campylobacter* flagellin. *J. Bacteriol.* **171**:3031–3038.

35. **Lohman, T. M., J. M. Green, and R. S. Beyer.** 1986. Large-scale overproduction and rapid purification of the *Escherichia coli ssb* gene product. Expression of the *ssb* gene under λPL control. *Biochemistry* **25**:21–25.
36. **Miller, J. F., W. J. Dower, and L. S. Tompkins.** 1988. High voltage electroporation of bacteria: genetic transformation of *Campylobacter jejuni* with plasmid DNA. *Proc. Natl. Acad. Sci. USA* **85**:856–860.
37. **Mulvey, M. R., P. A. Sorby, B. L. Triggs-Raine, and P. C. Loewen.** 1988. Cloning and physical characterization of *katE* and *katF* required for catalase HPII expression in *Escherichia coli. Gene* **73**:337–345.
38. **Nash, H. A., C. A. Robertson, E. Flamm, R. A. Weisberg, and H. I. Miller.** 1987. Overproduction of *Escherichia coli* integration host factor, a protein with nonidentical subunits. *J. Bacteriol.* **169**:4124–4127.
39. **Nuijten, P. J. M., C. Bartels, N. M. C. Bleumink-Pluym, W. Gastra, and B. A. M. van der Zeijst.** 1990. Size and physical map of the *Campylobacter jejuni* chromosome. *Nucleic Acids Res.* **18**:6211–6214.
40. **Nuijten, P. J. M., N. M. C. Bleumink-Pluym, W. Gaastra, and B. A. M. van der Zeijst.** 1989. Flagellin expression in *Campylobacter jejuni* is regulated at the transcriptional level. *Infect. Immun.* **57**:1084–1088.
41. **Nuijten, P. J. M., F. J. A. M. van Asten, W. Gaastra, and B. A. M. van der Zeijst.** 1990. Structural and functional analysis of two *Campylobacter jejuni* flagellin genes. *J. Biol. Chem.* **265**:17798–17804.
42. **Pearson, G. D. N., and J. Mekalanos.** 1982. Molecular cloning of *Vibrio cholerae* enterotoxin genes in *Escherichia coli* K-12. *Proc. Natl. Acad. Sci. USA* **79**:2976–2980.
43. **Post, L. E., and M. Nomura.** 1980. DNA sequence of the *str* operon of *Escherichia coli. J. Biol. Chem.* **255**:4660–4666.
44. **Post, L. E., G. D. Strycharz, M. Nomura, H. Lewis, and P. P. Dennis.** 1979. Nucleotide sequence of the ribosomal protein gene cluster adjacent to the gene for RNA polymerase β in *Escherichia coli. Proc. Natl. Acad. Sci. USA* **76**:1697–1701.
45. **Rashtchian, A., M. A. Abbott, and M. Shaffer.** 1987. Cloning and characterization of genes coding for ribosomal RNA in *Campylobacter jejuni. Curr. Microbiol.* **14**:311–317.
46. **Rashtchian, A., and M. Shaffer.** 1986. The nucleotide sequences of two tRNA genes from *Campylobacter jejuni. Nucleic Acids Res.* **14**:5560.
47. **Ritchie, A. E., J. H. Bryner, and J. W. Foley.** 1983. Role of DNA and bacteriophage in Campylobacter auto-agglutination. *J. Med. Microbiol.* **16**:333–340.
48. **Roca, A. I., and M. M. Cox.** 1990. The RecA protein: structure and function. *Crit. Rev. Biochem. Mol. Biol.* **25**:415–456.
49. **Salama, S., F. J. Bolton, and D. N. Hutchinson.** 1989. Improved method for the isolation of *Campylobacter jejuni* and *Campylobacter coli* bacteriophages. *Lett. Appl. Microbiol.* **8**:5–7.
50. **Salama, S., F. J. Bolton, and D. N. Hutchinson.** 1990. Application of a new phage typing scheme to campylobacters isolated during outbreaks. *Epidemiol. Infect.* **104**:405–411.
51. **Sancar, A., and W. D. Rupp.** 1979. Physical map of the *recA* gene. *Proc. Natl. Acad. Sci. USA* **76**:3144–3148.
52. **Shaw, J. H., and D. B. Clewell.** 1985. Complete nucleotide sequence of macrolide-lincosamide-streptogramin B-resistance transposon Tn*917* in *Streptococcus faecalis. J. Bacteriol.* **164**:782–796.
53. **Skirrow, M. B.** 1977. Campylobacter enteritis—a "new" disease. *Br. Med. J.* **2**:9–11.
54. **Smith, C. L., J. G. Econome, A. Schutt, S. Klco, and C. R. Cantor.** 1987. A physical map of the *Escherichia coli* K-12 genome. *Science* **236**:1448–1453.
55. **Su, C. J., and J. B. Baseman.** 1990. Genome size of *Mycoplasma genitalium. J. Bacteriol.* **172**:4705–4707.
56. **Taylor, D. E., E. C. Brose, S. Kwan, and W. Yan.** 1985. Mapping of transfer regions within incompatibility group HI plasmid R27. *J. Bacteriol.* **162**:1221–1226.
57. **Taylor, D. E., and N. Chang.** 1987. Immunoblot and enzyme-linked immunosorbent assays of *Campylobacter* major outer-membrane protein and application to the differentiation of *Campylobacter* species. *Mol. Cell. Probes* **1**:261–274.
58. **Taylor, D. E., N. Chang, R. S. Garner, R. Sherburne, and L. Mueller.** 1986. Incidence and antibiotic resistance and characterization of plasmids in *Campylobacter jejuni* isolated from clinical sources in Alberta, Canada. *Can. J. Microbiol.* **32**:28–32.
59. **Taylor, D. E., and P. Courvalin.** 1988. Mechanisms of antibiotic resistance in *Campylobacter* species. *Antimicrob. Agents Chemother.* **32**:1107–1112.
60. **Taylor, D. E., S. A. DeGrandis, M. A. Karmali, and P. C. Fleming.** 1980. Transmissible tetracycline resistance in *Campylobacter jejuni. Lancet* **ii**:797.
61. **Taylor, D. E., S. A. DeGrandis, M. A. Karmali, and P. C. Fleming.** 1981. Transmissible plasmids from *Campylobacter jejuni. Antimicrob. Agents Chemother.* **19**:831–835.
62. **Taylor, D. E., R. S. Garner, and B. J. Allan.** 1983. Characterization of tetracycline resistance plasmids from *Campylobacter jejuni* and *Campylobacter coli. Antimicrob. Agents Chemother.* **24**:930–935.
63. **Taylor, D. E., and K. Hiratsuka.** 1990. Use of non-radioactive DNA probes for detection of *Campylobacter jejuni* and *Campylobacter coli* in stool specimens. *Mol. Cell. Probes* **4**:261–271.
64. **Taylor, D. E., and K. Hiratsuka.** Unpublished data.
65. **Taylor, D. E., and R. Sherburne.** Unpublished data.

66. **Taylor, D. E., W. Yan, L.-K. Ng, E. K. Manavathu, and P. Courvalin.** 1988. Genetic characterization of kanamycin resistance in *Campylobacter coli. Ann. Inst. Pasteur Microbiol.* **139:**665–676.
67. **Taylor, D. E., W. Yan, and M. Eaton.** Unpublished data.
68. **Thomas, C. M., and C. A. Smith.** 1987. Incompatibility group P plasmids: genetics, evolution, and use in genetic manipulation. *Annu. Rev. Microbiol.* **41:**77–101.
69. **Triggs-Raine, B. L., and P. C. Loewen.** 1987. Physical characterization of *katG* encoding catalase HPI of *Escherichia coli. Gene* **52:**121–128.
70. **Vieira, J., and J. Messing.** 1982. The pUC plasmids, an M13mp7-derived system for insertion mutagenesis and sequencing in the synthetic universal primers. *Gene* **19:**259–268.
71. **Walker, R. I., M. B. Caldwell, E. C. Lee, P. Guerry, T. J. Trust, and G. M. Ruiz-Palacios.** 1986. Pathophysiology of *Campylobacter* enteritis. *Microbiol. Rev.* **50:**81–94.
72. **Wang, Y., and D. E. Taylor.** 1990. Natural transformation of *Campylobacter* species. *J. Bacteriol.* **172:**949–955.
73. **Wang, Y., and D. E. Taylor.** 1990. Chloramphenicol resistance in *Campylobacter coli:* nucleotide sequence, expression and cloning vector construction. *Gene* **94:**23–28.
74. **Wang, Y., and D. E. Taylor.** Unpublished data.
75. **Weitzmann, C. J., P. R. Cunningham, and J. Ofengand.** 1990. Cloning, *in vitro* transcription, and biological activity of *Escherichia coli* 23S ribosomal RNA. *Nucleic Acids Res.* **18:**3515–3520.
76. **Yan, W.** 1990. *Characterization of Erythromycin Resistance in Campylobacter spp.* Ph.D. thesis, University of Alberta, Edmonton.
77. **Yan, W., and D. E. Taylor.** 1991. Sizing and mapping of the genome of *Campylobacter coli* strain UA417R using pulsed-field gel electrophoresis. *Gene* **101:**117–120.

CHAPTER 30

Molecular and Structural Analysis of *Campylobacter* Flagellin

PATRICIA GUERRY, RICHARD A. ALM, MARY E. POWER, AND TREVOR J. TRUST

INTRODUCTION

Campylobacters are typically described as small, curved, S-shaped, or spiral bacteria with a single polar flagellum at one or both ends of the cell. This flagellum grows out of a characteristic cone-shaped depression or pit known as the flagella insertion point, and its rotation imparts high motility upon the *Campylobacter* cell. Indeed, the earliest observations of the association of *Campylobacter*-like organisms with human disease noted this characteristic motility (25).

Together with the spiral morphology of the *Campylobacter* cell, the motility imparted by the flagellum appears to play an important role in both the selection and ultimate colonization of their niche in the gastrointestinal tract, the viscous mucous blanket lining the tract. Ferrero and Lee (9) have shown that *C. jejuni* retains its motility in viscous solutions capable of immobilizing the majority of flagellated bacteria. Not surprisingly, Lee et al. (30) have also demonstrated that campylobacters are highly motile in intact mucus strands of mucosal scrapings taken from the ceca of infected mice. The motility observed in this environment was not the typical tumbles and runs seen with many bacteria, but involved rapid runs up and down the strands of mucus. The ability of the *Campylobacter* flagellum to impart such vigorous motility in this viscous and seemingly inimical environment is probably a reflection of both the strength of the motor driving the rotation of the flagella filament and perhaps a structural characteristic of the *Campylobacter* filament. The viscosity of the environment is known to cause conformational changes in the flagellar helix and so reduce the efficiency of propulsion of the flagella (48, 49). This presumably accounts for the decreased motility of conventional rod-shaped bacteria in high-viscosity solutions (24). Ferrero and Lee (9) have therefore suggested that *C. jejuni* may differ from other bacteria in that the torque generated by the *C. jejuni* flagellum may be regulated by alterations in the configuration of the flagellum brought on by increases in the viscosity of the medium. Certainly, it is clear that this motility suited to movement in a viscous environment provides campylobacters with a preferential ability to colonize gastrointestinal mucus, and it is not surprising that a loss of motility is inimical to the ability of campylobacters to colonize the gastrointestinal tract and produce disease (4, 7, 36). The best confirmation for motility as a virulence factor comes from the inability of true isogenic nonflagellated mutants described later in this chapter to colonize the gastrointestinal tract of experimental animals.

In addition to this virulence role, the flagellar protein is the predominant protein antigen of the *Campylobacter* cell. This is true both in natural infections, in which both secretory and circulating antibodies are produced in response to the gastrointestinal colonization, and in experimental situations such as parenteral immunization, in which antibody production is the objective (5, 6, 35, 42, 56). Early studies identified the flagellar protein as one with an apparent subunit molecular weight of 58,000 to 62,500. Western immunoblot analysis showed the presence of cross-reactive epitopes among the flagellins of *C. jejuni* and *C. coli* strains, the flagellins of other *Campylobacter* species, and

Patricia Guerry, Enteric Diseases Program, Naval Medical Research Institute, Bethesda, Maryland 20814. **Richard A. Alm, Mary E. Power, and Trevor J. Trust,** Department of Biochemistry and Microbiology, University of Victoria, Victoria, British Columbia, Canada V8W 3P6.

even *Helicobacter pylori* flagellin (26, 29, 33), indicating a degree of sequence conservation within the motility protein of this group of mucus-colonizing bacteria.

Subsequent studies involving absorption experiments against native flagella filaments, together with enzyme-linked immunosorbent assay, Western blot analysis, and immunoelectron microscopy, showed that a significant proportion of the cross-reactive epitopes were not exposed on the surface of the assembled *Campylobacter* flagella filament, but the filament possessed a sizable number of apparently serospecific surface-exposed epitopes (34). This confirmed the observations by Hébert et al. (17), using immunofluorescence, that certain of their typing antisera specifically bound the flagella of certain serotypes. Further evidence of the serospecificity of flagella was provided by the observation that in certain strains the loss of flagella appeared to be accompanied by a loss of ability to be serotyped in a heat-labile serotyping scheme (54, 55).

One puzzling observation in many of the earlier studies on *Campylobacter* flagella was the rather broad, diffuse character of the Coomassie blue staining reaction of flagellin in sodium dodecyl sulfate-polyacrylamide gel electrophoresis (SDS-PAGE) analysis and in Western blots. This hinted at the presence of flagellin molecules of different apparent subunit molecular weight (M_r), but in minor copy number compared with the predominant species. As more strains were examined, the presence of distinct flagellin bands of different subunit M_r in certain strains was confirmed. For example, a collection of strains of *C. coli* belonging to the LIO8 serogroup displayed this property (16). Since the Lior typing procedure is based on doubly cloned cultures, this suggested the possibility that a single strain of *C. coli* produced flagellin species of different subunit M_r. Immunoelectron-microscopic examination of certain of these cultures with the particular batch of typing antiserum available at the time further revealed within a single culture the presence of flagellum filaments which were capable of binding the typing antibodies and other flagellum filaments which apparently did not bind these antibodies. This suggested that the ability to produce flagellins of different subunit M_r might also be accompanied by an antigenic variation of flagella. When one of the LIO8 strains was examined in greater detail, this ability was confirmed (16).

Essentially, cultivation of cells of *C. coli* VC167 in the presence of antibodies capable of binding to the surface of one antigenic type of flagellum filament enabled isolation of cells producing a different antigenic type. This was possible from a single clone. Antibodies prepared against the second antigenic type of flagella allowed isolation of cells producing the original antigenic type of flagella. In cells producing antigenic type 1 (T1) flagella, a single flagellin band of apparent subunit M_r 61,500 was observed by SDS-PAGE. This protein was reactive with LIO8 antiserum, but not with an antiserum (LAH2 [16]) against antigenic type 2 (T2) flagella. Cells producing T2 flagella displayed a single flagellin band of apparent subunit M_r 59,500 by SDS-PAGE, and this flagellin was reactive with LAH2 antiserum but not with LIO8 antiserum. In addition to these serospecific epitopes, the two proteins shared cross-reactive flagellin epitopes. The proteins also shared identical N-terminal amino acid sequences to residue 30. These findings suggested that the flagellum filament of *C. coli* was composed of multiple copies of a single species of flagellin and that in *C. coli* VC167, the antigenic difference between the two flagellum filaments produced by this strain could perhaps be related to the difference in the subunit M_r of the species making up the filament. Similar changes in M_r were observed during animal passage (32). When nonimmune rabbits were infected with VC167-T1 cells, campylobacters isolated from the feces of these animals initially produced the 61,500 M_r flagellin characteristic of T1, but there was a gradual transition during the course of the infection such that isolates from most rabbits eventually produced only the M_r 59,500 flagellin characteristic of T2 cells. Rabbits infected with VC167-T2 cells consistently shed campylobacters producing only the M_r 59,500 flagellin. The variability between T1 and T2 flagellins has also been observed to be accompanied both in vitro and in vivo by an uncharacterized genomic rearrangement at a locus adjacent to one of the rRNA genes (15), as well as by sequence changes within the flagellin gene(s) (14).

A prerequisite for elucidating the molecular structure of campylobacter flagellin, as well as for determining the mechanism of antigenic variation in VC167, was to clone the flagellin gene from VC167. This was initially done by using a synthetic oligonucleotide probe specific for the N terminus of VC167 flagellin (33, 36). It was subsequently determined, as detailed below, that VC167 contained two flagellin genes organized in an unusual manner.

MOLECULAR CHARACTERIZATION OF FLAGELLIN GENES

Both VC167-T1 and VC167-T2 have been shown to contain two tandemly oriented flagellin genes, termed *flaA* and *flaB*, as seen diagramatically in Fig. 1 (15, 36). The *flaA* and *flaB* genes in both T1 and T2 cells are >93% homologous to one another and encode open reading frames of 572 amino acids. The DNA sequence of each is shown in Fig. 2, and the predicted protein sequences are compared in Fig. 3. The two campylobacter FlaA flagellins show a high degree of conservation with other bacterial flagellins. For example, at the N terminus of VC167-T1 FlaA, amino acid residues 3 to 169 (approximately encoded by region I in Fig. 1B) show 33.7% homology to *Salmonella typhimurium* flagellin (20) and 36.3% homology to *Bacillus subtilis* flagellin (8). At the C terminus of VC167-T1 FlaA flagellin, amino acid residues 474 to 572 (encoded by region V) show 41.9 and 36.4% identity with *S. typhimurium* and *B. subtilis*, respectively. In other bacterial flagellins these regions contain sequences essential for transport of the flagellin monomer and assembly of the monomers into the filament; the internal region, which lacks functional constraints, contains the antigenically variable region (20, 21, 22, 23, 27, 53). Not surprisingly, therefore, the small number of sequence differences between the antigenically distinct T1 and T2 flagellins occur in this central region of the flagellin molecule, in both *flaA* and *flaB*. The majority of sequence differences between *flaA* and *flaB* in both T1 and T2, however, occur within regions I and V of the molecule (Fig. 1). The two *flaB* gene products show a total of 30 common residue changes from the *flaA* gene products, 11 changes occurring in the N-terminal 75 residues, 6 changes in the central region from 260 to 272, and 13 changes in the C-terminal region from 504 to 572. The *flaB* gene product from T2 displays further changes from the T2 *flaA* gene product at the five amino acid residues 201, 202, 286, 287, and 301. The nucleotide sequence differences between the *flaA* gene of T1 and the *flaA* gene of T2 occur within region II, affecting residues 201 and 202; all sequence differences between the *flaB* gene of T1 and the *flaB* gene of T2 occur within region III, affecting residues 286, 287, and 301.

N-terminal amino acid sequencing of several internal peptides of VC167-T1 FlaA flagellin resulting from cyanogen bromide or trypsin cleavage suggested that certain residues were posttranslationally modified. The DNA sequence indicated that the blocked amino acids were serine residues, and these residues are indicated in Fig. 3. The most heavily modified region includes a duplication of a 9-amino-acid sequence separated by 34 amino acids. The most likely modification, at least of some of the serine residues in campylobacter flagellin, is phosphorylation, a common modification of this amino acid in eukaryotic systems. Indeed, treatment of purified flagellin from VC167 with acid phosphatase causes a reduction in its apparent M_r in SDS-PAGE gels (12). The presence of phosphorylated residues in a bacterial surface appendage is unusual. The most frequently observed modification of surface structures is methylation. For example, the flagellins of *S. typhimurium* and *Spirillum serpens* contain methyl-lysine residues (2, 11, 23), and the fimbrins of *Neisseria*, *Moraxella*, *Pseudomonas*, *Bacteroides*, and *Vibrio* species have methylated phenylalanine as the first residue (10, 19, 37, 47, 50). The biological significance of phosphorylated flagellin remains to be determined, but the charge imparted by the modified serines may contribute to the discrepancy between the apparent M_r on SDS-PAGE and the predicted M_r of each protein (Table 1) and may also be involved in the antigenic properties of the flagellin (see below).

Northern (RNA) blot analyses with synthetic oligonucleotide primers specific for each gene as probes indicated that the *flaA* and *flaB* genes were expressed concomitantly in both T1

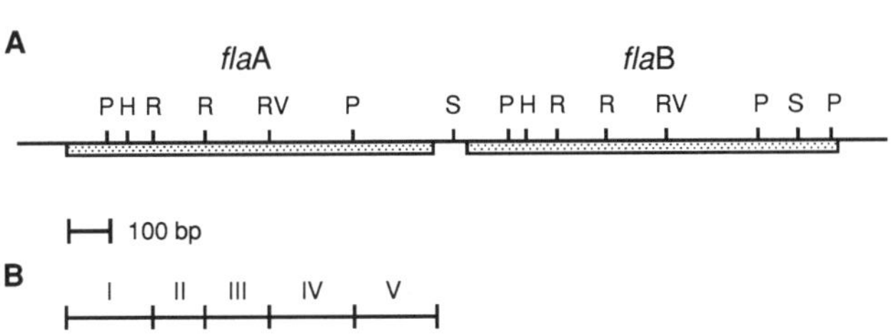

FIGURE 1. (A) Map of *C. coli* VC167 flagellin gene cluster. Transcription of the genes is from left to right as drawn. Restriction sites: P, *Pst*I; H, *Hin*dIII; R, *Eco*RI; RV, *Eco*RV; S, *Ssp*I. (B) Schematic representation of different regions of the *C. coli* VC167 flagellin gene based on restriction enzyme sites in *flaA*. The length of each region is as follows: region I, 435 bp; region II, 252 bp; region III, 324 bp; region IV, 408 bp; region V, 300 bp.

```
TTTTAGTGATGATAACTTTATACAGGTGGTATTTTAAAAGGGGTATTGTATTATCGTGGGAGTTTTTTATCTGAAGCTATAAAAAAAGATTTGAAAGATGAGGCGTATTATCTTTTAAAT  120
TTTATTAGCGCTTATCAAAAATGGCTTGAAAAGTTTATTGAGAGGCTAGAAATAAAAAATGCCATCATAAAAGATACAGTGTTAAAATATGGAAATTTGATATAAAATTTTATAAAACTC  240

-35             -10      mRNA                             rbs     flaA
TAAACTATTTTTCCTTTTAAACGATATAGTTTATAACAAGTTCATGGATGGACTTGAATTTATTTAAAAGGATTTAAAATGGGATTTCGTATTAACACAAATGTTGCAGCATTAAATGCT  360

AAAGCAAATTCGGATCTAAACAGCAGAGCATTAGATCAATCACTTTCAAGACTCAGTTCAGGTCTTAGAATCAACTCCGCAGCAGATGATGCTTCAGGGATGGCGATAGCAGATAGTTTA  480

AGATCTCAGGCAAATACTTTGGGTCAGGCTATATCTAATGGTAATGATGCTTTAGGTATCTTGCAAACTGCAGATAAGGCTATGGATGAGCAACTTAAAATCTTAGATACCATCAAGACT  600

AAAGCGACTCAAGCTGCTCAAGATGGTCAAAGCTTAAAAACAAGAACTATGCTTCAAGCAGACATCAACCGTTTGATGGAAGAACTTGATAATATCGCAAATACCACTTCATTTAATGGC  720

AAACAACTTTTAAGTGGTGGTTTTACCAATCAAGAATTCCAAATCGGTTCAAGTTCAAATCAAACTATTAAAGCAAGTATAGGAGCAACTCAGTCTTCTAAAATCGGTGTAACAAGATTT  840

                                                                                   G T G               A
GAAACAGGTTCACAAAGTTTTTCTTCAGGCACTGTAGGACTTACTATTAAAAACTACAACGGTATCGAAGATTTTAAATTTCAAAATGTAGTGATTTCTACTTCTGTAGGAACAGGTCTT  960

GGAGCTTTGGCTGAAGAGATCAACAGAAATGCAGATAAAACAGGAATTCGTGCAACTTTTGATGTAAAATCTGTAGGAGCCTATGCAATAAAAGCAGGAAATACTTCTCAGGATTTTGCT 1080

ATCAATGGGGTTGTTATAGGTAAGGTTGATTATTCAGATGGTGATGAGAATGGTTCTTTAATTTCAGCTATCAATGCTGTAAAAGATACAACTGGTGTTCAAGCCTCTAAAGATGAAAAT 1200

GGTAAACTTGTTCTTACTTCGGCCGATGGTAGAGGGATTAAAATCACAGGTAGCATAGGTGTAGGAGCTGGTATATTGCACACTGAAAATTATGGAAGGTTATCTTTAGTTAAAAATGAT 1320

GGTAGAGATATCAATATAAGTGGAACAGGTCTTTCAGCTATAGGTATGGGTGCTACAGACATGATTTCTCAATCTTCAGTATCTCTAAGAGAGTCAAAAGGGCAAATTTCAGCAGCCAAT 1440

GCTGATGCTATGGGCTTTAATGCTTATAATGGCGGCGGCGCTAAGCAAATTATTTTCGCTTCTAGTATTGCAGGATTTATGTCTCAGGCTGGTTCAGGCTTCTCTGCTGGTTCGGGATTT 1560

TCAGTAGGTAGTGGTAAAAATTATTCAGCCATTTTATCAGCTTCTATACAGATAGTATCTAGCGCACGTTCTATCAGTAGCACCTATGTTGTTTCTACTGGTTCAGGTTTCTCTGCTGGT 1680

TCAGGTAATTCTCAATTTGCAGCTTTAAGAATAAGTACAGTAAGTGCTCATGATGAAACTGCAGGTGTAACTACACTTAAGGGTGCAATGGCTGTGATGGATATAGCAGAAACTGCTATT 1800

ACCAATCTTGATCAAATCAGAGCGGATATAGGTTCTGTGCAAAATCAAATCACATCGACTATAAACAACATTACTGTAACCCAGGTAAATGTTAAATCAGCAGAATCACAAATCAGAGAT 1920
                                                                                                                    stop
GTAGATTTTGCAAGCGAGAGTGCAAATTACTCTAAAGCAAATATATTGGCTCAAAGTGGTTCTTATGCTATGGCTCAAGCAAATTCAAGCCAGCAAAATGTTTTAAGATTACTACAGTAG 2040
                            -82                                                                              -26
TATATAAAACATTCTTTAGCGTTTACTGTAATTTATACAAATCCAAGCCTAGTAGTAATACTAGGCTTTTTTTATTTCTAAATAAAATTTCAATTTGAATCAAAACTTGGAACACTTCTT 2160
-13        mRNA        rbs       flaB
GCTTTAATCTTTTCGATGCAATATTTTGAAAGGATTTAAAATGGGTTTTAGAATAAACACCAACATCGGTGCATTGAACGCACATGCAAATTCAGTTGTTAATGCTAGGGAGCTTGACAA 2280

GTCTTTAAGTAGACTTAGCTCAGGTCTTAGAATCAACTCCGCAGCAGATGATGCTTCAGGGATGGCGATAGCAGATTCTTTGCGTTCACAAGCAGCAACTTTAGGTCAAGCTATAAACAA 2400

TGGTAATGATGCTATAGGTATCTTGCAAACTGCAGATAAGGCTATGGATGAGCAACTTAAAATCTTAGATACCATCAAGACTAAAGCGACTCAAGCTGCTCAAGATGGTCAAAGCTTAAA 2520

AACAAGAACTATGCTTCAAGCAGACATCAACCGTTTGATGGAAGAACTTGATAATATCGCAAATACCACTTCATTTAATGGCAAACAACTTTTAAGTGGTGGTTTTACCAATCAAGAATT 2640

CCAAATCGGTTCAAGTTCAAATCAAACTATTAAAGCAAGTATAGGAGCAACTCAGTCTTCTAAAATCGGTGTAACAAGATTTGAAACAGGTTCACAAAGTTTTTCTTCAGGCACTGTAGG 2760

ACTTACTATTAAAAACTACAACGGTATCGAAGATTTTAAATTTGATAGTGTAGTGATTTCTACTTCAGTAGGAACAGGTCTTGGAGCTTTGGCTGAAGAGATCAACAGAAATGCAGATAA 2880

AACAGGAATTCGTGCAACTTTTGATGTAAAATCTGTAGGAGCCTATGCAATAAAAGCAGGAAATACTTCTCAGGATTTTGCTATCAATGGGGTTGTTATCGGACAAATAAATTATAATGA 3000

                                                           G  C                                     GGCC
CGGTGATAACAATGGTCAACTTATCTCAGCTATCAATGCTGTAAAAGATACAACTGGTATTGAAGCCTCTAAAGATGAAAATGGTAAACTTGTTCTTACTTCAAGAGATGGTAGAGGGAT 3120

TAAAATCACAGGTAGCATAGGTGTAGGAGCTGGTATATTGCACACTGAAAATTATGGAAGGTTATCTTTAGTTAAAAATGATGGTAGAGATATCAATATAAGTGGAACAGGTCTTTCAGC 3240

TATAGGTATGGGTGCTACAGACATGATTTCTCAATCTTCAGTATCTCTAAGAGAGTCAAAAGGGCAAATTTCAGCAGCCAATGCTGATGCTATGGGCTTTAATGCTTATAATGGCGGCGG 3360

CGCTAAGCAAATTATTTTCGCTTCTAGTATTGCAGGATTTATGTCTCAGGCTGGTTCAGGCTTCTCTGCTGGTTCGGGATTTTCAGTAGGTAGTGGTAAAAATTATTCAGCCATTTTATC 3480

AGCTTCTATACAGATAGTATCTAGCGCACGTTCTATCAGTAGCACCTATGTTGTTTCTACTGGTTCAGGTTTCTCTGCTGGTTCAGGTAATTCTCAATTTGCAGCTTTAAGAATAAGTAC 3600

AGTAAGTGCTCATGATGAAACTGCAGGTGTAACTACACTTAAGGGTGCAATGGCTGTGATGGATATAGCAGAAACTGCTATTACCAATCTTGATCAAATCAGAGCAGATATAGGTGCTGT 3720

GCAAAATCAGCTCCAAGTAACGATAAATAATATTACCGTAACCCAGGTAAATGTTAAAGCAGCAGAATCAACCATAAGAGATGTGGATTTCGCTGCAGAAAGTGCAAATTTTTCTAAGTA 3840
                                                                                    stop
CAATATCCTTGCGCAGTCGGGTTCATATGCTATGAGCCAACGTAACGCTGTGCAACAAAATGTCTTAAAACTTTTACAATAATTTTTCTAAAGAGCAAATTTTTGCTCTTTAGATTAAAT 3960

TTCTTTTTTCTAATTCATCTTGTAAAGGGATAATGGCTTTTTAATTCTTATGTTTTGACTTTCTATGAGATCAATTATAGTTTCAATTAAAGATTCGTTAGCATAAATCCAAGATAGAA 4080
TTTTATTTTGTCTTTGGCTTTCATTGTTAACACTTTGGATATAAATAGGGGCAATTAAACTTTCTTCATGATATAGACTAGGTCCTAAAATTTCATGTAAAAAAAAGTATCTTTTCTTGC 4200
```

FIGURE 2. DNA sequence of the *flaA* and *flaB* genes of *C. coli* VC167-T2. The initiation and termination codons for both genes are indicated in boldface type. The mRNA start sites determined by primer extension experiments (37) are indicated. Based on these mRNA start sites, putative promoters and ribosome-binding sites (rbs) for *flaA* and *flaB* have been indicated. The σ^{28} promoter regions (−35, −10) for *flaA* are shown in boldface type and double underlined. The σ^{54} promoter regions (−26, −13) for *flaB* are also in boldface and double underlined, and a potential upstream enhancer located 82 bp upstream of the ribosome-binding site is also indicated. The potential transcriptional terminator following the *flaA* coding region (nucleotides 2085 to 2108) is shown in underlined boldface type. The nucleotide changes above the *C. coli* VC167-T2 sequence shown in italics (*flaA:* 922, 924, 926, and 945; *flaB:* 3059, 3062, and 3103 to 3106) indicate the changes observed in the corresponding sequence of *C. coli* VC167-T1. This *C. coli* VC167-T1 sequence represents a revision of that previously published (36).

and T2 cells and that the mRNA for each size was unit length rather than polycistronic. Primer extension experiments confirmed the presence of independent promoters for each gene (Fig. 2). The *flaA* gene is transcribed from a typical σ^{28} promoter, as are flagellin genes from the family

```
                                                                 65
GFRINTNVAALNAKANSDLNSRALDQSLSRLSSGLRINSAADDASGMAIADSLRSQANTLGQAIS   T1 FLA A
:::::::::::::::::::::::::::::::::::::::::::::::::::::::::::::::::   T2 FLA A
:::::::IG:::H:::VV:A:E::K::::::::::::::::::::::::::::::::A::::::N   T1 FLA B
:::::::IG:::H:::VV:A:E::K::::::::::::::::::::::::::::::::A::::::N   T2 FLA B

                                                                130
NGNDALGILQTADKAMDEQLKILDTIKTKATQAAQDGQSLKTRTMLQADINRLMEELDNIANTTS   T1 FLA A
:::::::::::::::::::::::::::::::::::::::::::::::::::::::::::::::::   T2 FLA A
:::::I:::::::::::::::::::::::::::::::::::::::::::::::::::::::::::   T1 FLA B
:::::I:::::::::::::::::::::::::::::::::::::::::::::::::::::::::::   T2 FLA B

                                                                195
FNGKQLLSGGFTNQEFQIGSSSNQTIKASIGATQSSKIGVTRFETGSQSFSSGTVGLTIKNYNGI   T1 FLA A
:::::::::::::::::::::::::::::::::::::::::::::::::::::::::::::::::   T2 FLA A
:::::::::::::::::::::::::::::::::::::::::::::::::::::::::::::::::   T1 FLA B
:::::::::::::::::::::::::::::::::::::::::::::::::::::::::::::::::   T2 FLA B

                                                                260
EDFKFDSVVISTSVGTGLGALAEEINRNADKTGIRATFDVKSVGAYAIKAGNTSQDFAINGVVIG   T1 FLA A
:::::QN::::::::::::::::::::::::::::::::::::::::::::::::::::::::::   T2 FLA A
:::::::::::::::::::::::::::::::::::::::::::::::::::::::::::::::::   T1 FLA B
:::::::::::::::::::::::::::::::::::::::::::::::::::::::::::::::::   T2 FLA B

                                                                325
KVDYSDGDENGSLISAINAVKDTTGVQASKDENGKLVLTSADGRGIKITGSIGVGAGILHTENYG   T1 FLA A
:::::::::::::::::::::::::::::::::::::::::::::::::::::::::::::::::   T2 FLA A
QIN:N:::N::Q:::::::::::::::::::::::::::::::::::::::::::::::::::::   T1 FLA B
QIN:N:::N::Q:::::::::::::IE:::::::::::::R::::::::::::::::::::::::   T2 FLA B

                                                                390
RLSLVKNDGRDINISGTGLSAIGMGATDMISQSSVSLRESKGQISAANADAMGFNAYNGGGAKQI   T1 FLA A
:::::::::::::::::::::::::::::::::::::::::::::::::::::::::::::::::   T2 FLA A
:::::::::::::::::::::::::::::::::::::::::::::::::::::::::::::::::   T1 FLA B
:::::::::::::::::::::::::::::::::::::::::::::::::::::::::::::::::   T2 FLA B

                                                                455
IFASSIAGFMSQAGSGFSAGSGFSVGSGKNYSAILSASIQIVSSARSISSTYVVSTGSGFSAGSG   T1 FLA A
:::::::::::::::::::::::::::::::::::::::::::::::::::::::::::::::::   T2 FLA A
:::::::::::::::::::::::::::::::::::::::::::::::::::::::::::::::::   T1 FLA B
:::::::::::::::::::::::::::::::::::::::::::::::::::::::::::::::::   T2 FLA B

                                                                520
NSQFAALRISTVSAHDETAGVTTLKGAMAVMDIAETAITNLDQIRADIGSVQNQITSTINNITVT   T1 FLA A
:::::::::::::::::::::::::::::::::::::::::::::::::::::::::::::::::   T2 FLA A
:::::::::::::::::::::::::::::::::::::::::::::::::A::::LQV::::::::   T1 FLA B
:::::::::::::::::::::::::::::::::::::::::::::::::A::::LQV::::::::   T2 FLA B

                                                   572
QVNVKSAESQIRDVDFASESANYSKANILAQSGSYAMAQANSSQQNVLRLLQ                T1 FLA A
::::::::::::::::::::::::::::::::::::::::::::::::::::                T2 FLA A
:::::A:::T:::::::A::::F::Y::::::::::::::R:AV::::K:::                T1 FLA B
:::::A:::T:::::::A::::F::Y::::::::::::::R:AV::::K:::                T2 FLA B
```

FIGURE 3. Comparison of the gene products of the *flaA* and *flaB* genes of *C. coli* VC167-T1 and VC167-T2. The open reading frame encoded by *C. coli* VC167-T1 *flaA* is shown on the top line, and amino acids are designated by the single-letter code. Colons indicate identical residues, and changes are so indicated. The numbers on the right refer to the amino acid residues of the *C. coli* VC167-T1 *flaA* gene. The serine residues known to be modified in both T1 and T2 FlaA proteins are double underlined.

Enterobacteriaceae (3, 18) and *Bacillus* spp. (40), whereas the *flaB* gene is transcribed from a σ^{54} promoter. This latter class of highly specialized promoter controls nitrogen-regulated genes in the family *Enterobacteriaceae* (41, 46) and the temporally regulated flagellin genes of *Caulobacter crescentus* (38, 43). One of the characteristic features of σ^{54} promoters is the presence of an upstream enhancer sequence. A sequence resembling enhancers present in other σ^{54} promoters is present 82 bp upstream from the putative polymerase-binding site (Fig. 2). The signal strengths obtained in primer extension experiments indicated that more *flaA* transcript was present than *flaB* transcript under the conditions of growth used. This is consistent with previous observations from N-terminal amino acid sequencing of purified flagellin that the *flaA*

TABLE 1. Molecular weight of *C. coli* VC167 flagellins

Antigenic type	Apparent M_r (SDS-PAGE)	Predicted M_r	
		flaA	*flaB*
T1	61,500	58,844	58,955
T2	59,500	58,884	59,124

gene product was the major component of the filament. Nonetheless, several internal peptides specific for *flaB* were seen by chemical analyses, which suggested that the flagellar filament of VC167 might be a heteropolymer of *flaA* and *flaB* gene products.

MUTATIONAL ANALYSES OF THE *flaA* AND *flaB* GENES

To ascertain the role of the *flaA* and *flaB* genes in flagellar structure, site-specific mutations were made in each gene by using the gene replacement mutagenesis technique of Labigne-Roussel et al. (28). Initial mutations were constructed by insertion of a kanamycin resistance gene cartridge into a *Bgl*II site located 162 bp downstream of start of the *flaA* gene (14), and subsequent mutations were constructed by insertion of the same kanamycin resistance gene into an *Eco*RV site located 1 kb downstream of the start of the *flaA* gene (13). This mutated flagellin gene was conjugally transferred from *E. coli* into VC167 on a plasmid vector which was unable to replicate in the campylobacter recipient. Kanamycin-resistant campylobacter transconjugants represented events in which the kanamycin resistance gene was rescued by a crossover between the campylobacter sequences flanking the kanamycin resistance gene and the corresponding regions of homology in the chromosome. Such a crossover results in a transient duplication of sequences on the chromosome, and the subsequent excision of the vector DNA and one copy of the flagellin information should occur by the analogous single reciprocal crossover. Since *flaA* and *flaB* genes are highly homologous, crossovers inactivating both genes occurred. The genotypes of mutants were determined by Southern blot analysis and fell into the three possible classes: (i) *flaA flaB;* (ii) *flaA*$^+$ *flaB;* and (iii) *flaA flaB*$^+$. Mutants with mutations in both VC167-T1 and VC167-T2 were characterized for motility in semisolid agar, and their surface structure was examined by electron-microscopic analysis. The results are summarized in Table 2. Figure 4 shows that T2 wild-type cells are more motile that T1 wild-type cells and that both T1 and T2 cells are more motile at 42°C than at 37°C. Mutants with mutations in both genes (*flaA flaB*) were nonmotile (data not shown), and the cells were nonflagellated (Fig. 5), as expected. Cells which were defective in the *flaB* gene were slightly less motile than wild-type cells and produced a flagellar filament which was indistinguishable in length from the wild type (Fig. 5) (13). The mutant with the original *flaA flaB*$^+$ mutation, VC167-B2 (14), was nonflagellated and was shown to accumulate flagellin intracellularly, suggesting that the *flaB* gene product was not found in the filament (14).

TABLE 2. *C. coli* VC167 flagellin mutants

Antigenic type	Genotype	Filament	Motility
T2	*flaA*$^+$ *flaB*$^+$	+	4+
T2	*flaA*$^+$ *flaB*	+	3+
T2	*flaA flaB*$^+$	Truncated	1+
T2	*flaA flaB*	–	–
T1	*flaA*$^+$ *flaB*$^+$	+	3+
T1	*flaA*$^+$ *flaB*	+	2+
T1	*flaA flaB*$^+$	Truncated	+/–
T1	*flaA flaB*	–	–

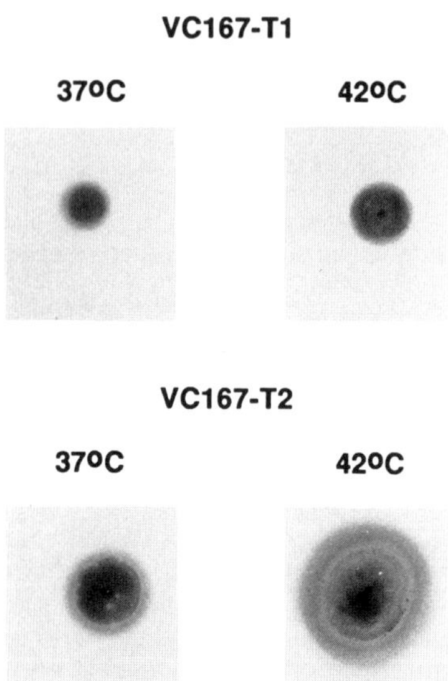

FIGURE 4. Comparison of the relative motility of *C. coli* VC167-T1 and *C. coli* VC167-T2 on 0.4% Mueller-Hinton agar at both 37 and 42°C. The higher temperature clearly increases the zone of bacterial growth.

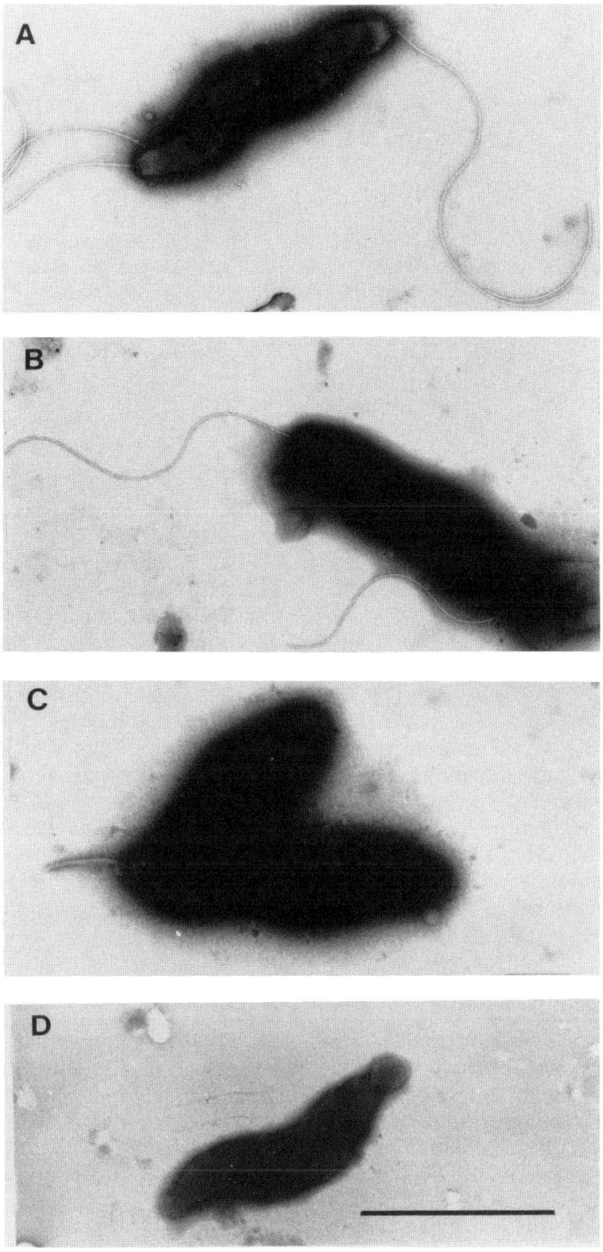

FIGURE 5. Electron micrographs of negatively stained VC167-T2 (A), the *flaA*⁺ *flaB* mutant (B), the *flaA flaB*⁺ mutant producing a truncated flagellar filament (C), and the bald *flaA flaB* mutant (D). Bar, 1 μm.

However, more recent data indicate that the VC167-B2 mutant contains a secondary defect in transport (1, 12). Additional, independently isolated *flaA flaB*⁺ mutants with mutations in both T1 and T2 cells consistently result in a partially motile phenotype (12, 13) and a severely truncated filament (Fig. 5). Figure 6 shows a Western blot analysis of flagellins purified from

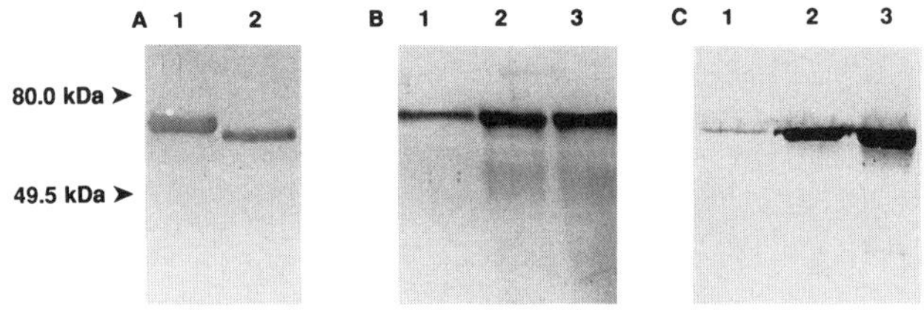

FIGURE 6. (A) Western blot analysis of *C. coli* VC167-T1 (lane 1) and *C. coli* VC167-T2 (lane 2) reacted with antiflagellin antiserum SML2. The M_r difference between the immunoreactive bands is evident. Molecular weights are indicated. (B) Western blot analysis of *C. coli* VC167-T1 *flaA flaB*⁺ (lane 1), *C. coli* VC167-T1 *flaA*⁺ *flaB* (lane 2), and *C. coli* VC167-T1 (lane 3) with antiserum SML2. *C. coli* VC167-T1 FlaA and FlaB are indistinguishable and have an M_r of 61,500. (C) Western blot analysis of *C. coli* VC167-T2 *flaA flaB*⁺ (lane 1), *C. coli* VC167-T2 *flaA*⁺ *flaB* (lane 2), and *C. coli* VC167-T2 (lane 3) with antiserum SML2. *C. coli* VC167-T2 FlaA and FlaB are indistinguishable and have an M_r of 59,500.

the various mutants. The *flaA* and *flaB* flagellins from VC167-T1 were indistinguishable in size, and both ran at an apparent M_r of 61,500; also, the *flaA* and *flaB* flagellins from VC167-T2 were also indistinguishable in size, and both ran at an apparent M_r of 59,500.

These results indicate that the native VC167 filament represents a complex flagellum composed of both *flaA* and *flaB* gene products. A filament composed of either gene product is functional, although the *flaA* filament confers much greater motility than the *flaB* filament does. The presence of both gene products in the filament confers maximum motility. This is similar to the situation for *Caulobacter crescentus,* which has a flagellar filament composed of three flagellin subunits. The absence of any one of the subunits in the filament results in reduced motility (39).

Immunogold electron microscopy was used in an effort to determine the distribution of the *flaB* flagellin in the wild-type filament. Antiserum LAH2 (16), which reacts with the *flaA* and *flaB* flagellins of VC167-T2 in Western blots, also reacts in immunogold electron microscopy with the VC167-T2 wild-type flagellar filament, the filament produced by a *flaA*⁺ *flaB* T2 mutant, and the truncated filament produced by a *flaA flaB*⁺ T2 mutant. When this antiserum is absorbed with *flaA*⁺ *flaB* cells to remove antibodies to the *flaA* gene product, the antiserum still reacts strongly with the truncated *flaB* filament, and it reacts sparsely along the entire length of the wild-type filament (Fig. 7). This suggests that the *flaB* product may be distributed throughout the length of the wild-type filament, although only a limited number of *flaB* epitopes seem to be exposed on the surface of the filament. This flagellar organization, with the *flaB* flagellin subunit intertwined among the *flaA* flagellin subunits, is distinctive from that seen in the complex flagellar filament of *Rhizobium meliloti* (45) and *Caulobacter crescentus* (39), in which different flagellins are assembled sequentially into distinct regions of the filament. This class of complex filament organization also seems to be that found in *H. pylori* (26).

It has been reported by Nuijten et al. (44) that the *flaB* gene of *C. jejuni* 81116 is not expressed, despite the fact that a full-length open reading frame preceded by a very similar σ^{54}-like promoter is present. This conclusion is based on the absence of detectable *flaB*-specific mRNA in Northern blots and primer extension experiments, but not by mutational analysis. We have constructed *flaA flaB*⁺ mutations in two other strains of *C. jejuni* and one additional strain of *C. coli,* and all three mutants display the truncated flagellar filament characteristic of a *flaB* filament (1, 12). This would suggest that a complex flagellar filament is not unique to *C. coli* VC167, but may be a common occurrence among *C. jejuni* and *C. coli* strains. This is also consistent with observations that most strains seem to have more than one copy of flagellin as determined by DNA hybridization analysis (51).

BIOLOGICAL SIGNIFICANCE OF TWO FLAGELLIN GENES

The tandem organization of flagellin genes on the campylobacter chromosome suggests that the two genes arose from a gene duplication event. The fact that the gene duplication, which in most bacteria would be unstable, has been maintained suggests that the advantages of two tandem flagellin genes must outweigh the re-

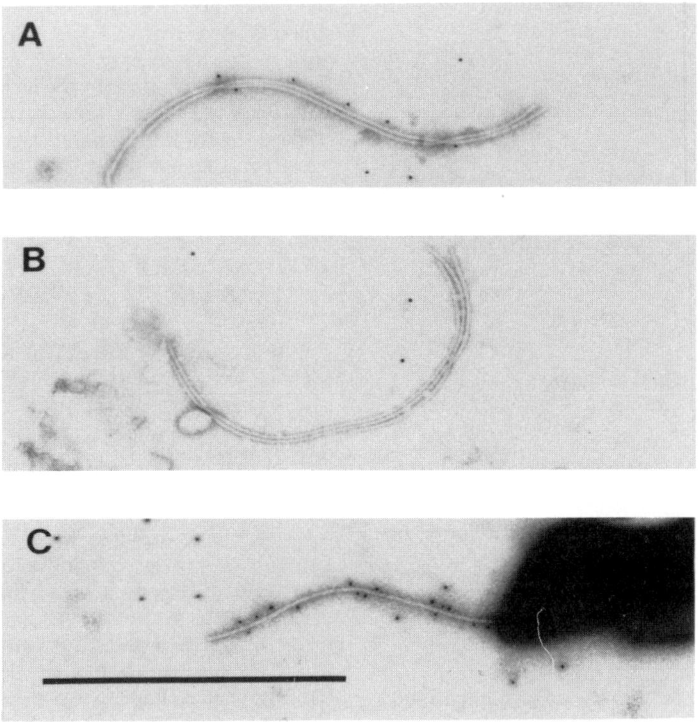

FIGURE 7. Immunoelectron microscopy of *C. coli* VC167-T2 flagella (A), *flaA⁺ flaB* flagella (B), and a cell harboring a truncated *flaA flaB⁺* filament (C) reacted with antiserum LAH2 absorbed with *C. coli* VC167-T2 *flaA⁺ flaB* whole cells. Bar, 1 μm.

sultant genetic instability for this organism. It is generally accepted that only motile campylobacters are capable of penetrating the mucous lining of the intestinal tract and establishing an infection. Clearly, a filament composed of both subunits confers greater motility than a filament of equal length composed of only the *flaA* subunit, although the reasons for this are unknown. This increased motility appears to enhance the ability of the organism to colonize the intestine. Under the in vitro growth conditions which we have examined, the *flaA* subunit is expressed at much higher levels than the *flaB* subunit. However, the presence of distinct, highly regulatable promoters offers the potential for varying the amounts of each subunit in the filament, in response to external stimuli, such that under certain signals the amount of *flaB* flagellin in the filament may increase. The biological advantage of possessing the *flaB* subunit may not be apparent until the regulation of the *flaB* gene is better elucidated.

The other major advantage to campylobacters in retaining two highly related flagellin genes may be to ensure that the flagellar filament can always be expressed, by virtue of maintaining a backup copy of the flagellin gene. Thus, if a mutation occurs in one copy, the lesion could be corrected by a recombinational event involving the alternate copy. We have observed such recombinational events occurring at relatively high frequencies among some classes of flagellin mutants (12). The process of repairing such mutations may in fact generate antigenic diversity as the two flagellin genes recombine. It is not clear whether such events occur intracellularly or by transformation of DNA released from lysed cells in the culture. Natural transformation among antigenically different *Campylobacter* strains may play a pivotal role in ensuring the antigenic diversity of the genus in general.

GENETIC RELATEDNESS AMONG *CAMPYLOBACTER* FLAGELLINS

In an effort to address the extent of antigenic variability of campylobacter flagellins, we have

TABLE 3. *Campylobacter* strains and flagellin mutants

Strain	Flagella	Serotype
C. coli		
VC167	Full length	LIO8
VC167-B3	Absent	LIO8
VC97	Full length	LIO20
VC97-3	Absent	LIO20
C. jejuni		
VC103	Full length	LIO17
VC103K	Absent	LIO17
VC104	Full length	LIO19
VC104K	Absent	LIO19
VC87	Full length	LIO1
VC87K	Absent	LIO1
VC83	Full length	LIO4
VC83K	Absent	Untypable
VC84	Full length	LIO6
VC84-1	Absent	LIO6

used DNA probes composed of various regions of the flagellin gene to examine nucleotide sequence similarities among strains of different Lior serogroups. A probe consisting of an intact flagellin gene from VC167 (51) or from the 3′ end of the gene (region V in Fig. 1) (12) hybridized strongly to strains of multiple serogroups. Probes from the internal region of the molecule showed various degrees of hybridization. The most specific probe was that taken from the region marked as region III in Fig. 1, which hybridized strongly to the parent VC167 *C. coli* strain and to two *C. jejuni* strains, also of serogroup LIO8 (51), but not to 27 other strains from 19 other serogroups. Similarly, the next most specific probe was from region IV in Fig. 1, which hybridized well only to three LIO8 strains and seven LIO77 strains. These data support the previously proposed structure of campylobacter flagellin, with conserved residues at the amino and carboxy ends and variable regions in the central portion, although there is considerable homology among serogroups within this region. This is most clearly seen in the comparison of the predicted protein sequences of the *C. coli* VC167 flagellins and those of *C. jejuni* 81116 (LIO6) (44), which are the only published DNA sequences of campylobacter flagellins. The overall protein similarity between the VC167-T1 *flaA* gene product and the *flaA* gene product of strain 81116 is 87.2%. If the five different regions of the molecule are compared, however, a greater range is seen: region 1 has 95.6% similarity, region II has 89.3%, region III has 83.3%, region IV has 72.8%, and region V has 97%. This comparison also suggests that the internal domains of flagellin contain variable regions and that the most variable are regions III and IV, coding for residues 229 to 473 of the protein.

INVOLVEMENT OF FLAGELLA IN LIOR HEAT-LABILE SEROSPECIFICITY

It has been a widely held notion among *Campylobacter* researchers that flagellin was the serodeterminant of the heat-labile serotyping scheme developed by Lior et al. (31). This is based on data that a nonflagellated phase variant of 81116 (a LIO6 strain) was untypable (54, 55) and that UV light-induced nonflagellated mutants in four serogroups (LIO5, LIO6, LIO7, and LIO17) were also unable to be typed in this scheme (55). However, for *C. coli* VC167, Harris et al. (16) showed that cells producing antigenically different T1 and T2 flagella both serotyped as LIO8, suggesting that a cell surface component other than flagella was the serodeterminant in this serogroup. This has been confirmed by serotypic analysis of the VC167 flagellin mutants described above. All classes of VC167 flagellin mutants, including bald mutants, serotype as LIO8, and this clearly implicates a nonflagellar cell surface antigen as the LIO8 serodeterminant.

To extend this study to other Lior serotypes, we exploited the previously observed high degree of homology among campylobacter flagellin genes to move flagellin mutations from the VC167 background into other strains of *C. jejuni* and *C. coli* by natural transformation (52). We used DNA from VC167 mutants in which one or more flagellin genes had been disrupted by

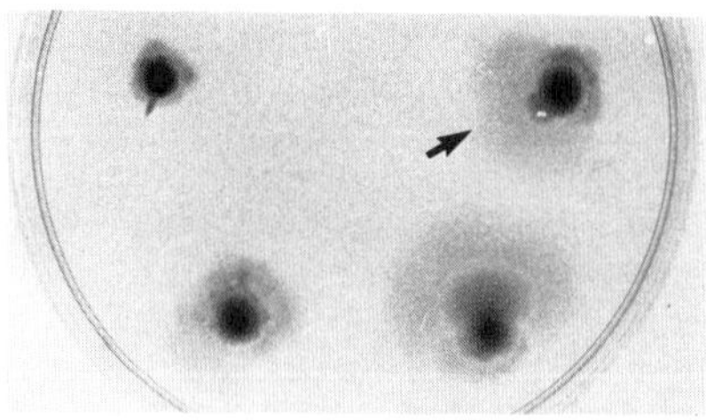

FIGURE 8. Single colonies of *C. coli* VC167 were inoculated onto 0.4% Mueller-Hinton motility agar and incubated at 42°C. After 36 to 48 h, spikes of increased motility were evident (arrow).

insertion of the kanamycin resistance cassette to transform other *Campylobacter* strains to kanamycin resistance. The high degree of homology between the incoming flagellin information and the resident flagellin genes should allow for the mutated VC167 flagellin gene to cross over into, and thereby disrupt, the resident flagellin information. The strains used and some of the mutants generated are summarized in Table 3 (1). In all cases examined, kanamycin-resistant transformants displayed motility defects as determined on semisolid agar. Most mutants generated by transformation with VC167-B3, the *flaA flaB* deletion mutation, displayed a totally bald, nonmotile phenotype (1). Most mutants of other serotypes generated with VC167-B2 DNA, the original *flaA flaB*+ mutant, displayed the bald, nonmotile phenotype typical of the original mutant. Southern blot analysis indicated that in one of these strains the resident flagellin information had been totally replaced with the VC167-B2 DNA. These data further suggest that the transport defect in this mutant resides either within the *flaB* structural gene itself or at a locus which maps very close to the structural gene. In two cases transformation with VC167-B2 led to mutants which were partially motile and produced the truncated filament characteristic of most *flaA* mutants. Southern analysis failed to detect VC167 genetic information, although rearrangements of the resident flagellin information had occurred. Most probably the crossover occurred between conserved flagellin information very close to the ends of the kanamycin cassette on the incoming DNA and the resident flagellin genes and resulted in disruption of only the resident *flaA* gene.

The serotyping results as performed by H. Lior, Laboratory Centre for Disease Control, Ottawa, Canada (summarized in Table 3) indicate that of the seven randomly selected serotypes in which flagellin mutations have been constructed, only in Lior serogroup 4 does flagellin seem to be involved in Lior serospecificity (1). LIO1, LIO6, LIO8, LIO17, LIO19, and LIO20 bald mutants still serotype as the parental wild types. Moreover, immunogold electron microscopy of these serotypes before and after serotyping confirm that the cell surface rather than the flagellar filament reacts with the appropriate typing sera. The discrepancy between these data and the previously published results may occur because the previously described mutants had been isolated following UV light mutagenesis and may have been affected at multiple loci. However, the fact that the phase variant of strain 81116 (LIO6) failed to serotype whereas the bald mutant of VC84 (LIO6) did serotype may indicate that phase variation is a phenomenon affecting multiple surface antigens and not just flagella.

It is interesting that even though flagellin is not the serodeterminant of the LIO8 serogroup, flagellin genes among LIO8 strains of *C. coli* and *C. jejuni* are highly conserved (see above). Presumably, although not involved in Lior serospecificity in most strains, *Campylobacter* flagellins do contain serospecific epitopes (16).

ANTIGENIC VARIATION OF VC167 FLAGELLINS

The described antigenic variation of VC167 from T1 to T2 has not been explained at the molecular level, but clearly does not involve alternate expression of the *flaA* and *flaB* structural genes. Previous studies suggested that the flagellar variation was associated with an uncharacterized genomic rearrangement adjacent to a ribosomal DNA locus, as well as with a rearrangement detected with the internal flagellin probe consisting of region II (51). In fact, there are minor DNA sequence differences in both the *flaA* and *flaB* genes in T1 and T2 (Fig. 2). There are four different residues between T1 and T2 in region II of the *flaA* gene. One of these is a silent change, and the others result in a change at amino acid residues 201 and 202 from aspartic acid and serine in T1 to glutamic acid and asparagine in T2 (Fig. 3). There are six different residues between T1 and T2 in region III of the *flaB* gene. These changes result in changes from valine and glutamine at residues 286 and 287, respectively, in T1 *flaB* to isoleucine and glutamic acid in T2 *flaB*. There is a silent base pair change 902 nucleotides into the open reading frame, as well as changes which result in a change at amino acid residue 301 from alanine in T1 *flaB* to arginine in T2 *flaB*. The T1 *flaB* gene contains a *Hae*III site at nucleotide 3104 in Fig. 2, but this site is not present in the T2 *flaB* gene. The above changes can be detected by Southern blot analyses with synthetic oligonucleotide probes (12) in DNAs from strains subjected to antibody selection as described by Harris et al. (16) or in cells passaged in animals (32). However, both of these types of variants have been subjected to quite extensive selective pressures that could have resulted in secondary changes unrelated to the flagellar antigenic variation. For this reason we have recently reexamined the question of chromosomal rearrangement. We took advantage of the ob-

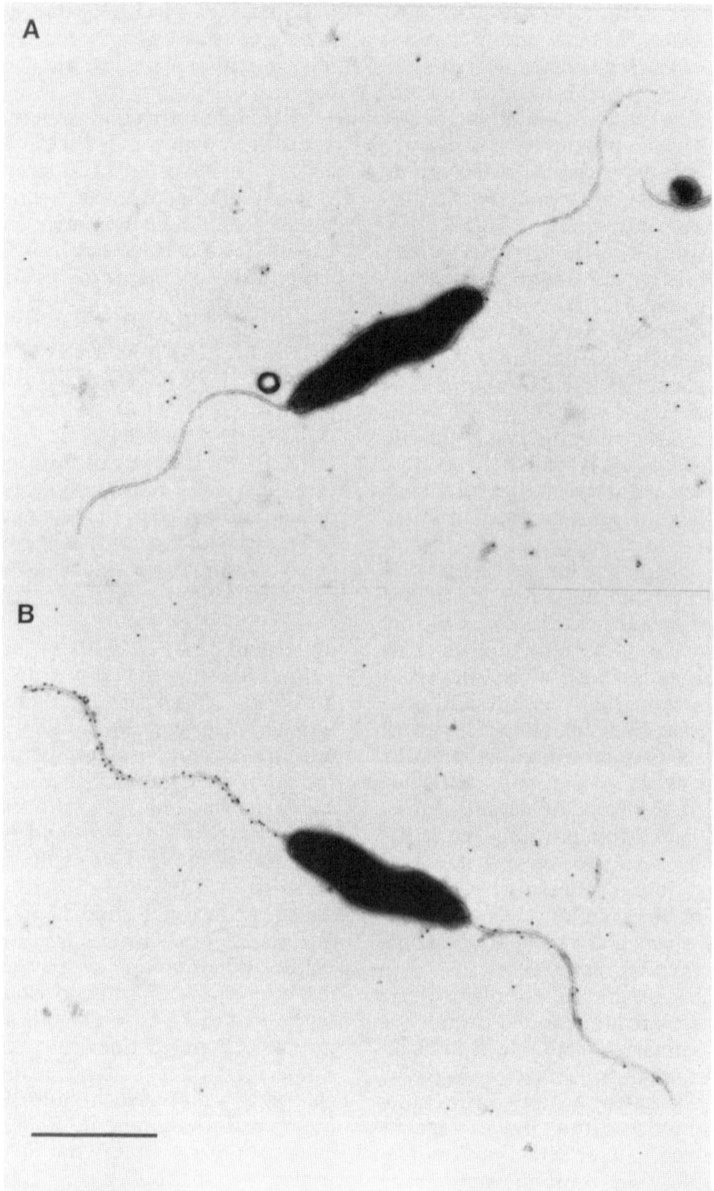

FIGURE 9. Immunoelectron microscopy of cells isolated from the less motile region (A) and a highly motile area (B) of a single clone of *C. coli* VC167 after growth on 0.4% agar at 42°C. The LAH2 antiserum used is serospecific for T2 flagellin and is seen reacting strongly with the flagella in panel B, but not to the flagella in panel A. Bar, 1 μm.

servation that cells producing T2 flagella were more motile than cells producing T1 flagella at 42°C (Fig. 4). When single colonies of VC167 were spotted on motility agar, a number of the resulting growths contained spikes of motility radiating from a central nonmotile region (Fig. 8). When cells from the more motile area are examined by immunoelectron microscopy and Western blot analysis with antiserum specific to T2 flagella (antiserum LAH2), antibody binding to the flagellar filament is clearly visible (Fig. 9B), and flagellin of subunit M_r 59,500 is produced and is immunoreactive (Fig. 10, lane 3). Cells from the edge of the less motile region of growth produce flagella which do not react with antiserum LAH2 (Fig. 9A), and the flagellin of these filaments has an M_r of 61,500 and is nonreactive with antiserum LAH2 by Western blotting (Fig. 10, lane 2). These antigenic variants have had minimal selective pressure and show none of the previously described DNA rearrangements (i.e., the sequence changes in *flaA* or *flaB* seen in Fig. 2 or the changes adjacent to the rRNA locus). This means that these previously observed rearrangements were unrelated to flagellar antigenic variation.

Since both the T2 *flaA* and T2 *flaB* gene products are reactive with antiserum LAH2, whereas the T1 *flaA* and T2 *flaB* gene products are nonreactive, it would appear that primary sequence differences cannot account for LAH2 serospecificity. At this point, we do not know whether there are differences in the degree of phosphorylation of the various flagellins, but acid phosphatase treatment of T2 flagellins appears not to interfere with their ability to bind LAH2 antibodies (12). The possibility exists, however, that some other as yet uncharacterized modification accounts for LAH2 serospecificity, and this possibility is under investigation.

What is obvious from this consideration of *Campylobacter* flagella is that the biochemistry, immunochemistry, and molecular genetics of this motility organelle and virulence factor are far more complex than originally envisioned. Clearly, much has still to be learned about the biochemical and immunochemical structure of the *Campylobacter* flagellar filament, especially the roles of the *flaA* and *flaB* gene products. The molecular basis for the observed antigenic variation of the flagella of *C. coli* VC167 still remains to be determined. This should include a consideration of the possible role of posttranslational modification in the process. Certainly, the role and regulation of the different promoters for the *flaA* and *flaB* genes must be determined. It is also clear that the other surface components which confer heat-labile serospecificity on the *Campylobacter* cell must be identified and characterized.

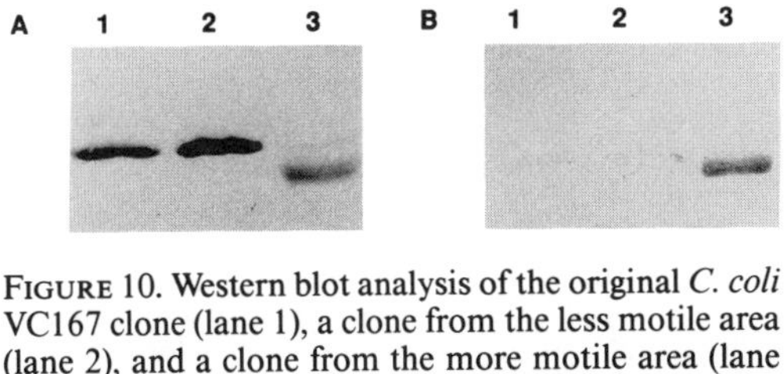

FIGURE 10. Western blot analysis of the original *C. coli* VC167 clone (lane 1), a clone from the less motile area (lane 2), and a clone from the more motile area (lane 3) of a motility ring. The blots were reacted with antisera SML2 (A) and LAH2 (B). The change in M_r and LAH2 immunoreactivity of the flagellin belonging to the cells with increased motility is clearly evident.

ACKNOWLEDGMENTS. Studies in the laboratory of T.J.T. are supported by the Medical Research Council of Canada, and studies by P.G. are supported by U.S. Navy Research and Development Command Research Work Unit no. 61102A3M161102BS13AK.111. We thank Gary Majam, Denny Cautivar, and Steve Martin for expert technical assistance.

REFERENCES

1. **Alm, R. A., P. Guerry, M. E. Power, H. Lior, and T. J. Trust.** 1991. Analysis of the role of flagella in the heat-labile Lior serotyping scheme of thermophilic campylobacters by mutant allele exchange. *J. Clin. Microbiol.* **29:**2438–2445.
2. **Ambler, R. P., and M. W. Rees.** 1959. N-methyllysine in bacterial flagellar protein. *Nature* (London) **184:**56–57.
3. **Arnosti, D. N., and M. J. Chamberlain.** 1989. Secondary sigma factor controls transcription of flagellar and chemotaxis genes in *Escherichia coli. Proc. Natl. Acad. Sci. USA* **86:**830–834.
4. **Black, R. E., M. M. Levine, M. L. Clements, T. P. Hughes, and M. J. Blaser.** 1988. Experimental *Campylobacter jejuni* infections in humans. *J. Infect. Dis.* **157:**472–479.
5. **Blaser, M. J., J. A. Hopkins, and M. L. Vasil.** 1984. *Campylobacter jejuni* outer membrane proteins are antigenic for humans. *Infect. Immun.* **43:**986–993.
6. **Burr, D. H., M. B. Caldwell, A. L. Bourgeois, H. R. Morgan, R. Wistar, Jr., and R. I. Walker.** 1988. Mucosal and systemic immunity to *Campylobacter jejuni* in rabbits after gastric inoculation. *Infect. Immun.* **56:**99–105.
7. **Caldwell, M. B., P. Guerry, E. C. Lee, J. P. Burans, and R. I. Walker.** 1985. Reversible expression of flagella in *Campylobacter jejuni. Infect. Immun.* **50:**941–943.
8. **Delange, R. J., J. Y. Chang, J. H. Sharper, and A. M. Glazer.** 1976. Amino acid sequence of flagellin of *Bacillus subtilis* 168. *J. Biol. Chem.* **254:**705–711.
9. **Ferrero, R. L., and A. Lee.** 1988. Motility of *Campylobacter jejuni* in a viscous environment: comparison with conventional rod shaped bacteria. *J. Gen. Microbiol.* **134:**53–59.
10. **Froholm, L. O., and K. Sletten.** 1977. Purification and N-terminal sequence of a fimbrial protein from *Moraxella nonliquefaciens. FEBS Lett.* **73:**29–32.
11. **Glaser, A. N., R. J. DeLange, and R. J. Martinez.** 1969. Identification of l-methyl-lysine in *Spirillum serpens* flagella and of dimethyl-lysine in *Salmo-*

nella typhimurium flagellum. *Biochim. Biophys. Acta* **188:**164–165.

12. **Guerry, P., R. A. Alm, M. E. Power, S. M. Logan, and T. J. Trust.** Unpublished data.
13. **Guerry, P., R. A. Alm, M. E. Power, S. M. Logan, and T. J. Trust.** 1991. Role of two flagellin genes in *Campylobacter* motility. *J. Bacteriol.* **173:**4757–4764.
14. **Guerry, P., S. M. Logan, S. Thornton, and T. J. Trust.** 1990. Genomic organization and expression of *Campylobacter* flagellin genes. *J. Bacteriol.* **172:**1853–1860.
15. **Guerry, P., S. M. Logan, and T. J. Trust.** 1988. Genomic rearrangements associated with antigenic variation in *Campylobacter coli. J. Bacteriol.* **170:**316–319.
16. **Harris, L. A., S. M. Logan, P. Guerry, and T. J. Trust.** 1987. Antigenic variation of *Campylobacter* flagella. *J. Bacteriol.* **169:**5066–5071.
17. **Hébert, G. A., D. G. Hollis, R. E. Weaver, A. G. Steigerwalt, R. M. McKinney, and D. J. Brenner.** 1983. Serogroups of *Campylobacter jejuni, Campylobacter coli,* and *Campylobacter fetus* defined by direct immunofluorescence. *J. Clin. Microbiol.* **17:**529–538.
18. **Helmann, J. D., and M. J. Chamberlain.** 1987. DNA sequence analysis suggests that expression of flagellar and chemotaxis genes in *Escherichia coli* and *Salmonella typhimurium* is controlled by an alternative sigma factor. *Proc. Natl. Acad. Sci. USA* **84:**6422–6424.
19. **Hermondson, M. A., K. C. S. Chen, and T. M. Buchanan.** 1978. *Neisseria* pili protein: amino terminal amino acid sequences and identification of an unusual amino acid. *Biochemistry* **17:**422–445.
20. **Homma, M., H. Fujita, S. Yamaguchi, and T. Iino.** 1987. Regions of *Salmonella typhimurium* flagellin essential for its polymerization and excretion. *J. Bacteriol.* **169:**291–296.
21. **Iino, T.** 1977. Genetics of structure and function of bacterial flagella. *Annu. Rev. Genet.* **11:**161–182.
22. **Joys, T. M.** 1985. The covalent structure of the phase-1 flagellar filament protein of *Salmonella typhimurium* and its comparisons with other flagellins. *J. Biol. Chem.* **247:**5180–5193.
23. **Joys, T. M., and H. Kim.** 1979. Identification of N-methyl-lysine residues in the phase-1 flagellar protein of *Salmonella typhimurium. Microbios Lett.* **7:**65–68.
24. **Kaiser, G. E., and R. N. Doetsch.** 1975. Enhanced translational motion of leptospira in viscous environments. *Nature* (London) **255:**656–657.
25. **Kist, M.** 1985. The historical background to *Campylobacter* infections: new aspects, p. 23–27. *In* A. D. Pearson, M. B. Skirrow, H. Lior, and B. Rowe (ed.), *Campylobacter III.* Public Health Laboratory Service, London.
26. **Kostrzynska, M., J. D. Betts, J. W. Austin, and T. J. Trust.** 1991. Identification, characterization, and spatial localization of two flagellin species of *Helicobacter pylori* flagella. *J. Bacteriol.* **173:**937–946.
27. **Kuwajima, G., I. Kawagishi, M. Homma, J.-I. Asaka, E. Kondo, and R. M. Macnab.** 1989. Export of an N-terminal fragment of *Escherichia coli* flagellin by a flagellum-specific pathway. *Proc. Natl. Acad. Sci. USA* **86:**4953–4957.
28. **Labigne-Roussel, A., P. Courcoux, and L. Tompkins.** 1988. Gene disruption as a feasible approach for mutagenesis of *Campylobacter jejuni. J. Bacteriol.* **170:**1704–1708.
29. **Lee, A., S. M. Logan, and T. J. Trust.** 1987. Demonstration of a flagella antigen shared by a diverse group of spiral-shaped bacteria that colonize intestinal mucus. *Infect. Immun.* **55:**828–831.
30. **Lee, A., J. L. O'Rourke, P. J. Barrington, and T. J. Trust.** 1986. Mucus colonization by *Campylobacter jejuni:* a mouse cecal model. *Infect. Immun.* **51:**536–546.
31. **Lior, H., D. L. Woodward, J. A. Edgar, L. J. Laroche, and P. Gill.** 1982. Serotyping of *Campylobacter jejuni* by slide agglutination based on heat-labile antigenic factors. *J. Clin. Microbiol.* **15:**761–768.
32. **Logan, S. M., P. Guerry, D. M. Rollins, D. H. Burr, and T. J. Trust** 1989. In vivo antigenic variation of *Campylobacter* flagellin. *Infect. Immun.* **57:**2583–2585.
33. **Logan, S. M., L. A. Harris, and T. J. Trust.** 1987. Isolation and characterization of *Campylobacter* flagellins. *J. Bacteriol.* **169:**5072–5077.
34. **Logan, S. M., and T. J. Trust.** 1983. Molecular identification of surface protein antigens of *Campylobacter jejuni. Infect. Immun.* **42:**675–682.
35. **Logan, S. M., and T. J. Trust.** 1986. Location of epitopes on *Campylobacter jejuni* flagella. *J. Bacteriol.* **168:**739–745.
36. **Logan, S. M., T. J. Trust, and P. Guerry.** 1989. Evidence for posttranslational modification and gene duplication of *Campylobacter* flagellin. *J. Bacteriol.* **171:**3031–3038.
37. **McKern, N. M., I. J. O'Donnell, A. S. Inglis, D. J. Stewart, and B. L. Clark.** 1983. Amino acid sequence of pilin from *Bacteroides nodosus* (strain 198), the causative organism of ovine footrot. *FEBS Lett.* **164:**149–153.
38. **Minnich, S. A., and A. Newton.** 1987. Promoter mapping and cell cycle regulation of flagellin gene transcription in *Caulobacter crescentus. Proc. Natl. Acad. Sci. USA* **84:**1142–1146.
39. **Minnich, S. A., N. Ohta, N. Taylor, and A. Newton.** 1988. Role of the 25-, 27-, and 29-kilodalton flagellins in *Caulobacter crescentus* cell motility: method for construction of deletion and Tn*5* insertion mutants by gene replacement. *J. Bacteriol.* **170:**3953–3960.
40. **Mirel, D. B., and M. J. Chamberlain.** 1989. The *Bacillus subtilis* flagellin gene (*hag*) is transcribed by the σ^{28} form of RNA polymerase. *J. Bacteriol.* **171:**3095–3101.
41. **Mullin, D. A., and A. Newton.** 1989. Ntr-like promoters and upstream regulatory sequence *ftr* are required for transcription of a developmentally regulated *Caulobacter crescentus* flagellar gene. *J. Bacteriol.* **171:**3218–3227.
42. **Nachamkin, I., and A. M. Hart.** 1985. Western blot analysis of the human antibody response to

Campylobacter jejuni cellular antigens during gastrointestinal infection. *J. Clin. Microbiol.* **21:**33–38.

43. **Ninfa, A. J., D. A. Mullin, G. Ramakrishnan, and A. Newton.** 1989. *Escherichia coli* σ^{54} RNA polymerase recognizes *Caulobacter crescentus flbG* and *flaN* flagellar gene promoters in vitro. *J. Bacteriol.* **171:**383–391.
44. **Nuijten, P. J. M., A. J. A. M. van Asten, W. Gaastra, and B. A. M. van der Zeijst.** 1990. Structural and functional analysis of two *Campylobacter jejuni* flagellin genes. *J. Biol. Chem.* **265:**17798–17804.
45. **Pleier, E., and R. Schmitt.** 1991. Expression of two *Rhizobium meliloti* flagellin genes and their contribution to the complex filament structure. *J. Bacteriol.* **173:**2077–2085.
46. **Sasse-Dwight, S., and J. D. Gralla.** 1990. Role of eukaryotic-type functional domains found in the prokaryotic enhancer receptor factor sigma^{54}. *Cell* **62:**945–954.
47. **Sastry, P. A., B. B. Finlay, B. L. Pasloske, W. Paranchych, J. R. Pearlstone, and L. B. Smillie.** 1985. Comparative studies of the amino acid and nucleotide sequences of pilin derived from *Pseudomonas aeruginosa* PAK and PAO. *J. Bacteriol.* **164:**571–577.
48. **Schneider, W. R., and R. N. Doetsch.** 1974. Effect of viscosity on bacterial motility. *J. Bacteriol.* **117:**696–701.
49. **Shimada, K., R. Kamiya, and S. Asakura.** 1975. Left-handed to right-handed helix conversion in *Salmonella* flagella. *Nature* (London) **254:**330–334.
50. **Taylor, R. K., V. L. Miller, D. B. Furlong, and J. J. Mekalanos.** 1987. Use of *phoA* fusions to identify a pilus colonization factor coordinately regulated with cholera toxin. *Proc. Natl. Acad. Sci. USA* **84:**2833–2837.
51. **Thornton, S. A., S. M. Logan, T. J. Trust, and P. Guerry.** 1990. Polynucleotide sequence relationships among flagellin genes of *Campylobacter jejuni* and *Campylobacter coli*. *Infect. Immun.* **58:**2686–2689.
52. **Wang, Y., and D. E. Taylor.** 1990. Natural transformation in *Campylobacter* species. *J. Bacteriol.* **172:**949–955.
53. **Wei, L.-N., and T. M. Joys.** 1985. Covalent structure of three phase-1 flagellar filament proteins of *Salmonella*. *J. Mol. Biol.* **186:**791–803.
54. **Wenman, W. M., J. Chai, T. J. Louie, C. Goudreau, H. Lior, D. G. Newell, A. Pearson, and D. E. Taylor.** 1985. Antigenic analysis of *Campylobacter* flagellar protein and other proteins. *J. Clin. Microbiol.* **21:**108–112.
55. **Wenman, W. M., D. E. Taylor, and H. Lior.** 1985. The flagellar protein determines *Campylobacter jejuni* heat labile serotype, p. 212. *In* A. D. Pearson, M. B. Skirrow, H. Lior, and B. Rowe (ed.), *Campylobacter III*. Public Health Laboratory Service, London.
56. **Winsor, D. K., Jr., J. J. Mathewson, and H. L. Dupont.** 1986. Western blot analysis of intestinal secretory immunoglobulin A response to *Campylobacter jejuni* antigens in patients with naturally acquired *Campylobacter* enteritis. *Gastroenterology* **90:**1217–1222.

CHAPTER 31

Molecular Characterization and Analysis of *Campylobacter jejuni* Flagellin Genes and Proteins

PIET J. M. NUIJTEN, TRUDY M. WASSENAAR, DIANE G. NEWELL, AND BERNARD A. M. VAN DER ZEIJST

INTRODUCTION

Enteric *Campylobacter jejuni* infections of humans are widespread in both developed and developing countries. *C. jejuni* is also prevalent in healthy and sick animals; the bacterium can be transmitted from these animals to humans through contaminated food and water. The complex epidemiology of this pathogen makes it difficult to effectively intervene in its spread. Therefore, prevention of *Campylobacter* infections requires more data on its pathogenesis. This will help to develop vaccines, circumventing the use of antibiotics and the resulting antibiotic resistance (58).

Studies at the molecular level are most suited to enhance the understanding of bacterial virulence. Flagella are the best-characterized potential virulence factors of *Campylobacter* spp.; the spontaneous occurrence of aflagellate, nonmotile variants (phase variation) has been a useful tool in studying the role of flagella in *Campylobacter* colonization and pathogenesis. Flagellin is the major protein subunit of the flagellar filament. This filament and the other structural components of the flagellum are lacking in aflagellate variants. However, it is not clear how other proteins or bacterial components, which are coregulated with flagellum synthesis, contribute to virulence. *Campylobacter* flagella have been studied in conjunction with different aspects of *Campylobacter* virulence, pathogenesis, and diagnosis. They are needed to colonize the intestines of mice (32, 38), rabbits (3), and hamsters (1), and they have been implicated as adhesins (28, 38). Flagellin and flagella are immunodominant during infections (29, 30). They probably contain Lior serotype-specific antigens (25, 61); cross-protection can be achieved in animal models when strains have the same Lior serotype (Walker et al., this volume). *C. coli* flagella can undergo antigenic variation (13), whereas *C. jejuni* flagellum synthesis is subject to phase variation (3).

Direct genetic evidence to support flagellin-associated virulence has been lacking. Therefore, we have focused on the molecular biology of the *Campylobacter* flagellin and the regulation of its synthesis. In this chapter we describe the flagellin gene organization, function, and expression in *C. jejuni* 81116, which was isolated from an outbreak of *Campylobacter* infections in 1984 (48).

FLAGELLIN GENE STRUCTURE AND ORGANIZATION

Cloning Strategy

Several reports on the molecular biology of *Campylobacter* spp. have described the difficulties encountered in attempting to clone and express *Campylobacter* genes in *Escherichia coli* (23, 24). Therefore, we used an approach which was not dependent on the expression of the complete flagellin protein (41). Polyvalent rabbit hyperimmune serum against denatured flagellin, isolated as a 62-kDa band from a sodium dodecyl sulfate (SDS)-polyacrylamide gel, was prepared. Further, we constructed a λgt11

Piet J. M. Nuijten, Trudy M. Wassenaar, and Bernard A. M. van der Zeijst, Department of Bacteriology, Institute of Infectious Diseases and Immunology, University of Utrecht, 3508 TD Utrecht, The Netherlands. **Diane G. Newell,** Central Veterinary Laboratory, Ministry of Agriculture, Fisheries and Food, New Haw, Weybridge, Surrey KT15 3NB, United Kingdom.

expression library of randomly sheared chromosomal DNA fragments. We screened approximately 150,000 isopropyl-β-D-thiogalactopyranoside (IPTG)-induced plaques of this library with the flagellin-specific antiserum. Only one clone, with an insert of 850 bp, reacted with the antiserum; it contained the 3′ end of the flagellin gene, expressing the C-terminal part of the flagellin as a fusion protein with the β-galactosidase of λgt11. The small number of clones and the small insert size may reflect the difficulties other investigators have experienced in attempting to express *Campylobacter* genes in *E. coli.*

Flagellin Gene Organization

We used the flagellin-specific DNA probe (850-bp insert) to detect the entire flagellin gene. For this purpose we screened plasmid (Bluescript) libraries containing chromosomal DNA digested with *Hin*dIII or *Bgl*II or partially digested with *Sau*3A1 (44). In this way, five independent, overlapping clones were isolated. Restriction mapping yielded the relative positions of these clones as depicted in Fig. 1. There are two highly similar (strong cross-hybridization) regions, encoding flagellins A and B (see below), each containing similar restriction sites.

We tested several other *C. jejuni* strains for duplicated flagellin gene sequences. Southern blots with DNA of strains from Canada, the United Kingdom, and the Netherlands were hybridized to the 1.2-kb *Pst*I fragment of region B; at least 75% of these strains were found to have duplicated flagellin sequences (44).

Nucleotide Sequence of the Flagellin Locus

Sequence analysis identified two virtually identical flagellin genes (*flaA* and *flaB*) of 1,731 bp each. The open reading frames are 95% identical at the nucleotide level. Differences between *flaA* and *flaB* were found mainly in the 5′ and 3′ ends and in a small region in the middle of the genes. Not all substitutions resulted in an altered amino acid residue in the putative protein products.

The genes are arranged in a head-to-tail repeat separated by an intergenic region of 170 bp; the length of the intergenic region makes it less likely that the two genes are part of one operon. Furthermore, the intergenic region contains two inverted repeats that could function as transcription terminators for *flaA,* and therefore both genes may be transcribed or expressed separately. The genes are similar only within the coding regions; their upstream regions show no

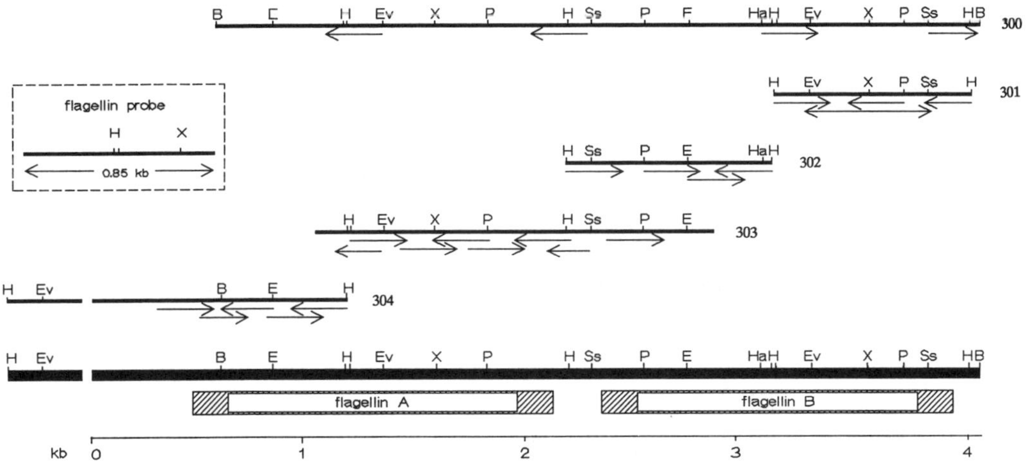

Figure 1. Organization of flagellin genes in *C. jejuni* 81116. A flagellin-specific probe isolated from a λgt11 library (dashed-lined box) (41) was used to isolate clones pIVB3–300 to pIVB3–304. Clones pIVB3–301 (0.84 kb), pIVB3–302 (0.9 kb), and pIVB3–304 (2.7 kb) were isolated from a *Hin*dIII library. Clones pIVB3–300 (3.4 kb) and pIVB3–303 (2.1 kb) were isolated from a *Bgl*II library and a *Sau*3A1 library, respectively. The location of the two flagellin genes, *flaA* and *flaB*, is indicated; transcription of the genes proceeds from left to right. Arrows below each clone indicate the sequencing strategy. Abbreviations: B, *Bgl*II; E, *Eco*RI; Ev, *Eco*RV; H, *Hin*dIII; Ha, *Hae*III; P, *Pst*I; Ss, *Ssp*I; and X, *Xba*I.

significant similarity. These data suggest that if both genes are expressed, their transcription is regulated by different promoter signals.

Remarkably, the *Xba*I recognition sites in both open reading frames (bp 1582 and 3485 [Fig. 2]) predicted from the nucleotide sequence could not be confirmed experimentally. This was observed both with DNA isolated from *Campylobacter* spp. and with DNA cloned in *E. coli.* We were not able to identify specific secondary structures in the DNA in this region, and therefore the explanation of this phenomenon has not been determined. The G+C content of this locus (33%) is close to the average G+C content of *C. jejuni* (35%) (47).

Location of the Flagellin Locus on the Chromosome

In another study we constructed a physical map of the *C. jejuni* chromosome (42), locating a limited number of genes which have now been determined. The map was prepared by using rare-cutting restriction enzymes, such as *Sal*I, *Bss*HII, and *Nci*I, and pulsed-field agarose gel electrophoresis to separate large restriction fragments, ranging in size from 25 to 1,000 kb. The *C. jejuni* chromosome was found to be approximately 1,700 kb in length. This is small compared with other enteropathogens such as *E. coli,* which has a 4,700-kb chromosome (18). Our data correlate well with those of Chang and Taylor (6). Southern blot hybridizations were used to construct the physical map of the chromosome (Fig. 3). The flagellin and rRNA genes were mapped on the chromosome.

Flagellum Structure and Flagellin Genes in Other Bacteria

Campylobacter spp. contain unsheathed (naked) flagella, of which the filament is one major protein component. Some bacteria, e.g., *Vibrio cholerae, Helicobacter pylori,* and *Treponema* spp., have sheathed flagella, and in these species the sheath is continuous with the bacterial membrane and envelops the flagellar filament. This implies that proteins other than flagellin are part of the flagellar structure. As opposed to sheath proteins, which are probably exposed to the surface of the bacterium, species with unsheathed flagella have flagellins with surface-exposed domains.

Flagellins fulfill similar structural functions and therefore possibly contain conserved regions. However, the size of flagellin proteins varies from 27 kDa in *Caulobacter* spp. to 62 kDa in *Campylobacter* spp.

Flagellin gene multiplication (31) has also been found in a number of other bacteria including *Salmonella* spp. (60), *Caulobacter crescentus* (triplication) (31), *Rhizobium meliloti* (50), and *Treponema* spp. (5). Other bacteria have just one flagellin gene (27, 54). The function of amplification of flagellin genes varies. In *Salmonella* spp. one or two, and sometimes three (one copy on a plasmid [51]), flagellin genes are located on different positions on the chromosome. The *Salmonella* bacterium expresses only one gene at a time and is able to switch the expression from one flagellin gene to another, thereby changing the antigenic properties of the flagellum (H-antigen antigenic variation). In *Caulobacter crescentus* (31) and *R. meliloti* (49) flagellin genes are simultaneously expressed and fulfill a structural function. In *C. coli* two flagellin genes are present, organized in a similar way as in *C. jejuni* (Guerry et al., this volume).

STRUCTURE AND ANTIGENICITY OF FLAGELLIN PROTEINS

Primary and Secondary Structure

The two *C. jejuni* 81116 flagellin genes, *flaA* and *flaB,* code for very similar but not identical proteins of 576 residues; 32 amino acids are different (Fig. 4). The substitutions are clustered in three regions: both termini and the middle. The FlaA and FlaB proteins have predicted molecular weights of 59,538 and 59,909 and pI values of 5.32 and 5.53, respectively. During SDS-polyacrylamide gel electrophoresis of whole-cell extracts, flagellins migrate at approximately 62 kDa (39, 41). However, high-resolution gel electrophoresis can distinguish two flagellin-specific bands, migrating at 62 and 60 kDa (37). These two bands do not represent the protein products of *flaA* and *flaB.*

The amino acid sequences of the FlaA and FlaB proteins were compared with the available sequences of other bacterial flagellins; only the amino- and carboxyl-terminal ends were homologous. The amino terminus of the *E. coli* flagellin is needed for transport (16), and both ends of the *Salmonella* (15) and *E. coli* (22) flagellins are necessary for assembly. By analogy, the conserved terminal ends of *C. jejuni* flagellin seem to contain essential functions for filament formation. Since it was impossible to find a significant consensus in the primary sequence of these proteins (16), we investigated the possible conservation of secondary structure. Earlier reports mentioned the presence, in the flagellin termini, of alpha-helical structures which might be

```
          -35                       -10                 mRNA                                    RBS
0001 GGTATAAATTTTTAAAAAAAAGTAACGATATAGCATTTAACAAGCTCATGGATGAGTTTGAAATTATTTAAAAGGATTTAAA
        =====                   ========             *--->                                  -------              oligonucleotide A
0083 ATG GGA TTT CGT ATT AAC ACA AAT GTT GCA GCA TTG AAT GCA AAA GCA AAC TCT GAT CTT AAT GCT AAA AGT TTA GAT GCT TCT
                                                                                                 - --- --- --- --- --- ---
0167 TTA AGC AGA CTT AGT TCA GGT CTT AGA ATT AAC TCA GCA GCA GAT GAT GCT TCA GGG ATG GCG ATA GCA GAT AGC TTA AGA TCT
0251 CAA GCA AAT ACT TTA GGT CAA GCT ATA TCA AAT GGT AAT GAT GCT TTA GGT ATC TTA CAA ACC GCA GAT AAA GCT ATG GAT GAG
0335 CAA TTA AAA ATT CTT GAT ACT ATC AAG ACT AAA GCT ACT CAA GCA GCT CAA GAT GGA CAA AGT TTA AAA ACA AGA ACT ATG CTT
0419 CAA GCA GAT ATT AAT AAA TTA ATG GAA GAG CTT GAT AAT ATC GCT AAT ACT ACT TCA TTT AAT GGT AAG CAA CTT TTA AGT GGA
0503 AAT TTT ACC AAT CAA GAA TTC CAA ATC GGC GCA AGT TCA AAC CAA ACT GTG AAA GCA ACT ATC GGT GCT ACT CAA TCT TCT AAA
0587 ATC GGT GTT ACA AGA TTT GAA ACC GGT GCT CAA AGT TTT ACT TCA GGT GTG GTT GGT CTT ACT ATT AAA AAC TAC AAT GGT ATA
0671 GAA GAT TTT AAA TTT GAT AAT GTT GTG ATT TCA ACT TCA GTT GGA ACA GGA CTT GGA GCT TTG GCT GAA GAG ATC AAT AAA AGC
0755 GCT GAT AAA ACA GGA GTT CGC GCA ACT TAC GAT GTA AAA ACA ACT GGC GTT TAT GCT ATA AAA GAA GGA ACT ACT TCT CAA GAC
0839 TTT GCC ATT AAT GGA GTA ACT ATA GGA AAA ATT GAA TAC AAA GAC GGA GAT GGT AAC GGC TCT TTG ATT TCA GCT ATC AAT GCG
0923 GTT AAA GAT ACC ACA GGA GTT CAA GCT TCT AAA GAT GAA AAC GGC AAG CTT GTT CTT ACA TCG GCT GAT GGC AGG GGT ATT AAA
1007 ATT ACT GGA GAT ATA GGT GTT GGT TCT GGT ATT TTG GCA AAT CAA AAA GAA AAC TAT GGG CGA TTA TCT TTA GTT AAA AAT GAT
1091 GGT AGA GAT ATC AAT ATA AGT GGA ACC AAT CTT AGT GCT ATA GGT ATG GGT ACA ACA GAT ATG ATT TCT CAA TCT TCA GTG TCT
1175 TTA AGA GAA TCA AAA GGT CAA ATT TCA GCA ACC AAT GCC GAT GCT ATG GGA TTT AAT TCT TAT AAA GGT GGT GGA AAA TTT GTT
1259 TTT ACT CAA AAT GTA AGT TCA ATT TCT GCA TTT ATG AGT GCA CAA GGT TCA GGA TTT TCT AGA GGT TCA GGA TTT TCT GTG GGT
1343 AGT GGT AAA AAT TTA TCT GTT GGA TTG AGT CAA GGA ATA CAA ATT ATT TCA AGT GCG GCT TCA ATG AGC AAT ACT TAT GTT GTT
1427 TCA GCA GGT TCA GGA TTT TCT TCT GGC TCA GGA AAT TCT CAA TTT GCA GCC CTT AAA ACT ACT GCT GCT AAT ACA ACT GAT GAG
1511 ACT GCA GGT GTA ACC ACT CTT AAA GGT GCA ATG GCG GTT ATG GAT ATA GCA GAA ACT GCT ATA ACA AAT CTA GAT CAA ATC AGA
1595 GCA GAT ATT GGT TCT ATA CAA AAT CAA GTT ACA TCA ACT ATA AAT AAC ATT ACT GTA ACT CAA GTT AAT GTT AAA GCA GCA GAA
1679 TCG CAA ATC AGA GAT GTA GAC TTT GCA AGT GAG AGT GCA AAC TAC TCT AAA GCT AAC ATC TTA GCC CAA AGT GGT TCT TAT GCA
1763 ATG GCT CAA GCA AAT TCT AGT CAG CAA AAT GTT TTA AGA TTA TTA CAA TAG
                                                 IR                                               IR
1814 TTAAATCTTAAAATCACTTTACATTCTTTTAAGAATGCTGCAATTTATACAAATCCAAGCCTAGTTTAAATACTAGGCTTTTTATTTATAAGCTTAAAATTTTTAATCAA
                                         ------->< -------                          --------->     <---------
              -24              -12                               RBS
1925 ATTAAAACTTGGAACACTTCTTGCTTTAATCTTTTCGATGCAATATTTTGAAAGGATTTAAA
               =======         =====                           -------                         oligonucleotide B
1987 ATG GGT TTT AGG ATA AAC ACC AAC ATC GGT GCA TTA AAT GCA CAT GCA AAT TCA GTT GTT AAC TCT AAT GAA CTT GAC AAG TCT
                                                                                                 - --- --- --- --- --- ---
2071 TTA AGT AGA CTT AGT TCA GGT CTT AGA ATT AAC TCA GCA GCA GAT GAT GCT TCA GGG ATG GCG ATA GCA GAT TCT TTG CGT TCA
2155 CAA GCA GCA ACT TTA GGT CAA GCT ATA AAC AAT GGT AAT GAT GCC ATA GGT ATT TTG CAA ACT GCA GAT AAA GCT ATG GAT GAG
2239 CAA TTA AAA ATT CTT GAT ACT ATC AAG ACT AAA GCT ACT CAA GCA GCT CAA GAT GGA CAA AGT TTA AAA ACA AGA ACT ATG CTT
2323 CAA GCA GAT ATT AAC CGC TTG ATG GAA GAG CTT GAT AAT ATC GCA AAT ACA ACT TCA TTT AAC GGC AAA CAA CTT TTA AGT GGA
2407 AAT TTT ACC AAT CAA GAA TTC CAA ATC GGC GCA AGT TCA AAC CAA ACT ATA AAA GCA ACT ATC GGT GCT ACT CAA TCT TCT AAA
2491 ATC GGT GTT ACA AGA TTT GAA ACC GGT GCT CAA AGT TTT ACT TCA GGT GTG GTT GGT CTT ACT ATT AAA AAC TAC AAT GGT ATA
2575 GAA GAT TTT AAA TTT GAT AAT GTT GTG ATT TCA ACT TCA GTT GGA ACA GGA CTT GGA GCT TTG GCT GAA GAG ATC AAT AAA AGC
2659 GCT GAT AAA ACA GGA GTT CGC GCA ACT TAC GAT GTA AAA ACA ACT GGC GTT TAT GCT ATA AAA GAA GGA ACT ACT TCT CAA GAC
2743 TTT GCC ATT AAT GGA GTT GTA ATT GGT CAG ATT AAT TAT AAA GAT GGT GAT AAT AAC GGC CAA TTG GTT TCA GCT ATC AAT GCG
2827 GTT AAA GAT ACC ACA GGA GTT CAA GCT TCT AAA GAT GAA AAC GGC AAG CTT GTT CTT ACA TCG GCT GAT GGC AGG GGT ATT AAA
2911 ATT ACT GGA GAT ATA GGT GTT GGT TCT GGT ATT TTG GCA AAT CAA AAA GAA AAC TAT GGG CGA TTA TCT TTA GTT AAA AAT GAT
2995 GGT AGA GAT ATC AAT ATA AGT GGA ACC AAT CTT AGT GCT ATA GGT ATG GGT ACA ACA GAT ATG ATT TCT CAA TCT TCA GTG TCT
3079 TTA AGA GAA TCA AAA GGT CAA ATT TCA GCA ACC AAT GCC GAT GCT ATG GGA TTT AAT TCT TAT AAA GGT GGT GGA AAA TTT GTT
3163 TTT ACT CAA AAT GTA AGT TCA ATT TCT GCA TTT ATG AGT GCA CAA GGT TCA GGA TTT TCT AGA GGT TCA GGA TTT TCT GTG GGT
3247 AGT GGT AAA AAT TTA TCT GTT GGA TTG AGT CAA GGA ATA CAA ATT ATT TCA AGT GCG GCT TCA ATG AGC AAT ACT TAT GTT GTT
3331 TCA GCA GGT TCA GGA TTT TCT TCT GGC TCA GGA AAT TCT CAA TTT GCA GCC CTT AAA ACT ACT GCT GCT AAT ACA ACT GAT GAG
3415 ACT GCA GGT GTA ACC ACT CTT AAA GGT GCA ATG GCG GTT ATG GAT ATA GCA GAA ACT GCT ATA ACA AAT CTA GAT CAA ATC AGA
3499 GCA GAT ATT GGT TCT GTA CAA AAT CAA CTT CAA GTT ACT ATA AAC AAT ATT ACT GTA ACT CAG GTA AAT GTT AAA GCA GCC GAA
3583 TCA ACC ATA AGA GAT GTA GAC TTT GCA AGT GAG AGT GCG AAT TTT TCT AAA TAT AAC ATT CTT GCA CAA TCA GGC TCA TAT GCT
3667 ATG AGT CAA CGT AAC GCT GTA CAG CAA AAT GTT TTA AAA CTA TTA CAA TAA
                             IR
3718 TCTTTCTAAAGAGCAATTTTGCTCTTTAGTTTTAGATTAAGCTTCTTTTTTCTAGCTCATCCTGTAAGGGAATAATAGCTTTTTTTAATCTTGTATTTTGACTTTCTATAA
          ----------->< -----------
3829 GATC
```

FIGURE 2. Nucleotide sequence of the *C. jejuni* flagellin genes. Coding sequences are given in triplets. Flagellins A and B are separated by an intergenic region of 173 bp. Flagellin A- and B-mRNA-specific oligonucleotides, ribosome-binding sites (RBS), and the 5′ end of the *flaA* mRNA (*--->) are indicated. Putative transcription termination signals (inverted repeats [IR]) are shown. The −35 and −10 boxes of σ^{28} and −24 and −12 boxes of σ^{54} promoter consensus sequences are underlined twice.

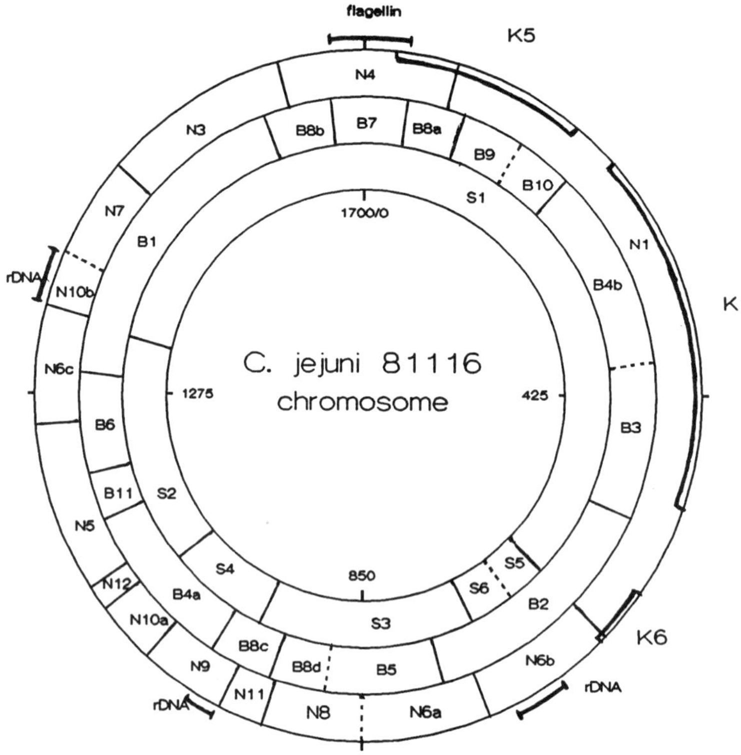

FIGURE 3. Physical map of the *C. jejuni* 81116 chromosome. The locations of the restriction fragments were determined by using the data from Table 2 in reference 42; in the inner circle the map positions are indicated in kilobases, corresponding to the length of the chromosome. The middle of B7 was chosen as the zero position. The locations of flagellin and rRNA genes were determined by hybridization experiments.

involved in stabilization of the filament upon polymerization of the flagellins (17, 35, 57). Alignment of the amino acid sequences of the termini of 12 flagellins showed conservation of nonpolar residues at certain sites. When these domains of the proteins are displayed as an alpha-helix, the nonpolar residues are located at one side of the helix (Fig. 5). We have suggested that the nonpolar backbones of two alpha-helices interact during filament assembly, thereby stabilizing the filamental structure (44). The involvement of hydrophobic interactions between helices in building a supramolecular model for filament structure has been suggested in an independent study by others (9). Despite sequence differences between FlaA and FlaB in the terminal regions of the *C. jejuni* and *C. coli* flagellins, the above-mentioned nonpolar backbone is conserved.

Further analysis revealed a direct repeat of five amino acids, GSG(F/N)S, which was separated by 30 residues that are identical in the two proteins (Fig. 4). A similar repeat has been reported for the flagellin gene of *S. typhi* H1-d. In that case, DNA recombination between the nucleotide repeats led to the excision of a part of the flagellin gene and the appearance of a new H serotype, H1-j (10). However, so far there is no evidence for recombination in *Campylobacter* flagellin genes.

Antigenic Regions on Flagellins in *C. jejuni* 81116

As described above and in other chapters of this volume, flagellar antigens are candidates for vaccines as well as suitable antigens for diagnostic purposes (25, 30, 34, 36). However, the antigenicity of flagella is complex.

Antibodies may recognize conformation-dependent or conformation-independent epitopes, and intact flagella or flagellin subunits can

```
MGFRINTNVAALNAKANSDLNAKSLDASLSRLSSGLRINSAADDASGMAIADSLR -55
        **    *   ** ***  *
MGFRINTNIGALNAHANSVVNSNELDKSLSRLSSGLRINSAADDASGMAIADSLR -55

SQANTLGQAISNGNDALGILQTADKAMDEQLKILDTIKTKATQAAQDGQSLKTRT -110
   *      *     *
SQAATLGQAINNGNDAIGILQTADKAMDEQLKILDTIKTKATQAAQDGQSLKTRT -110

MLQADINKLMEELDNIANTTSFNGKQLLSGNFTNQEFQIGASSNQTVKATIGATQ -165
       *                                      *
MLQADINRLMEELDNIANTTSFNGKQLLSGNFTNQEFQIGASSNQTIKATIGATQ -165

SSKIGVTRFETGAQSFTSGVVGLTIKNYNGIEDFKFDNVVISTSVGTGLGALAEE -220

SSKIGVTRFETGAQSFTSGVVGLTIKNYNGIEDFKFDNVVISTSVGTGLGALAEE -220

INKSADKTGVRATYDVKTTGVYAIKEGTTSQDFAINGVTIGKIEYKDGDGNGSLI -275
                                      *  * *     *  * *
INKSADKTGVRATYDVKTTGVYAIKEGTTSQDFAINGVVIGQINYKDGDNNGQLV -275

SAINAVKDTTGVQASKDENGKLVLTSADGRGIKITGDIGVGSGILANQKENYGRL -330

SAINAVKDTTGVQASKDENGKLVLTSADGRGIKITGDIGVGSGILANQKENYGRL -330

SLVKNDGRDINISGTNLSAIGMGTTDMISQSSVSLRESKGQISATNADAMGFNSY -385

SLVKNDGRDINISGTNLSAIGMGTTDMISQSSVSLRESKGQISATNADAMGFNSY -385

KGGGKFVFTQNVSSISAFMSAQGSGFSRGSGFSVGSGKNLSVGLSQGIQIISSAA -440

KGGGKFVFTQNVSSISAFMSAQGSGFSRGSGFSVGSGKNLSVGLSQGIQIISSAA -440

SMSNTYVVSAGSGFSSGSGNSQFAALKTTAANTTDETAGVTTLKGAMAVMDIAET -495

SMSNTYVVSAGSGFSSGSGNSQFAALKTTAANTTDETAGVTTLKGAMAVMDIAET -495

AITNLDQIRADIGSIQNQVTSTINNITVTQVNVKAAESQIRDVDFASESANYSKA -550
              *   ***                 *            *  *
AITNLDQIRADIGSVQNQLQVTINNITVTQVNVKAAESTIRDVDFASESANFSKY -550

NILAQSGSYAMAQANSSQQNVLRLLQ -576
           * * **     *
NILAQSGSYAMSQRNAVQQNVLKLLQ -576
```

Figure 4. Alignment of amino acid sequences of FlaA (upper line) and FlaB (lower line) of *C. jejuni* 81116. Differences between the two proteins are indicated by asterisks. The GSG(F/N)S sequence, repeated four times, is underlined.

be used as antigens (25, 30, 36, 37). In this respect it is necessary to mention that flagellum epitopes are thought to be involved as antigenic determinants in the heat-labile Lior serotyping scheme (61). The Lior antibodies should bind to intact flagella, because they agglutinate intact bacteria. A number of monoclonal antibodies that have been prepared against *C. jejuni* 81116 (Lior 6) are Lior serotype specific, whereas other are broadly cross-reactive (36). However, all of these antibodies reacted only to denatured flagellin, which means that they recognized conformation-independent epitopes, whereas none of them was able to label the flagellum (Table

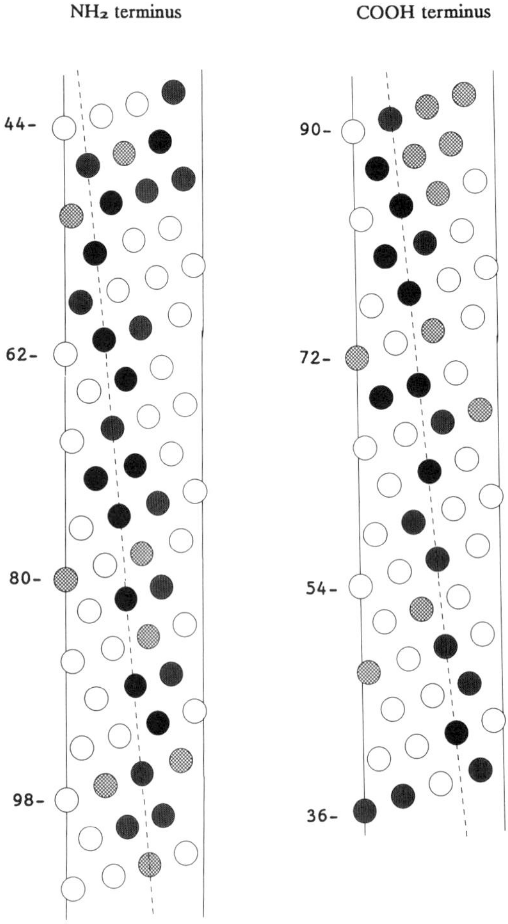

FIGURE 5. Conservation of nonpolar residues in the NH_2- and COOH-terminal regions of bacterial flagellins. The amino- and carboxy-terminal amino acid sequences were aligned (data not shown). This showed a conservation of nonpolar residues (A, G, I, L, M, F, V, and W). The figure represents a flattened helix projection, which shows both sides of the helix, of both termini, showing residues 41 to 106 of the amino terminus and residues 81 to 36 of the carboxy terminus, both in *C. jejuni* numbering; the dashed line indicates the direction of the nonpolar backbone. Positions where all (12 of 12) residues are nonpolar are shown in black; positions where 9 to 11 residues are nonpolar are indicated in dark grey; positions where 6 to 8 residues are nonpolar are indicated in light grey; and positions where fewer than 6 residues are nonpolar are indicated in white. Flagellins used in the compilation are *C. jejuni flaA* and *flaB, C. coli, E. coli, B. subtilis, Roseburia cecicola, Serratia marcescens, S. typhimurium* H1-a, *R. meliloti flaA* and *flaB, Treponema pallidum,* and *Borrelia burgdorferi* (see reference 44).

1). Thus epitopes that are hidden in intact flagella become immunogenic after immunization. This could be caused by dissociation of the flagellar filament into smaller segments or into flagellin subunits.

The location of conformation-independent epitopes can be mapped by using the bacterial expression system pEX (19, 53). Segments of the gene to be expressed are inserted in the correct reading frame in the pEX vector. Expression results in fusion proteins containing the amino-terminal part of the vector-encoded protein Cro-LacZ linked to the carboxy-terminal part of the inserted protein. The expression of the fusion gene can be easily controlled; the gene is silent at 30°C and strongly expressed at 42°C, owing to the inactivation of the *c*I repressor at 42°C. This minimizes toxic effects on the *E. coli* host cell. Furthermore, the fusion proteins are partly protected against proteolysis since they are insoluble and precipitate within the bacteria.

To compare the antigenicity of the predicted protein products of the *flaA* and *flaB* genes of *C. jejuni* 81116, we expressed parts of both genes in pEX (Fig. 6). Five overlapping gene segments were cloned and expressed from each gene. The protein products were reacted with monoclonal antibodies which were raised against *C. jejuni* 81116 flagella (36, 37, 45). In this way we could broadly localize the epitopes recognized by these monoclonal antibodies (Table 1). Three immunogenic regions were found: in both termini and in the center of the protein. CF17 reacted to NH_2-terminal region II and CF16 to COOH-terminal region VII of both proteins. However, the middle of the FlaA protein was antigenically different from that of the FlaB protein (region IV); some antibodies (CF1, CF2, CF3, CF4, CF5, and CF13) reacted only with FlaA protein products, whereas others (CF6 and CF15) also recognized the FlaB products. No FlaB-specific monoclonal antibodies were found.

We studied the localization of the epitopes in the center of flagellin A in more detail by means of competitive radioimmunoassays (45). In combination with other data obtained from immunogold labeling (37) and serotype specificity (36) studies, we concluded that the middle of FlaA contains at least three different serotype-specific epitopes. In addition, a second area in the center of FlaA could be distinguished; this was located directly adjacent to the previous one and contains epitopes for CF6 and CF15 that are less serotype specific.

In conclusion, the central part of the flagellin genes (54), and therefore also the center of the proteins (45), contain serotype- and species-

TABLE 1. Properties of monoclonal antibodies against *Campylobacter* flagellin

Antibody	Serotype (no. of Lior serotypes reacting)[a,b]	Reaction with flagellin fragment[c]	Reaction with *flaA* and/or *flaB* region[b]	Immunogold electron microscopy
CF1	1	A2 A3	A IV	BS
CF2	1	A2 A3	A IV	NR
CF3	2	A2 A3	A IV	TBF
CF4	2	A2 A3	A IV	TBF
CF5	13	A2 A3	A IV	NR
CF6	9	A2 A3 B2	A IV, B II–VI	NR
CF7	13	All	Several	NR
CF13	1	A2 A3	A IV	TBF
CF15	18	A2 A3 B2	A IV, B II–VI	NR
CF16	18	A4 A5 B4 B5	A+B VII	NR
CF17	18	A2 B2	A+B II	NR

[a] See reference 36.
[b] Data from reference 45; each gene was divided into seven regions as shown in Fig. 6.
[c] The locations of the flagellin fragments are indicated in Fig. 6.
[d] Abbreviations: BS, bacterial surface; TBF, tips and broken pieces of flagella; NR, no reaction. Data from reference 37.

specific sequences, which is in agreement with results of studies on the localization of H-antigen-specific regions of *Salmonella* (60) and *E. coli* (21) flagellins.

Posttranslational Modification of Flagellins

No amino-terminal methionine residue was found by amino acid sequence analysis of *C. jejuni* flagellin. Apparently, this methionine is cleaved off posttranslationally. Isoelectrofocusing of *Campylobacter* flagellins has revealed a charge heterogeneity; flagellin-specific antisera and monoclonal antibodies recognized about six different flagellin subspecies (33). Thus more than the two possible protein products of the *flaA* and *flaB* genes must be accounted for. So far, two different explanations for this phenomenon have been given: (i) translational errors causing amino acid substitutions which lead to differences in charge (7), and (ii) posttranslational modifications, which possibly involve the phosphorylation of serine residues in several regions of the protein (26). Furthermore, flagellin microheterogeneity is not restricted to charge; we have demonstrated the presence of two flagellin bands in high-resolution gel systems, as mentioned above (37). Since the two flagellin proteins of *C. jejuni* 81116 are very similar in molecular weight, it is possible that molecular weight heterogeneity is related to the expression of these two genes. However, monoclonal antibody CF1, which reacts to FlaA flagellin only, recognized all flagellin subspecies: both molecular weight bands and all acidic spots (45). Therefore it seems likely that flagellin is subject to posttranslational modifications, as has been reported for *C. coli* flagellin (26). Preparation of monoclonal antibodies that specifically react to modified or unmodified flagellin epitopes would greatly improve the detection and our understanding of the function of this posttranslational event. In conclusion, the available data suggest that posttranscriptional modifications occur, at least on the FlaA protein. Whether the *flaB* gene is or can be expressed is discussed below.

STRUCTURE AND FUNCTION OF FLAGELLA

Inactivation of Flagellin Genes

Deletions were introduced into the *flaA* and *flaB* genes to determine the function of these genes. A simple method was developed to obtain these deletion mutants. Briefly, a *Campylobacter* kanamycin resistance gene was inserted into a cloned fragment of one flagellin gene in the vector Bluescript and electroporated directly into *C. jejuni* 81116. The Bluescript plasmid is unable to replicate in campylobacters; therefore, selection for kanamycin-resistant colonies should yield recombinants in which *flaA*, *flaB*, or both

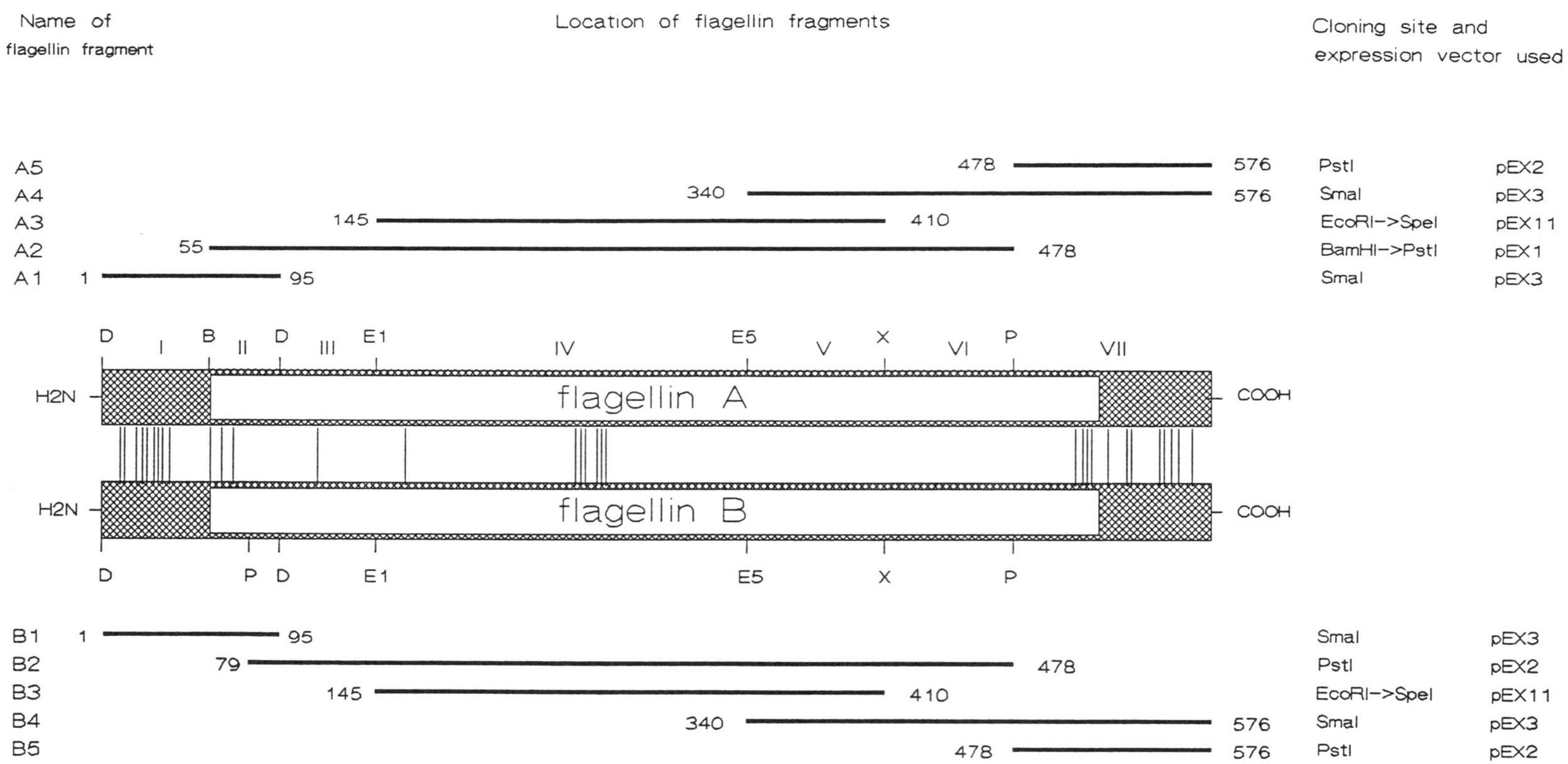

FIGURE 6. Construction of *C. jejuni* 81116 flagellin gene fusion proteins in pEX. The subcloning strategy was as follows. Restriction enzyme fragments were isolated from the available flagellin clones (44) and ligated in pEX vectors as indicated. Each flagellin protein was thereby divided in seven regions (I to VII). Fusion products A2 and B2 are different because of the use of different restriction enzymes. The locations of amino acids at junctions between regions are indicated with each restriction site. Abbreviations: B, *Bgl*II; D, *Dra*I; E1, *Eco*RI; E5, *Eco*RV; P, *Pst*I; X, *Xba*I. Differences in amino acid sequences between FlaA and FlaB proteins are shown as lines connecting the two flagellins.

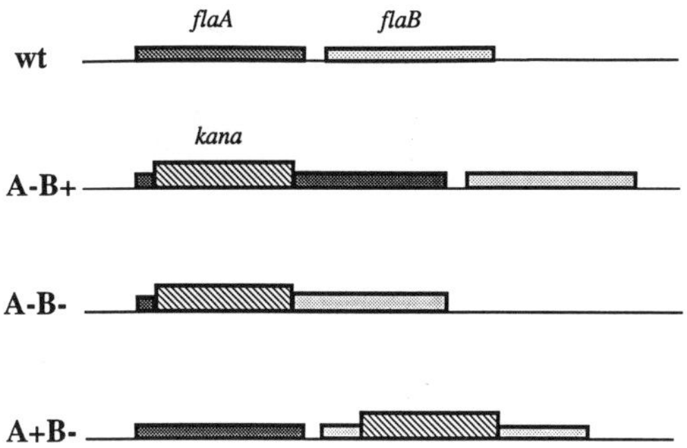

FIGURE 7. Flagellin gene inactivation. Flagellin genes *flaA, flaB,* or both were inactivated by insertion of a kanamycin resistance gene in flagellin gene constructs in *E. coli* (59). *C. jejuni* was electroporated with these constructs. Homologous recombination between the introduced plasmid and chromosomal DNA yielded kanamycin-resistant *C. jejuni* colonies carrying destroyed *flaA* (A^- B^+) or *flaB* (A^+ B^-) genes, or both (A^- B^-). A^+ B^+ is the genotype for Fla^+ and for Fla^- variants.

were disrupted. Since the *flaA* and *flaB* genes are 95% identical, various recombinants were expected after two crossover recombinational events: (i) the flagellin-kanamycin construct could recombine in the *flaA* gene, leaving the *flaB* gene undisturbed (A^- B^+); (ii) the same construct would inactivate only the *flaB* gene, leaving an intact *flaA* gene (A^+ B^-); or (iii) the construct could recombine with the 5′ region of the *flaA* gene and the 3′ region of the *flaB* gene, thereby inactivating both genes (A^- B^-). Indeed, all three recombinants were obtained; by Southern hybridization analysis, they lacked vector sequences (59) (Fig. 7).

Effect of Flagellin Gene Inactivation on Flagellum Formation and Motility

The three recombinants described above were tested together with the motile, flagellated wild type (Fla^+, A^+ B^+) and a naturally occurring nonmotile, aflagellated variant (Fla^-; also with the A^+ B^+ genotype [see below]) for (i) the presence of flagella and motility, (ii) agglutination by Lior 6 antiserum, and (iii) the production of flagellin A (as detected with monoclonal antibody CF1) or A plus B (as detected with monoclonal antibody CF17). The results are summarized in Table 2. Mutants in which *flaB* but not *flaA* was inactivated remained motile; the A^+ B^- genotype produced normal flagella. The A^- B^+ genotype was nonmotile, but produced nonfunctional, short, truncated flagella consisting of FlaB protein. These results indicate that the *flaB* gene was expressed in the A^- B^+ mutant. The Fla^- variant lacked flagella but made minor amounts of FlaB. The agglutination of the A^+ B^- mutant by Lior 6 antiserum (absorbed antiserum kindly provided by H. Lior) showed that the FlaB protein is not required for Lior serotype determination. The FlaB protein also contained the conserved nonpolar backbone structure in both termini, although many differences with the FlaA protein are found in these regions. These differences may account for structural changes in the protein, causing a short, truncated, and more fragile FlaB flagellum in the A^- B^+ genotype. Another explanation for the shorter FlaB flagellum in this mutant could be the low expression level of the *flaB* gene, causing a shortage of the filamental protein subunit.

Role of Flagella in Pathogenesis

The five different phenotypes (Table 2) were used to study the effect of flagellin gene inactivation on virulence. We used an in vitro assay measuring the invasion of *C. jejuni* into INT 407 cells, which were derived from human intestinal epithelium. Penetration of *C. jejuni* into intestinal cells has been used as a measurement of

TABLE 2. Properties of *C. jejuni* 81116 flagellin mutants

Genotype	Flagellin production: CF1 (FlaA)	Flagellin production: CF17 (FlaA + FlaB)	Motility	Type of flagella	Invasion (%)[b]	Lior 6 serotypic reaction
A^+ B^+[a]	++	++	+	Long	100	+
A^- B^+	−	+	−	Short	1	−
A^+ B^-	++	++	+	Long	98	+
A^- B^-	−	−	−	None	0.5	−
Fla^-	−	+[c]	−	None	0.06	−

[a] A^+ B^+ is motile wild type (Fla^+).
[b] The ability to invade was compared with that of the wild type (A^+ B^+ = 100%).
[c] The amount of protein reacting is smaller than in A^{-1} B^+ mutants.

virulence (40). This invasion assay measures the final result of motility, attachment, and penetration.

The mutants lacking a functional *flaA* gene and the Fla⁻ variant have a highly reduced (5,000-fold) invasive capacity (Table 2). FlaB did not functionally substitute for FlaA. Centrifugation of the bacteria onto the eukaryotic cells improved invasion of Fla⁻, A⁻ B⁻, and A⁻ B⁺ mutants 5- to 500-fold (59), showing that motility contributes to invasion. However, after centrifugation the nonmotile phenotypes still had reduced levels of invasion compared with motile bacteria. These experiments suggest that a functional flagellin is required for invasion and possibly also a positive chemotactic behavior towards the eukaryotic cells. Previous data described diminished virulence of the aflagellated variant, which, in fact, could have been less virulent through the coregulation of other proteins. Indications that the motility rather than adhesive properties of *Campylobacter* flagella is important come from the above-mentioned centrifugation experiments and from experiments in which purified flagella were added to the INT 407 cells before inoculation with *C. jejuni*. We found, as also described by others (28), that this had no effect on invasiveness (59).

REGULATION OF FLAGELLIN GENE EXPRESSION

Transcriptional Analysis

The results presented above indicate that mainly FlaA protein was produced in wild-type *C. jejuni*. However, FlaB flagellin was found in minor amounts in A⁻ B⁺ and the Fla⁻ variant (Table 2). A further analysis of the nucleotide sequence of the promoter regions of both flagellin genes provided a clue concerning the regulation of expression. Many bacterial flagellin gene promoter regions contain typically σ^{28}-controlled sequences (11, 37, 55). This means that these promoters are transcribed by an RNA polymerase complex containing an alternative sigma factor (14, 20). In *C. jejuni*, however, the σ^{28} consensus was present in front of the *flaA* gene only (Fig. 2) and was absent in front of the *flaB* gene. The *flaA* and *flaB* genes are separated by 170 bp, and in this region a σ^{54}-specific *flaB* promoter sequence was detected (20) (Fig. 2). Experimental data regarding the transcription of the *flaA* and *flaB* genes was obtained by using *flaA* and *flaB* mRNA-specific oligonucleotide probes. We could demonstrate the presence of a single monocistronic *flaA* mRNA of 1,800 nucleotides in motile bacteria. Primer extension experiments with the same oligonucleotides confirmed this observation: the *flaA* mRNA has a 5′ end at 43 nucleotides upstream from the ATG start codon (Fig. 2), whereas no *flaB* mRNA could be detected. The *flaA* and *flaB* promoter activities were tested by in vitro transcription with σ^{28}- and σ^{54}-dependent transcription systems; clones pIVB3-304 and pIVB3-302, encoding *flaA* and *flaB* promoters, respectively (Fig. 1), were used as templates. The results of such in vitro assays are supposed to reflect the expression of the flagellin genes in vivo. Only σ^{28} holoenzyme was able to activate the *flaA* promoter (43). These data suggest that *flaA* is expressed at a much higher level compared with *flaB*. Thus, flagella consist mainly of FlaA protein, although the presence of a low level of FlaB cannot be excluded.

Mechanism of Flagellar Phase Variation

Caldwell et al. (3) showed that certain *Campylobacter* strains were able to switch flagellum formation on and off (phase variation). This raised several questions: what is the trigger for phase variation, and what might be its biological significance? Furthermore, we were interested in the molecular mechanism by which *C. jejuni* is able to switch the production of this virulence factor on and off. To answer some of these questions we isolated nonmotile, aflagellated variants (Fla⁻), which were then cultured in a stable and pure form. Flagellar phase variation appeared to be reversible, and the frequency of switching was affected by growth conditions (unpublished data); however, so far we have been unable to determine the exact nature of the stimuli causing a switch or the factors that control the direction of the switch. The presence of flagellin mRNA in Fla⁺ and Fla⁻ variants was determined by Northern (RNA) blot analysis with the λgt11 insert probe and the *flaA*- and *flaB*-specific oligonucleotides. Very low levels of flagellin mRNA could be detected in aflagellated cells with the λgt11 flagellin probe, but no signal was observed with the oligonucleotide probes. Since minor amounts of FlaB protein were found in the aflagellated variant, there probably was a very low concentration of *flaB* mRNA. We conclude from these experiments that reversible *flaA* gene expression is regulated at the transcriptional level and that this expression is required for functional flagella. In this respect it is interesting that Aguero-Rosenfeld et al. (1) demonstrated a microheterogeneity of flagellin in a motile variant of *C. jejuni* IN1 (Lior 7) that was absent in an aflagellated variant. The aflagellated bacteria contained minute amounts of a homogeneous (one-dot) flagellin. This resembles the situation in *C. jejuni* 81116. However, we have not yet analyzed the nature of the C. *jejuni* 81116 flagellin present in Fla⁻ variants. Our hypothesis is that during phase variation in strain 81116 only one flagellin gene, the *flaA* gene, is switched off.

Posttranslational modification of the flagellin protein in the aflagellated variant seems to be absent (1); this can be caused by the protein itself (FlaB type) or by the absence of modifying enzymes coregulated with switch off of flagellum synthesis. We have studied in more detail the mechanism by which the expression of the *flaA* gene in the aflagellated variant is curtailed. As discussed above, σ^{28} is needed for *flaA* transcription. There are several ways in which transcription of the *flaA* gene can be switched off, including, for example, differences between motile and nonmotile bacteria at the DNA level. To this end the nucleotide sequence of the complete flagellin locus of the Fla⁻ variant was determined and found to be identical to the sequence of the wild type. Therefore, DNA rearrangements or mutations in the flagellin locus are not responsible for switching off flagellin gene expression. In addition, we have studied DNA-protein interactions by using the technique of Southwestern (DNA-protein) blotting and have shown that the Fla⁻ but not the Fla⁺ strain has a strong DNA-binding capacity (55), indicating the possible presence of a repressor in the Fla⁻ variant.

DISCUSSION AND PROSPECTS

The importance of flagella as virulence factors of pathogenic bacteria is well established for several of the better-studied systems. By means of their motility, bacteria are able to move actively toward the intestinal surfaces or crypts, in this way promoting colonization, adherence, or invasion. However, no unifying function of flagella in bacterial pathogenesis can be stated, and direct proof of their role in infection is difficult to obtain. Yet, evidence is accumulating that flagella help pathogens to establish infection (2, 4, 8, 12, 52). The construction of genetically manipulated *C. jejuni* 81116 mutants that lack one or both flagellin genes has provided important evidence for the role of the flagellum, and the motility it provides, in virulence. Now these mutants are available, it is possible to test them in animal models or in human volunteers for their pathogenic properties and potential as a vaccine. Although the ability to inactivate specific *Campylobacter* genes is a great step forward, it would be an enormous advantage to have a transposon mutant library, each mutant having one inactivated gene. So far, all attempts to make such a library have failed.

The role of flagella on virulence and pathogenesis can be studied by making use of flagellar antigenic variation and phase variation. Both types of variation give the bacterium an opportunity to escape a flagellum-specific immune response of the host. Furthermore, phase variation will switch off a number of energy-consuming processes such as flagellum formation, motility, and chemotaxis. Despite substantial efforts, we were unable to demonstrate antigenic variation in *C. jejuni* 81116 flagella. It seems possible that both phase variation and antigenic variation exist within one *Campylobacter* strain; for example, *C. coli* VC167 shows phase variation in addition to antigenic variation (13). Therefore, it is likely that both types of variation are regulated by different mechanisms.

The expression of both flagellin genes noted in *C. coli* was not observed in *C. jejuni* 81116. The absence of *flaB* expression in *C. jejuni* may be due to a weaker promoter activity; there are indeed differences between the *flaB* promoters of *C. jejuni* and *C. coli* (44). Another explanation is the lack of additional transcription factors required for the expression of the *C. jejuni flaB* gene. However, the FlaB protein is clearly produced by the A⁻ B⁺ genotype and assembled into a filament. With respect to the function of the *flaB* gene and FlaB protein, it is interesting that it is not needed for motility and invasion. It is still unclear whether gene *flaB* can serve as a source of antigenic variability within strain 81116, thereby producing new flagellar serotypes either by differential expression or by means of recombinational events between the two flagellin genes.

Alternative sigma factors have been recognized as important regulatory proteins that control gene expression. Several alternative sigma factors have been identified and studied (14, 20). σ^{28}-dependent expression seems to be a generally observed mechanism for the regulation of chemotaxis and flagellin gene transcription in many bacteria. It is well known that in *Salmonella* spp., *E. coli, B. subtilis,* and *Caulobacter* spp. (see references 27 and 46 and references therein) motility and chemotaxis demand the coordinately regulated expression of more than 40 genes, controlled within one regulon. This regulon contains several operons of different transcriptional levels. Some of the gene products within this regulon have a regulatory function and control the transcription of lower-level operons, thus making it possible to express genes when needed. The σ^{28} factor has been shown to be such a regulator and is located within the transcriptional level above (and before) the flagellin genes and genes of other flagellar structural components. We were able to confirm σ^{28}-dependent *flaA* transcription by using an in vitro *B. subtilis* σ^{28} RNA polymerase. The presence and expression of this alternative sigma factor may be a clue to understanding the on-off switch of the *flaA* gene. However, so far we were not able to identify a σ^{28}-like protein or gene in *C. jejuni* 81116. Reversible flagellin gene expression may also be controlled at a higher level of the motility-chemotaxis regulon.

DNA-protein interactions of the *flaA* promoter region with proteins of the Fla⁻ variant and wild type indicated that the aflagellate variant produced additional DNA-binding proteins. It is not yet clear whether these proteins specifically repress *flaA* transcription or whether they cover more DNA regions, thereby repressing the expression of several more genes involved in flagellum synthesis, motility, and chemotaxis.

REFERENCES

1. **Aguero-Rosenfeld, M. E., X.-H. Yang, and I. Nachamkin.** 1990. Infection of adult Syrian hamsters with flagellar variants of *Campylobacter jejuni*. *Infect. Immun.* **58:**2214–2219.
2. **Attridge, S. R., and D. Rowley.** 1983. The role of the flagellum in the adherence of Vibrio cholerae. *J. Infect. Dis.* **147:**864–872.
3. **Caldwell, M. B., P. Guerry, E. C. Lee, J. P. Burans, and R. I. Walker.** 1985. Reversible expression of flagella in *Campylobacter jejuni*. *Infect. Immun.* **50:**941–943.
4. **Canale-Parola, E.** 1978. Motility and chemotaxis of spirochetes. *Annu. Rev. Microbiol.* **32:**69–99.
5. **Champion, C. I., J. N. Miller, M. A. Lovett, and D. R. Blanco.** 1990. Cloning, sequencing, and expression of two class B endoflagellar genes of *Treponema pallidum* subsp. *pallidum* encoding the 34.5- and 31.0-kilodalton proteins. *Infect. Immun.* **58:**1697–1704.
6. **Chang, N., and D. E. Taylor.** 1990. Use of pulsed-field agarose gel electrophoresis to size *Campylobacter* species genomes and to construct a *Sal*I map of *Campylobacter jejuni* UA580. *J. Bacteriol.* **172:**5211–5217.
7. **Dunn, B. E., M. J. Blaser, and E. L. Snyder.** 1987. Two-dimensional gel electrophoresis and immunoblotting of *Campylobacter* outer membrane proteins. *Infect. Immun.* **55:**1564–1572.
8. **Drake, D., and T. C. Montie.** 1988. Flagella, motility and invasive virulence of Pseudomonas aeruginosa. *J. Gen. Microbiol.* **134:**43–52.
9. **Fedorov, O. V., and A. V. Efimov.** 1990. Flagellin as an object for supramolecular engineering. *Protein Eng.* **3:**411–413.
10. **Frankel, G., S. M. C. Newton, G. K. Schoolnik, and B. A. D. Stocker.** 1989. Intragenic recombination in a flagellin gene: characterization of the H1-j gene of Salmonella typhi. *EMBO J.* **8:**3149–3152.
11. **Guerry, P., S. M. Logan, S. Thornton, and T. J. Trust.** 1990. Genomic organization and expression of *Campylobacter* flagellin genes. *J. Bacteriol.* **172:**1853–1860.
12. **Harmon, R. C., R. L. Rutherford, H.-M. Wu, and M. S. Collins.** 1989. Monoclonal antibody-mediated protection and neutralization of motility in experimental *Proteus mirabilis* infection. *Infect. Immun.* **57:**1936–1941.
13. **Harris, L. A., S. M. Logan, P. Guerry, and T. J. Trust.** 1987. Antigenic variation of *Campylobacter* flagella. *J. Bacteriol.* **169:**5066–5071.
14. **Helmann, J. D., and M. J. Chamberlin.** 1988. Structure and function of bacterial sigma factors. *Annu. Rev. Biochem.* **57:**839–872.
15. **Homma, M., H. Fujita, S. Yamaguchi, and T. Iino.** 1987. Regions of *Salmonella typhimurium* flagellin essential for its polymerization and excretion. *J. Bacteriol.* **169:**291–296.
16. **Kawajima, G., I. Kawagishi, M. Homma, J.-I. Asaka, E. Kondo, and R. M. Macnab.** 1989. Export of an N-terminal fragment of Escherichia coli flagellin by a flagellum-specific pathway. *Proc. Natl. Acad. Sci. USA* **86:**4953–4957.
17. **Kostyukova, A. S., M. G. Pyatibratov, V. V. Filimonov, and O. V. Fedorov.** 1988. Flagellin parts acquiring a regular structure during polymerization are disposed on the molecular ends. *FEBS Lett.* **241:**141–144.
18. **Kohara, Y., K. Akiyama, and K. Isono.** 1987. The physical map of the whole E. coli chromosome: application of a new strategy for rapid analysis and sorting of a large genomic library. *Cell* **50:**495–508.
19. **Kusters, J. G., J. Jager, and B. A. M. van der Zeijst.** 1989. Improvement of the cloning linker of the bacterial expression vector pEX. *Nucleic Acids Res.* **17:**8007.
20. **Kustu, S., E. Santero, J. Keener, D. Popham, and D. Weiss.** 1989. Expression of σ^{54} *(ntrA)*-dependent genes is probably united by a common mechanism. *Microbiol. Rev.* **53:**367–376.
21. **Kuwajima, G.** 1988. Flagellin domain that affects H antigenicity of *Escherichia coli* K-12. *J. Bacteriol.* **170:**485–488.
22. **Kuwajima, G.** 1988. Construction of a minimum-size functional flagellin of *Escherichia coli*. *J. Bacteriol.* **170:**3305–3309.
23. **Labigne-Roussel, A., P. Courcoux, and L. Tompkins.** 1988. Gene disruption and replacement as a feasible approach for mutagenesis of *Campylobacter jejuni*. *J. Bacteriol.* **170:**1704–1708.
24. **Labigne-Roussel, A., J. Harrel, and L. Tompkins.** 1987. Gene transfer from *Escherichia coli* to *Cam-*

pylobacter species: development of shuttle vectors from genetic analysis of *Campylobacter jejuni*. *J. Bacteriol.* **169:**5320–5323.

25. **Lior, H.** 1984. Serotyping of *Campylobacter jejuni* and *Campylobacter coli* by slide agglutination based on heat-labile antigenic factors, p. 61–76. *In* J.-P. Butzler (ed.), *Campylobacter Infection in Man and Animals*. CRC Press, Inc., Boca Raton, Fla.
26. **Logan, S. M., T. J. Trust, and P. Guerry.** 1989. Evidence for posttranslational modification and gene duplication of *Campylobacter* flagellin. *J. Bacteriol.* **171:**3031–3038.
27. **Macnab, R. M.** 1987. Flagella, p. 70–83. *In* F. C. Neidhardt, J. L. Ingraham, K. B. Low, B. Magasanik, M. Schaechter, and H. E. Umbarger (ed.), *Escherichia coli and Salmonella typhimurium: Cellular and Molecular Biology,* vol. 1. American Society for Microbiology, Washington, D.C.
28. **McSweegan, E., and R. I. Walker.** 1986. Identification and characterization of two *Campylobacter jejuni* adhesins for cellular and mucous substrates. *Infect. Immun.* **53:**141–148.
29. **Mills, S. D., and W. C. Bradbury.** 1984. Human antibody response to outer membrane proteins of *Campylobacter jejuni* during infection. *Infect. Immun.* **43:**739–743.
30. **Mills, S. D., L. A. Kurjanczyk, and J. L. Penner.** 1988. Identification of an antigen common to different species of the genus *Campylobacter*. *J. Clin. Microbiol.* **26:**1411–1413.
31. **Minnich, S. A., N. Ohta, N. Taylor, and A. Newton.** 1988. Role of the 25-, 27-, and 29-kilodalton flagellins in *Caulobacter crescentus* cell motility: method for construction of deletion and Tn*5* insertion mutants by gene replacement. *J. Bacteriol.* **170:**3953–3960.
32. **Morooka, T., A. Umeda, and K. Amako.** 1985. Motility as an intestinal colonization factor for *Campylobacter jejuni*. *J. Gen. Microbiol.* **131:**1973–1980.
33. **Nachamkin, I., and X.-H. Yang.** 1988. Isoelectric focusing of *Campylobacter jejuni* flagellin: microheterogeneity and restricted antigenicity of charged species with a monoclonal antibody. *FEMS Microbiol. Lett.* **49:**235–238.
34. **Nachamkin, I., and X.-H. Yang.** 1989. Human antibody response to *Campylobacter jejuni* flagellin protein and a synthetic N-terminal flagellin peptide. *J. Clin. Microbiol.* **27:**2195–2198.
35. **Namba, K., I. Yamashita, and F. Vonderviszt.** 1989. Structure of the core and central channel of bacterial flagella. *Nature* (London) **342:**648–654.
36. **Newell, D. G.** 1986. Monoclonal antibodies directed against the flagella of *Campylobacter jejuni:* cross-reacting and serotypic specificity and potential use in diagnosis. *J. Hyg.* **96:**377–384.
37. **Newell, D. G.** 1986. Monoclonal antibodies directed against the flagella of *Campylobacter jejuni:* production, characterization and lack of effect on colonization of infant mice. *J. Hyg.* **96:**131–141.
38. **Newell, D. G., H. McBride, and J. M. Dolby.** 1985. Investigations on the role of flagella in the colonization of infant mice with *Campylobacter jejuni* and attachment of *Campylobacter jejuni* to human epithelial cell lines. *J. Hyg.* **95:**217–227.
39. **Newell, D. G., H. McBride, and A. D. Pearson.** 1984. The identification of outer membrane proteins and flagella of *Campylobacter jejuni*. *J. Gen. Microbiol.* **130:**1201–1208.
40. **Newell, D. G., and A. Pearson.** 1984. The invasion of epithelial cell lines and the intestinal epithelium of infant mice by *Campylobacter jejuni*. *J. Diarhoeal Dis. Res.* **2:**19–26.
41. **Nuijten, P. J. M., N. M. C. Bleumink-Pluym, W. Gaastra, and B. A. M. van der Zeijst.** 1988. Flagellin expression in *Campylobacter jejuni* is regulated at the transcriptional level. *Infect. Immun.* **84:**1084–1088.
42. **Nuijten, P. J. M., C. Bartels, N. M. C. Bleumink-Pluym, W. Gaastra, and B. A. M. van der Zeijst.** 1990. Size and physical map of the *Campylobacter jejuni* chromosome. *Nucleic Acids Res.* **18:**6211–6214.
43. **Nuijten, P. J. M., L. Màrquez Magaña, A. Wedel, and B. A. M. van der Zeijst.** Submitted for publication.
44. **Nuijten, P. J. M., A. J. A. M. van Asten, W. Gaastra, and B. A. M. van der Zeijst.** 1990. Structural and functional analysis of two *Campylobacter jejuni* flagellin genes. *J. Biol. Chem.* **265:**17798–17804.
45. **Nuijten, P. J. M., B. A. M. van der Zeijst, and D. G. Newell.** 1991. Localization of immunogenic regions of the flagellin proteins of *Campylobacter jejuni* 81116. *Infect. Immun.* **59:**1100–1105.
46. **Ohta, N., L.-S. Chen, D. A. Mullin, and A. Newton.** 1991. Timing of flagellar gene expression in the *Caulobacter* cell cycle is determined by a transcriptional cascade of positive regulatory genes. *J. Bacteriol.* **173:**1514–1522.
47. **Owen, R. J., and S. Leaper.** 1981. Base composition, size, and nucleotide sequence similarities of genome deoxyribonucleic acids from species of the genus *Campylobacter*. *FEMS Microbiol. Lett.* **12:**395–400.
48. **Palmer, S. R., P. R. Gully, J. M. White, A. D. Pearson, W. G. Suckling, D. M. Jones, J. C. L. Rawes, and J. L. Penner.** 1983. Water-borne outbreak of *Campylobacter* gastroenteritis. *Lancet* **i:**287–290.
49. **Pleier, E., and R. Schmitt.** 1991. Expression of two *Rhizobium meliloti* flagellin genes and their contribution to the complex filament structure. *J. Bacteriol.* **173:**2077–2085.
50. **Pleier, E., and R. Schmitt.** 1989. Identification and sequence analysis of two related flagellin genes in *Rhizobium meliloti*. *J. Bacteriol.* **171:**1467–1475.
51. **Smith, N. H., and R. K. Selander.** 1991. Molecular genetic basis for complex flagellar antigen expression in a triphasic serovar of Salmonella. *Proc. Natl. Acad. Sci. USA* **88:**956–960.
52. **Smyth, C. J.** 1988. Flagella: their role in virulence, p. 3–11. *In* P. Owen and T. J. Foster (ed.), *Immunochemical and Molecular Genetic Analysis of Bacterial Pathogens*. Elsevier Scientific Publishers, Amsterdam.

53. **Stanley, K. K., and J. P. Luzio.** 1984. Construction of a new family of high efficiency bacterial expression vectors: identification of cDNA clones coding for human liver proteins. *EMBO J.* **3:**1429–1434.
54. **Thornton, S. A., S. M. Logan, T. J. Trust, and P. Guerry.** 1990. Polynucleotide sequence relationships among flagellin genes of *Campylobacter jejuni* and *Campylobacter* coli. *Infect. Immun.* **58:**2686–2689.
55. **Totten, P. A., and S. Lory.** 1990. Characterization of the type a flagellin gene from *Pseudomonas aeruginosa* PAK. *J. Bacteriol.* **172:**7188–7199.
56. **Van 't Hoog, A. I.** Unpublished data.
57. **Vonderviszt, F., S. Kanto, S.-I. Aizawa, and K. Namba.** 1989. Terminal regions of flagellin are disordered in solution. *J. Mol. Biol.* **209:**127–133.
58. **Walker, R. I., M. B. Caldwell, E. C. Lee, P. Guerry, T. J. Trust, and G. M. Ruiz-Palacios.** 1986. Pathophysiology of *Campylobacter* enteritis. *Microbiol. Rev.* **50:**81–94.
59. **Wassenaar, T. M., N. M. C. Bleumink-Pluym, and B. A. M. van der Zeijst.** 1991. Inactivation of *Campylobacter jejuni* flagellin genes by homologous recombination demonstrates that *flaA* but not *flaB* is required for invasion. *EMBO J.* **10:**2055–2061.
60. **Wei, L.-N., and T. M. Joys.** 1985. Covalent structure of three phase-1 flagellar filament proteins of Salmonella. *J. Mol. Biol.* **186:**791–803.
61. **Wenman, W. M., J. Chai, T. J. Louie, C. Goudreau, H. Lior, D. G. Newell, A. D. Pearson, and D. E. Taylor.** 1985. Antigenic analysis of *Campylobacter* flagellar protein and other proteins. *J. Clin. Microbiol.* **21:**108–112.

INDEX